Social Anxiety

Social Anxiety

Clinical, Developmental, and Social Perspectives

Second Edition

Edited by

Stefan G. Hofmann and Patricia M. DiBartolo

ELSEVIER

AMSTERDAM • BOSTON • HEIDELBERG • LONDON
NEW YORK • OXFORD • PARIS • SAN DIEGO
SAN FRANCISCO • SINGAPORE • SYDNEY • TOKYO

Academic Press is an Imprint of Elsevier

Academic Press is an imprint of Elsevier
32 Jamestown Road, London NW1 7BY, UK
30 Corporate Drive, Suite 400, Burlington, MA 01803, USA
525 B Street, Suite 1800, San Diego, CA 92101-4495, USA

Second edition

British Library Cataloguing-in-Publication Data
A catalogue record for this book is available from the British Library

Library of Congress Cataloging-in-Publication Data
A catalog record for this book is available from the Library of Congress

ISBN : 978-0-12-375096-9

For information on all Academic Press publications
visit our website at www.elsevierdirect.com

Typeset by MPS Limited, a Macmillan Company, Chennai, India
www.macmillansolutions.com

Printed and bound in the United States of America

10 11 12 13   10 9 8 7 6 5 4 3 2 1

Contents

Part III
Treatment Approaches

Contributors

Anne Marie Albano, *NYS Psychiatric Institute, New York, NY 10032*

Lynn E. Alden, *Department of Psychology, University of British Columbia, Vancouver, Canada*

Danielle Amado, *Department of Psychology, University of Montreal, QC, Canada*

Nader Amir, *Joint Doctoral Program, San Diego State University/University of California, San Diego, CA, USA*

Carlos Blanco, *Department of Psychiatry, Columbia University, New York, NY 10032*

Jessica Bomyea, *Joint Doctoral Program, San Diego State University/University of California, San Diego, CA, USA*

Lynn L. Brandsma, *Department of Psychology, Drexel University, Philadelphia, PA 90102*

Faith A. Brozovich, *Adult Anxiety Clinic of Temple University, Philadelphia, PA 19122*

Michelle C. Capozzoli, *Center for the Treatment and Study of Anxiety, University of Pennsylvania, Philadelphia, PA 19104*

Leslie G. Cohn, *Private Practice, Seattle, WA, USA*

Jonathan S. Comer, *NYS Psychiatric Institute, New York, NY 10032*

Michael F. Detweiler, *USAF Educational, Developmental, and Intervention Services (EDIS) Program, RAF Lakenheath, UK*

Randy O. Frost, *Department of Psychology, Clark Science Center, Smith College, Northampton, MA 01060*

Joel Gelernter, *Yale University School of Medicine, VA CT Healthcare Center, West Haven, CT 06516*

Katharine Glossner, *Department of Psychology, Clark Science Center, Smith College, Northampton, MA 01060*

Pamela Handelsman, *Anxiety Research and Treatment Program, Southern Methodist University, Dallas, TX 75205*

Bridget A. Hearon, *Center for Anxiety and Related Disorders, Boston University, MA 02215*

Richard G. Heimberg, *Adult Anxiety Clinic of Temple University, Philadelphia, PA 19122*

Lynne Henderson, *The Shyness Institute, Palo Alto, CA 94306; Stanford University Continuing Studies, Stanford, CA, 94305*

James D. Herbert, *Department of Psychology, Drexel University, Philadelphia, PA 90102*

Debra A. Hope, *Department of Psychology, University of Nebraska–Lincoln, NE 68588*

Jerome Kagan, *Department of Psychology, Harvard University, Cambridge, MA 02138*

Todd B. Kashdan, *Department of Psychology, George Mason University, Fairfax, VA 22030*

Heide Klumpp, *Department of Psychiatry, University of Michigan, Ann Arbor, MI 48109*

Angela Kyparissis, *Department of Psychology, University of Montreal, QC, Canada*

Mark R. Leary, *Department of Psychology, Duke University, Durham, NC 27708*

C.W. Lejuez, *Department of Psychology, University of Maryland, MD 20742*

Michael R. Liebowitz, *Department of Psychology, Columbia University, New York, NY 10032*

Sarah Maxner, *Department of Psychology, Clark Science Center, Smith College, Northampton, MA 01060*

Daniel W. McNeil, *Anxiety, Psychophysiology, and Pain Research Laboratory, Department of Psychology, West Virginia University, Morgantown, WV 26506*

Rowland S. Miller, *Department of Psychology and Philosophy, Sam Houston State University, Huntsville, TX 77341*

Mayumi Okuda, *Department of Psychiatry, Columbia University, New York, NY 10032*

Michael W. Otto, *Center for Anxiety and Related Disorders, Boston University, MA 02215*

K. Luan Phan, *Department of Psychiatry, University of Michigan, Ann Arbor, MI 48109; Mental Health Service, VA Ann Arbor Healthcare System, MI 48105*

Mark B. Powers, *Center for the Treatment and Study of Anxiety, University of Pennsylvania, Philadelphia, PA 19104*

Ronald M. Rapee, *Centre for Emotional Health, Macquarie University, Sydney, NSW, Australia*

Marci J. Regambal, *Department of Psychology, University of British Columbia, Vancouver, BC, Canada*

James Reich, *Department of Psychiatry, UCSF Medical School, and Department of Psychiatry and Behavioral Health, Stanford Medical School, San Francisco, CA 94123*

Alyssa A. Rheingold, *Department of Psychiatry, Drexel University, Philadelphia, PA 90102*

Steven A. Safren, *Center for Anxiety and Related Disorders, Boston University, MA 02215*

Franklin R. Schneier, *Department of Psychiatry, Columbia University, New York, NY 10032*

Jasper A.J. Smits, *Anxiety Research and Treatment Program, Southern Methodist University, Dallas, TX 75205*

John T. Sorrell, *Department School of Medicine, Department of Anaesthesia, Stanford University, CA 94305*

Murray B. Stein, *University of California, San Diego La Jolla, CA 92093*

Ariel Stravynski, *Department of Psychology, University of Montreal, QC, Canada*

Justin W. Weeks, *Department of Psychology, Ohio University, Athens, OH 45701*

Brandon J. Weiss, *Department of Psychology, University of Nebraska–Lincoln, NE 68588*

Amy Wenzel *Department of Psychiatry*, *University of Pennsylvania, Philadelphia, PA 19104*

Philip Zimbardo *The Shyness Institute, Palo Alto, CA 94306; Palo Alto University, Palo Alto, CA, 94304*

Introduction

Toward an Understanding of Social Anxiety Disorder

Stefan G. Hofmann and Patricia M. DiBartolo

Humans are social creatures. We have a strong need to be liked, valued, and approved of by others. As a result, we have generated sophisticated social structures and hierarchies that greatly determine an individual's value. Ostracism from these social groups negatively impacts a variety of health-related variables, and social exclusion is experienced as a punishment. For example, violations of social norms can lead to imprisonment, which limits an individual's social contacts. Moreover, violating prison rules can lead to a further restriction of social relationships and even solitary confinement. Due to the importance of our social structures, humans naturally fear negative evaluation by their peers.

The clinical expression of this evolutionarily adaptive concern is social anxiety disorder (SAD). In Western cultures, the lifetime prevalence rates of SAD range between 7 and 12% of the population (Furmark, 2002; Kessler, Berglund, Demler, Jin, & Walters, 2005). This disorder affects men and women relatively equally, with the average gender ratio (female : male) ranging between 1 : 1 (Moutier & Stein, 1999) and 3 : 2 (Kessler et al., 2005) in community studies. During childhood, SAD is often associated with shyness and behavioral inhibition (BI). If the problem is left untreated, it typically follows a chronic, unremitting course and can lead to substantial impairments in vocational and social functioning (Stein & Kean, 2001).

When reading the existing literature of social anxiety, one is struck by the lack of integration of the research findings that have been gathered by the various scientific disciplines, including social psychology, clinical psychology, psychiatry, developmental psychology, and behavior genetics. For example, clinical psychologists and psychiatrists tend to know relatively little about the relationship between social anxiety, shyness, and embarrassment or about contributions from behavior genetics. Conversely, social and developmental psychologists know relatively little about SAD subtypes, biological theories

Social Anxiety: Clinical, Developmental, and Social Perspectives. DOI: 10.1016/B978-0-12-375096-9.00028-6

of SAD, and cognitive behavioral or pharmacological treatment outcome studies. In order to address these gaps in knowledge, we (Hofmann & DiBartolo, 2001) recruited some of the most distinguished theorists and researchers from the various fields to initiate an interdisciplinary dialogue in one edited volume almost 10 years ago. The field has progressed considerably since that first book was published. This current volume updates the status of the scientific findings across a variety of diverse disciplines with contributors providing data and theory from their own conceptual perspectives relevant to their area of expertise.

DELINEATION OF SOCIAL ANXIETY

Chapter 1 by McNeil reviews the evolution of the terms social anxiety, SAD, and related constructs. Constructs such as shyness, introversion, BI, social anxiety, and SAD all share very similar meanings and are often used interchangeably, which can complicate things enormously. Choosing the right terminology is not a trivial thing. It reflects, and possibly determines, our understanding and conceptualization of the issue under investigation. McNeil proposes a number of specific ways in which these terms may inter-relate. He concludes that different forms of "social anxieties" exist along a continuum, and that related constructs, such as shyness, span from "normal" and "high normal" to pathological levels of social anxiety.

A similar dimensional approach towards psychopathology is the implicit model of many psychological assessment procedures for social anxiety and social SAD. Consistent with this notion, Herbert and colleagues (Chapter 2) start from the basic premise that social anxiety and SAD do not differ qualitatively but rather quantitatively. Therefore, the various assessment methods (which should include a multimodal approach) can be used for assessing social anxiety as well as SAD. However, as we note below, other theorists believe that such a dimensional perspective toward SAD and shyness is problematic (e.g., see Chapter 12).

The aforementioned terminology problem becomes even more complex when we consider the construct of shyness, which is covered by Henderson and Zimbardo (Chapter 3). As their chapter shows, it seems almost impossible to discuss the psychopathology of shyness without referring to social anxiety or related constructs. Their chapter notes the overlap between shyness and SAD while recognizing that individuals who label themselves as shy often express heterogeneous behavioral and symptom profiles. A little clearer seems to be the distinction between social anxiety/SAD and embarrassment, which is discussed by Miller (Chapter 4). Unlike SAD, the experience of embarrassment is something ordinary, normal, and adaptive because it provides an effective way to overcome minor and inevitable mishaps that occur in interactions with other people. Miller points to one important commonality between social anxiety/SAD and embarrassment: both constructs include the fear of negative evaluation by others. Neither SAD nor embarrassment would exist if people did not care what others thought of them.

Does this mean that socially anxious individuals are overly perfectionistic when it comes to social interactions? This hypothesis is investigated in the chapter by Frost, Glossner, and Maxner (Chapter 5). They conclude that certain characteristics of perfectionism, and in particular the maladaptive evaluative concern dimensions, are in fact associated with social anxiety and related constructs. A review of the literature suggests that, compared to nonanxious controls, individuals with clinical levels of social anxiety are more perfectionistic. The central features of perfectionism related to SAD are an excessive concern over mistakes, doubts about the quality of one's actions, and the perception that other people have excessively high expectations. Although similar differences in perfectionism dimensions can also be found when comparing nonclinical participants with other anxiety-disordered groups, certain of these dimensions are elevated in samples with SAD relative to other anxiety patients.

The next chapter, by Stravynski, Kyparissis, and Amado (Chapter 6), deals in detail with the relationship between social anxiety/SAD and social skills, and more specifically with the (once) popular assumption that SAD is caused by a deficit in social skills. Based on a critical review of the literature, Stravynski et al. conclude that there is very little empirical evidence to suggest that SAD is caused by, or even consistently linked with, deficits in social skills. They argue that the main problem lies in the conceptualization and operational definition of the construct of social skills. The authors encourage researchers to take a fresh look at the "social" aspect of SAD by investigating the pattern of social behaviors characterizing SAD in real-life situations.

Two of the remaining chapters of the first part of the volume deal with contemporary diagnostic controversies, namely with the relationship between SAD and other DSM (Diagnostic and statistical manual of mental disorders) Axis I disorders in adulthood (Chapter 7 by Wenzel), and Axis II disorders (Chapter 8 by Reich). Comorbidity, which refers to the co-occurrence of two or more mental disorders in one person, is an inevitable "side effect" of our existing categorical diagnostic classification system (the DSM). Based on the existing literature, Wenzel concludes that comorbidity is common, even typical, for individuals with SAD. Rates of comorbidity between SAD and other anxiety and mood disorder are high and there is growing evidence of heightened risk for substance use disorders as well. Wenzel also notes emerging evidence indicating increased risk of comorbidity for SAD and a variety of other conditions (e.g., eating disorders, bipolar disorder). She urges the field to begin to identify the pathogenesis of these comorbidities, rather than merely document their co-occurrence.

Among the Axis II disorders, the most highly comorbid (and most controversial) diagnostic category is avoidant personality disorder (APD). The empirical evidence, as reviewed by Reich, suggests that SAD and APD probably relate to the same disorder with different subtypes. SAD and APD cannot be distinguished on the basis of symptomatology or treatment response. Although individuals with both SAD and APD seem to report a greater degree of distress in social situations, they respond equally well to treatment to those without this additional Axis II diagnosis. Reich points out that this raises the question of whether APD is in fact a viable Axis II diagnosis because our diagnostic system defines a personality disorder as an enduring, inflexible, and pervasive problem. Reich offers a creative solution to this problem by creating a subcategory in Axis II for chronic Axis I disorders "with significant personality features."

The final chapter of Part I, by Detweiler, Comer, and Albano (Chapter 9), examines the risks, phenomenology, etiology, and empirically supported treatments for socially anxious children and adolescents. Their review reveals the considerable social, occupational, and emotional tolls associated with SAD in developing youth. Furthermore, Detweiler et al. present the latest research on the biological, social, and developmental risks associated with SAD in youth and describe a model to guide clinicians considering a SAD diagnosis in this demographic. Throughout the chapter, their work emphasizes the importance of sensitivity to developmental expectations, as well as appreciation of the persistence and functional interference associated with social anxiety. Fortunately, there are options for effective treatments for youth with social anxiety. Nonetheless, they argue continued attention needs to be paid to the developmental pathways of socially anxious youth in order to identify children at risk for clinical diagnosis and to continue the development of effective prevention and treatment programs for this costly disorder.

THEORETICAL PERSPECTIVES

This next section of this book deals with the most prominent theoretical perspectives on social anxiety and SAD discussed by social psychologists, developmental psychologists, behavior geneticists, clinical psychologists, and psychiatrists. These different theoretical perspectives emphasize different factors that might contribute to the etiology and/or maintenance of social anxiety/SAD. They can be classified into the following four broad categories: (1) biological mechanisms, including temperamental factors (Chapters 10–12); (2) behavioral factors (Chapter 13); (3) cognitive variables (Chapters 14–17); and (4) interpersonal processes that are relevant in social interactions (Chapter 18). As pointed out by a number of our contributors, these perspectives are not mutually exclusive; the "real world" is probably a combination of all of these theories.

In a new contribution to this edition, Phan and Klumpp (Chapter 10) review the emerging findings from two areas of science – neuroimaging and neuroendocrinology – that help inform our understanding of the physiology of SAD. Although evidence from neuroendocrinology studies sometimes finds cortisol dysregulation in individuals with SAD, this finding has been inconsistent, indicating the need for future research on how to predict and understand the role of this apparent vulnerability. Neuroimaging studies suggest that the symptoms of SAD may be related to two separate abnormalities: hyper-reactivity of limbic and paralimbic areas as well as hypoactivation of frontal regions of the cortex involved in emotion regulation and cognitive appraisal. These functional abnormalities in brain areas involved in affect and cognition intersect well with the observed emotional and cognitive symptoms of social anxiety.

As noted by Stein and Gelernter (Chapter 11), there seems to exist strong evidence for a genetic contribution to the SAD diagnosis. Their review of the literature on the molecular genetics of SAD explores relationships between specific genes and related intermediate phenotypes, such as BI. What preliminary evidence suggests using recent twin studies is that there appear to be common genetic risks across the anxiety disorders, an important area for future research.

Kagan (Chapter 12) further hypothesizes that a person's temperament, such as the behavioral response to unfamiliar and unexpected events (BI), may be directly related to the threshold of excitability of the amygdala. Kagan presents convincing evidence from his own longitudinal work with behaviorally inhibited children (now followed up through adolescence) suggesting that temperamental bias (e.g., high vs. low reactivity) "constrains" the possibility of developing particular behavioral profiles, and is associated with distinct psychophysiological response patterns. These first three chapters of Part II all suggest that there may be biological, neurophysiological, and possibly genetic "markers" that distinguish individuals with and without social anxiety/SAD, which is inconsistent with the idea that social anxiety and related constructs are "dimensional" variables (e.g., Chapters 1–3). This is clearly an important area for future research.

The next chapter, by McNeil, Lejuez, and Sorrell (Chapter 13), also acknowledges the contribution of biological and genetic factors, but focuses primarily on a variety of behavioral principles (including but not limited to operant and respondent conditioning events) as important factors for the development and maintenance of social anxiety/SAD. Cognitive variables, on the other hand, are not considered to be causal agents within this theoretical framework.

This is in contrast with the following three chapters. The first of this series, by Amir (Chapter 14), reviews the literature on information processing biases (i.e., the preferential cognitive processing of threat-relevant information) in individuals with social anxiety/SAD. He concludes that attention biases, sporadic memory biases, and interpretation biases seem to be responsible for the development and maintenance of social anxiety. More specifically, Amir suggests that socially anxious individuals show a "vigilance–avoidance" pattern of information processing of threat-relevant information, which may contribute to the maintenance of the problem.

The chapter by Heimberg, Brozovich, and Rapee (Chapter 15) also emphasizes the importance of cognitive factors in the etiology and maintenance of social anxiety/SAD. They present a revision of their integrative cognitive behavioral model of SAD, based on the research examining new areas of cognitive vulnerability, including imagery, post-event processing, fear of positive evaluation, and combined or interactive cognitive biases.

Another new addition to this volume is the chapter by Kashdan and Weeks (Chapter 17), which examines the relationship of social anxiety with the biobehavioral system associated with positive emotions and approach behaviors. Although much of the research on the phenomenology of social anxiety focuses on negative emotions and their concomitant avoidance behaviors, Kashdan and Weeks's review indicates that social anxiety is also related to impairments associated with the positive biobehavioral system, including fewer positive life events, inhibited positive emotionality, and a poorer quality of life. Interestingly, they note that diminishment of positive experiences in social anxiety is not explained by concomitant depressive symptomatology, indicating the importance of examining these two separable systems in future social anxiety research.

When reviewing the literature, one is struck by the number and diversity of self-related constructs that appear in the discussion of social anxiety and SAD, such as self-consciousness, self-evaluation, self-blame, self-esteem, self-focused attention, self-criticism, etc. But what exactly is the "self," and how does it relate to social behavior and anxiety? This question dates back to the very beginnings of psychology (James, 1890), and it is also the question that is addressed in the chapter by Alden and Regambal (Chapter 16). In theories of social anxiety, which have been predominantly developed by social and personality psychologists, conceptualizations of the self center around the self as relational, malleable, and multidimensional. In contrast, in models of SAD typically developed by clinical psychologists and psychiatrists, the self is stable and unidimensional with relatively less emphasis on the self in relation to others. The authors conclude that these conceptualizations of the self have necessarily focused, and perhaps limited, scientists in their research efforts and that additional work in the future should be directed toward integrating these theories.

One important social psychological theory of social anxiety that emphasizes the role of the self is self-presentation theory (Leary, Chapter 18). In principle, this theory states that people experience social anxiety when they want to make a desired impression on other people but doubt that they will successfully do so. Leary offers a refinement and extension of this original theory. According to his revised theory, the "sociometer theory," social anxiety can arise well in advance of actual rejection if the "sociometer," which is an early-warning system, detects potential relational devaluation. Therefore, social anxiety primarily arises when one's impressions have implications for relational devaluation, given the strong drive we have to forge and protect interpersonal bonds.

TREATMENT APPROACHES

At the same time that researchers are gaining a more sophisticated understanding of the phenomenology of social anxiety and SAD and are creating complex etiological models, the field has also made significant strides in developing and evaluating treatments for chronic and debilitating social anxiety. For example, the number of pharmacological studies has increased substantially in recent years. Some of the most common drug treatments for SAD include monoamine oxidase inhibitors (MAOIs), which include both reversible (e.g., moclobemide) and irreversible (e.g., phenelzine) compounds; selective serotonin reuptake inhibitors, which include paroexetine, the first Food and Drug Administration FDA-approved drug for SAD; benzodiazepines; antidepressants; and beta blockers. Blanco, Schneier, Okuda, and Liebowitz (Chapter 19) conclude that the SSRIs are the first-line medications for the treatment of SAD. Nonetheless, they note that there are still a number of unexplored research areas in this field, including predicting pharmacotherapy response, addressing treatment resistance to drugs, and determining how best to administer maintenance treatments.

Weiss, Hope, and Cohn's review (Chapter 20) of the psychotherapy literature of SAD is uniquely organized around specific features of SAD in an attempt to determine which treatments address which symptoms most effectively. We currently have available a number of effective psychological treatments for SAD. Although most treatments (e.g., CBT, exposure intervention, social skills training) lead to a reduction of social anxiety, some symptoms seem to improve more under certain modalities than others. For example, cognitive restructuring alone does not seem to be the treatment of choice to reduce behavioral avoidance and improve performance. The authors note in their review that recent SAD treatment research has moved in the direction of more sophisticated questions, including elucidating mechanisms of action, augmenting exposure therapy's effects, and employing newly developed measures of cognitive change.

Powers, Capozzoli, Handelsman and Smits (Chapter 21) compare outcomes associated with empirically supported psychological versus pharmacological treatments for SAD. Given treatment data for SAD indicating that each of these treatments as well as their combination yield generally equivalent outcomes, they provide a fine-grained analysis of other indices to be considered (e.g., cost, durability, availability of trained practitioners) when making decisions about treatment order, choice, or combinations, based on the best available theoretical, analogue, and applied research.

The final chapter, by Otto, Safren, and Hearon (Chapter 22), investigates the mechanisms of action in pharmacotherapy and CBT (including exposure-based therapy). The authors hypothesize that these two modalities intervene at different points in this cycle. According to Otto et al.'s analysis, pharmacotherapy is successful because it blocks the pathological anxiety reactions that are experienced by individuals with SAD. In contrast, CBT is hypothesized to be effective because graduated and repeated exposure of clients to anxiety-provoking situations allows active relearning that these situations are safe.

CONCLUSION

We believe that it is clear from the proliferation of knowledge represented in this volume that our understanding of social anxiety and SAD has burgeoned dramatically in the years since our first edited volume was published. These important and complex phenomena have captured the interest of researchers from a multitude of disciplines who have been committed to expanding our insight into the continuum of human experience as it relates to our fears of interpersonal rejection and inadequacy. This explosion of research interest and theoretical development has provided much-needed understanding of universal and transient feelings of social anxiety as well as the less common, but unremitting and debilitating, condition of SAD. We hope that this updated volume will help to consolidate the latest evidence and conceptual theories that are available for social anxiety and its disorder. We believe that a review of the data and theoretical knowledge included in this volume represents some of the best thinking in the field. We hope that the breadth of perspective represented in this volume will help foster continued interdisciplinary dialogue and efforts toward cross-fertilization. Despite the tremendous burst of knowledge in our understanding of the phenomenology, etiology, and treatment of SAD, it is clear that we have a great deal of work left to accomplish. This is an exciting time in the field and we are looking forward to the future with the hope that we will be increasingly able to help those individuals whose lives can be so dramatically affected by chronic social anxiety.

In conclusion, we have invited distinguished experts to summarize their unique expertise in an attempt to provide a resource that will allow the reader to appreciate the breadth of the perspectives that have been taken on the study of social anxiety and SAD. As a whole, we hope that this volume will help to foster crossfertilization across disciplines as the field continues to make significant advances in our understanding, conceptualization, and treatment of chronic and debilitating social anxiety.

REFERENCES

Furmark, T. (2002). Social phobia: Overview of community surveys. *Acta Psychiatrica Scandinavica*, *105*, 84–93.

James, W. (1890). *The principles of psychology*. New York: Holt.

Kessler, R. C., Berglund, P. A., Demler, O., Jin, R., & Walters, E. E. (2005). Lifetime prevalence and age-of-onset distributions of DSM-IV disorders in the National Comorbidity Survey Replication (NCS-R). *Archives of General Psychiatry*, *62*, 593–602.

Moutier, C. Y., & Stein, M. B. (1999). The history, epidemiology, and differential diagnosis of social anxiety disorder. *Journal of Clinical Psychiatry*, *60*, 4–8.

Stein, M. B., & Kean, Y. M. (2001). Disability and quality of life in social phobia: Epidemiologic findings. *American Journal of Psychiatry*, *157*, 1606–1613.

Part I

Delineation of Social Anxiety

Chapter 1

Evolution of Terminology and Constructs in Social Anxiety and its Disorders

Daniel W. McNeil
Anxiety, Psychophysiology, and Pain Research Laboratory, Department of Psychology, West Virginia University, Morgantown, WV 26506

INTRODUCTION

Unpleasant emotional states and nonadaptive behaviors associated with social situations have historically been known as significant, life-affecting problems for many people. Given the social nature of human beings, and the functional nature of social relationships (e.g., social support), discomfort associated with interacting with others is particularly difficult, as socialization cannot be easily avoided, unlike other anxiety problems such as some phobias. Social anxieties and fears were described by Hippocrates and began to be systematically delineated with other phobias in the 1870s (Marks, 1970, 1985). In the recent past, the social psychological focus on shyness (e.g., Zimbardo, 1977), the work of Marks and others in the 1960s and 1970s, and the identification of social phobia (SP) as a distinct disorder in the *Diagnostic and statistical manual of mental disorders* (DSM)–III (e.g., American Psychiatric Association, 1980) and subsequent revisions, heralded a massive growth in the related scientific and self-help literatures.

This general arena of problems likely includes several somewhat overlapping constructs; the scientific language has many different terms that apply or relate, including shyness, social anxiety, social withdrawal, SP, social anxiety disorder (SAD), behavioral inhibition (BI), communication apprehension, and introversion. In both everyday and scientific language, these states have been described in a myriad of ways. Leitenberg (1990, p.2), in introducing his book on the area, states:

Social anxiety has been studied in various guises. Shyness, performance anxiety, social phobia, avoidant personality disorder, social withdrawal, social isolation, public speaking anxiety, speech anxiety, communication apprehension, fear of interpersonal rejection, dating anxiety, separation anxiety, stage fright, fear of strangers, shame,

Social Anxiety: Clinical, Developmental, and Social Perspectives. DOI: 10.1016/B978-0-12-375096-9.00001-8

embarrassment, social inhibition, social timidity – all of these and more fall under the umbrella of social anxiety.

Other anxiety-related syndromes, such as test anxiety and selective mutism, also likely have a strong social component, and may be instantiations of SAD (Bögels et al., 2010). Body dysmorphic disorder (BDD), highly comorbid with SAD, similarly is socially determined, at least in part, in that the perception of others regarding (imagined) defects may be an underlying feature.

There also are a variety of terms that suggest, at least in part, deficient social skills, such as "nerd," "geek," and "wallflower." Masia and Morris (1998) identify terms related to social distress in children across areas of psychology: developmental (i.e., peer neglect, social withdrawal), personality (i.e., shyness), and clinical (i.e., SP, avoidant personality disorder (APD)). Stranger anxiety and separation anxiety likely are related constructs as well (Thompson & Limber, 1990). Masia and Morris note that this varying "psychological language" (p. 212) creates problems in investigating phenomena (e.g., parental behavior and its relation to child social anxiety) that spans across subdisciplines in psychology, and presumably across related disciplines (e.g., psychiatry).

It should be noted that comparative psychology has contributions to this area as well. Social anxieties are not solely human phenomena; such social/emotional problems are shared by other primates (Mineka & Zinbarg, 1995; Suomi, 1997) and lower animals. Social dominance and submissiveness hierarchies have been suggested as important as determinants of socially anxious behavior across species of primates, including humans (Schneier & Welkowitz, 1996; Trower & Gilbert, 1989). Facial expressions, for example, provide important social interactional cues in both humans and other primates, including both aggression and appeasement related to anxiety (Öhman, 1986).

One of the issues that is an albatross for the field concerns the everyday language basis of the most frequently used terms: shyness, stage fright, and social anxiety. Some years ago, Harris (1984) detailed a number of problems inherent in using the lay language of "shyness" in scientific discourse, problems that still exist today. Clinically oriented scientists may try to "distance" SAD from shyness, perhaps to emphasize that individuals who meet criteria for the disorder suffer with impairment in social and occupational functioning that can be quite terrible, leading to chronic misery. Adding further complexity, some degree of social anxiety can be adaptive (Schneier & Welkowitz, 1996). Moreover, the social consequences of some socially anxious behaviors are quite positive. One example is a "bashful" child who hides his face by planting it directly in some part of one of his parents' bodies, resulting in adult laughter and encouragement to socialize. A further example is a distant, detached person who is regarded as "coy," "interesting," or even "mysterious" (or conversely, as "stuck up") as a result of their lack of social initiation or response.

This chapter provides a perspective on conceptual, definitional, and diagnostic nosology issues for the field. It is proposed that social anxieties and

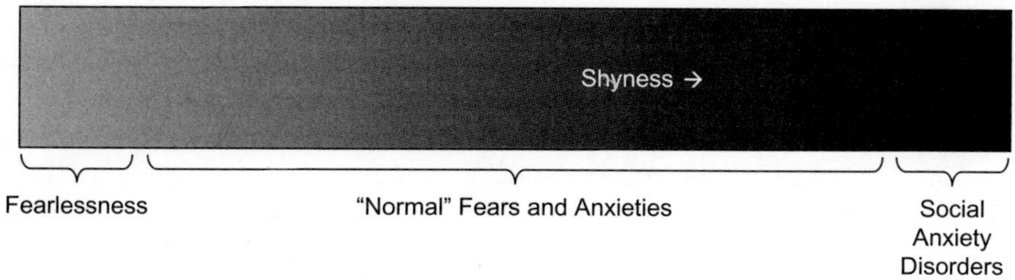

FIGURE 1.1 Model of the continuum of social anxieties and fears across the general population.

fears, like other phobic disorders, exist along a continuum across the general population, as explicated later in this chapter and as shown in Figure 1.1. The range of social anxieties/fears along this continuum is from no anxiety/fear to "normal" levels to psychopathological extremes. The debate (e.g., Campbell-Sills & Stein, 2005; Wakefield, Horowitz, & Schmitz, 2005a; Wakefield, Horowitz, & Schmitz, 2005b) on "overpathologizing" socially anxious people then may be somewhat addressed by a conceptualization that acknowledges both "normal" social anxieties that are mildly to moderately intense, or transient, and also their potential connectedness to SAD, depending on potentially contributing environmental and individual factors.

This chapter also reviews the evolution of constructs important to the area. Finally, it re-emphasizes the need for a multidisciplinary approach to studying and understanding distress and dysfunction related to social situations. This chapter, similarly to other work (Masia & Morris, 1998), uses the term "social anxiety" in an attempt to broadly encompass the various constructs emanating from the various disciplines and subdisciplines. Given the recognized differences between anxiety and fear states generally (Bouton, Mineka, & Barlow, 2001; McNeil, Turk, & Ries, 1994), the term "social fear" is incorporated into this lexicon and will be further elaborated in this chapter. Consistently with the evolving literature (Bögels et al., 2010), the term "social anxiety disorder" (SAD) (and, more properly, in the plural to emphasize the heterogeneity of problems in this area) is used to describe psychopathological levels of such anxieties or fears, although "SP" is used when describing historical designations.

OVERLAPPING AND CONTRASTING EMOTIONAL STATES

Anxiety and fear are not "lumps" (Lang, 1968) and are not, in and of themselves, disease states. Rather, they exist along continua across the population. At the extreme, high levels of social fears and anxiety are psychopathological, and can be classified as clinical syndromes such as SAD. Depending on the type of anxiety or fear, as well as other factors such as gender (Craske, 2003), the distributions vary.

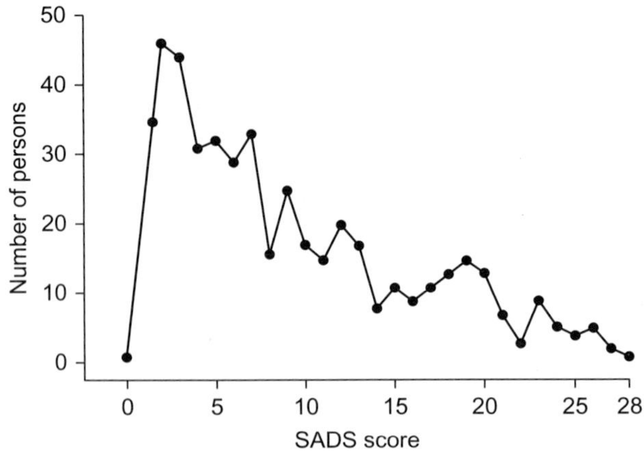

FIGURE 1.2 Number of individuals having each total score, reflecting general social anxiety using the Social Avoidance and Distress Scale (SADS; Watson & Friend, 1969; *top panel*), and public speaking fear based on the Personal Report of Confidence as a Speaker Scale (PRCS; Paul, 1966; *bottom panel*). The possible range of scores is 0–28 for the SADS and 0–30 for the PRCS. Higher scores for both instruments are indicative of greater anxiety. The total sample consists of 477 male and female undergraduates.

Figure 1.2 illustrates the distributions of general social anxiety based on Social Avoidance and Distress Scale (SADS; Watson & Friend, 1969) scores of 477 male (n = 214) and female (n = 263) university undergraduates. The mean age of the sample was 19.9 (SD = 3.1). Score distributions also are provided for specific public speaking fear using the Personal Report of Confidence as a Speaker scale (PRCS; Paul, 1966) for these same individuals. The SADS distribution is positively skewed toward lower scores, which are associated with less anxiety, but kurtosis was unremarkable (skewness and kurtosis coefficients are 0.79 and −0.39, respectively). In contrast, the PRCS is more normally distributed, but has a rectangular distribution in which each score has the same frequency of occurrence (skewness and kurtosis coefficients are −0.04 and −1.1, respectively).

Self-reported social fears and anxieties are unique in that females and males typically differ less (or not at all), unlike many other types of anxiety and fear, in which females report higher scores and males report lower ones (Craske, 2003). In fact, it has been suggested that there may be a higher incidence of a social skill deficit type of SP in males, while other types of the syndrome may be displayed equally between the sexes (Marks, 1985), although the literature is equivocal in this regard. Given the size of the present sample, substantively small differences (i.e., less than 2 points on 28- and 30-item scales) were statistically significant. The varying directionality of the sex differences, however, is interesting. For general social anxiety measured by the SADS, males (M = 9.9, SD = 7.3) had higher scores, indicating more anxiety, than females ($M = 8.4$, $SD = 6.3$), $t(475) = 2.40$, $p < 0.05$. Conversely, for specific public speaking fear on the PRCS, females ($M = 16.2$, $SD = 7.7$) indicated more anxiety than males ($M = 14.8$, $SD = 7.6$), $t(475) = 1.97$, $p < 0.05$. These differences provide suggestive evidence of the differences between general social anxieties and specific public speaking fears. While there may be differences in SADS and PRCS total scores between the sexes, the shape of the distributions were relatively consistent, except for kurtosis on the SADS, as evidenced by coefficients for skewness (SADS: males = 0.60 and females = 0.95; PRCS: males = −0.02 and females = −0.06) and kurtosis (SADS: males = −0.79 and females = 0.06; PRCS: males = −1.1 and females = −1.0).

These unique features of public speaking fear as measured by the PRCS, relative to general social anxieties, are consistent with prior research (Klorman, Weerts, Hastings, Melamed, & Lang, 1974) that compared the PRCs to other specific-fear questionnaires, although not a general social anxiety instrument. The different distribution shapes for the SADS and PRCS are interesting, particularly since general social anxiety and public speaking fear seem intrinsically related. Regardless of the distribution shapes, these data clearly demonstrate that both general social anxiety and public speaking fear exist along continua, albeit different ones, in a general population. The more normal distribution of public speaking fear scores, with a greater number of individuals at the right tail of the distribution (associated with higher scores and greater anxiety), is consistent with reports of their high prevalence in the general population, relative to general social anxiety (Kessler, Stein, & Berglund, 1998; Pollard & Henderson, 1988; Stein, Torgrud, & Walker, 2000).

Not only do social anxieties and fears exist across the general population, but significant features of social anxiety are present across various psychological disorders, including but not limited to anxiety disorders in addition to SAD. The comorbidity of anxiety disorders with one another is well documented (Barlow, 2002) and argues for a more dimensional classification scheme. High levels of social anxiety, and perhaps other anxieties, also exist across clinical syndromes such as schizophrenic disorders, affective disorders, and substance use disorders (Hall & Goldberg, 1977).

DEFINITIONS

In 1966, Marks and Gelder described patients with "social anxieties" as having "phobias of social situations, expressed variably as shyness, fears of blushing in public, of eating meals in restaurants, of meeting men or women, of going to dances or parties, or of shaking when the center of attention" (p. 218). A few years later, Marks (1970) further elucidated the classification of "SPs," distinguishing them from animal phobias and agoraphobia. He noted that the SP group of patients had "fears of eating, drinking, shaking, blushing, speaking, writing or vomiting in the presence of other people" (p. 383). Even at that point, however, Marks noted that "We need to know more about social phobics before definitely classifying them on their own" (p. 383). From these early scientific descriptions has grown a myriad of definitions; the evolution of our understanding of SAD continues with the recommended changes for the forthcoming DSM–V (Bögels et al., 2010; Lewis-Fernandez et al., 2010).

Most researchers in Western nations adopt the most current DSM definition (e.g., DSM-IV-TR, American Psychiatric Association, 2000). Presently, that definition includes, as an essential feature, "clinically significant anxiety provoked by exposure to certain types of social or performance situations, often leading to avoidance behavior" (American Psychiatric Association, 2000, p.429); it is further described in the next section. Aside from this definition, there is little consensus in the field, either about the definitions themselves or the underlying constructs. In each of the other areas, a different label (describing a slightly different construct) is used, with a correspondingly different definition. In fact, even within subdisciplines, there are different definitions depending on the model from which the researcher is working.

DIAGNOSTIC NOSOLOGY CLASSIFICATIONS

SP first was recognized as a separate diagnostic entity in the DSM system with the advent of DSM-III (American Psychiatric Association, 1980). DSM-II (American Psychiatric Association, 1968), for example, did not even specifically mention SPs under the phobic neurosis category. Nor was APD specifically detailed in that DSM version. In DSM-III, however, there were two fairly simple sets of criteria for SP, and an exclusionary category. Both fear and a desire to avoid were required in the first set of criteria. Significant distress and a recognition of the excess or unreasonableness of the fear were both necessary for the second criteria set. DSM-III descriptions implied that SP had discrete manifestations in one of four areas: public speaking/performing, using public bathrooms, eating in public, and writing in front of others. APD was one of the exclusionary criteria for SP, so patients might meet criteria for both disorders but only could be diagnosed with APD, thus making it the more predominant categorization. Children and adolescents with psychopathological social anxiety typically would be diagnosed with avoidant disorder of childhood or adolescence (AVD), which was in the DSM categorization of disorders usually first evident in infancy, childhood, or adolescence. There were, however, no stated criteria that would specifically prohibit diagnosis of a child or adolescent with SP. Conversely to adult classification, if the patient was under 18 years old, AVD was an exclusionary criterion for APD, and so took precedence over it.

The publication of DSM-III-R (American Psychiatric Association, 1987) represented a significant shift in the conceptualization of SP as a syndrome. In addition to a greater number of separate diagnostic criteria, and more specificity in these criteria, a generalized type of SP was allowed as a specifier "if the phobic situation includes most social situations" (p. 243), although it was noted that the disorder could be circumscribed. Also, APD was allowed as a comorbid diagnosis with SP. AVD was a formal exclusionary diagnosis for SP in individuals under age 18.

In DSM-IV (American Psychiatric Association, 1994), the SP diagnosis was slightly changed once again. For the first time, the term "SAD" was parenthetically listed along with "SP," apparently representing a conceptual shift to differentiate it from other phobic disorders. Perhaps this evolving change could also help in discriminating the extreme of psychopathological behaviors from "normal" social anxieties that affect most people in certain situations. In DSM-IV, AVD was subsumed into the SP diagnosis.

The text revision of the DSM-IV (i.e., DSM-IV-TR; American Psychiatric Association, 2000) of course retained the same criteria as the DSM-IV, and incorporated relatively minor wording changes and additions (e.g., noting that SAD may be associated with suicidal ideation). In the recommended changes (Bögels et al., 2010; Lewis-Fernandez et al., 2010) that may be incorporated in the DSM-V, what may result, among other potential changes, is dropping the "generalized" specifier but adding a "predominantly performance" specifier. "Social anxiety disorder" (SAD) would replace SP as the predominant wording, with the latter term in parentheses secondary to the former term. Interaction fears would be added to criterion A, along with the existing two (i.e., social and performance) core types of feared social situations. Additionally, the requirement for at least six months' duration may be extended to include all age groups, not just adults as in the DSM-IV-TR. Criterion A may be changed to include reference to concern about offending others, to be sensitive to cross-cultural differences in SAD. In a related way, Criterion C may be slightly altered to include one's social reference group in determining whether one recognizes that the fear is out of proportion to reality. What ultimately will be implemented as changes in DSM-V remains to be decided at the time of writing this chapter.

This evolution of criteria for SP and APD, while representing advances in some ways, also has hampered the literature in terms of historical comparisons. A group of individuals diagnosed with DSM-defined SP in 1985, for example, would differ from an analogous group so classified in 1995, and both likely would differ from a group classified in 2015, making comparisons across these studies of limited and uncertain value.

While virtually all clinically based SAD research in the United States presently uses the DSM system, lest we fall victim to national imperialism, it should be remembered that there is an International Classification of Diseases (ICD) diagnostic nomenclature (e.g., World Health Organization, 2007), which exists in its most current instantiation as ICD-X (version for 2007); there are other methodologies for classifying and understanding psychopathology as well. The ICD and DSM systems are different, and SAD/SP provides an important example. In the ICD-X "SP" classification, the criteria are more general and structured differently from the six inclusionary criteria in DSM-IV-TR. There is no generalized type or subtype in the ICD-X, although there is mention of the possibility of "more pervasive SP." Perhaps most importantly, relative to DSM-IV-TR, the ICD-X has considerable focus on physiologically related symptoms regarded as being unique to SP (i.e., blushing, hand tremor, nausea, and urgency of micturition). The ICD-X also suggests that symptoms of SP may evolve into panic attacks. Individuals classified with SP by one of these systems may well not be diagnosed in the same category by the other system. The diagnostic concordance rate between these two systems may only range between 39 and 66%, which certainly is troubling (Andrews, Slade, Peters, & Beard, 1998). Finally, it is important to note that social anxiety exists cross-culturally, albeit in varying forms (Hong & Woody, 2007; Kleinknecht, Dinnel, Kleinknecht, Hiruma, & Harada, 1997; McNeil, Porter, Zvolensky, Chaney, & Kee, 2000), as discussed later in this chapter, so an international classification or descriptive system is imperative.

The DSM system dominates the field and its utilization in both research and clinical settings in the United States is almost universal. While immensely helpful in a variety of ways, the DSM is limiting in terms of discouraging cross-disciplinary work with non-service-delivery disciplines. Also, the focus on categorical diagnoses is artificial, given the comorbidity across anxiety disorders. Individualized, functional analyses of behavior, followed by theory-driven therapy, seem almost antithetical to the DSM system (Eifert, 1996). Nevertheless, there are attempts to move the field away from syndromal classification to functional classification (Hayes, Wilson, Strosahl, Gifford, & Follette, 1996). In the case of SAD, for example, analysis of function (e.g., of poor social skills) is of great importance because the same behavior across individuals may have widely different antecedents (e.g., lack of knowledge about appropriate social responses vs. inhibited display of social behaviors due to anxiety).

RELATION OF PERFORMANCE DEFICITS AND SOCIAL ANXIETY

Because of the strong contribution of performance-related issues in some social anxieties, social skill and social anxiety in the past often were (inaccurately) viewed as always being one and the same problem, or as inextricably intertwined issues. Making public speeches is one prominent example, in which a high degree of anxiety displayed by the speaker may negatively affect skill level, and vice versa: poor public speaking skills may be one antecedent to anxiety in speech situations. Sometimes, however, performance anxieties have been considered separately, as in the cases of males experiencing sexual dysfunction (e.g., Bruce & Barlow, 1990), musical performance (e.g., Clark & Agras, 1991), and athletes in competitive sport situations (e.g., Smith & Smoll, 1990). Nevertheless, the relation of social skill and social anxiety is complex and inconsistently addressed in the literature (Hopko, McNeil, Zvolensky, &

Eifert, 2001). Intersecting relationships between social skill and anxiety have been suggested (Lewin, McNeil, & Lipson, 1996). Such a conceptualization may help to explain the curious (but relatively common) cases of clinical patients who have a sophisticated set of social skills but are extremely anxious nonetheless and who evaluate their performance negatively. The literature suggests individuals with SAD regard their own social performance harshly, more than less anxious persons do, and more so than independent observers (Hofmann & Barlow, 2002). Alternatively, it has been suggested that performance problems in generalized social anxiety might best be thought of as inhibitions rather than deficits (Rapee, 1995). Clearly, in this area particularly, more research is needed to clarify the relations between these constructs. From a clinical perspective, it is important to know whether a problem with social performance has a primary deficit (i.e., the ability was never learned), a secondary deficit (i.e., anxiety disrupts performance, in spite of the ability being present), or a tertiary deficit (i.e., the ability is absent and there is anxiety about performing the skill as well) (Hopko et al., 2001). The relation of skill and anxiety in the social arena must be better explained for the literature in the area to more fully and properly evolve.

SUBTYPES OF SAD

The literature on subtypes of SAD, sometimes referred to as types, is considerable (Hofmann, Heinrichs, & Moscovitch, 2004). Over two decades, considerable progress has been made in understanding and conceptualizing SAD, as well as treating it, but some fundamental questions remain. Current data strongly suggest there are unique variations of SAD, and that the DSM- and ICD-designated disorders are not homogenous ones. The semantic issue is actually quite important: Is there one major type of SAD, with some slight variants, or are there several SADs? At this point in the field, the idea that the disorder varies along a severity continuum enjoys considerable support (Bögels et al., 2010; McNeil, 2001). The conception of "subtypes" (e.g., Kessler et al., 1998) remains viable, with strong evidence for the existence of predominantly performance-based instantiations of the disorder (Bögels et al., 2010). The most common of the performance subtypes involves public speaking (e.g., Boone et al., 1999). There are performance fears in other areas, as earlier identified in DSM-III-R (American Psychiatric Association, 1980): public eating, writing, and use of lavatories. The circumscribed public speaking fears have even been suggested as being equally like specific phobias relative to other social Phobias (Boone et al., 1999). Individuals with more generalized fears certainly often have strong public speaking fears as part of the constellation of distressing social situations, but there is a separate group having social fears exclusively or almost so in this one domain. These latter persons are not often seen in behavioral health facilities, particularly in major health care centers, because public speaking fears are not viewed as "mental health" problems but rather are perceived as "normal" even when at high levels (Booth-Butterfield & Cottone, 1991; West, 1988). Distress about public speaking situations may most appropriately be regarded as fear rather than anxiety given the high degree of situation specificity, robust psychophysiological response, prevalence of avoidance behavior, and prevalence of traumatic conditioning histories in individuals who have circumscribed concerns about public speaking (Boone et al., 1999). Test anxiety is in many ways similar to other social anxieties, and may in fact best be considered a form of evaluation anxiety (Bögels et al., 2010). Similarly, test anxiety in its extreme forms may be phobic in nature, although lesser forms are more typical and considered "normal" based on situational demands. In psychopathological extremes, these problems are phobic in nature, and thus would be considered as DSM phobic disorders, although they may functionally be more similar to specific phobias than other SADs (Boone et al., 1999).

In the DSM-IV-TR (American Psychiatric Association, 2000), there is a "generalized" specifier that designates individuals who fear "most social situations." Nevertheless, there has been a lack of a clear, generally accepted operational definition of this generalized type of SAD, which has hampered progress in the literature. Given the idea of a continuum of severity for SAD, the generalized specifier does not appear to add much to the demarcation of this disorder (Bögels et al., 2010).

Additionally, a "nongeneralized" SP has been suggested (Heimberg, Holt, Schneier, Spitzer, & Liebowitz, 1993). These individuals may represent the "typical" types and severities of SAD encountered in clinical settings. Their problems are not so pervasive as to warrant a classification of "generalized," not so severe as also to be consistent with APD, and not restricted to one (or one type) of social situation so as to be considered circumscribed. Interaction anxiety in a broad range of situations has been suggested as an important feature of "nongeneralized" SADs. Rather than specifying generalized or nongeneralized types of SAD, currently there is consideration of DSM-V having a specifier that denotes "predominantly performance" fears (Bögels et al., 2010), such as public speaking. Also, the identification of other core fears within SAD, such as social interaction, being observed, and displaying anxiety symptoms (particularly blushing) is of some interest (Bögels et al., 2010). This conceptual approach would seem to have particular heuristic value for future dimensional classifications, which might assess, among other points, the functional aspects of social situations that engender anxiety.

The relation of SP and APD has been the subject of great interest; the relation of these states has had more focus in the APD literature than any other (Mendlowicz, Braga, Cabizuca, Land, & Figueira, 2006). Of the seven criteria for APD in the DSM-IV-TR (American Psychiatric Association, 2000), six describe a social interactional component. While comorbidity rates for SAD and APD vary (Alden, Laposa, Taylor, & Rider, 2002; Bögels et al., 2010; Heimberg et al., 1993), they are generally substantial. It should not be expected, however, that a high percentage of individuals with SAD also would be classified with APD, given the likelihood of a continuum of severity in SAD. Only a minor percentage of those individuals with (severe) instantiations of SAD also would meet criteria for APD. While most studies find substantial overlap between SAD and APD (e.g., Hofmann, Newman, Becker, Taylor, & Roth, 1995), including an early collection of three studies and an overview devoted specifically to the topic (Herbert, Hope, & Bellack, 1992; Holt, Heimberg, & Hope, 1992; Turner, Beidel, & Townsley, 1992; Widiger, 1992), as well as a more recent review (Alden et al., 2002), there are some inconsistencies (Tran & Chambless, 1995).

Overall, there appears to be relatively little support for the idea that APD describes a disorder that is qualitatively different from SAD (e.g., Boone et al., 1999; Hofmann et al., 2004). At this point in time, APD primarily seems to describe a distinction that is quantitative in nature (Alden et al., 2002): Individuals who meet criteria for APD in addition to SAD are more severely affected by social fears and anxieties. Nevertheless, that conception may not paint a complete picture, in that other qualities, even features of the schizophrenia spectrum disorders (Bögels et al., 2010), may demarcate APD. Additionally, other distinguishing features of APD may be the likelihood of using avoidance as a coping strategy (Taylor, Laposa, & Alden, 2004), personality patterns such as degree of rigidity, and ambivalence about the positive aspects of interpersonal interactions. The approach–avoidance gradient in social anxieties and fears may be a particularly important one, given that it is much more difficult to entirely avoid certain core aspects of social anxieties and fears, primarily interactional fears and secondarily observational fears. (Performance-based fearful situations may be somewhat easier to avoid, in general.) It is the perseverative avoidance, in spite of social costs (e.g., lack of social support and even outright rejection) and at the same time the difficulty or impossibility of completely avoiding the target of social anxiety and fear, that distinguishes SAD from other DSM phobic disorders and that may distinguish the severity of APD from other SAD(s).

Understanding the types of SAD and their relation to one another depends in part upon a broader conceptualization of both nonpathological and psychopathological forms of such behavior in social anxiety. Hofmann et al. (2004) introduce important dimensions to consider in conceptualizing SAD, including fearfulness and anxiousness, shyness and self-consciousness, and submissiveness and anger. Figure 1.1, as noted earlier, presents a proposed model of a continuum of social anxieties and fears across the population. Related constructs such as shyness span across "normal" to high "normal" to psychopathological levels of social anxiety, with the assumption that there is overlap across a gradient (cf. Turner, Beidel, & Townsley, 1990). The most severe instantiations of this behavior are labeled as SADs, which exist in various forms and themselves differ along a continuum of severity, based in large part on the number of social situations that are feared and cause anxiety. While the idea of a continuum of SADs has intuitive appeal, related to the distribution of social anxieties and fears in the general population, possible qualitative differences within SADs should be further considered (Hofmann et al., 2004).

CULTURAL AND DEVELOPMENTAL CONSIDERATIONS

Social anxieties and SADs exist internationally (Hong & Woody, 2007), across cultures, broadly defined. While there are many similarities across groups, there are disparate aspects as well, and unique manifestations that go beyond DSM and other Western society conceptualizations. The Māori of New Zealand, for example, have the concept of *whakamā*, which involves shyness, embarrassment, and feelings of inadequacy, but also feelings of shame and being unsettled (Metge & Kinloch, 1978; Sachdev, 1990). A severe variant of this condition involves *whakapeke*, which is running away and hiding (Metge & Kinloch, 1978); this latter response may be akin to avoidant behavior observed in SAD in other cultural groups.

Epidemiological investigations have focused on various factors, such as nationality, race/ethnicity, sex, age, socioeconomic status, and urban–rural distinctions, both in terms of social anxieties and related disorders. One of the important distinctions is whether social anxiety is being evaluated (typically through self-reports), or whether impairment and life disruption due to social anxiety is being assessed (to diagnose an SAD). Uncertainty about how social anxieties are socially conceived and scientifically measured, as well as insufficient information, currently disallow a complete picture of uniqueness across cultures. Nevertheless, social anxieties are more frequently indicated on self-report scales in East Asia relative to the United States and Europe, while the rate of SAD is higher in the United States than in other non-European countries (Lewis-Fernández et al., 2010). Collectivist cultural orientations in East Asia (vs. individualism in the latter areas) may help explain the functions of nonpathological social anxiety in these cultures in promoting sensitivity to others and awareness of one's social impact.

Such allocentric anxieties, focused on one's social effect on others, is observed in *taijin kyofusho* (TKS) in East Asian cultural groups (Lewis-Fernández et al., 2010). TKS has been of great interest in the SAD literature, given its similarities to and general consistency with DSM and ICD classifications. TKS appears to be of two subtypes, one of which partially overlaps with SAD but that also has more allocentric qualities. In the other variant, the offensive subtype, there is anxiety about offending or embarrassing another person by one's appearance or behavior, including physiologically based bodily functions such as emitting intestinal gas. An associated olfactory response syndrome has been specifically identified, in which there is concern about emanating noxious body odor (Lewis-Fernández et al., 2010).

In terms of other epidemiological considerations, there are data to suggest that people in rural areas report more social anxiety than their urban counterparts (Grant et al., 2005; Pakriev, Vasar, Aluoja, & Shlik, 2000), which may be testimony to learned responses (see Chapter 13 on basic behavioral mechanisms and processes), perhaps through social skill development on the basis of experience, through exposure that reduces anxiety, or other mechanisms. Greater and lesser population density may impact opportunities for such social learning to occur.

As noted earlier in this chapter, possible sex differences in the epidemiology of social anxieties, SAD, and treatment-seeking related to SAD are inconsistent and uncertain in the literature. It seems fairly clear, however, that the sex differences observed in many other anxiety disorders, with females reporting higher anxiety and males indicating less anxiety, and more diagnoses and treatment-seeking among females relative to males, is much less pronounced in social anxieties and SAD than other anxiety disorders, and may even be nonexistent (Craske, 2003).

SAD often begins early in life, in the mid-teens or even early childhood (Hofmann & Barlow, 2002). The diagnosis of SAD likely can be reliably rendered down to age six (Bögels et al., 2010). As explicated in the DSM-IV-TR, childhood and adolescence may be particular developmental periods in which transient social anxieties appear. To restrict the diagnosis of SAD to children and adolescents whose problems are enduring, it has been suggested that the criterion of at least six months' duration be inclusive of all age groups and not just those 18 years of age and older, as in the DSM-IV-TR (Bögels et al., 2010).

COVERAGE ACROSS DISCIPLINES AND SUBDISCIPLINES

Hope, Gansler, and Heimberg (1989), focusing on SP, noted that the high degree of specialization in psychology and related areas deters "cross fertilization" (p. 49) across disciplines and subdisciplines. Contributions from personality psychology and social psychology are obvious, even when their terms (e.g., "shyness") differ from those popular in clinical and counseling psychology arenas. Psychiatry certainly brings important perspectives, particularly the emphases on biological antecedents and approaches. Other areas, such as "communication apprehension" in the communications area, are less often considered, but still deal with much of the same subject matter (e.g., Booth-Butterfield & Cottone, 1991; Richmond & McCroskey, 1998). Other behavioral/mental health disciplines such as social work and counseling also figure importantly in terms of the treatment of individuals with social anxiety that is of problematic proportions. Moreover, evolutionary biology and ethology have contributed immensely to this area, focusing on dominance/submission behavioral patterns, defensive systems, and gaze. These constructs have been extremely provocative in terms of understanding present-day human social behavior (Mineka & Zinbarg, 1995; Trower, Gilbert, & Sherling, 1990). Finally, anthropology, sociology, and cultural studies can bring an important perspective in terms of the behavior of groups, which has obvious implications for understanding social anxieties in individuals. The knowledge base, theoretical perspectives, and methods for acquiring information from each of these fields, when considered together, offer a tremendous opportunity for a comprehensive conceptualization and understanding of social anxieties and fears, broadly defined. There are strong arguments, therefore, supporting multidisciplinary approaches, and a cross-disciplinary nomenclature, in the area of social anxieties and fears, as well as their psychopathological disorders.

SUMMARY AND CONCLUSIONS

Social anxieties, fears, and their disorders have many faces. Since the early writings of Marks (e.g., 1970; Marks & Gelder, 1966), behavioral and health scientists have studied the varied dimensions of these problems, which can be debilitating and severely limiting in the extreme. Conversely, situationally restricted and mild to moderate levels of social anxiety can be highly transient, and even pleasurable, such as when one is about to give a speech in accepting an award or when a young person telephones to ask for a date with someone he or she finds attractive. These gradients of social anxieties also give us glimpses of what it is that makes us uniquely human.

This area of investigation has long since arrived as a *bona fide*, accepted, and independent area of study. No longer do clinicians and researchers have to justify that SAD accounts for more than everyday problems of living. At the same time, trying to entirely divorce SAD from shyness may not be so critical if one appreciates the continuum of severity that characterizes social anxieties and fears across people. SAD once was dubbed the "neglected" anxiety disorder (Liebowitz, Gorman, Fyer, & Klein, 1985), and the relative coverage was considered less than some other problems with anxiety. While it was no longer considered "neglected" over two decades ago (Heimberg, 1989), significant conceptual and diagnostic work remains.

Changes are needed in the DSM and ICD diagnostic systems, particularly to include dimensional characteristics. A "predominantly performance" designator in DSM-V would do much to acknowledge the existence of "circumscribed" SAD in describing public speaking phobia and other specific SPs. The relation between SAD and APD is unlikely to be resolved with the DSM-V; much work remains in clarifying the conceptualizations of these disorders; perhaps APD is unnecessary as a categorization (Hofmann et al., 2004). Avoidant behaviors of all kinds are of great importance; such manifestations should be investigated in their own right, independently of the personality disorder designation (Hayes et al., 1996).

Volumes such as this one help to organize, synthesize, and advance the state of knowledge about social anxieties, social fears, and SAD(s). The accumulated knowledge base in the social anxieties and fears area over 40 or more years is considerable. It clearly is time, therefore, for the evolution of a common nomenclature (Gray, 1991) that can be used across disciplines and theoretical and other orientations, as well as a dimensional classification scheme for SAD. While the DSM diagnostic nomenclature likely will be enhanced with the forthcoming DSM-V, undoubtedly further conceptual work on the diagnosis of SAD will be necessary. Multinational, multicultural, and transdisciplinary approaches are needed, prompting greater sharing of knowledge throughout related fields, and more collaborative work across disciplines.

ACKNOWLEDGMENTS

Preparation of this revised chapter was supported in part by a Fulbright New Zealand Senior Scholar Fellowship to the author.

Patrick F. Riley, John T. Sorrell, and Kevin E. Vowles provided helpful assistance in the preparation of an earlier version of this chapter. Michael R. Lewin, Avie J. Rainwater, and other research assistants and associates in the Anxiety and Psychophysiology Research Laboratory at Oklahoma State University participated in collecting the SADS and PRCS data. These efforts are acknowledged with gratitude.

REFERENCES

Alden, L. E., Laposa, J. M., Taylor, C. T., & Rider, A. G. (2002). Avoidant personality disorder: Current status and future directions. *Journal of Personality Disorders, 16*, 1–29.

American Psychiatric Association. (1968). *Diagnostic and statistical manual of mental disorders* (2nd ed.), (DSM-II). Washington, DC: Author.

American Psychiatric Association. (1980). *Diagnostic and statistical manual of mental disorders* (3rd ed.), (DSM-III). Washington, DC: Author.

American Psychiatric Association. (1987). *Diagnostic and statistical manual of mental disorders* (3rd ed.), (DSM-III). Washington, DC: Author rev.).

American Psychiatric Association. (1994). *Diagnostic and statistical manual of mental disorders* (4th ed.), (DSM-IV). Washington, DC: Author.

American Psychiatric Association. (2000). *Diagnostic and statistical manual of mental disorders* (4th ed., text rev.) (DSM-IV-TR). Washington, DC: Author.

Andrews, G., Slade, T., Peters, L., & Beard, J. (1998). Generalized anxiety disorder, obsessive-compulsive disorder and social phobia: Sources of dissonance between ICD-10 and DSM-IV. *International Journal of Methods in Psychiatry Research, 7*, 110–115.

Barlow, D. G. (2002). *Anxiety and its disorders: The nature and treatment of anxiety and panic* (2nd ed.). New York: Guilford.

Bögels, S. M., Alden, L., Beidel, D. C., Clark, L. A., Pine, D. S., Stein, M. B., et al. (2010). Social anxiety disorder: Questions and answers for the DSM-V. *Depression and Anxiety, 27*, 168–189.

Boone, M. L., McNeil, D. W., Masia, C. L., Turk, C. L., Carter, L. E., Ries, B. J., et al. (1999). Multimodal comparisons of social phobia subtypes and avoidant personality disorder. *Journal of Anxiety Disorders, 13*, 271–292.

Booth-Butterfield, S., & Cottone, R. R. (1991). Ethical issues in the treatment of communication apprehension and avoidance. *Communication Education, 40*, 172–179.

Bouton, M. E., Mineka, S., & Barlow, D. E. (2001). A modern learning theory perspective on the etiology of panic disorder. *Psychological Review, 108*, 4–32.

Bruce, T. J., & Barlow, D. G. (1990). The nature and role of performance anxiety in sexual dysfunction. In H. Leitenberg (Ed.), *Handbook of social anxiety* (pp. 357–384). New York: Plenum.

Campbell-Sills, L., & Stein, M. B. (2005). Justifying the diagnostic status of social phobia: A reply to Wakefield, Horowitz, and Schmitz. *Canadian Journal of Psychiatry, 50*, 320–323.

Clark, D. B., & Agras, W. S. (1991). The assessment and treatment of performance anxiety in musicians. *American Journal of Psychiatry, 148*, 598–605.

Craske, M. G. (2003). *Origins of phobias and anxiety disorders: Why more women than men?* Oxford, UK: Elsevier.

Eifert, G. H. (1996). More theory-driven and less diagnosis-based behavior therapy. *Journal of Behavior Therapy and Experimental Psychiatry, 27*, 75–86.

Grant, B. F., Hasin, D. S., Blanco, C., Stinson, F. S., Chou, S. P., Goldstein, R. B., et al. (2005). The epidemiology of SAD in the United States: Results from the National Epidemiologic Survey on alcohol and related conditions. *Journal of Clinical Psychiatry, 66*, 1351–1361.

Gray, J. A. (1991). Fear, panic, and anxiety: What's in a name? *Psychological inquiry, 2*, 77–78.

Hall, R., & Goldberg, D. (1977). The role of social anxiety in social interaction difficulties. *British Journal of Psychiatry, 131*, 610–615.

Harris, P. R. (1984). Shyness and psychological imperialism; on the dangers of ignoring the ordinary language roots of the terms we deal with. *European Journal of Social Psychology, 14*, 169–181.

Hayes, S. C., Wilson, K. G., Strosahl, K., Gifford, E. V., & Follette, V. M. (1996). Experiential avoidance and behavioral disorders: A functional dimensional approach to diagnosis and treatment. *Journal of Consulting and Clinical Psychology, 64*, 1152–1168.

Heimberg, R. G. (1989). Social phobia: No longer neglected. *Clinical Psychology Review, 9*, 1–2.

Heimberg, R. G., Holt, C. S., Schneier, F. R., Spitzer, R. L., & Liebowitz, M. R. (1993). The issue of subtypes in the diagnosis of social phobia. *Journal of Anxiety Disorders, 7*, 249–269.

Herbert, J. D., Hope, D. A., & Bellack, A. S. (1992). Validity of the distinction between generalized social phobia and avoidant personality disorder. *Journal of Abnormal Psychology, 101*, 332–339.

Hofmann, S. G., & Barlow, D. G. (2002). Social phobia (social anxiety disorder). In D. G. Barlow (Ed.), *Anxiety and its disorders: The nature and treatment of anxiety and panic* (2nd ed.). (pp. 454–476). New York: Guilford Press.

Hofmann, S. G., Heinrichs, N., & Moscovitch, D. A. (2004). The nature and expression of social phobia: Toward a new classification. *Clinical Psychology Review, 24*, 769–797.

Hofmann, S. G., Newman, M. G., Becker, E., Taylor, C. B., & Roth, W. T. (1995). Social phobia with and without avoidant personality disorder: Preliminary behavior therapy outcome findings. *Journal of Anxiety Disorders, 9*, 427–438.

Holt, C. S., Heimberg, R. G., & Hope, D. A. (1992). Avoidant personality disorder and the generalized subtype in social phobia. *Journal of Abnormal Psychology, 101*, 318–325.

Hong, J., & Woody, S. (2007). Cultural mediators of self-reported social anxiety. *Behaviour Research and Therapy, 45*, 1779–1789.

Hope, D. A., Gansler, D. A., & Heimberg, R. G. (1989). Attentional focus and causal attributions in social phobia: Implications from social psychology. *Clinical Psychology Review, 9*, 49–60.

Hopko, D., McNeil, D. W., Zvolensky, M. J., & Eifert, G. E. (2001). The relation between anxiety and skill in performance-based anxiety disorders: A behavioral formulation of social phobia. *Behavior Therapy, 32*, 185–207.

Kessler, R. C., Stein, M. B., & Berglund, P. (1998). Social phobia subtypes in the national comorbidity survey. *American Journal of Psychiatry, 155*, 613–619.

Kleinknecht, R. A., Dinnel, D. L., Kleinknecht, E. E., Hiruma, N., & Harada, N. (1997). Cultural factors in social anxiety: A comparison of social phobia symptoms and taijin kyofusho. *Journal of Anxiety Disorders, 11*, 157–177.

Klorman, H., Weerts, T. C., Hastings, J. E., Melamed, B. G., & Lang, P. J. (1974). Psychometric description of some specific-fear questionnaires. *Behavior Therapy, 5*, 401–409.

Lang, P. J. (1968). Fear reduction and fear behavior: Problems in treating a construct. In J. M. Shlien (Series Ed.) *Research in psychotherapy: Vol 3*. Washington, DC: American Psychological Association.

Leitenberg, H. (1990). Introduction. In H. Leitenberg (Ed.), *Handbook of social and evaluation anxiety* (pp. 1–8). New York: Plenum.

Lewin, M. R., McNeil, D. W., & Lipson, J. M. (1996). Enduring without avoiding: Pauses and verbal dysfluencies in public speaking fear. *Journal of Psychopathology and Behavioral Assessment, 18*, 387–402.

Lewis-Fernandez, R., Hinton, D. E., Laria, A. J., Patterson, E. H., Hofmann, S. G., Craske, M. G., et al. (2010). Culture and the anxiety disorders: Recommendations for DSM-V. *Depression and Anxiety, 27*, 212–229.

Liebowitz, M. R., Gorman, J. M., Fyer, A. J., & Klein, D. F. (1985). Social phobia: Review of a neglected anxiety disorder. *Archives of General Psychiatry, 42*, 729–736.

Marks, I. M. (1970). The classification of phobic disorders. *British Journal of Psychiatry, 116*, 377–386.

Marks, I. M. (1985). Behavioral treatment of social phobia. *Psychopharmacology Bulletin, 21*, 615–618.

Marks, I. M., & Gelder, M. G. (1966). Different ages of onset in varieties of phobia. *American Journal of Psychiatry, 123*, 218–221.

Masia, C. L., & Morris, T. L. (1998). Parental factors associated with social anxiety: Methodological limitations and suggestions for integrated behavioral research. *Clinical Psychology: Science and Practice, 5*, 211–228.

McNeil, D. W. (2001). Terminology and evolution of constructs related to social phobia. In S. G. Hofmann & P. M. DiBartolo (Eds.), *Social phobia and social anxiety: An integration* (pp. 8–19). Needham Heights, MA: Allyn & Bacon.

McNeil, D. W., Porter, C. A., Zvolensky, M. J., Chaney, J. M., & Kee, M. (2000). Assessment of culturally related anxiety in American Indians and Alaska Natives. *Behavior Therapy, 31*, 301–325.

McNeil, D. W., Turk, C. L., & Ries, B. J. (1994). Anxiety and fear. In V. S. Ramachandran (Series Ed.), *Encyclopedia of human behavior: Vol. 1*. New York: Academic Press.

Mendlowicz, M. V., Braga, R. J., Cabizuca, M., Land, M. G., & Figueira, I. L. (2006). A comparison of publication trends on avoidant personality disorder and social phobia. *Psychiatry Research, 144*, 205–209.

Metge, J., & Kinloch, P. (1978). *Talking past each other: Problems of cross-cultural communication*. Wellington, NZ: Victoria University Press.

Mineka, S., & Zinbarg, R. (1995). Conditioning and ethological models of social phobia. In R. G. Heimberg, M. R. Liebowitz, D. A. Hope, & F. R. Schneier (Eds.), *Social phobia: Diagnosis, assessment, and treatment* (pp. 134–162). New York: Guilford.

Öhman, A. (1986). Face the beast and fear the face: Animal and social fears as prototypes for evolutionary analyses of emotion. *Psychophysiology, 23*, 123–145.

Pakriev, S., Vasar, V., Aluoja, A., & Shlik, J. (2000). Prevalence of social phobia in the rural population of Udmurtia. *Nordic Journal of Psychiatry*, *54*, 109–112.

Paul, G. L. (1966). *Insight versus desensitization in psychotherapy*. Stanford, CA: Stanford University Press.

Pollard, C. A., & Henderson, J. G. (1988). Four types of social phobia in a community sample. *Journal of Nervous and Mental Disease*, *176*, 440–445.

Rapee, R. M. (1995). Descriptive psychopathology of social phobia. In R. G. Heimberg, M. R. Liebowitz, D. A. Hope, & F. R. Schneier (Eds.), *Social phobia: Diagnosis and treatment* (pp. 41–66). New York: Guilford.

Richmond, V. P., & McCroskey, J. C. (1998). *Communication: Apprehension, avoidance, and effectiveness* (5th ed.). Needham, MA: Allyn & Bacon.

Sachdev, P. S. (1990). Whakamā: Culturally determined behaviour in the New Zealand Maori. *Psychological Medicine*, *20*, 433–444.

Schneier, F., & Welkowitz, L. (1996). *The hidden face of shyness: Understanding and overcoming social anxiety*. New York: Avon.

Smith, R. E., & Smoll, F. L. (1990). Sport performance anxiety. In H. Leitenberg (Ed.), *Handbook of social anxiety* (pp. 417–454). New York: Plenum.

Stein, M. B., Torgrud, L. J., & Walker, J. (2000). Social phobia symptoms, subtypes, and severity. *Archives of General Psychiatry*, *57*, 1046–1052.

Suomi, S. J. (1997). Nonverbal communication in nonhuman primates: Implications for the emergence of culture. In U. C. Segerstrale & P. Molnar (Eds.), *Nonverbal communication: Where nature meets culture* (pp. 131–150). Mahway, NJ: Lawrence Erlbaum.

Taylor, C. T., Laposa, J. M., & Alden, L. E. (2004). Is avoidant personality disorder more than just social avoidance?. *Journal of Personality Disorders*, *18*, 571–594.

Thompson, R. A., & Limber, S. P. (1990). "Social anxiety" in infancy: Stranger and separation reactions. In H. Leitenberg (Ed.), *Handbook of social and evaluation anxiety* (pp. 85–137). New York: Plenum.

Tran, G. Q., & Chambless, D. L. (1995). Psychopathology of social phobia: Effects of subtype and of avoidant personality disorder. *Journal of Anxiety Disorders*, *9*, 489–501.

Trower, P., & Gilbert, P. (1989). New theoretical conceptions of social anxiety and social phobia. *Clinical Psychology Review*, *9*, 19–35.

Trower, P., Gilbert, P., & Sherling, G. (1990). Social anxiety, evolution, and self-presentation. In H. Leitenberg (Ed.), *Handbook of social and evaluation anxiety* (pp. 11–45). New York: Plenum.

Turner, S. M., Beidel, D. C., & Townsley, R. M. (1990). Social phobia: Relationship to shyness. *Behaviour Research and Therapy*, *28*, 497–505.

Turner, S. M., Beidel, D. C., & Townsley, R. M. (1992). Social phobia: A comparison of specific and generalized subtypes and avoidant personality disorder. *Journal of Abnormal Psychology*, *102*, 326–331.

Wakefield, J. C., Horowitz, A. V., & Schmitz, M. R. (2005a). Are we overpathologizing the socially anxious? Social phobia from a harmful dysfunction perspective. *Canadian Journal of Psychiatry*, *50*, 317–319.

Wakefield, J. C., Horowitz, A. V., & Schmitz, M. R. (2005b). Social disadvantage is not mental disorder: Response to Campbell-Sills and Stein. *Canadian Journal of Psychiatry*, *50*, 324–326.

Watson, D., & Friend, R. (1969). Measurement of social-evaluative anxiety. *Journal of Consulting and Clinical Psychology*, *33*, 448–457.

West, L. J. (1988). Distinguishing normal fears from abnormal anxiety. *Journal of Clinical Psychiatry*, *49*(10), 5–6.

Widiger, T. A. (1992). Generalized social phobia versus avoidant personality disorder. *Journal of Abnormal Psychology*, *102*, 340–343.

World Health Organization. (2007). The international classification of mental and behavioural disorders – 10 (*Version for 2007*). Geneva: Author. Retrieved April 30, 2010 from http://apps.who.int/classifications/apps/icd/icd10online/.

Zimbardo, P. G. (1977). *Shyness: What it is, what to do about it*. Reading, MA: Addison–Wesley.

Chapter 2

Assessment of Social Anxiety and Social Phobia

James D. Herbert, Alyssa A. Rheingold, and Lynn L. Brandsma
Department of Psychology, Drexel University, Philadelphia, PA 90102

Social anxiety is a universal phenomenon. At any given time, for any given individual, one's degree of social anxiety may vary from fearlessness at one extreme to debilitating anxiety and avoidance at the other. When the level of anxiety, avoidance, and impairment in functioning reaches clinical proportions, a diagnosis of SAD (also known as SP) – and possibly APD – is made. Unfortunately, such diagnostic categories are often reified, and the underlying dimensional continuity of social anxiety is overlooked. At this time, there is no compelling reason to believe that social anxiety and SP differ qualitatively (Jørstad-Stein & Heimberg, 2009; Rapee, 1995). Hence, the assessment methods described here can be used for assessing subdiagnostic social anxiety as well as SAD *per se*.

Careful and thorough assessment is critical to treatment planning and clinical research. Assessment measures for social anxiety have typically been divided into two broad groups: behavioral assessment methods (Glass & Arnkoff, 1989; McNeil, Ries, & Turk, 1995), which include role-playing procedures and self-monitoring, and cognitive assessment procedures (Arnkoff & Glass, 1989; Elting & Hope, 1995; Heimberg, 1994), including thought-listing and information-processing paradigms. Although this is a useful organization scheme, it also has its drawbacks. Primary among these is the fact that whether any given measure is considered a behavioral or a cognitive assessment procedure is more a function of one's theoretical perspective than of the measure itself. Depending on one's perspective, self-report questionnaires, for example, may be viewed as measures of behavioral symptoms comprising a clinical syndrome or of a cognitive theoretical construct central to the etiology of that syndrome.

In this chapter we have elected to organize the various assessment procedures according to the methodology of the procedure. Many of the tools described can be used for different purposes depending upon one's goals (e.g., treatment planning in a clinical context, psychopathology research) and

Social Anxiety: Clinical, Developmental, and Social Perspectives. DOI: 10.1016/B978-0-12-375096-9.00002-X

one's theoretical orientation (e.g., behaviorist, mediational, cognitivist). The first section describes the clinical interview, with particular attention to structured clinical interviews. This is followed by a review of the most commonly used self-report questionnaires for social anxiety. Role-playing procedures are then described, followed in turn by self-monitoring and thought-listing techniques. Finally, psychophysiological assessment is discussed briefly. We limit our review to instruments and procedures that are commonly used either in clinical settings or in treatment outcome research. Procedures developed specifically to test hypotheses in experimental psychopathology research are beyond the scope of this chapter. For example, in addition to measuring cognitive content through questionnaires or thought-listing procedures, there has recently been a growing emphasis on the measurement of cognitive processes. This literature employs various information-processing paradigms in an effort to elucidate cognitive processing anomalies unique to social anxiety (e.g., Amir, Beard, Burns, & Bomyea, 2009; Schmidt, Richey, Buckner, & Timpano, 2009). Interested readers are referred to Elting and Hope (1995) and Heimberg (1994) for reviews of such procedures. Although our primary focus is on adults, we briefly review issues pertaining to the assessment of social anxiety in children and adolescents, as well as instruments developed specifically for these populations.

THE CLINICAL INTERVIEW

The clinical interview is by far the most common assessment method of SAD, or any other form of psychopathology for that matter. Clinical interviews vary along as many dimensions as there are interviewers. For example, some clinicians use a highly directive, structured format, whereas others prefer a more unstructured, free-flowing approach.

Regardless of style, there are typically three goals of the clinical interview when working with persons with social anxiety: (1) establishing rapport, (2) accurate diagnosis, and (3) assessment of symptom patterns, phobic stimuli, and impairment in functioning. The clinical interview is typically the first contact the patient has with the therapist or researcher, and as such the development of a good working rapport is critical. Although this is true with any patient, the nature of social anxiety presents special challenges to this task. It is difficult to overstate how difficult the first interview is for most persons with high social anxiety. These persons rarely realize how common their problems are, believing they are unique and perhaps even "crazy." In addition, they often fear being judged negatively by the interviewer and are vigilant for signs of disapproval. Given the chronic, unremitting nature of SP, individuals frequently have come to view the condition as simply part of who they are and, therefore, have difficulty recognizing the ways in which their functioning has become impaired.

We recommend several strategies for interviewing persons with social anxiety. First, the clinician may begin the interview with a period of small talk to break the ice. Although open-ended questions are often preferred in clinical interviews (Greist, Kobak, Jefferson, Katzelnick, & Chene, 1995), we suggest frequently using simple closed-ended questions to help put at ease persons with social anxiety. It is especially important, however, that the interview not be perceived as an interrogation. The pace of the interview often needs to be slowed; we typically allot at least two hours for an initial interview. It is critical that the interviewer avoid signs that he or she is disapproving of something the patient says. Initial interviews with socially anxious children and adolescents can be especially challenging. We recommend beginning the initial session with some naturalistic activity away from the consultation office (e.g., an impromptu walk to purchase a drink from a vending machine), a strategy that often provides a valuable entrée into the interview process.

For adults, obtaining sufficient and reliable information to make a diagnosis according to standard criteria outlined in the DSM-IV (1994) is typically not problematic, because socially anxious adults are generally adequate informants regarding their own symptoms and the DSM-IV criteria for SAD are relatively straightforward. Such is not the case with children and adolescents, however, because they tend to under-report symptoms. Obtaining information from parents and teachers is often helpful once the child has been identified as having a problem. Unfortunately, initial identification of social anxiety in children is often difficult. In fact, SAD in children and adolescents frequently goes unnoticed by parents and school personnel alike, not being recognized unless it results in frequent school absences or outright school refusal (Kashdan & Herbert, 2001; Kearney & Albano, 2004).

The most common diagnostic dilemmas involve misdiagnosing SAD as agoraphobia and failing to recognize comorbid conditions. SAD is often misdiagnosed as agoraphobia when socially anxious individuals (SAIs) avoid so many situations that they spend a great deal of time at home. Although there is some evidence that the pattern of physiological symptoms tends to differ between the two conditions (Amies, Gelder, & Shaw, 1983), the critical distinction is made on the basis of the nature of the underlying fear: In the case of social anxiety the primary fear is of humiliation and negative evaluation by others, whereas in the case of agoraphobia it is the fear of having a panic attack. Diagnostic comorbidity with SAD is the rule rather than the exception (Schneier, Johnson, Hornig, Liebowitz, & Weissman, 1992). Among the most common comorbid diagnoses are major depression, substance abuse, and APD. In the case of depression, it is important to clarify the relationship between the two conditions over time. If the symptoms of anxiety clearly preceded the onset of depression, a separate diagnosis of SP may be warranted. If the anxiety covaries with the other symptoms of depression, the anxiety may be conceptualized as part of the depressive episode. Alcohol abuse among individuals with social anxiety is common, as many have learned to use alcohol prior to and during social situations to alleviate anxiety. Finally, the relationship between SAD and APD has been the subject of much debate (Huppert, Strunk, Ledley, Davidson, & Foa, 2008; Widiger, 1992). Although there appears to be little theoretical or empirical justification for qualitative distinctions between the two diagnostic categories, the DSM-IV rules permit both diagnoses to be made concurrently when their respective criteria are met.

Accurate diagnosis is only the beginning of the assessment process. There is substantial heterogeneity among persons with social anxiety, which is reflected in patterns of cognitive and physiological symptoms and behavioral avoidance, the stimulus parameters that elicit anxiety, and the degree of social and vocational functional impairment. A good clinical interview reviews each of these areas to generate a complete picture of the individual's clinical status. The construction of a fear hierarchy – a list of phobic social situations in order of degree of anxiety elicited and degree of avoidance – is especially important as a prelude for behaviorally oriented treatments.

Structured Interviews

Unstructured interviews are most commonly used in clinical practice, whereas structured interviews are more commonly used in research contexts. There is, however, a growing awareness of the utility of structured interviews in non-research clinical settings. Zimmerman and Mattia (1999) found that diagnostic rates of SAD based on structured interviews were nine times higher than rates based on unstructured interviews, suggesting that the former greatly reduce the rates of false-negative judgments. Structured interviews function as a template to guide the interviewer's questions and make decision rules explicit, thereby greatly enhancing the reliability of assessment information. Although some clinicians believe that structured interviews render the interview process awkward and rigid, in our experience, in the hands of a skilled interviewer, the process can be as smooth and seamless as traditional unstructured approaches.

The most commonly used structured interviews for social anxiety are the Anxiety Disorders Interview Schedule for DSM-IV (ADIS-IV) (Brown, DiNardo, & Barlow, 1994) and the Structured Clinical Interview for DSM-IV (SCID-IV) (First, Spitzer, Williams, & Gibbon, 1997). Another well-known structured clinical interview is the Schedule for Affective Disorders and Schizophrenia (Spitzer & Endicott, 1978), although it is rarely used as the primary diagnostic tool for anxiety disorders. Both the ADIS-IV and the SCID-IV were designed to yield diagnoses compatible with the DSM-IV. Although the ADIS-IV also yields mood disorder diagnoses and screens for somatoform, psychotic, and substance use disorders, it is designed primarily to make distinctions among the various mood and anxiety disorders. The ADIS-IV is especially useful in evaluating social anxiety because it provides symptomatic information beyond that required to make a diagnosis. For example, the interviewer makes ratings of fear and avoidance related to various common social situations (e.g., speeches, initiating conversations). Child and parent versions of the ADIS have also been developed (Albano & Silverman, 1996; Silverman & Nelles, 1988). The SCID-IV covers the full range of DSM-IV major psychiatric syndromes. DSM-IV criteria are built directly into the structure of the interview. The SCID-IV organizes classes of disorders into separate modules and is geared toward eliciting sufficient information to make accurate diagnoses across all psychiatric syndromes, without special attention to any particular spectrum of psychopathology. The SCID-IV does not prompt the interviewer to routinely query about as many social situations as the ADIS-R, and there is some evidence that supplementing the SCID-IV with additional prompts regarding more social situations can improve diagnostic accuracy, particularly in the reduction of false-negative judgments (Dalrymple & Zimmerman, 2008). Both the ADIS-IV and the SCID-IV require training to ensure proper administration and interpretation. The SCID-IV is widely viewed as the gold standard for diagnostic purposes in clinical research studies of anxiety disorders (e.g., Kessler et al., 2006; Shear et al., 2000; Steiner, Tebes, Sledge, & Walker, 1995).

Several studies have evaluated the test-retest and inter-rater reliability of the SCID and the ADIS, although most of these were conducted with earlier versions of the instruments that were linked to the DSM-III or DSM-III-R. One exception is a study of the SCID-IV by Ventura, Liberman, Green, Shaner, and Mintz (1998), which found excellent inter-rater reliability on assessments of symptoms across a variety of disorders (overall kappa = 0.85) following extensive training of interviewers. In addition, a telephone version of the social anxiety module of the SCID-IV was found to be comparable to the in-person interview, and demonstrated good test–retest reliability (Crippa et al., 2008). Several other studies examining the differential diagnosis of various disorders have found moderate to high test–retest and inter-rater reliability for the SCID-III-R (Malow, West, Williams, & Sutker, 1989; Riskind, Beck, Berchick, Brown, & Steer, 1987; Segal, Hersen, & Van Hassalt, 1994; Stukenberg, Dura, & Kiecolt-Glaser, 1990; Williams et al., 1992). Good test–retest reliability of DSM-IV ADIS-C/P diagnoses has been demonstrated in a clinical sample of adolescents (Silverman, Saavedra, & Pina, 2001). Regarding the diagnosis of SAD specifically, Skre, Onstand, Torgersen, and Kringlen (1991) obtained a kappa of 0.72 for inter-rater reliability using the SCID-III-R. Williams et al. (1992) obtained a more modest kappa of 0.47 for test–retest reliability of SP using the DSM-III-R.

Few studies have evaluated the psychometric properties of the ADIS-IV. However, good inter-rater reliability has been found for the ADIS-IV SP module (kappa = 0.77), as well as for dimensional ratings of SP symptoms on scales of fear and avoidance (Pearson $r = 0.86$ for both dimensions; Brown, DiNardo, Lehman, & Campbell, 2001). Di Nardo, Moras, Barlow, Rapee, and Brown (1993) evaluated the reliability of an earlier version of the instrument, the ADIS-R, which is based on the DSM-III-R. Di Nardo et al. (1993) found excellent diagnostic inter-rater reliability in a sample of

267 anxiety clinic outpatients. Furthermore, excellent inter-rater reliability was found for the diagnosis of SP (kappa = 0.66). The Parent and Child versions of the ADIS-R have been demonstrated to have excellent test–retest and inter-rater reliability across anxiety disorder diagnoses, including SP (Rapee, Barrett, Dadds, & Evans, 1994; Silverman & Eisen, 1992; Silverman & Nelles, 1988; Silverman & Rabian, 1995).

INTERVIEWER-RATED SCALES

Liebowitz (1987) developed an interviewer-rated scale for measuring the severity of SP symptoms: the Liebowitz Social Phobia Scale (LSPS). This 24-item scale requires the interviewer to make separate ratings of fear and avoidance for a range of social situations. Items are divided into social/interactional situations (13 items) and performance situations (11 items). Each item is rated for fear and avoidance on a 4-point Likert scale. The interview yields five scores: an overall severity rating, performance fear, performance avoidance, social fear, and social avoidance. The scale has become an increasingly popular assessment instrument in clinical trials of SAD, particularly pharmacological trials, and has been shown to demonstrate good treatment sensitivity (e.g., Adler et al., 2009; Book, Thomas, Randall, & Randall, 2008; Koszycki, Benger, Shlik, Bradwejn, 2007; Lipsitz et al., 2008). The scale has been shown to have good internal consistency (Heimberg & Holaway, 2007; Heimberg et al., 1999) and good concurrent validity with other measures of social anxiety (Davidson et al., 1991). Despite now being the most widely used interviewer-rated scale of social anxiety, however, the LSPS was not developed empirically, nor was the derivation of the two subscales. In fact, it is not clear on what basis many of the items were categorized as "social" versus "performance," and this distinction appears to lack face validity for some items. Indeed, research indicates that the two subscales are highly correlated, calling into question their distinctiveness and clinical utility (Heimberg & Holaway, 2007; Heimberg et al., 1999; Oakman, Van Ameringen, Mancini, & Farvolden, 2003). Moreover, Safren et al. (1999) found the original subscales to be a poor fit to the data and proposed four factor-analytically derived subscales: public speaking, social interaction, observation by others, and eating/drinking in public. Heimberg and Holaway (2007) found that two of these subscales (public speaking and social interaction) discriminated between patients with SAD, patients with generalized anxiety disorder (GAD), and nonpatients.

The LSPS is a useful clinician-rated measure of the severity of social anxiety symptoms. Further research is needed to clarify the instrument's factor structure and to assess the clinical utility of resulting subscales. Although the LSPS was originally designed as a clinician-rated measure, it has also been used as a self-report questionnaire. This application of the LSPS is described below.

Davidson et al. (1991) developed the Brief Social Phobia Scale (BSPS), another observer-rated instrument. The scale consists of seven items describing common social situations that are rated on both fear and avoidance, and four items measuring physiological symptoms. All ratings are made on 5-point Likert scales. Davidson et al. (1991) reported initial data supporting the test–retest reliability, internal consistency, and convergent validity of the instrument in a clinical population. Davidson et al. (1997) provided further evidence for the psychometric properties of the BSPS in a sample of 275 individuals diagnosed with SAD. Like the LSPS, the BSPS has been used in a number of clinical trials of both pharmacotherapy (e.g., Emmanuel et al., 2000) and psychotherapy (e.g., Ledley et al., 2005), and is sensitive to treatment effects. Its strengths lie in its brevity and ease of administration, and its assessment of physiological symptoms.

The assessment of functional impairment has gained increased attention over the past few years. The most commonly used instrument for anxiety disorders is the Sheehan Disability Scale (SDS; Leon, Olfson, Portera, Farbert, & Sheehan, 1997). This instrument consists of 11-point Likert ratings made by interviewers of current impairment in vocational, social/leisure, and family/home domains; the SDS is also sometimes used in a self-report format. It is widely used in pharmacological trials of SAD. Despite its common use, there is a paucity of data on its psychometric properties.

Other measures of functional impairment include the clinician-rated Disability Profile (DP) and its sister self-report scale, the Liebowitz Self-Rated Disability Scale (LSRDS; Schneier et al., 1994). Both of these instruments are designed to assess both current and lifetime impairment across multiple domains resulting from a specific disorder. The LSRDS consists of 4-point Likert scales that are rated for 11 domains of functioning, whereas the DP consists of 5-point Likert ratings of 8 of the 11 domains assessed by the LSRDS. Like the SDS, there is little psychometric data on either the DP or the LSRDS. A potential drawback of these measures is the difficulty distinguishing impairment associated with a specific disorder from impairment resulting from other factors; this concern is even more problematic in the case of chronic conditions such as SAD.

Hambrick et al. (2004) examined the psychometric properties of the SDS, DP, and LSRDS in a sample of patients with SAD ($n = 153$). All three scales demonstrated good internal consistency, and all three were correlated not only with one another but with symptom measures of depression, social anxiety, and quality of life. In addition, social anxiety accounted for variability in the scales above and beyond that attributable to depression.

SELF-REPORT MEASURES

Self-report questionnaires are extremely useful in the assessment of social anxiety. On a practical level, questionnaires are efficient, requiring little time to administer and score. They can be administered repeatedly over time to evaluate the ongoing effects of treatment. Theoretically, questionnaires reduce an important source of error variance by eliminating the need for the clinician to interpret patient responses.

Several self-report instruments have been developed specifically to assess social anxiety. These can be divided into three broad groups. The first consists of instruments designed to measure directly specific symptoms of social anxiety or SP. The second group is comprised of measures of theoretically derived components of social anxiety. Finally, instruments have been recently developed to assess social anxiety and related constructs among children and adolescents. The most commonly used of each of these three groups of instruments are reviewed next.

GENERAL MEASURES OF SOCIAL ANXIETY AND SOCIAL PHOBIA

The Liebowitz Social Phobia Scale – Self-Report

As noted above, although originally designed as a clinician-administered instrument, the LSPS has been increasingly used in a self-report format. Research indicates that the clinician-administered LSPS and the self-report version (LSPS-SR) are highly correlated and yield comparable means for both clinical and nonclinical groups (Baker, Heinrichs, Kim, & Hofmann, 2002; Fresco et al., 2001). Rytwinski and colleagues (2009) found that the LSPS-SR could distinguish patients with the generalized versus nongeneralized subtypes of SAD, and both of these from nonpatient controls, using the same cut-off scores as the clinician-administered LSPS, derived by Mennin et al. (2002).

The Social Phobia and Anxiety Inventory

Turner, Beidel, Dancu, and Stanley (1989) developed the Social Phobia Anxiety Inventory (SPAI), an empirically derived 45-item self-report instrument to assess the critical features of SP. The SPAI was systematically constructed according to the behavioral-analytic model of Goldfried and D'Zurilla (1969). The measure assesses specific somatic symptoms, thoughts, and behaviors – including avoidance and escape behaviors – across a range of potentially distressing social situations. A 7-point Likert-scale format is used to assess severity of distress and functional impairment. Higher scores represent higher levels of distress and functional impairment.

The instrument consists of two subscales: a 32-item SP subscale and a 13-item agoraphobia subscale. Twenty-one of the 32 SP subscale items assess degree of distress in various social settings, requiring four separate ratings based on the presence of four different audience groups (strangers, authority figures, opposite sex, and people in general). The SP subscale assesses the specific symptoms of social anxiety, whereas the agoraphobia subscale assesses fear in situations typically avoided by agoraphobics (e.g., crossing streets, waiting in lines, public transportation). Subtracting the agoraphobia subscale from the SP subscale determines a difference subscale score. The necessity of calculating this difference score is based upon theoretical and empirical findings of the overlap among anxiety disorders, particularly the overlap between agoraphobia and SP (Turner, Beidel et al., 1989). However, the issue of how best to score the SPAI has been a matter of debate. Herbert, Bellack, and Hope (1991) argue that the SP subscale may be a better index of social anxiety symptoms than the difference subscale, and they caution that using the difference score may produce false negatives in individuals with symptoms of both agoraphobia and SP (Herbert, Bellack, Hope, & Mueser, 1992). Beidel and Turner (1992), however, maintain the superiority of the difference subscale.

In their initial description of the instrument's development, Turner, Beidel et al. (1989) present data supporting the test–retest reliability and internal consistency of the SPAI over a two-week period. In addition, the SPAI was found to successfully discriminate social phobic individuals from individuals with other anxiety disorders. In a following study investigating concurrent and external validity, Beidel, Turner, Stanley, and Dancu (1989) found that the SPAI was capable of discriminating social phobic patients from nonsocial phobics and accurately predicting distress in daily social encounters. In fact, Peters (2000) found that the SPAI showed the best predictive and discriminative properties compared to other widely used SAD measures. Beidel, Turner, Stanley et al. (1989) also found a moderate correlation between the ratings of a significant other and the individual's own rating of distress. In addition, the SPAI has been shown to demonstrate adequate concurrent validity and specificity with respect to other measures of social anxiety and related constructs and measures of other forms of psychopathology in a clinic sample (Herbert et al., 1991; Turner, Stanley, Beidel, & Bond, 1989). The SPAI shows adequate concurrent validity with respect to the self-monitoring of daily social behaviors, somatic responding, and avoidance behaviors of a clinic sample of social phobics when engaged in an anxiety-producing task (Beidel, Borden, Turner, & Jacob, 1989).

The SPAI has been demonstrated to be a useful measure of treatment outcome (Beidel, Turner, & Cooley, 1993). Taylor, Woody, McLean, and Koch (1997) found the SPAI to be more sensitive to treatment effects relative to several other measures. In addition to its usefulness as a research tool, the SPAI is especially useful in clinical contexts because it not only provides a global index of social phobic symptomatology but also reviews distress and avoidance associated with various common social situations. Such specificity is useful in determining targets for treatment. In addition, the SPAI has been shown to be sensitive to treatment effects (Beidel et al., 1993; Herbert et al., 2005; Hofmann et al., 2006). Use of the SPAI has spread worldwide as non-English versions have been developed, including Portuguese and Spanish language versions (Picon et al., 2006; Olivares et al., 2002; respectively). Strengths of the SPAI include its strong psychometric properties and detailed assessment of specific phobic situations. The primary limitation is its relatively long length, which precludes its use as a screening tool (Tharwani & Davidson, 2001).

Social Interaction Anxiety Scale

The Social Interaction Anxiety Scale (SIAS) and its companion scale, the Social Phobia Scale (SPS), were developed in response to the need for instruments that assess various commonly feared social situations (Mattick & Clark, 1998). The development of the SIAS was based on the conceptualization that social anxiety occurs in two types of situations: those involving social interaction with others (e.g., initiating and maintaining conversation) and those involving being observed or scrutinized by others (e.g., giving a speech or eating in public) (Liebowitz, 1987; Mattick & Clark, 1998). Each type of situation requires somewhat different skills on the part of the individual, and, therefore, a person with SP may fear one, the other, or both types of situations (Heimberg, Mueller, Holt, Hope, & Liebowitz, 1992). The SIAS attempts to measure the first of the two concepts, social interactional anxiety. The SIAS consists of 20 items that are rated on a 5-point Likert scale ranging from "not at all characteristic of me" to "extremely characteristic of me." Items are self-statements describing reactions to social interactions in dyads or groups. A total SIAS score is generated by summing the ratings after reverse scoring three positively worded items.

The SIAS is supported by a variety of psychometric data. Mattick and Clark (1998) reported good test–retest reliability and internal consistency across five patient and control groups. Heimberg et al. (1992) reported similar test–retest reliability and internal consistency figures in a study with undergraduate students, community volunteers, and patients with SP. The SIAS has also been found to be positively correlated with other anxiety measures (Habke, Hewitt, Norton, & Asmundson, 1997; Heimberg et al., 1992; Mattick & Clark, 1998). Scores on the SIAS were most highly correlated with indexes of social interactional anxiety (Heimberg et al., 1992). Discriminant validity of the SIAS has been examined in a number of studies. Socially anxious patients scored higher on the SIAS than undergraduates and community controls as well as patients with a range of anxiety disorders (Heimberg et al., 1992; Holt, Heimberg, & Hope, 1992; Mattick & Clark, 1998; Rapee, Brown, Antony, & Barlow, 1992). Furthermore, comorbid diagnoses of mood or panic disorder (PD) did not affect SIAS scores among social phobic patients; an additional diagnosis of GAD, however, was associated with higher SIAS scores (Brown et al., 1997). Rodebaugh, Woods, Heimberg, Liebowitz, & Schneier (2006) and Rodebaugh, Woods, & Heimberg (2007) present data suggesting that the reverse-scored items actually hinder the psychometric properties of the SIAS, and suggest omitting these items.

Social Phobia Scale

As noted previously, the SPS was developed by Mattick and Clark (1998) to measure anticipatory anxiety associated with being observed by others, anxiety when actually being observed, and anxiety felt when engaging in activities in the presence of others (e.g., eating, writing). The format of the SPS is similar to the SIAS: 20 items are rated on a 5-point Likert scale, with a total score being derived by summing the ratings. The psychometric properties of the SPS were investigated simultaneously with the SIAS. The SPS has been shown to demonstrate good test–retest reliability and internal consistency across various clinical and nonclinical groups (Mattick & Clark, 1998; Heimberg et al., 1992). The SPS also shows good concurrent validity among patients with SP, being positively correlated with various social anxiety scales and highly correlated with measures of performance fear (Brown et al., 1997; Habke et al., 1997; Heimberg et al., 1992; Mattick & Clark, 1998). Excellent discriminant validity of the scale has been shown in various studies. Social phobic patients scored higher on the SPS than undergraduates and community controls as well as patients with a range of anxiety disorders (Mattick & Clark, 1998; Heimberg et al., 1992; Holt et al., 1992; Rapee et al., 1992). Clinician-rated severity of SP was moderately related to SPS scores, and additional diagnoses of mood or PD did not affect SPS scores among social phobic patients (Brown et al., 1997).

Both the SPS and the SIAS are sensitive to treatment effects (Mattick & Peters, 1988; Mattick, Peters, & Clark, 1989), although they appear to be less useful than the SPAI in reliably discriminating patients with versus without SAD (Peters, 2000). They are both clinically useful due to ease of administration and scoring and their survey of a range of commonly feared social situations. The SPS and SIAS were developed concurrently based upon the concept that social anxiety is comprised of the fear of two types of situations (interaction and being observed), so the two measures can be considered to be subscales of one larger measure and are most useful when employed together. The SPS and SIAS have been translated into several languages (Sica et al., 2007; Ye, Qian, Lu, & Chen, 2007; Zubeidat, Salinas, Sierra, & Fernandez-Parra, 2007).

Fear Questionnaire

The Fear Questionnaire (FQ), developed by Marks and Mathews (1979), has been widely used both within the United States and internationally as a screening tool for anxiety. Like the other measures described in this section, the FQ has been translated into several languages (e.g., Eguchi et al., 2005; Kasvikis, Sotiropoulou, Mitskidou, Livanou, & Poulou, 2006). Technically, the FQ is comprised of three sections. First, one is asked to list one's primary fear and to rate how much situations associated with that fear are avoided. The second section, the Anxiety–Depression scale, consists of five items assessing general affective disturbances. The third section, also known as the Fear Questionnaire, is the main section of the measure and has the same name as the overall instrument. This has caused some confusion in the literature. Generally, the term FQ in the literature refers to this latter scale alone rather than the overall instrument.

The FQ consists of 15 items designed to assess avoidance behaviors associated with social situations, agoraphobia, and blood/injury phobia. Although a total phobia score can be derived from the sum of the items, the use of individual subscale scores is more common (Arrindell, Emmelkamp, & van der Ende, 1984).

The FQ demonstrates high test–retest reliability and good internal consistency (Marks & Mathews, 1979; Michelson & Mavissakalian, 1983; van Zuuren, 1988). The FQ also has shown good discriminate validity, with agoraphobics and social phobics being discriminated by their respective subscales, and both groups being distinguished from nonanxious individuals and persons representing other diagnostic groups (Cox, Swinson, & Shaw, 1991; Oei, Gross, & Evans, 1989; Oei, Moylan, & Evans, 1991). Confirmatory factor analyses of the FQ conducted in both social anxiety and agoraphobia samples also supported the discriminative validity of the measure (Cox, Parker, & Swinson 1996; Cox, Swinson, & Parker, 1993; Lelliott, McNamee, & Marks, 1991). However, the instrument showed marginal diagnostic power to distinguish patients with anxiety disorders in a representative epidemiological sample (Hoyer, Becker, Neumer, Soeder, & Margraf, 2002).

The FQ has been used as a treatment outcome measure in multiple studies with various clinical samples. It is a brief and easy questionnaire to administer and score, leading to its wide clinical appeal. However, the FQ SP subscale only has five items and does not cover the broad range of situations that individuals with social anxiety may fear; nor does it incorporate all the DSM-V criteria for SAD (Heimberg et al., 1992). Moreover, the FQ only assesses degree of avoidance, rather than degree of distress. This distinction is important because many SAIs do not actually avoid certain phobic situations but instead endure them despite extreme distress.

Social Phobia Inventory

The Social Phobia Inventory (SPIN) was developed as a self-report companion to the interviewer-based BSPS (Connor et al., 2000). Like the latter instrument, the SPIN was designed to assess three components of social anxiety: subjective fear, avoidance behavior, and physiological symptoms. Each of 17 items is rated on a 5-point Likert scale. In their initial report on the SPIN, Connor and colleagues (2000) found that the scale demonstrated good internal consistency and test–retest reliability. It had good convergent validity, as demonstrated by high correlations with other measures of social anxiety (i.e., the Liebowitz Social Anxiety Scale (LSAS), BSPS, and the FQ SP subscale), and discriminant validity was supported by findings of no correlation with a measure of health status (i.e., the Medical Outcomes Study Short-Form 36). Furthermore, the SPIN reliably distinguished between patients with and without a diagnosis of SAD. Antony, Coons, McCabe, Ashbaugh, and Swinson (2006) provided further psychometric support for the SPIN, finding excellent internal consistency, test–retest reliability, and convergent and discriminant validity. The scale reliably distinguished patients with SAD from those with PD or obsessive compulsive disorder (OCD).

A number of studies have found the SPIN to be sensitive to treatment effects from both pharmacotherapy (e.g., Liebowitz, Mangano, Bradwejn, & Asnis, 2005) and cognitive behavioral therapy (CBT) (e.g., Antony et al., 2006). The advantages of the SPIN are its brevity, ease of scoring, and specific assessment of physiological symptoms.

Mini-SPIN

Connor, Kobak, Churchill, Katzelnick, and Davidson (2001) derived a brief, three-item version of the SPIN as a screening instrument for generalized social anxiety disorder (GSAD). The three items ("Fear of embarrassment causes me to avoid doing things or speaking to people; I avoid activities in which I am the center of attention; Being embarrassed or looking stupid are among my worse fears") were chosen among those from the SPIN that demonstrated the biggest mean difference between patients diagnosed with SAD and non-socially anxious controls. Each item is rated on a 5-point Likert scale and ratings are summed to create a total score. In a large sample of managed care patients, Connor et al. (2001) demonstrated that the Mini-SPIN demonstrated strong sensitivity, specificity, and positive and negative predictive value in identifying patients with GSAD. Weeks, Spokas, & Heimberg (2007) extended these findings in a sample of individuals seeking cognitive behavioral treatment for social anxiety. They found that the Mini-SPIN had strong internal consistency, convergent and discriminant validity, and diagnostic sensitivity and efficiency. Discriminant validity was also found for the Mini-SPIN with a Brazilian university sample (De Lima Osorio, Crippa, & Laureiro, 2007). Although more research is needed, preliminary data suggest that the Mini-SPIN is a useful brief screening tool for GSAD.

MEASURES OF THEORETICALLY DERIVED COMPONENTS OF SOCIAL ANXIETY

The second group of self-report measures includes instruments that were developed to assess specific components of social anxiety. These measures are typically not used in either clinical or research settings as primary indices of symptom severity, but rather as measures of theoretical constructs central to social anxiety.

Fear of Negative Evaluation Scale

The Fear of Negative Evaluation Scale (FNE) is a 30-item true–false self-report measure. The construction of the FNE was based on a theoretical understanding of the principle features comprising social anxiety (Watson & Friend, 1969). According to the authors, social anxiety encompasses the experience of fear of and distress about social situations, avoidance of social situations, and a fear of provoking negative evaluations from others. The FNE was specifically designed to assess this concern over negative evaluation by others. Fear of negative evaluation was defined as "apprehension about others' evaluations, avoidance of evaluative situations, and the expectation that others would evaluate oneself negatively" (Watson & Friend, 1969, p. 499). This fear can also be characterized as the fear of loss of social approval. Examples of FNE items include "I rarely worry about seeming foolish to others" (scored negatively) and "I am frequently afraid of other people noticing my shortcomings."

Through three experimental studies and one correlational study in college student populations, Watson and Friend (1969) showed that the FNE had sufficient test–retest reliability and concurrent validity. Subsequent studies provided further support for the validity of the FNE (Friend & Gilbert, 1973; Smith & Sarason, 1975). The FNE has been frequently used in studies of social anxiety and SP. Improvement in SP symptoms following cognitive behavioral treatment has been associated with a reduction in FNE scores (Heimberg, Dodge et al., 1990; Hope, Herbert, & White, 1995). Nevertheless, as noted by Heimberg (1994), treatment-related changes in FNE scores are typically modest and not specific to type of treatment, owing to both the instrument's true–false format and the confounding of concern over negative evaluation with other symptoms of social anxiety in several items.

A brief version of the FNE scale was developed by Leary (1983) to increase the scale's utility. The Brief-FNE consists of 12 of the original 30 items from the FNE. The response format was modified from the original true–false format to a 5-point Likert scale ranging from "not at all" to "extremely characteristic of me." The Brief-FNE correlates very highly ($r = 0.96$, $p < 0.001$) with the original FNE and demonstrates good test–retest reliability and internal consistency (Leary, 1983). The Brief-FNE continues to be used in outcome studies of SAD (e.g., Lipsitz et al., 2008). It is especially useful in clinical contexts because its brevity facilitates repeated administration and its Likert-response format may make it more sensitive to treatment effects.

Recent years have witnessed a resurgence of research on the Brief-FNE, which was sparked by concerns that the four reverse-scored items formed a second factor, undermining the scale's theoretical unitary factor structure (Rodebaugh et al., 2004). Various modifications to the scale have been recommended, including dropping the reverse-keyed items (Rodebaugh et al., 2004) and rewording them in various ways (Carleton, McCreary, Norton, & Asmundson, 2006; Collins, Westra, Dozois, & Stewart, 2005; Taylor, 1993).

Carleton, Collimore, & Asmundson (2007) recently found that optimal fit with a unitary factorial structure was obtained with an eight-item version of the scale, which is composed of a combination of some of the original items plus some reworded items.

Although there is growing consensus that the reversed-scored items of the Brief-FNE are problematic, the field has yet to settle on which of the various alternatives is the preferred version. The eight-item version proposed by Carleton et al. (2007) is promising and is noteworthy for its parsimony, but needs further evaluation in clinical samples. In the meantime, we recommend using the Collins et al. (2005) version, which maintains all of the scale's original items while straightforwardly rephrasing the reverse-keyed items.

Social Avoidance and Distress Scale

The SADS was constructed concurrently with the FNE (Watson & Friend, 1969) and was developed to encompass the authors' theoretical view of two of the three aspects that comprise social anxiety: the experience of distress and the deliberate avoidance of social situations. Physiological signs of anxiety or impaired performance were excluded from the scale. The SADS consists of 28 true–false items. Although the authors described two subscales (social avoidance and social distress), these are rarely used in practice. Typical items include "I try to avoid talking to people unless I know them well" and "I often think up excuses in order to avoid social engagements" (Watson & Friend, 1969). Watson and Friend (1969) report data supporting the test–retest reliability and concurrent validity of the SADS.

Turner, McCanna, and Beidel (1987) administered both the SADS and the FNE to a large group of patients diagnosed with various anxiety disorders and found that persons with SAD could not be distinguished from those with other anxiety disorders by either instrument, thereby questioning their discriminative validity. Turner et al. (1987) concluded that, although both the SADS and the FNE appeared to be sensitive to anxiety and emotional distress as indicated by significant correlations with specific measures of depression and anxiety and general indexes of emotional distress, they lacked the ability to discriminate social anxiety from other types of anxiety. Heimberg, Hope, Rapee, and Bruch (1988), however, argued that these results do not necessarily lead to the conclusion that the SADS and FNE measure general distress rather than social anxiety because social anxiety may be manifested in other anxiety disorders and individuals with social anxiety are highly heterogeneous. Turner and Beidel (1988) responded by reaffirming their position that the SADS and FNE lack discriminative validity. Hofmann, DiBartolo, Holaway, and Heimberg (2004) discovered an error in the original scoring instructions of the SADS; specifically, the key for one of the items (number 19) was incorrectly reverse-scored. Hofmann et al. found that this error resulted in higher scores of central tendency relative to the correctly scored version, although the error does not appear to have significantly biased prior studies that have used the SADS.

The popularity of the SADS has declined over the past decade, most likely due to the development of arguably better measures of social anxiety symptoms, and questions regarding its discriminant validity. Users of the SADS should obviously be aware of the error in scoring instructions in the original publication.

Cognitive-Somatic Anxiety Questionnaire

The Cognitive-Somatic Anxiety Questionnaire (CSAQ) is a 14-item self-report measure designed to assess both cognitive and somatic symptoms of anxiety (Schwartz, Davidson, & Goleman, 1978). Individuals are asked to rate on a 5-point Likert scale the degree to which they typically experience a specific symptom when they are feeling anxious. The measure consists of a cognitive scale and a somatic scale, each of which is comprised of seven items. The cognitive scale describes unpleasant thoughts or ruminations about a feared situation, whereas the somatic scale is characterized by physical symptoms of anxiety. Scoring involves the summation of items for each scale and combining both scale scores to obtain a total score.

The CSAQ has received only limited psychometric support. Schwartz et al. (1978) developed the CSAQ to address the lack of face validity that existed in other cognitive and somatic anxiety self-report measures during that time. Initial evidence of the utility of the CSAQ was shown in a retrospective study comparing CSAQ scores of individuals taking an exercise class with individuals taking a meditation class (Schwartz et al., 1978). The authors found that meditators reported less cognitive and more somatic anxiety than did those in the exercise class. Later studies have shown the utility of the CSAQ in assessing the effects of relaxation treatments as well as in characterizing the patterns of symptomatology in chronic pain patients (DeGood, Buckalew, & Tait, 1985; Tercilla, 1981). Tamaren, Carney, and Allen (1985) found that the cognitive scale correlated with other cognitive self-report measures, whereas the somatic scale was associated with skin conductance levels produced in response to stress, thereby supporting the construct validity of the measure. DeGood and Tait (1987) found that, for males, CSAQ scores correlated significantly with several anxiety-related measures, but, for females, CSAQ scale scores correlated less consistently with other test scores. Results from two separate factor-analytic procedures support the cognitive and somatic dimensions of the CSAQ (Crits-Christoph, 1986; Steptoe & Kearsley, 1990). The two studies differed significantly, however, in the degree to which the two scales were correlated. The two-dimensional factor structure of the CSAQ is challenged by results of a factor analysis in an anxious sample in which four factors emerged: fear-laden cognitions, autonomic arousal, general worries, and indecision/agitation (Freeland & Carney, 1988).

Heimberg, Gansler, and Dodge (1987) found the CSAQ to have good convergent and discriminant validity in a sample of individuals with SAD. The cognitive scale was associated with measures of anxiety and self-evaluation, thought-listing scores, and self-rated anxiety during a behavioral test. The somatic scale was related to heart rate during a four-minute behavioral simulation. The behavioral simulations were individualized to induce greater arousal. The two scales, as in previous studies with nonclinical populations, were significantly correlated. Although the CSAQ has been used in various clinical studies with social anxiety, its popularity has declined in recent years. The instrument may prove to be useful if further refinements result in less overlap between the scales.

SELF-REPORT MEASURES FOR CHILDREN AND ADOLESCENTS

Recent years have witnessed a growing interest in children and adolescents who suffer from social anxiety (Kashdan & Herbert, 2001). Several clinical rating scales and self-report measures have been developed specifically for pediatric populations and used in treatment-outcome studies.

Liebowitz Social Anxiety Scale for Children and Adolescents

The Liebowitz Social Anxiety Scale for Children and Adolescents (LSAS-CA), based on the adult LSAS, was designed to assess a range of social situations and performance interactions that children and adolescents may fear (Masia-Warner et al., 2003). The measure consists of 24 items: 12 social interactions and 12 performance situations, which are rated on 0–3 Likert scales. Separate fear and avoidance ratings are assessed. Six subscale scores are computed including Total Anxiety, Social Anxiety, Performance Anxiety, Total Avoidance, Social Avoidance, and Performance Avoidance. The LSAS-CA has show high internal consistency and test–retest reliability (Masia-Warner et al., 2003). However, factor analyses indicate that anxiety and avoidance ratings are best explained by a two-factor solution named Social and School Performance (Storch et al., 2006). The LSAS-CA has been used in several treatment outcome studies with children and adolescents and demonstrated sensitivity to treatment effects (Masia-Warner et al., 2005; Wagner et al., 2004).

Social Phobia and Anxiety Inventory for Children

Beidel, Turner, and Morris (1995) developed a version of the SPAI to be used with children older than seven and with adolescents – the Social Phobia and Anxiety Inventory for Children (SPAI-C). The SPAI-C is a 26-item self-report measure designed to assess distress in a range of potentially anxiety-producing situations, as well as the physiological, cognitive, and behavioral avoidance manifestations of anxiety. Like the SPAI, there are a number of items in the

SPAI-C in which individuals rate their distress in various situations based on characteristics of the audience. The SPAI-C has been shown to have high two-week test–retest reliability, adequate reliability at 10 months, and high internal consistency (Beidel et al., 1995; Storch, Masia-Warner, Dent, Roberti, & Fisher, 2004). Confirmatory factor analyses supported the five-factor structure proposed by the original theoretical model (Storch et al., 2004). Scores on the SPAI-C successfully differentiate socially anxious children from children with externalizing disorders or no disorders (Beidel, Turner, & Fink, 1996; Beidel, Turner, Hamlin, & Morris, 2000). Beidel et al. (1996) further found that the SPAI-C demonstrates adequate convergent validity as determined by comparing scores to daily diary ratings of distress. In addition, the scale has been shown to have adequate concurrent validity, internal consistency, and test–retest reliability within a non-American sample (Aune, Stiles, & Svarva, 2008). The SPAI-C has been used in several clinical trials (Beidel, Turner, Young, & Paulson, 2005; Compton et al., 2001; Herbert et al., 2009; Isolan et al., 2007; Masia-Warner, Fisher, Shrout, Rathor, & Klein, 2007; Wagner et al., 2004).

Social Anxiety Scale for Children

The Social Anxiety Scale for Children or Adolescents – Revised (SASC-CA) is an 18-item self-report measure assessing social-evaluative anxiety, with separate child (LaGreca & Stone, 1993) and adolescent versions (Ginsburg, LaGreca, & Silverman, 1997). The SASC-CA items are derived from two adult measures: the SADS and the FNE. The SASC-CA also yields three factors: fear of negative evaluation, social avoidance and distress in new situations (SAD-N), and general social avoidance and inhibition (SAD-G). Normative data have been reported for adolescents in grades 4 through 11 (Walters, Caster, & Inderbitzen, 1996). The SAS-CA has been found to discriminate adolescents with and without SAD (Ginsburg, LaGreca, & Silverman, 1998) and to show good discriminate validity (Kristensen & Torgersen, 2006). It has also been shown to have good internal consistency and 12-month test–retest reliability (Storch et al., 2004). The SAS-CA has also been used in several clinical trials to assess treatment outcome with noticeable sensitivity (March, Entusah, Rynn, Albano, & Tourian, 2007; Masia-Warner et al., 2005; Wagner et al., 2004).

Social Skills Questionnaires

Three self-report measures of social skills have been developed. The Social Skills Questionnaire (SSQ-P) (Spence, 1995) is a 30-item scale that assesses a parent's perception of their child's social skills. A 3-point Likert scale is used. The SSQ-P has good internal consistency and split-half reliability (Spence, 1995). The Teenage Inventory of Social Skills (TISS) (Inderbitzen & Foster,

1992) was designed to identify adolescents in grades 7 through 12 with problematic peer relationships and to help target specific problematic behaviors for intervention. It is a 40-item self-report scale with initial reports demonstrating good test–retest reliability and convergent and discriminant validity (Inderbitzen & Foster, 1992). The Matson Evaluation of Social Skills with Youngsters (MESSY) (Matson, Rotatori, & Helsel, 1983) is another self-report measure of social skills in children. It is a 62-item questionnaire that consists of five factors: overconfident, impulsive/recalcitrant, jealous/withdrawal, inappropriate assertiveness, and appropriate social skills.

Spence Children's Anxiety Scale

The Spence Children's Anxiety Scale (SCAS) (Spence, 1998) is a self-report instrument for various anxiety disorders to be used with children aged 8 to 12. The instrument consists of 38 clinical items and 6 filler items; the SP subscale consists of 6 items. The frequency of each item is rated on a 4-point Likert scale. Spence (1998) provided data supporting the psychometric properties of the SCAS and supporting the factor structure of the instrument. The SCAS is unique in that it assesses symptoms consistent with several childhood anxiety disorders rather than general anxiety, and it was developed with sensitivity to developmental factors rather than as a downward extension of an adult measure. Although the SCAS may prove useful as a screening tool for anxiety disorders in children, the SP subscale provides relatively little information, limiting its clinical utility as a measure of social anxiety *per se*.

Kutcher Generalized Social Anxiety Scale for Adolescents

Brooks and Kutcher (2004) developed a measure to assess social anxiety symptoms and treatment outcome in adolescents aged 11–17. The Kutcher Generalized Social Anxiety Scale for Adolescents (K-GSADS-A) is a clinician-administered measure with four subscales: Fear and Anxiety, Avoidance, Affective Distress, and Somatic Distress. The K-GSADS-A demonstrates adequate internal consistency, convergent validity with other severity measures, and divergent validity with respect to depression (Brooks & Kutcher, 2004). The K-GSADS-A also demonstrates good sensitivity to changes in severity. It has been used in several clinical trials (Brooks & Kutcher, 2004; Wagner et al., 2004).

In addition, there are several other self-report measures that assess a broad range of anxiety symptoms and that include social anxiety subscales. These include the Multi-Dimensional Anxiety Scale for Children (MASC; March, Parker, Sullivan, Stallings, & Conners, 1997), the Screen for Child Anxiety Related Emotional Disorders (SCARED; Birmaher, Khetarpal, & Brent, 1997), and the Revised Children's Manifest Anxiety Scale (RCMAS; Reynolds & Richmond; 1978).

ROLE-PLAYING PROCEDURES

A primary goal of any clinical assessment procedure is to obtain a reliable sample of behavior that is representative of the individual's functioning outside the clinic or laboratory context so valid inferences can be made about the person's behavior in naturalistic settings. Social anxiety by its very nature involves social settings and interactions, so *in vivo* naturalistic observations of social encounters would be ideal. Such observations are generally precluded on both practical and theoretical grounds, however. Although naturalistic observation may be feasible for socially anxious children in some cases (e.g., in the classroom, on the playground), it is very difficult to observe adults unobtrusively in their natural environments. Moreover, established avoidance patterns may preclude assessment of precisely the situations that are most problematic for any individual. A SAI with a primary fear of heterosocial interactions, for example, may avoid all such situations, and naturalistic observations alone would therefore fail to capture this domain. Finally, naturalistic observations make comparisons among individuals difficult, because each individual largely determines the stimulus parameters to which he or she responds, thereby resulting in a loss of standardization.

For all of these reasons, role-playing procedures, in which various situations are enacted with trained confederates in the clinic or laboratory, have become quite popular in the assessment of social anxiety. In our experience, even clients who express initial skepticism about how realistic such simulations will be are quickly surprised to find how psychologically realistic they become. Although role-playing procedures can be used for treatment purposes (Butler & Wells, 1995), the following discussion is limited to their use as assessment tools.

Role-Play Test

The Role-Play Test (RPT) is the most common procedure in the behavioral assessment of SP (Glass & Arnkoff, 1989). RPTs are used to obtain a representative sample of the patient's behavior and are particularly helpful when attempting to identify specific social skills deficits. The RPT is not, strictly speaking, a standardized test, but rather a series of procedures focusing on the enactment of simulated social situations in the therapist's office or the research laboratory. Two types of role-plays have emerged: structured and unstructured. These types of role-plays are not qualitatively different, but rather vary in the degree of structure imposed on the stimulus. In both situations, patients are aware that they are being observed and usually videotaped. In the structured approach, patients are presented with a series of descriptions of social situations, with a confederate delivering a prompt line at the end of each description. The confederate typically responds as minimally as possible in order to keep the focus on the patient, and the interaction goes on for a predetermined period of time, typically 2 to 5 minutes. In the unstructured role-play, patients interact with a confederate for a period of time, typically 2 to 12 minutes, and they are instructed to behave as they typically would in social interactions. Confederates are trained to behave as naturalistically as possible while permitting the patient ample opportunity to talk. Structured role-plays are preferred in research settings, and they have the advantage of providing a sample of behavior in response to a standard stimulus. Unstructured role-plays may be more externally valid, but the ability to make normative comparisons among patients is more limited. Unlike RPTs traditionally used with chronic psychiatric patients, which tend to be very brief and highly structured (e.g., Bellack, Morrison, Mueser, Wade, & Sayers, 1990), the RPTs used with persons with social anxiety are typically of longer duration and permit the confederate greater leeway in interacting with the patient. This method establishes a more natural social context, thereby increasing the representativeness of the resulting behavior. Ratings of skill and anxiety can be derived from patient reports, confederate reports, and ratings of videotapes by external raters. Depending upon one's purposes, behavioral ratings can be micro (e.g., exact duration of eye contact) or macro (overall quality of social skills) in level of analysis.

In addition to their use to assess social skills, RPTs can be used to assess cognitive processes associated with social anxiety. For example, Greenberg-Saluck and Herbert (2005) found that self-focused attention among individuals with SAD (but not among nonclinical controls) was associated with poorer recall of interpersonal information about a confederate following a RPT.

The validity of RPTs for assessing social skills of initiating and maintaining a conversation was tested in one study by comparing structured and unstructured role-plays with a naturalistic interaction (Merluzzi & Biever, 1987). Social skill ratings by judges, confederates, and subjects did not differ as a function of type of interaction. Extended RPTs have been shown to be sensitive to change associated with treatment in dating-anxious individuals and have distinguished confident from shy students (Arkowitz, Lichtenstein, McGovern, & Hines, 1975; Twentyman & McFall, 1975). RPTs have also been shown to be sensitive to treatment effects in adults with SAD (e.g., Herbert et al., 2005). Similarly, RPTs have also been successfully used with child and adolescent samples in treatment outcome research to assess social skills and anxiety (Beidel et al., 2005; Compton et al., 2001; Herbert et al., 2009). Further research is needed to investigate both the reliability and validity of the RPT in greater detail.

Along with RPTs, impromptu speeches are also useful behavioral assessment paradigms for social anxiety, because public speaking is by far the single most common phobic situation identified by social phobics. Impromptu speeches require the patient to speak for a given length of time (typically 3 to 10 minutes) to a small audience (usually two to three confederates). Patients can be given a set of topics to choose from or can pick topics of their choice. Little research has been done on the validity and reliability of the impromptu speech task. In a study by Beidel, Turner, Jacob, and Cooley (1989), a 10-minute impromptu speech in which the patient was given a set of topics to choose from was found to be a reliable method for determining the physiological, cognitive, and behavioral parameters of SP. In our laboratory, we use both a structured RPT and an impromptu speech in our assessment of persons with SP (e.g., Herbert, Hope, & Bellack, 1992; Herbert et al., 2005). We rate video recordings on overall social skills, as well as the quality of verbal content, nonverbal behavior, and paralinguistic features (e.g., speech rate, volume, tone, etc.).

Simulated Social Interaction Test

Curran et al. (1980, 1982) developed the Simulated Social Interaction Test (SSIT), a highly standardized RPT. The SSIT is a behavioral RPT that consists of trained judges' ratings of subjects' performance in various simulated social situations. The interactions comprising the SSIT are based on different types of problematic social situations drawn from the factor-analytic work of Richardson and Tasto (1976). These types of interactions include (1) disapproval or criticism, (2) social visibility and assertiveness, (3) confrontation and anger expression, (4) heterosexual contact, (5) interpersonal warmth, (6) conflict with or rejection by parent or relative, (7) interpersonal loss, and (8) receiving compliments. Each SSIT simulation involves a narrator who reads a script describing a social situation and a confederate who provides verbal prompts. Four of the simulations involve a male confederate and the other involves a female. The individual's anxiety response and social skills are then evaluated by a rater on an 11-point Likert scale.

The SSIT is one of the best validated behavioral tests for the measurement of social skills. It has been shown to have high test–retest reliability, good inter-rater reliability, and high internal consistency of both anxiety and performance scores (Curran, 1982; Curran et al., 1980; Farrell, Curran, Zwick, & Monti, 1983). The construct validity of the anxiety and skill components of the SSIT has been supported in various populations, including psychiatric outpatients (Curran et al., 1980), psychiatric inpatients, and a control of National Guard members (Farrell et al., 1983) and college students (Monti, Wallander, Ahern, Abrams, & Munroe, 1983). Mersch, Breukers, and Emmelkamp (1992) investigated the utility of the SSIT with a Dutch socially anxious population. The study supports the cross-national usefulness of the SSIT as well as the generalizability of the measure with social phobic populations. They found that the anxiety reported by individuals during the SSIT was correlated with distress reported on self-report measures and that subjective anxiety ratings on the SSIT were correlated with the frequency of negative self-statements measured immediately afterward. They did, however, find that the convergent validity of the SSIT is questionable, because the SSIT was poorly correlated with other supposed measures for the same constructs.

The SSIT was found to be sensitive to change in a treatment outcome study of individuals with social anxiety (Mersch, Emmelkamp, & Lips, 1991). Although the SSIT provides a wealth of behavioral data, its utility in clinical settings is limited by the high degree of structure required and the need for highly trained judges.

Self-Monitoring

Self-monitoring involves the client recording the frequency, and at times the intensity and quality, of targeted thoughts, feelings, and overt behaviors that may be present during anxiety-provoking situations. (It is noteworthy that this clinical use of the term is distinct from its use in social psychology, where it refers to the tailoring of one's behavior to specific social situations for self-presentational purposes; see, for example, Hofmann, 2006). The primary advantage of self-monitoring is that it can be used in naturalistic settings and, therefore, provides data with a high degree of external validity. Observations are recorded in various diaries, daily logs, and other recording forms. Frequency and duration of social interactions, content of conversations, thoughts evoked by phobic situations, and degree of anxiety experienced are all examples of common target behaviors. Self-monitoring can be used as a method to assist in identifying anxiety-provoking situations for the purpose of planning and monitoring the effects of treatment. In addition, the well-known reactivity effects of self-monitoring, in which merely engaging in the procedure tends to increase the frequency of positive behaviors and decrease negative behaviors, makes self-monitoring a useful therapeutic tool in and of itself (Herbert & Nelson-Gray, 1997; Nelson, Hay, Devany, & Koslow-Green, 1980; Nietzel, Bernstein, & Russell, 1988).

Self-monitoring is an integral part of most cognitive behavioral treatment programs for social anxiety, and the procedure has been used as an outcome measure in treatment studies of SP (Butler, Cullington, Munby, Amies, & Gelder, 1984; Mattick & Peters, 1988). However, little research has examined the psychometrics of self-monitoring in socially anxious samples.

THOUGHT-LISTING AND THOUGHT-ENDORSEMENT PROCEDURES

With the increasing prominence of information-processing conceptualizations of social anxiety (Clark & Wells, 1995; Rapee & Heimberg, 1997) and the development of effective cognitively based intervention protocols (Heimberg, Hope, Dodge, & Becker, 1990), procedures designed to assess the content of dysfunctional cognitions have grown in popularity. The self-report questionnaires described previously are designed to assess one aspect of cognitive content: the individual's beliefs about socially relevant situations. That is, persons are essentially asked to infer general beliefs from their experience. A less inferential approach is to have socially anxious persons directly report their thoughts in response to some relevant stimulus, such as a social task, then possibly to rate the frequency or impact of each thought. As with role-playing procedures, thought-listing has become an integral part of cognitive behavioral treatment programs for SP, although the current discussion will focus on its use as an assessment tool.

Social Interaction Self-Statement Test

The Social Interaction Self-Statement Test (SISST) (Glass, Merluzzi, Biever, & Larsen, 1982), the best-known cognitive endorsement procedure, combines elements of a self-rating measure with an RPT. The SISST is a 30-item scale in which individuals rate on 5-point Likert scales the frequency of 15 positive and 15 negative thoughts after a role-play of a heterosocial interaction. Positive and negative subscale scores are then derived. The SISST was initially developed and validated with a socially anxious college student sample (Glass et al., 1982). It was found to correlate with social anxiety questionnaires and with self-report inventories of social skill.

Studies have yielded mixed results regarding the extent to which the SISST and other protocol measures of self-statements yield a consistent picture of a person's internal dialogue (Glass & Furlong, 1990). Some data suggest that alternative cognitive assessment procedures may yield discrepant results (Johnson & Glass, 1989; Myszka, Galassi, & Ware, 1986). Dodge, Hope, Heimberg, and Becker (1988) found that negative thought statements on the SISST were related to various measures of anxiety and depression as well as to negative thoughts reported after an individualized behavioral test. Furthermore, the negative thoughts subscale of the SISST discriminated between socially anxious persons whose primary fear involved social interactions and those whose anxiety was related to public speaking. Similarly, Glass and Furlong (1990) found that negative thoughts on a thought-listing prior to an actual conversation were related to negative self-statements on the SISST completed after the interaction in a sample of socially anxious adults. In the same study, thoughts on the SISST were also related to various self-report measures of social anxiety, irrational beliefs, and negative evaluation, as well as global ratings of skill and anxiety made by judges.

The SISST has shown that high SAIs endorse more negative and fewer positive thoughts than low anxious individuals (Beidel, Turner, & Dancu, 1985; Glass et al., 1982). Moreover, SISST negative subscale scores have been shown to be sensitive to situational factors (Beazley, Glass, Chambless, & Arnkoff, 2001; Turner, Beidel, & Larkin, 1986). Both the positive and negative subscales significantly discriminated patients with SAD from patients with other anxiety disorders in a treatment-seeking sample (Becker, Namour, Zayfert, & Hegel, 2001). Similarly, Cho and Telch (2005) found that the content of both positive and negative self-statements distinguished symptoms of social anxiety and depression.

The SISST has been used in treatment outcome research and has been shown to be sensitive to treatment effects in SAD (Heimberg, Dodge et al., 1990; Turner, Beidel, & Jacob, 1994). It is a resourceful questionnaire to use in cognitive interventions when a client is having difficulty spontaneously generating thoughts. A limitation of the SISST, however, is that the thoughts are limited to those involving heterosexual interactions and do not cover other social situations that a person with SP may fear (Elting & Hope, 1995). Further research is needed to assess the validity of the SISST with other types of situations or possibly to develop other self-statement measures specifically for certain situations.

The SISST has been modified to assess typical fearful thoughts associated with public speaking (Hofmann & DiBartolo, 2000). This instrument, the Self-Statements during Public Speaking Scale (SSPS), is a 10-item questionnaire consisting of two 5-item subscales, the positive self-statements and the negative self-statements subscales. In contrast to the SISST, no role-play is required to assess fearful thoughts. Preliminary data reveal that both the positive and negative subscales of the SSPS are supported by factor analyses in both clinical and nonclinical samples, and have good internal consistency and test–retest reliability (Hofmann & DiBartolo, 2000). The factor structure of a German version of the scale was subsequently supported (Gerlach, Heinrichs, Bandl, & Zimmermann (2007).

Thought-Listing and Thought-Recall

Along with the SISST, thought-listing is a common practice of cognitive assessment in social anxiety research. Thought-listing, sometimes referred to as thought-recall, is a method in which patients are asked to record the thoughts that they recall having in a given time period (Cacioppo & Petty, 1981). Thought-listing is often used in conjunction with RPTs. After a role-play is completed, patients are instructed to write thoughts they remember having during the role-play. Thought-listing can be used while anticipating an upcoming situation (for example, listing thoughts about having to ask a person out on a date). Patients can also be asked to keep a diary and list thoughts after real-life interactions. Through protocol analysis, these thoughts are scored according to criteria such as content (themes) or valence (positive, negative, and neutral) (Arnkoff & Glass, 1989).

Social anxiety studies that use thought-listings have generally coded the thoughts for valence, specifically focusing on the frequency of positive versus negative thoughts. A few studies have focused on coding thoughts according to focus of thought (self vs. other or task) (Glass & Furlong, 1990; Hope, Heimberg, Zollo, Nyman, & O'Brien, 1987). Regarding psychometric properties, inter-rater reliability for coding thoughts has usually been high, especially when raters have been trained. Mixed results have been found regarding the construct validity of thought-listing. Cacioppo, Glass, and Merluzzi (1979) have shown that thought-listing is able to differentiate high and low socially anxious subjects. However, these findings were not found in a study by Hope et al. (1987). Socially anxious subjects have been found to report fewer positive thoughts and more negative thoughts during interactions relative to nonphobic controls (Heimberg, Acerra, & Holstein, 1985; Turner et al., 1986). Thought-listing has also shown mixed results for concurrent validity. Hope et al. (1987) showed that thoughts written after interactions through the use of a daily diary were related to anxiety, length, and frequency of the interaction. This study suggests that one's thoughts are related to the level of anxiety felt in a given situation. In contrast, Glass and Furlong (1990) did not find a relationship between thought-listing scores written before a role-play and fear of negative evaluation or public-consciousness in severely socially anxious adults, suggesting thought-listing may not always be related to other types of cognitive assessments. Sturmer, Bruch, Haase, and Amico (2002) found superior convergent validity for the more structured SISST relative to a thought-listing procedure among college students.

Negative thoughts scores on thought-listings have differentiated social anxious individuals from normal controls but not from heterosocially anxious college students (Nyman & Heimberg, 1985). Thought-listing has also been used as a dependent variable in treatment outcome studies of SP (e.g., Heimberg & Liebowitz, 1992; Heinrichs & Hofmann, 2005), and both positive and negative thoughts have been found to change as a function of treatment (Heimberg, Dodge et al., 1990).

Other thought-production or endorsement methods have occasionally been employed, primarily in studies of subclinical social anxiety, but none has garnered widespread acceptance. For example, the Articulated Thoughts during Simulated Situations procedure requires subjects to report their thoughts at predetermined intervals in response to audiotaped descriptions of various social situations.

PSYCHOPHYSIOLOGICAL ASSESSMENT

Physiological arousal is a hallmark of anxiety. A growing body of research addresses the assessment of physiological responses to anxiety-provoking stimuli. The autonomic nervous system (ANS) is divided into two branches: the sympathetic system and the parasympathetic system. The sympathetic nervous system responds to threat by increasing autonomic arousal, resulting in the so-called fight-or-flight response. Common changes include increases in respiration, cardiovascular activity, and muscle tension, with corresponding decreases in peripheral blood flow and gastrointestinal activity. The parasympathetic nervous system has essentially the opposite effects, resulting in decreased arousal. Although the vast majority of work on the physiological assessment of anxiety has focused on sympathetic arousal, Leary and Kowalski (1995) argue that parasympathetic effects may also be involved in some anxiety-related reactions, such as embarrassment.

There has been some controversy over the degree of importance to place on psychophysiological assessment in social anxiety. McNeil et al. (1995) believe that physiological measures are essential to thorough assessment. Scholing and Emmelkamp (1990), in contrast, raise questions about the value of such assessment, including concerns about the test–retest reliability of cardiovascular measures in particular. Another problem is the overall lack of specificity of arousal patterns across the various anxiety disorders. Although some research has found differences in patterns of physiological arousal across different forms of anxiety (e.g., Liebowitz et al., 1985), most studies have found wide variability across individuals within any given diagnostic group and few consistent differences across the anxiety disorders. It is also unclear how physiological data relate to treatment choice and treatment outcome. Unlike assessment of cognitive content or social skills, which relate directly to the manner in which one conducts cognitive restructuring or social skills training, physiological data are not clearly related to treatment decisions – including pharmacological treatment – given currently available interventions. Finally, most phobic situations in the case of social anxiety (e.g., holding a conversation, giving a speech) involve motoric responses of some kind, and such task demands may mask differences across groups or otherwise interfere with physiological measurement (McNeil et al., 1995). Despite these concerns, psychophysiological data may eventually hold the key to the elusive question of meaningful subtypes of social anxiety.

Cardiovascular Assessment

Cardiovascular responses can be assessed by measures of heart rate and blood pressure. Heart rate has been the most commonly used physiological measure in SP research because it is easily measured and relatively insensitive to measurement artifacts (Neitzel & Bernstein, 1981). Heart rate is typically measured by assessing the subject's pulse at regular intervals across a specific time period, although it can also be recorded continuously with a plethysmograph. Heart rate and blood pressure have been assessed during simulations of phobic social situations using role-playing procedures (Beidel et al., 1985; Heimberg, Hope et al., 1990; Hofmann, Newman, Ehlers, & Roth, 1995). For example, a person's pulse rate and systolic blood pressure can be recorded after that person is told about the role-play task, immediately before the task, at regular intervals during the role-play, and immediately afterward. Although there is consensus on the importance of baseline measurement, there is currently no standard for the parameters of baseline recordings.

Heart rate and blood pressure measurements have demonstrated good test–retest reliability during an impromptu speech task (Beidel, Turner, Jacob et al., 1989). Heart rate and systolic blood pressure have been found to differentiate between patients with SP and normal controls during role-play interactions and public speaking tasks (Beidel et al., 1985; Hofmann et al., 1995). Heimberg, Hope et al. (1990) found higher heart rates during a public speaking task in social phobics with specific public speaking fears relative to generalized social phobics and normal controls, although no differences were found between the latter two groups. Similar results were reported by Levin et al. (1993). Heart rate recordings during role-play procedures have been shown to be sensitive to treatment effects in outcome studies of SP (Emmelkamp, Mersch, Vissia, & Van Der Helm, 1985; Turner, Beidel, Long, & Greenhouse, 1992). Of interesting note is that there has been little research examining resting cardiovascular responses or other psychophysiology in SP. Most cardiovascular data, for example, has been derived from studies using phobic provocations.

Electrodermal Recordings

Recordings of dermatologic electrical activity can be assessed by skin conductance and skin resistance; Palmar Sweat Prints and Finger Sweat Prints are examples of skin conductance and skin resistance measures. Individuals with SP have been found to exhibit a slower habituation rate of electrodermal activity and greater range of response than normal controls in response to both social and nonsocial stimuli (Lader, 1967; Dimberg, Fredrikson, & Lundquist, 1986). Electrodermal activity, however, is very reactive to both environmental and psychological artifacts.

Other Physiological Assessments

Several studies have begun to examine the psychobiology of social anxiety. Research has examined both central and ANS functioning, as well as neuroendocrine responses to biological challenges. For example, in a classic study, Liebowitz et al. (1985) found that social phobics did not experience an exacerbation of symptoms after lactate infusions, but PD patients did react. Davidson and colleagues (1993) used magnetic resonance spectroscopy (MRS) to compare a sample of social phobics with a sample of normal control subjects and found lower central nervous system (CNS) activity in both cortical and subcortical regions for the social phobic group. Stein, Asmundson, and Chartier (1994) found no differences in plasma bioamine levels between social phobics and normal controls. Stein and Stein (2008) provide an overview of several neuroimaging studies in their review of the current research on SAD. It is difficult to draw general conclusions from the literature on the psychobiology of social anxiety at this time because most studies have used small samples, testing procedures have not been uniform across studies, and, not surprisingly, results have been inconsistent.

SUMMARY

The hallmark of a comprehensive assessment of social anxiety and SP is a multimodal approach. Assessment using a single measure or procedure is unlikely to provide adequate depth and breadth of information. The specific strategy employed will vary as a function of the assessment goals. In clinical settings, a comprehensive clinical interview followed by one or more standardized self-report questionnaires and an RPT provide a solid foundation for treatment planning. Further assessment may be required depending upon the type of treatment employed. For example, further assessment of cognitions using thought-listing procedures may be necessary before beginning cognitive restructuring, and further self-monitoring and role-play procedures may be required to identify specific targets for social skills training. At this time, physiological assessment does not play a central role in the clinical setting because such assessment is not central to any of the empirically supported treatments (ESTs) for social anxiety.

By their very nature, self-report questionnaires yield data that are readily comparable across clinicians and researchers. By comparing scores from instruments such as the SPAI, LSAS, or SPIN, for example, one can quickly judge the overall comparability of symptom severity of samples of SAIs. Similarly, the advent of structured clinical interviews has resulted in increased diagnostic reliability. Unfortunately, despite their increased use, such standardization has generally not occurred with thought-listing and role-play procedures, making comparisons of research findings across groups difficult. Future work aimed at standardizing such procedures by combining the most useful elements across investigators would facilitate progress.

A striking limitation of virtually all of the measures related to social interactions is the assumption of heterosexuality. The SISST, for example, assesses only heterosocial situations. Many RPTs require the individual to interact with an opposite-sex confederate, on the assumption that the situation will elicit fears associated with dating or romantic interests. Without explicit recruitment efforts, we have found that a surprisingly large number of the persons presenting for our treatment programs for SP are bi- or homosexual. When possible, we have modified extant assessment instruments accordingly, but more explicit attention to this issue is clearly warranted.

In clinical contexts, the ultimate value of any assessment measure lies in the degree to which it contributes to decisions that positively impact treatment outcome, a concept that Hayes, Nelson, and Jarrett (1986) refer to as "treatment utility." Given its importance, surprisingly little research has directly addressed this topic. Instead, instruments are typically evaluated solely according to traditional psychometric criteria. The past three decades have witnessed a proliferation of self-report questionnaires measuring some aspect of social anxiety, and detailed psychometric data are routinely provided. Notwithstanding the importance of psychometrics, greater emphasis on the clinical utility of instruments would be helpful to clinicians and researchers alike.

REFERENCES

Adler, L. A., Liebowitz, M., Kronenberger, W., Qiao, M., Rubin, R., Hollandbeck, M., et al. (2009). Atomoxetine treatment in adults with attention-deficit/hyperactivity disorder and comorbid social anxiety disorder. *Depression & Anxiety*, *26*, 212–221.

Albano, A. M., & Silverman, W. K. (1996). *The anxiety disorders interview schedule for DSM-IV – Child version*. San Antonio: The Psychological Corporation.

American Psychiatric Association. (1994). *Diagnostic and statistical manual of mental disorders* (4th ed.). (DSM-IV) Washington, DC: Author.

Amies, P. L., Gelder, M. G., & Shaw, P. M. (1983). Social phobia: A comparative clinical study. *British Journal of Psychiatry*, *142*, 174–179.

Amir, N., Beard, C., Burns, M., & Bomyea, J. (2009). Attention modification program in individuals with generalized anxiety disorder. *Journal of Abnormal Psychology*, *118*, 28–33.

Antony, M. M., Coons, M. J., McCabe, R. E., Ashbaugh, A., & Swinson, R. P. (2006). Psychometric properties of the social phobia inventory: Further evaluation. *Behaviour Research and Therapy*, *44*, 1177–1185.

Arkowitz, H., Lichtenstein, E., McGovern, K., & Hines, P. (1975). The behavioral assessment of social competence in males. *Behaviour Therapy*, *6*, 3–13.

Arnkoff, D. B., & Glass, C. R. (1989). Cognitive assessment in social anxiety and social phobia. *Clinical Disorders Psychology Review*, *9*, 61–74.

Arrindell, W. A., Emmelkamp, P. M. G., & van der Ende, J. (1984). Phobic dimensions: I. Reliability and generalizability across samples, gender and nations. *Advances in Behaviour Research and Therapy*, *6*, 207–254.

Aune, T., Stiles, T. C., & Svarva, K. (2008). Psychometric properties of the Social Phobia and Anxiety Inventory for Children using a non-American population-based sample. *Journal of Anxiety Disorders*, *22*, 1075–1086.

Baker, S. L., Heinrichs, N., Kim, H. J., & Hofmann, S. G. (2002). The Liebowitz Social Anxiety Scale as a self-report instrument: A preliminary psychometric analysis. *Behaviour Research and Therapy*, *40*, 701–715.

Becker, C. B., Namour, N., Zayfert, C., & Hegel, M. T. (2001). Specificity of the Social Interaction Self-Statement Test in social phobia. *Cognitive Therapy and Research*, *25*, 227–233.

Beazley, M. B., Glass, C. R., Chambless, D. L., & Arnkoff, D. B. (2001). Cognitive self-statements in social phobia: A comparison across three types of social situations. *Cognitive Therapy and Research*, *25*, 781–799.

Beidel, D. C., Borden, J. W., Turner, S. M., & Jacob, R. G. (1989). The Social Phobia Anxiety Inventory: Concurrent validity with a clinic sample. *Behaviour Research and Therapy*, *27*, 573–576.

Beidel, D. C., & Turner, S. M. (1992). Scoring the Social Phobia and Anxiety Inventory: Comments on Herbert et al. (1991). *Journal of Psychopathology and Behavioral Assessment*, *14*, 377–379.

Beidel, D. C., Turner, S. M., & Cooley, M. R. (1993). Assessing reliable and clinically significant change in social phobia: Validity of the Social Phobia and Anxiety Inventory. *Behaviour Research and Therapy*, *31*, 149–158.

Beidel, D. C., Turner, S. M., & Dancu, C. V. (1985). Physiological, cognitive, and behavioral aspects of social anxiety. *Behaviour Research and Therapy*, *23*, 109–117.

Beidel, D. C., Turner, S. M., & Fink, C. M. (1996). Assessment of childhood social phobia: Construct, convergent, and discriminative validity of the Social Phobia and Anxiety Inventory for Children (SPAI-C). *Psychological Assessment*, *8*, 235–240.

Beidel, D. C., Turner, S. M., Hamlin, K., & Morris, T. L. (2000). The social phobia and anxiety inventory: External and discriminative validity. *Behaviour Therapy, 31*, 75–87.

Beidel, D. C., Turner, S. M., Jacob, R. G., & Cooley, M. R. (1989). Assessment of social phobia: Reliability of an impromptu speech task. *Journal of Anxiety Disorders, 3*, 149–158.

Beidel, D. C., Turner, S. M., & Morris, T. L. (1995). A new inventory to assess childhood social anxiety and phobia: The social phobia and anxiety inventory for children. *Psychological Assessment, 7*(1), 73–79.

Beidel, D. C., Turner, S. M., Stanley, M. A., & Dancu, C. V. (1989). The Social Phobia and Anxiety Inventory: Concurrent and external validity. *Behaviour Therapy, 20*, 417–427.

Beidel, D. C., Turner, S. M., Young, B., & Paulson, A. (2005). Social effectiveness therapy for children: Three-year follow-up. *Journal of Consulting and Clinical Psychology, 73*, 721–725.

Bellack, A. S., Morison, R. L., Mueser, K. T., Wade, J. H., & Sayers, S. L. (1990). Role play for assessing the competence of psychiatric patients. *Psychological Assessment: A Journal of Consulting and Clinical Psychology, 2*, 248–255.

Birmaher, B., Khetarpal, S., & Brent, D. (1997). The Screen for Child Anxiety Related Emotional Disorders (SCARED): Scale construction and psychometric characteristics. *Journal of American Academy of Child and Adolescent Psychiatry, 36*, 545–553.

Book, S. W., Thomas, S. E., Randall, P. K., & Randall, C. L. (2008). Paroxetine reduces social anxiety in individuals with a co-occurring alcohol use disorder. *Journal of Anxiety Disorders, 22*, 310–318.

Brooks, S. J., & Kutcher, S. (2004). The Kutcher Generalized Social Anxiety Disorder Scale for Adolescents: Assessment of its evaluative properties over the course of a 16-week pediatric psychopharmacology trial. *Journal of Child and Adolescent Psychopharmacology, 14*, 273–286.

Brown, E. J., Turovsky, J., Heimberg, R. G., Juster, H. R., Brown, T. A., & Barlow, D. H. (1997). Validation of the Social Interaction Anxiety Scale and the Social Phobia Scale across the anxiety disorders. *Psychological Assessment, 9*, 21–27.

Brown, T. A., DiNardo, P. A., & Barlow, D. H. (1994). *Anxiety disorders interview schedule for DSM-IV (ADIS-IV)*. Albany, NY: Graywind.

Brown, T. A., DiNardo, P. A., Lehman, C. L., & Campbell, L. A. (2001). Reliability of DSM-IV anxiety and mood disorders: Implications for the classification of emotional disorders. *Journal of Abnormal Psychology, 110*, 49–58.

Butler, G., Cullington, A., Munby, M., Amies, P., & Gelder, M. (1984). Exposure and anxiety management in the treatment of social anxiety. *Journal of Consulting and Clinical Psychology, 52*, 642–650.

Butler, G., & Wells, A. (1995). Cognitive behavioral treatments: Clinical applications. In R. G. Heimberg, M. R. Liebowitz, D. A. Hope, & F. R. Schneier (Eds.), *Social phobia: Diagnosis, assessment, and treatment* (pp. 310–333). New York: Guilford Press.

Cacioppo, J. T., Glass, C. R., & Merluzzi, T. V. (1979). Self-statements and self-evaluations: A cognitive response analysis. *Cognitive Therapy and Research, 3*, 249–262.

Cacioppo, J. T., & Petty, R. (1981). Social psychological procedures for cognitive response assessment: The thought-listing technique. In T. V. Merluzzi, C. R. Glass, & M. Genest (Eds.), *Cognitive Assessment* (pp. 309–342). New York: Guilford Press.

Carleton, R. N., Collimore, K. C., & Asmundson, G. J. (2007). Social anxiety and fear of negative evaluation: Construct validity of the BFNE-II. *Journal of Anxiety Disorders, 2*, 131–141.

Carleton, R. N., McCreary, D., Norton, P. J., & Asmundson, G. J. G. (2006). The Brief Fear of Negative Evaluation Scale, Revised. *Depression and Anxiety, 23*, 297–303.

Cho, Y., & Telch, M. J. (2005). Testing the cognitive content-specificity hypothesis of social anxiety and depression: An application of structural equation modeling. *Cognitive Therapy and Research*, *29*, 399–416.

Clark, D. M., & Wells, A. (1995). A cognitive model of social phobia. In R. G. Heimberg, M. R. Liebowitz, D. A. Hope, & F. R. Schneier (Eds.), *Social phobia: Diagnosis, assessment, and treatment* (pp. 69–93). New York: Guilford Press.

Collins, K. A., Westra, H. A., Dozois, D. J. A., & Stewart, S. H. (2005). The validity of the brief version of the fear of negative evaluation scale. *Journal of Anxiety Disorders*, *19*, 345–359.

Compton, S. N., Grant, P. J., Chrisman, A. K., Gammon, P. J., Brown, V. L., & March, J. S. (2001). Sertraline in children and adolescents with social anxiety disorder: An open trial. *Journal of American Academy of Child and Adolescent Psychiatry*, *40*, 564–571.

Connor, K. M., Davidson, J. R. T., Churchill, L. E., Sherwood, A., Foa, E., & Weisler, R. H. (2000). Psychometric properties of the Social Phobia Inventory (SPIN): New self rating scale. *British Journal of Psychiatry*, *176*, 379–386.

Connor, K. M., Kobak, K. A., Churchill, L. E., Katzelnick, D., & Davidson, J. R. (2001). Mini-SPIN: A brief screening assessment for generalized social anxiety disorder. *Depression and Anxiety*, *14*, 137–140.

Cox, B. J., Parker, J. D. A., & Swinson, R. P. (1996). Confirmatory factor analysis of the Fear Questionnaire with social phobia patients. *British Journal of Psychiatry*, *168*, 497–499.

Cox, B. J., Swinson, R. P., & Parker, J. D. A. (1993). Confirmatory factor analysis of the Fear Questionnaire in panic disorder with agoraphobia. *Psychological Assessment*, *5*, 235–237.

Cox, B. J., Swinson, R. P., & Shaw, B. F. (1991). Value of the Fear Questionnaire in differentiating agoraphobia and social phobia. *British Journal of Psychiatry*, *159*, 842–845.

Crippa, J. A., de Lima Osorio, F., Del-Ben, C. M., Filho, A. S., de Silva Freitas, M. C., & Laureiro, S. R. (2008). Comparability between telephone and face-to-face structured clinical interview for DSM-IV in assessing social anxiety disorder. *Perspectives in Psychiatric Practice*, *44*, 241–247.

Crits-Christoph, P. (1986). The factor structure of the Cognitive Anxiety Questionnaire. *Journal of Psychosomatic Research*, *30*(6), 685–690.

Curran, J. P. (1982). A procedure for the assessment of social skills: The Simulated Social Skills Interaction Test. In J. P. Curran & P. M. Monti (Eds.), *Social skills training: A practical handbook for assessment and treatment*. New York: Guilford Press.

Curran, J. P., Monti, P. M., Corriveau, D. P., Hay, L. R., Hagerman, S., Zwick, W. R., et al. (1980). The generalizability of a procedure for assessing social skills and social anxiety in a psychiatric population. *Behavioral Assessment*, *2*, 389–401.

Curran, J. P., Wessberg, H. W., Farrell, A. D., Monti, P. M., Corriveau, D. P., & Coyne, N. A. (1982). Social skills and social anxiety: Are different laboratories measuring the same construct? *Journal of Consulting and Clinical Psychology*, *50*, 396–406.

Dalryple, K. L., & Zimmerman, M. (2008). Screening for social fears and social anxiety disorder in psychiatric outpatients. *Comprehensive Psychiatry*, *49*, 399–406.

Davidson, J. R. T., Krishnan, K. R. R., Charles, H. C., Boyko, O., Potts, N. L. S., Ford, S. M., et al. (1993). Magnetic resonance spectroscopy in social phobia: Preliminary findings. *Journal of Clinical Psychiatry*, *54*, 19–25.

Davidson, J. R. T., Miner, C. M., De Veaugh-Geiss, J., Tupler, L. A., Colket, J. T., & Potts, N. L. S. (1997). The Brief Social Phobia Scale: A psychometric evaluation. *Psychological Medicine*, *27*, 161–166.

Davidson, J. R. T., Potts, N. L. S., Richichi, E. A., Ford, S. M., Krishnan, R. R., Smith, R. D., et al. (1991). The Brief Social Phobia Scale. *Journal of Clinical Psychiatry*, *52*, 48–51.

DeGood, D. E., Buckalew, S. P., & Tait, R. C. (1985). Cognitive-somatic anxiety response patterning in chronic pain patients and nonpatients. *Journal of Consulting and Clinical Psychology*, *53*, 137–138.

DeGood, D. E., & Tait, R. C. (1987). The cognitive-somatic anxiety questionnaire: Psychometric and validity data. *Journal of Psychopathology and Behavioral Assessment*, *9*(1), 75–87.

De Lima Osorio, F., Crippa, J. A., & Laureiro, S. R. (2007). A study of the discriminative validity of a screening tool (Mini-SPIN) for social anxiety disorder applied to Brazilian university students. *European Psychiatry: The Journal of the Association of European Psychiatrists*, *22*, 239–243.

Dimberg, U., Fredrikson, M., & Lundquist, O. (1986). Autonomic reactions to social and neutral stimuli in subjects high and low in public speaking fear. *Biological Psychology*, *23*, 223–233.

Di Nardo, P. A., Moras, K., Barlow, D. H., Rapee, R. M., & Brown, T. A. (1993). Reliability of DSM-III-R anxiety disorder categories using the Anxiety Disorders Interview Schedule – Revised (ADIS-R). *Archives of General Psychiatry*, *50*, 251–256.

Dodge, C. S., Hope, D. A., Heimberg, R. G., & Becker, R. E. (1988). Evaluation of the Social Interaction Self-Statement Test with a social phobic population. *Cognitive Therapy and Research*, *12*, 209–220.

Eguchi, M., Noda, Y., Nakano, Y., Kanai, T., Yamamoto, I., Watanabe, N., et al. (2005). Quality of life and social role functioning in Japanese patients with panic disorder. *Journal of Nervous and Mental Disease*, *193*, 686–689.

Elting, D. T., & Hope, D. A. (1995). Cognitive assessment. In R. G. Heimberg, M. R. Liebowitz, D. A. Hope, & F. R. Schneier (Eds.), *Social phobia: Diagnosis, assessment, and treatment* (pp. 232–258). New York: Guilford Press.

Emmanuel, N. P., Brawman-Mintzer, O., Morton, W. A., Book, S. W., Johnson, M. R., Lorberbaum, J. P., et al. (2000). Bupropion-SR in treatment of social phobia. *Depression & Anxiety*, *12*, 111–113.

Emmelkamp, P. G., Mersch, P. E, Vissia, E., & Van Der Helm, M. (1985). Social phobia: A comparative evaluation of cognitive and behavioral interventions. *Behaviour Research and Therapy*, *23*, 365–369.

Farrell, A. D., Curran, J. P., Zwick, W. R., & Monti, P. M. (1983). Generalizability and discriminant validity of anxiety and social skills ratings in two populations. *Behavioral Assessment*, *6*, 1–14.

First, M. B., Spitzer, R. L., Williams, J. B. W., & Gibbon, M. (1997). Structured Clinical Interview for DSM-IV (SCID). Washington, DC: American Psychiatric Association.

Freeland, K., & Carney, R. (1988). Factor analysis of the Cognitive-Somatic Anxiety Questionnaire. *Journal of Psychopathology and Behavioral Assessment*, *10*(4), 367–375.

Fresco, D. M., Coles, M. E., Heimberg, R. G., Liebowitz, M. R., Hami, S., Stein, M. B., et al. (2001). The Liebowitz Social Anxiety Scale: A comparison of the psychometric properties of self-report and clinician-administered formats. *Psychological Medicine*, *31*, 1025–1035.

Friend, R., & Gilbert, J. (1973). Threat and fear of negative evaluation as determinants of locus of social comparison. *Journal of Personality*, *41*, 328–340.

Gerlach, A. L., Heinrichs, N., Bandl, C., & Zimmermann, T. (2007). Ein fragebogen zur erfassung der kognitiven komponente von redeangst. *Zeitschrift fur Klinische Psychologie und Psychotherapie: Forschung und Praxis*, *36*, 112–120.

Ginsburg, G. S., LaGreca, A. M., & Silverman, W. K. (1997). *Social anxiety in adolescents with anxiety disorders: Utility of the Social Anxiety Scale for Adolescents.* Paper presented at the annual meeting of the Association for Advancement of Behavior Therapy, Miami Beach, FL.

Ginsburg, G. S., LaGreca, A. M., & Silverman, W. K. (1998). Social anxiety in children with anxiety disorders: Relation with social and emotional functioning. *Journal of Abnormal Child Psychology*, *26*, 175–185.

Glass, C. R., & Arnkoff, D. B. (1989). Behavioral assessment of social anxiety and social phobia. *Clinical Psychology Review*, *9*, 75–90.

Glass, C. R., & Furlong, M. (1990). Cognitive assessment of social anxiety: Affective and behavioral correlates. *Cognitive Therapy and Research*, *14*(4), 365–384.

Glass, C. R., Merluzzi, T. V., Biever, J. L., & Larsen, K. H. (1982). Cognitive assessment of social anxiety: Development and validation of a self-statement questionnaire. *Cognitive Therapy and Research*, *6*, 37–55.

Goldfried, M. R., & D'Zurilla, T. J. (1969). A behavioral-analytic model for assessing competence. In C. D. Spielberger (Series Ed.), *Current topics in clinical psychology: Vol. 1* (pp. 151–196). New York: Academic Press.

Greenberg-Saluck, R., & Herbert, J. D. (2005). *Attentional demands and recall of interpersonal information in social anxiety disorder.* Paper presented at the meeting of the Association of Behavioral and Cognitive Therapies, Washington, DC.

Greist, J. H., Kobak, K. A., Jefferson, J. W., Katzelnick, D. J., & Chene, R. L. (1995). The clinical interview. In R. G. Heimberg, M. R. Liebowitz, D. A. Hope, & F. R. Schneier (Eds.), *Social phobia: Diagnosis, assessment, and treatment* (pp. 185–201). New York: Guilford Press.

Habke, A. M., Hewitt, P. L., Norton, R., & Asmundson, G. (1997). The Social Phobia and Social Interaction Anxiety Scales: An exploration of the dimensions of social anxiety and sex differences in structure and relations and pathology. *Journal of Psychopathology and Behavioral Assessment*, *19*(1), 21–39.

Hambrick, J. P., Turk, C. L., Heimberg, R. G., Schneier, F. R., & Liebowitz, M. R. (2004). Psychometric properties of disability measures among patients with social anxiety disorder. *Anxiety Disorders*, *18*, 825–839.

Hayes, S. C., Nelson, R. O., & Jarrett, R. B. (1986). Evaluating the quality of behavioral assessment. In R. O. Nelson & S. C. Hayes (Eds.), *Conceptual foundations of behavioral assessment* (pp. 463–503). New York: Guilford Press.

Heimberg, R. G. (1994). Cognitive assessment strategies and the measurement of outcome of treatment for social phobia. *Behaviour Research and Therapy*, *32*, 269–280.

Heimberg, R. G., Acerra, M. C., & Holstein, A. (1985). Partner similarity mediates interpersonal anxiety. *Cognitive Therapy and Research*, *9*, 443–453.

Heimberg, R. G., Dodge, C. S., Hope, D. A., Kennedy, C. R., Zollo, L., & Becker, R. E. (1990). Cognitive behavioral group treatment of social phobia: Comparison to a credible placebo control. *Cognitive Therapy and Research*, *14*, 1–23.

Heimberg, R. G., Gansler, D., & Dodge, C. S. (1987). Convergent and discriminant validity of the Cognitive-Somatic Anxiety Questionnaire in a social phobic population. *Behavioral Assessment*, *9*, 379–388.

Heimberg, R. G., & Holaway, R. M. (2007). Examination of the known-groups validity of the Liebowitz Social Anxiety Scale. *Depression & Anxiety*, *24*, 447–454.

Heimberg, R. G., Hope, D. A., Dodge, C. S., & Becker, R. E. (1990). *DSM-III-R* subtypes of social phobia: Comparison of generalized social phobics and public speaking phobics. *Journal of Nervous and Mental Disease*, *178*, 172–179.

Heimberg, R. G., Hope, D. A., Rapee, R. M., & Bruch, M. A. (1988). The validity of the Social Avoidance and Distress Scale and the Fear of Negative Evaluation Scale with social phobic patients. *Behaviour Research and Therapy*, *26*, 407–410.

Heimberg, R. G., Horner, K. J., Juster, H. R., Safren, S. A., Brown, E. J., Schneier, F. R., et al. (1999). Psychometric properties of the Liebowitz Social Phobia Scale. *Psychological Medicine*, *29*, 199–212.

Heimberg, R. G., & Liebowitz, M. R. (1992). *A multi-center comparison of the efficacy of phenelzine and cognitive behavioral group treatment for social phobia*. Paper presented at the annual meeting of the Anxiety Disorders Association of America, Houston, TX.

Heimberg, R. G., Mueller, G. P., Holt, C. S., Hope, D. A., & Liebowitz, M. R. (1992). Assessment of anxiety on social interaction and being observed by others: The Social Interaction Anxiety Scale and the Social Phobia Scale. *Behaviour Therapy*, *23*, 53–73.

Heinrichs, N., & Hofmann, S. G. (2005). Cognitive assessment of social anxiety: A comparison of self-report and thought-listing methods. *Cognitive Behaviour Therapy*, *34*, 3–15.

Herbert, J. D., Bellack, A. S., & Hope, D. A. (1991). Concurrent validity of the Social Phobia and Anxiety Inventory. *Journal of Psychopathology and Behavioral Assessment*, *13*(4), 357–369.

Herbert, J. D., Bellack, A. S., Hope, D. A., & Mueser, K. T. (1992). Scoring the Social Phobia and Anxiety Inventory: Reply to Beidel and Turner. *Journal of Psychopathology and Behavioral Assessment*, *14*, 381–383.

Herbert, J. D., Gaudiano, B. A., Rheingold, A., Harwell, V., Dalrymple, K., & Nolan, E. M. (2005). Social skills training augments the effectiveness of cognitive behavior group therapy for social anxiety disorder. *Behaviour Therapy*, *36*, 125–138.

Herbert, J. D., Gaudiano, B. A., Rheingold, A. A., Moitra, E., Myers, V. H., Dalrymple, K. L., et al. (2009). Cognitive behavior therapy for generalized social anxiety disorder in adolescents: A randomized controlled trial. *Journal of Anxiety Disorders*, *23*, 167–177.

Herbert, J. D., Hope, D. A., & Bellack, A. S. (1992). Validity of the distinction between generalized social phobia and avoidant personality disorder. *Journal of Abnormal Psychology*, *101*, 332–339.

Herbert, J. D., & Nelson-Gray, R. O. (1997). La autoobservación. In G. Buela-Casa & J. Carlos Sierra (Eds.), *Manual de evaluación psicológica: Fundamentos, técnicas y aplicaciones*. Madrid: Siglo XXI de España Editores, SA.

Hofmann, S. G. (2006). The emotional consequences of social pragmatism: The psychophysiological correlates of self-monitoring. *Biological Psychology*, *73*, 169–174.

Hofmann, S. G., & DiBartolo, P. M. (2000). An instrument to assess self-statements during public speaking: Scale development and preliminary psychometric properties. *Behaviour Therapy*, *31*, 499–515.

Hofmann, S. G., DiBartolo, P. M., Holaway, R. M., & Heimberg, R. G. (2004). Scoring error of Social Avoidance and Distress Scale and its psychometric implications. *Depression and Anxiety*, *19*, 197–198.

Hofmann, S. G., Meuret, A. E., Smits, J. A. J., Simon, N. M., Pollack, M. H., Eisenmenger, K., et al. (2006). Augmentation of exposure therapy with D-Cycloserine for social anxiety disorder. *Archives of General Psychiatry*, *63*, 298–304.

Hofmann, S. G., Newman, M. G., Ehlers, A., & Roth, W. T. (1995). Psychophysiological differences between subgroups of social phobia. *Journal of Abnormal Psychology*, *104*, 224–231.

Holt, C. S., Heimberg, R. G., & Hope, D. A. (1992). Avoidant personality disorder and the generalized subtype of social phobia. *Journal of Abnormal Psychology*, *101*, 318–325.

Hope, D. A., Heimberg, R. G., Zollo, L. J., Nyman, D. J., & O'Brien, G. T. (1987). *Thought-listing in the natural environment: Valence and focus of listed thoughts among socially anxious and nonanxious subjects*. Paper presented at the Association for Advancement of Behavior Therapy, Boston, MA.

Hope, D. A., Herbert, J. D., & White, C. (1995). Social phobia subtype, avoidant personality disorder, and psychotherapy outcome. *Cognitive Therapy and Research*, *19*, 339–417.

Hoyer, J., Becker, E. S., Neumer, S., Soeder, U., & Margraf, J. (2002). Screening for anxiety in an epidemiological sample: Predictive accuracy of questionnaires. *Journal of Anxiety Disorders*, *16*, 113–134.

Huppert, J. D., Strunk, D. R., Ledley, D. R., Davidson, J. R., & Foa, E. B. (2008). Generalized social anxiety disorder and avoidant personality disorder: Structural analysis and treatment outcome. *Depression & Anxiety*, *25*, 441–448.

Inderbitzen, H. M., & Foster, S. L. (1992). The Teenage Inventory of Social Skills: Development, reliability, and validity. *Psychological Assessment*, *4*, 451–459.

Isolan, L., Pheula, G., Abrahao Salum, G., Oswald, S., Rohde, L. A., & Manfro, G. G. (2007). An open-label trial of escitalopram in children and adolescents with social anxiety disorder. *Journal of Child and Adolescent Psychopharmacology*, *17*, 751–759.

Johnson, R. L., & Glass, C. R. (1989). Heterosexual anxiety and focus of attention in high school boys. *Cognitive Therapy and Research*, *13*, 509–526.

Jørstad-Stein, E. C., & Heimberg, R. G. (2009). Social phobia: An update on treatment. *Psychiatric Clinics of North America*, *32*, 641–663.

Kashdan, T. B., & Herbert, J. D. (2001). Social anxiety disorder in childhood and adolescence: Current status and future directions. *Clinical Child and Family Psychology Review*, *4*, 37–61.

Kasvikis, Y., Sotiropoulou, V., Mitskidou, P., Livanou, M., & Poulou, P. (2006). Psychometric properties of the Greek translation of the Marks and Mathews' Fear Questionnaire. *Psychiatriki*, *17*, 314–324.

Kearney, C. A., & Albano, A. M. (2004). The functional profiles of school refusal. *Behaviour Modification*, *28*, 147–168.

Kessler, R., Akiskal, H., Angst, J., Guyer, M., Hirschfeld, R., Merikangas, K., et al. (2006). Validity of the assessment of bipolar spectrum disorders in the WHO CIDI 3.0. *Journal of Affective Disorders*, *96*, 259–269.

Koszycki, D., Benger, M., Shlik, J., & Bradwejn, J. (2007). Randomized trial of a meditation-based stress reduction program and cognitive behavior therapy in generalized social anxiety disorder. *Behaviour Research and Therapy*, *45*, 2518–2526.

Kristensen, H., & Torgersen, S. (2006). Social anxiety disorder in 11–12-year-old children: The efficacy of screening and issues in parent–child agreement. *European Child Adolescent Psychiatry*, *15*, 163–171.

Lader, M. H. (1967). Palmer skin conductance measures in anxiety and phobic states. *Journal of Psychosomatic Research*, *11*, 271–281.

LaGreca, A. M., & Stone, W. L. (1993). Social Anxiety Scale for Children – Revised: Factor structure and concurrent validity. *Journal of Clinical Child Psychology*, *22*, 17–27.

Leary, M. R. (1983). A brief version of the Fear of Negative Evaluation Scale. *Personality and Social Psychology Bulletin*, *9*, 371–375.

Leary, M. R., & Kowalski, R. M. (1995). *Social anxiety*. New York: Guilford Press.

Ledley, D. R., Huppert, J. D., Foa, E. B., Davidson, J. R., Keefe, F. J., & Potts, N. L. (2005). Impact of depressive symptoms on the treatment of generalized social anxiety disorder. *Depression & Anxiety*, *22*, 161–167.

Lelliott, P., McNamee, G., & Marks, I. (1991). Features of agora-, social, and related phobias and validation of the diagnoses. *Journal of Anxiety Disorders*, *5*, 313–322.

Leon, A. C., Olfson, M., Portera, L., Farbert, L., & Sheehan, D. V. (1997). Assessing psychiatric impairment in primary care with the Sheehan Disability Scale. *International Journal of Psychiatry in Medicine*, *27*, 93–105.

Levin, A. P., Saoud, J. B., Strauman, T., Gorman, J. M., Fyer, A. J., Crawford, R., et al. (1993). Responses of "generalized" and "discrete" social phobics during public speaking. *Journal of Anxiety Disorders*, *7*, 207–221.

Liebowitz, M. R. (1987). Social phobia. *Modern Problems in Pharmacopsychiatry*, *22*, 141–173.

Liebowitz, M. R., Fyer, A. J., Gorman, J. M., Dillon, D., Davies, S., Stein, J. M., et al. (1985). Specificity of lactate infusions in social phobia versus panic disorder. *American Journal of Psychiatry*, *142*, 947–950.

Liebowitz, M. R., Mangano, R. M., Bradwejn, J., & Asnis, G. (2005). SAD Study Group. A randomized controlled trial of venlafaxine extended release in generalized social anxiety disorder. *Journal of Clinical Psychiatry*, *66*, 238–247.

Lipsitz, J. D., Gur, M., Vermes, D., Petkova, E., Cheng, J., Miller, N., et al. (2008). A randomized trial of interpersonal therapy versus supportive therapy for social anxiety disorder. *Depression and Anxiety*, *25*, 542–553.

Malow, R. M., West, J. A., Williams, J. L., & Sutker, P. B. (1989). Personality disorders classification and symptoms in cocaine and opioid addicts. *Journal of Consulting and Clinical Psychology*, *57*, 765–767.

March, J. S., Entusah, A. R., Rynn, M., Albano, A. M., & Tourian, K. A. (2007). A randomized controlled trial of venlafaxine ER versus placebo in pediatric social anxiety disorder. *Biological Psychiatry*, *62*, 1149–1154.

March, J., Parker, J., Sullivan, K., Stallings, P., & Conners, C. K. (1997). The Multidimensional Anxiety Scale for Children (MASC): Factor structure, reliability, and validity. *Journal of the American Academy of Child and Adolescent Psychiatry*, *36*, 554–565.

Marks, I. M., & Mathews, A. M. (1979). Brief standard rating for phobic patients. *Behaviour Research and Therapy*, *17*, 263–267.

Masia-Warner, C., Fisher, P. H., Shrout, P. E., Rathor, S., & Klein, R. G. (2007). Treating adolescents with social anxiety disorder in school: An attention control trial. *Journal of Child Psychology and Psychiatry*, *48*, 676–686.

Masia-Warner, C., Klein, R. G., Dent, H., Fisher, P. H., Alvir, J., Albano, A. M., et al. (2005). School-based intervention for adolescents with social anxiety disorder: Results of a controlled study. *Journal of Abnormal Child Psychology*, *33*, 707–722.

Masia-Warner, C., Storch, E. A., Pincus, D. B., Klein, R. G., Heimberg, R. G., & Liebowitz, M. R. (2003). The Liebowitz Social Anxiety Scale for Children and Adolescents: An initial psychometric investigation. *Journal of the American Academy of Child and Adolescent Psychiatry*, *42*, 1076–1084.

Matson, J. L., Rotatori, A. F., & Helsel, W. J. (1983). Development of a rating scale to measure social skills in children: The Matson Evaluation of Social Skills with Youngsters (MESSY). *Behaviour Research and Therapy*, *21*, 335–340.

Mattick, R. P., & Clark, J. C. (1998). Development and validation of measures of social phobia scrutiny fear and social interaction anxiety. *Behavioral Research and Therapy*, *36*, 455–470.

Mattick, R. P., & Peters, L. (1988). Treatment of severe social phobia: Effects of guided exposure with and without cognitive restructuring. *Journal of Consulting and Clinical Psychology*, *56*, 251–260.

Mattick, R. P., Peters, L., & Clark, J. C. (1989). Exposure and cognitive restructuring for social phobia: A controlled study. *Behaviour Therapy*, *20*, 3–23.

McNeil, D. W., Ries, B. J., & Turk, C. L. (1995). Behavioral assessment: Self-report, physiology, and overt behavior. In R. G. Heimberg, M. R. Liebowitz, D. A. Hope, & F. R. Schneier (Eds.), *Social phobia: Diagnosis, assessment, and treatment* (pp. 202–231). New York: Guilford Press.

Mennin, D. S., Fresco, D. M., Heimberg, R. G., Schneier, F. R., Davies, S. O., & Liebowitz, M. R. (2002). Screening for social anxiety disorder in the clinical setting using the Liebowitz Social Anxiety Scale. *Journal of Anxiety Disorders*, *16*, 661–673.

Merluzzi, T. V., & Biever, J. (1987). Role-playing procedures for the behavioral assessment of social skill: A validity study. *Behavioral Assessment*, *9*, 361–377.

Mersch, P. P. A., Breukers, P., & Emmelkamp, P. M. G. (1992). The simulated social interaction test: A psychometric evaluation with Dutch social phobic patients. *Behavioral Assessment, 14,* 133–151.

Mersch, P. P. A., Emmelkamp, P. M. G., & Lips, C. (1991). Social phobia: Individual response patterns and the long-term effects of behavioral and cognitive interventions. A follow-up study. *Behaviour Research and Therapy, 29,* 357–362.

Michelson, L., & Mavissakalian, M. (1983). Temporal stability of self-report measures in agoraphobia research. *Behaviour Research and Therapy, 21*, 695–698.

Monti, P. M., Wallander, J. L., Ahern, D. K., Abrams, D. B., & Munroe, S. M. (1983). Multimodal measurement of anxiety and social skills in a behavioral role-play test: Generalizability and discriminant validity. *Behavioral Assessment*, *6*, 15–25.

Myszka, M. T., Galassi, J. P., & Ware, W. B. (1986). Comparison of cognitive assessment methods with heterosexually anxious college women. *Journal of Counseling Psychology*, *33*, 401–407.

Nelson, R. O., Hay, L. R., Devany, J., & Koslow-Green, L. (1980). The reactivity and accuracy of children's self-monitoring: Three experiments. *Child Behavior Therapy*, *2*, 1–24.

Nietzel, M. T., & Bernstein, D. A. (1981). Assessment of anxiety and fear. In M. Hersen & A. S. Bellack (Eds.), *Behavioral assessment: A practical handbook* (2nd ed.). New York: Pergamon Press.

Nietzel, M. T., Bernstein, D. A., & Russell, R. L. (1988). *Assessment of anxiety and fear* (3rd ed.). Elmsford, NY: Pergamon Press.

Nyman, D., & Heimberg, R. G. (1985). *Heterosocial anxiety among college students: A reasonable analogue to social phobia?* Paper presented at the Association for Advancement of Behaviour Therapy, Houston, TX.

Oakman, J., van Ameringen, M., Mancini, C., & Farvolden, P. (2003). A confirmatory factor analysis of a self-report version of the Liebowitz Social Anxiety Scale. *Journal of Clinical Psychology*, *59*, 149–161.

Oei, T. P. S., Gross, P. R., & Evans, L. (1989). Phobic disorders and anxiety states: How do they differ? *Australian and New Zealand Journal of Psychiatry*, *23*(81-88).

Oei, T. P. S., Moylan, A., & Evans, L. (1991). Validity and clinical utility of the Fear Questionnaire for anxiety-disorder patients. *Psychological Assessment*, *3*(3), 391–397.

Olivares, J., Garcia-Lopez, L. J., Hidalgo, M. D., La Greca, A. M., Turner, S. M., & Beidel, D. C. (2002). A pilot study on normative data for two social anxiety measures: The Social Phobia and Anxiety Inventory and the Social Anxiety Scale for Adolescents. *International Journal of Clinical and Health Psychology*, *2*, 467–476.

Peters, L. (2000). Discriminant validity of the Social Phobia and Anxiety Inventory (SPAI), the Social Phobia Scale (SPS) and the Social Interaction Anxiety Scale (SIAS). *Behaviour Research and Therapy*, *38*, 943–950.

Picon, P., Gauer, G. J. C., Fachel, J. M. G., Beidel, D. C., Seganfredo, A. C., & Manfro, G. G. (2006). The Portuguese language version of the Social Phobia and Anxiety Inventory: Analysis of items and internal consistency in a Brazilian sample of 1014 undergraduate students. *Journal Brasileiro de Psiquiatria*, *55*, 114–119.

Rapee, R. M. (1995). Descriptive psychopathology of social phobia. In R. G. Heimberg, M. R. Liebowitz, D. A. Hope, & F. R. Schneier (Eds.), *Social phobia: Diagnosis, assessment, and treatment* (pp. 41–66). New York: Guilford Press.

Rapee, R. M., Barrett, P. M., Dadds, M. R., & Evans, L. (1994). Reliability of the *DSM-III-R* childhood anxiety disorders using structured interview: Inter-rater and parent–child agreement. *Journal of the American Academy of Child and Adolescent Psychiatry*, *33*, 984–992.

Rapee, R. M., Brown, T. A., Antony, M. M., & Barlow, D. H. (1992). Response to hyperventilation and inhalation of 5.5% carbon dioxide enriched air across the *DSM-III-R* anxiety disorders. *Journal of Abnormal Psychology*, *101*, 538–552.

Rapee, R. M., & Heimberg, R. G. (1997). A cognitive behavioral model of anxiety in social phobia. *Behaviour Research and Therapy*, *35*, 741–756.

Reynolds, C. R., & Richmond, B. (1978). What I think and feel: A revised measure of children's manifest anxiety. *Journal of Abnormal Child Psychology*, *6*, 271–280.

Richardson, F. C., & Tasto, D. L. (1976). Development and factor analysis of a social anxiety inventory. *Behavior Therapy*, *7*, 453–462.

Riskind, J. H., Beck, A. T., Berchick, R. J., Brown, G., & Steer, R. A. (1987). Reliability of *DSM-III* diagnoses for major depression and generalized anxiety disorder using the Structured Clinical Interview for *DSM-III*. *Archives of General Psychiatry*, *44*, 817–820.

Rodebaugh, T. L., Woods, C. M., & Heimberg, R. G. (2007). The reverse of social anxiety is not always the opposite: The reverse-scored items of the social interaction anxiety scale do not belong. *Behaviour Therapy*, *38*, 192–206.

Rodebaugh, T. L., Woods, C. M., Heimberg, R. G., Liebowitz, M. R., & Schneier, F. R. (2006). The factor structure and screening utility of the Social Interaction Anxiety Scale. *Psychological Assessment*, *18*, 231–237.

Rodebaugh, T. L., Woods, C. M., Thissen, D. M., Heimberg, R. G., Chambless, D. L., & Rapee, R. M. (2004). More information from fewer questions: The factor structure and item properties of the original and Brief Fear of Negative Evaluation Scale. *Psychological Assessment*, *2*, 169–181.

Rytwinski, N. K., Fresco, D. M., Heimberg, R. G., Coles, M. E., Liebowitz, M. R., Cissell, S., et al. (2009). Screening for social anxiety disorder with the self-report version of the Liebowitz Social Anxiety Scale. *Depression and Anxiety*, *26*, 34–38.

Safren, S. A., Heimberg, R. G., Horner, K. J., Juster, H. R., Schneier, F. R., & Liebowitz, M. R. (1999). Factor structure of social fears: The Liebowitz Social Anxiety Scale. *Journal of Anxiety Disorders*, *13*, 253–270.

Schneier, F. R., Heckelman, L. R., Garfinkel, R., Campeas, R., Fallon, B. A., Gitow, A., et al. (1994). Functional impairment in social phobia. *Journal of Clinical Psychiatry*, *55*, 322–331.

Schneier, F. R., Johnson, J., Hornig, C. D., Liebowitz, M. R., & Weissman, M. M. (1992). Social phobia: Comorbidity and morbidity in an epidemiological sample. *Archives of General Psychiatry*, *49*, 282–288.

Scholing, A., & Emmelkamp, P. M. G. (1990). Social phobia: Nature and treatment. In H. Leitenberg (Ed.), *Handbook of Social and Evaluation Anxiety* (pp. 269–324). New York: Plenum Press.

Schmidt, N. B., Richey, J. A., Buckner, J. D., & Timpano, K. R. (2009). Attention training for generalized social anxiety disorder. *Journal of Abnormal Psychology*, *118*, 5–14.

Schwartz, G. E., Davidson, R. J., & Goleman, D. J. (1978). Patterning of cognitive and somatic processes in the self-regulation of anxiety: Effects of meditation versus exercise. *Psychosomatic Medicine*, *40*, 321–328.

Segal, D. L., Hersen, M., & Van Hassalt, V. B. (1994). Reliability of the Structured Clinical Interview for DSM-III-R: An evaluative review. *Comprehensive Psychiatry*, *35*, 316–327.

Shear, M. K., Greeno, C., Kang, J., Ludewig, D., Frank, E., Swartz, H. A., et al. (2000). Diagnosis of nonpsychotic patients in community clinics. *American Journal of Psychiatry*, *157*, 581–587.

Sica, C., Musoni, I., Chiri, L. R., Bisi, B., Lolli, V., & Sighinolfi, C. (2007). Social Phobia Scale (SPS), Social Interaction Anxiety Scale (SIAS): Traduzione ed adattamento Italiano. *Bollettino di Psicologia Applicata*, *252*, 59–71.

Silverman, W. K., & Eisen, A. R. (1992). Age differences in the reliability of parent and child reports of child anxious symptomatology using a structured interview. *Journal of the American Academy of Child and Adolescent Psychiatry*, *31*, 117–124.

Silverman, W. K., & Nelles, W. B. (1988). The Anxiety Disorders Interview Schedule for Children. *Journal of the American Academy of Child and Adolescent Psychiatry*, *27*(6), 772–778.

Silverman, W. K., & Rabian, B. (1995). Test–retest reliability of the DSM-III-R childhood anxiety disorders symptoms using the Anxiety Disorders Interview Schedule for Children. *Journal of Anxiety Disorders*, *9*, 139–150.

Silverman, W. K., Saavedra, L. M., & Pina, A. A. (2001). Test–retest reliability of anxiety symptoms and diagnoses with the Anxiety Disorders Interview Schedule for DSM-IV: Child and parent versions. *Journal of the American Academy of Child & Adolescent Psychiatry*, *40*, 937–944.

Skre, I., Onstand, S., Torgersen, S., & Kringlen, E. (1991). High interrater reliability for the Structured Clinical Interview for DSMI-III-R Axis I (SCID-I). *Acta Psychiatrica Scandinavica*, *84*, 167–173.

Smith, R. E., & Sarason, I. G. (1975). Social anxiety and the evaluation of negative interpersonal feedback. *Journal of Consulting and Clinical Psychology*, *43*, 429.

Spence, S. H. (1995). In *Social Skills Training: Enhancing Social Competence with Children and Adolescents*. Windsor, UK: NFER-NELSON Publishing Co.

Spence, S. H. (1998). A measure of anxiety symptoms among children. *Behaviour Research and Therapy*, *36*, 545–566.

Spitzer, R. L., & Endicott, J. (1978). *Schedule for affective disorders and schizophrenia*. New York: New York State Psychiatric Institute, Biometrics Research Division.

Stein, M. B., Asmundson, G. J. G., & Chartier, M. (1994). Autonomic responsivity in generalized social phobia. *Journal of Affective Disorders*, *31*, 211–221.

Stein, M. B., & Stein, D. J. (2008). Social anxiety disorder. *Lancet*, *371*, 115–125.

Steiner, J. L., Tebes, J. K., Sledge, W. H., & Walker, M. L. (1995). A comparison of the Structured Clinical Interview for DSMIII-R and clinical diagnoses. *Journal of Nervous and Mental Disease*, *183*, 365–369.

Steptoe, A., & Kearsley, N. (1990). Cognitive and somatic anxiety. *Behaviour Research and Therapy*, *28*(1), 75–81.

Storch, E. A., Masia-Warner, C., Dent, H. C., Roberti, J. W., & Fisher, P. H. (2004). Psychometric evaluation of the Social Anxiety Scale for Adolescents and the Social Phobia and Anxiety Inventory for Children: Construct validity and normative data. *Anxiety Disorders*, *18*, 665–679.

Storch, E. A., Masia-Warner, C., Heidgerken, A. D., Fisher, P. H., Pincus, D. B., & Liebowitz, M. R. (2006). Factor structure of the Liebowitz Social Anxiety Scale for Children and Adolescents. *Child Psychiatry Human Development*, *37*, 25–37.

Sturmer, P. J., Bruch, M. A., Haase, R. F., & Amico, K. R. (2002). Convergent validity in cognitive assessment of social anxiety: Endorsement versus production methods in deriving states of mind ratio. *Cognitive Therapy and Research*, *26*, 487–503.

Stukenberg, K. W., Dura, J. R., & Kiecolt-Glaser, J. K. (1990). Depression screening scale validation in an elderly community dwelling population. *Psychological Assessment*, *2*, 134–138.

Tamaren, A. J., Carney, R. M., & Allen, T. W. (1985). Assessment of cognitive and somatic anxiety: A preliminary validity study. *Behavioral Assessment*, *7*, 197–202.

Taylor, S. (1993). The structure of fundamental fears. *Journal of Behavior Therapy and Experimental Psychiatry*, *24*, 289–299.

Taylor, S., Woody, S., McLean, P. D., & Koch, W. J. (1997). Sensitivity of outcome measures for treatments of generalized social phobia. *Assessment*, *4*(2), 181–191.

Tercilla, R. (1981). Efficacy of relaxation techniques in the attenuation of cognitive versus somatic anxiety. *Dissertation Abstracts International*, *41*, 27–83.

Tharwani, H. M., & Davidson, J. R. T. (2001). Symptomatic and functional assessment of social anxiety disorder in adults. *The Psychiatric Clinics of North America*, *24*, 643–659.

Turner, S. M., & Beidel, D. C. (1988). Some further comments on the measurement of social phobia. *Behaviour Therapy*, *16*, 384–392.

Turner, S. M., Beidel, D. C., Dancu, C. V., & Stanley, M. A. (1989). An empirically derived inventory to measure social fears and anxiety: The social phobia and anxiety inventory. *Psychological Assessment*, *1*(1), 35–40.

Turner, S. M., Beidel, D. C., & Jacob, R. G. (1994). Social phobia: A comparison of behavior therapy and atenolol. *Journal of Consulting and Clinical Psychology*, *62*, 350–358.

Turner, S. M., Beidel, D. C., & Larkin, K. T. (1986). Situational determinants of social anxiety in clinic and non-clinic samples: Physiological and cognitive correlates. *Journal of Consulting and Clinical Psychology*, *54*, 523–527.

Turner, S. M., Beidel, D. C., Long, P. J., & Greenhouse, J. (1992). Reduction of fear in social phobics: An examination of extinction patterns. *Behaviour Therapy*, *23*, 389–403.

Turner, S. M., McCanna, M., & Beidel, D. C. (1987). Discriminant validity of the Social Avoidance and Distress and Fear of Negative Evaluation Scales. *Behaviour Research and Therapy*, *25*, 113–115.

Turner, S. M., Stanley, M. A., Beidel, D. C., & Bond, L. (1989). The Social Phobia and Anxiety Inventory: Construct validity. *Journal of Psychopathology and Behavioral Assessment*, *11*(3), 221–234.

Twentyman, C. T., & McFall, R. M. (1975). Behavioral training of social skills in shy males. *Journal of Consulting and Clinical Psychology*, *43*, 384–395.

van Zuuren, F. J. (1988). The fear questionnaire, some data on validity, reliability, and layout. *British Journal of Psychiatry*, *153*, 659–662.

Ventura, J., Liberman, R. P., Green, M. F., Shaner, A., & Mintz, J. (1998). Training and quality assurance with the Structured Clinical Interview for DSM-IV (SCID-I/P). *Psychiatry Research*, *79*, 163–173.

Wagner, K. D., Berard, R., Stein, M. B., Wetherhold, E., Carpenter, D. J., Perera, P., et al. (2004). A multicenter, randomized, double-blind, placebo-controlled trial of paroxetine in children and adolescents with social anxiety disorder. *Archives of General Psychiatry*, *61*, 1153–1162.

Walters, K. S., Caster, J. B., & Inderbitzen, H. M. (1996). *The Social Anxiety Scale for Children—Revised: Normative data for an adolescent population.* Paper presented at the annual meeting of the Association for Advancement of Behaviour Therapy, New York.

Watson, J., & Friend, R. (1969). Measurement of social-evaluative anxiety. *Journal of Consulting and Clinical Psychology*, *33*, 448–457.

Weeks, J. W., Spokas, M. E., & Heimberg, R. G. (2007). Psychometric evaluation of the mini-social phobia inventory (Mini-SPIN) in a treatment-seeking sample. *Depression and Anxiety*, *24*, 382–391.

Widiger, T. A. (1992). Generalized social phobia versus avoidant personality disorder: A commentary on three studies. *Journal of Abnormal Psychology*, *101*, 340–343.

Williams, J. B., Gibbon, M., First, M. B., Spitzer, R. L., Davies, M., Borus, J., et al. (1992). The Structured Clinical Interview for DSM-III-R (SCID). *Archives of General Psychiatry*, *49*, 630–636.

Ye, D-M., Qian, M-Y., Liu, X-H., & Chen, X. (2007). Revision of Social Interaction Anxiety Scale and Social Phobia Scale. *Chinese Journal of Clinical Psychology*, *15*, 115–117.

Zimmerman, M., & Mattia, J. I. (1999). Psychiatric diagnosis in clinical practice: Is comorbidity being missed? *Comprehensive Psychiatry*, *40*, 182–191.

Zubeidat, I., Salinas, J. M., Sierra, J. C., & Fernandez-Parra, A. (2007). Psychometric properties of the Social Interaction Anxiety Scale and separation criterion between Spanish youths with and without subtypes of social anxiety. *Journal of Anxiety Disorders*, *21*, 603–624.

Chapter 3

Shyness, Social Anxiety, and Social Anxiety Disorder

Lynne Henderson[1] and Philip Zimbardo[2]

[1]*The Shyness Institute, Palo Alto, CA 94306; Stanford University Continuing Studies, Stanford, CA, 94305,* [2]*The Shyness Institute, Palo Alto, CA 94306; Palo Alto University, Palo Alto, CA, 94304*

INTRODUCTION

In 1971, one of us conducted the now well-known Stanford Prison Experiment (Zimbardo, 1977). The purpose of the study was to examine the role of situational factors in producing behaviors, thoughts, and feelings typically assumed to manifest themselves as dispositional attributes of the person, such as sadism or submissiveness. Preselected normal college students, randomly assigned to play the roles of prisoner or guard in a simulated prison, were having such extreme stress reactions that they had to be released early – as prisoners – or were behaving brutally and sadistically – as guards. The study demonstrated how powerful context and situation are in producing the syndrome of affect, behavior, and cognition relating to authoritarianism, aggression, submission, and despair. Upon reflection, the coercive control that typified the guard mentality and the passive-reactive mentality of the prisoners seemed to be combined in the mental makeup of the shy person. The "guard self" issued constraining demands that limited the freedoms of the behaving aspect of the "shy self" the shy person reluctantly submitted, and thereby lost personal autonomy and a sense of personal esteem. That conceptualization led to considering the situational and personal determinants of shyness in adults, and, in turn, to a long-term research program, the Stanford Shyness Program (Zimbardo, 1977). The Stanford Clinic was founded in 1977 and later renamed the Shyness Clinic.

From the outset, the Shyness Clinic's programs were designed to meet the expressed needs of people in our community. Responses to the initial Stanford Shyness Survey (see appendix in Zimbardo, 1977) served as guidelines for selecting techniques to help shy individuals who sought its services. Therapists helped clients implement strategies that addressed their concerns about their negative thoughts, inhibited or overactive behaviors, painful emotions, and difficulty regulating uncomfortable physiological arousal. Over the three decades

Social Anxiety: Clinical, Developmental, and Social Perspectives. DOI: 10.1016/B978-0-12-375096-9.00003-1

that followed, we have learned much from our interactions with clients, our own empirical research, and emerging relevant developments in the fields of social psychology, personality theory, and clinical psychology.

During the personal growth movement, which straddled the 1970s, many people adopted the posture that it was up to us individually to make our lives better. "I can do it" captured the directives of the day: self-responsibility and self-efficacy. Following that period, psychology became increasingly medicalized. Extreme shyness was conceptualized as a psychological disorder, Social Anxiety Disorder (SAD), a relatively rare but serious problem located in the person that could be treated by doctors/professionals acting on the person. Unfortunately, this scheme would logically serve to increase the passivity and pessimism of those already feeling that they are helpless and passive observers of life. Our overarching treatment mission at the clinic – one about which we are both passionate – has been to guide individuals in ways that empower them to help themselves. We have sought to promote in our clients the idea that they can overcome their inhibitions and become more socially comfortable and competent; indeed, even that they should do so, given that each of us, as social beings, has important and valuable contributions to make to the general community.

As part of directing the Shyness Clinic for over 25 years, one of us developed a new model to guide our treatment program (Henderson, 1994). Currently, we operate our clinic based on the belief that shyness, even extreme shyness, is best conceptualized as a state of "social fitness," analogous to physical fitness. We deem this analogy useful in several ways and on several levels. It allows an ecological analysis that takes into account the fit between characteristics of the individual, the individual's goals, and the demands and expectations of the social environment, as each varies over time and across situations. Rather than dichotomizing people into categories of "socially phobic" or "not socially phobic," "socially anxious" or "not socially anxious," "shy" or "not shy," the model admits to a continuum for each dimension, which we believe better accords with reality: Few of us may be considered world-class social athletes, just as few are world-class physical athletes. Moreover, the model accommodates varying definitions of "world-class" across cultures and across situations within a given culture. An example of the usefulness of the metaphor is illustrated by the fact that social fitness, like physical fitness, is importantly determined by the amount of time and effort spent exercising social skills (working out) and learning (through observation and instruction) the social norms and expectations (rules) of various socio-cultural niches (sports or games).

In the time since we contributed to the first edition of this book we have added an emphasis in our work with groups on resisting the negative social stereotyping of ordinary shyness, which has grown during the past 50 years. The research of Claude Steele and others has taught us about the power of negative stereotyping on a target's level of self-consciousness (whether inside or outside awareness) and on a person's well-being in general (Davies, Spencer, & Steele, 2005; Eagly & Karau, 2002; Steele, 1997). Recent research has revealed the effects of the negative stereotyping of shyness as a personality trait and the assigning of moral blame to individuals, reframing the problem, if there is one, as outside society (Lane, 2007; Scott, 2006).

We believe that it is important to help clients not only to recognize stereotyping when it is happening, and to counter it, at least internally, but also to contribute to educating the larger society regarding both the strengths of some aspects of shyness and the harmful effects of stereotyping any temperament or personality style, all of which have particular strengths and weaknesses. Given the recent statistics that 50–60% of college student samples report being shy, one has to wonder to what degree the trait is adaptive, given that it occurs not only more frequently in the population, but also now constitutes more than half of college student samples. A recent study of 1194 college students revealed that 36% of 57.7% self-reported shy people did not see it as a problem. In contrast to earlier studies, only 1.3% denied ever having been shy. Strangers, people of the opposite sex, and individual authority continue to remain the biggest challenges, as they were in our earlier surveys (Carducci, Stubbins, & Bryant, 2007). It appears that we may be increasing people's awareness of shyness, allowing people to be more open to acknowledging it, but we are not sufficiently distinguishing between ordinary "garden variety" shyness and problematic shyness, or acknowledging the negative stereotyping of shyness due to a more extreme emphasis in the United States on personal dominance and extraversion, particularly in males.

Clinicians and researchers alike continue to struggle with definitional problems and problems of convergent and discriminant validity between the constructs "shyness," "social anxiety," and "SAD." Each of these constructs shares similarities: continua of severity are seen in each, ranging from mild, infrequent, and transitory difficulty to severe, chronic, and debilitating problems. Yet, each has been used to define distinct aspects of psychological life vis-à-vis interpersonal functioning. The challenge in agreeing on definitions related to shyness will be creating and clarifying shared definitions that neither omit important components of a construct nor generalize to the extent that terms are interchangeable and thus devoid of precise meaning.

DEFINITIONS

The constructs of social anxiety, SAD, and shyness obviously share much common ground, but the following definitions focus on the unique features of each of them. Social anxiety is defined as a cognitive and affective experience that is triggered by the perception of possible evaluation by others (Schlenker & Leary, 1982). It includes unpleasant physiological arousal and fear of psychological harm (Leary & Kowalski, 1995). The definition focuses on a *feeling* or state of *arousal* that is centered on interactions with others.

SAD is defined as a "marked and persistent fear of one or more situations in which the person is exposed to possible scrutiny by others and fears that he or she may do something or act in a way that will be humiliating or embarrassing" (American Psychiatric Association, 1994, p. 416). Although there are exceptions, a diagnosis of SAD usually involves marked behavioral avoidance of one or more social situations. By definition, a phobia, such as a snake phobia, requires the notion of an avoidance response. A phobic response is the behavior of avoiding a feared stimulus or situation of a particular kind.

Shyness has been defined as "a heightened state of individuation characterized by excessive egocentric preoccupation and over concern with social evaluation, . . . with the consequence that the shy person inhibits, withdraws, avoids, and escapes" (Zimbardo, 1982, pp. 467–468). William James considered shyness a basic human instinct, following Darwin (James, 1890). Izard described shyness as a discrete, fundamental emotion (1972). In an emotion profile in a "shy" situation, shyness is a blend of fear and interest (Izard, 1972; Mosher & White, 1981). Carver and Scheier defined shyness in self-regulation terms, with unfavorable social outcome expectancies leading to disengagement in task efforts (Carver & Scheier, 1986).

While most definitions of these constructs involve discomfort and the motivation to escape situations that contribute to it, we need to acknowledge that shyness *per se* does not necessarily involve problematic emotion or avoidance of goals important to the shy person. One distinction to be made is that shyness may include social anxiety as an emotional component, but social anxiety does not necessarily lead to shyness behaviorally. Shyness may combine both feeling and behavior, but need not. Shy extraverts do not avoid and shy introverts may be phobic and not socially anxious. The avoidant behavior has already been conditioned to external stimuli and is not triggered by feelings of anxiety.

Although social phobics have been described as more avoidant than the shy, these comparisons were based on samples of normal college students, and the authors pointed to the dearth of empirical studies of shyness treatment samples (Turner, Beidel, & Townsley, 1990). They also reported that SAD was defined by specific criteria while shyness was not. Although shyness is part of common language and described both as an emotional state and trait, specific criteria for chronic problematic shyness were delineated when treatment at the Stanford Shyness Clinic was initiated in 1977. Chronic shyness was defined as "a fear of negative evaluation that was sufficient to inhibit participation in desired activities and that significantly interfered with the pursuit of personal or professional goals" (Henderson, 1992).

Recent research has supported our belief and the early findings of Turner et al. (1990) that shyness is heterogeneous. Interestingly, many people who say they were excessively or extremely shy as children do not meet criteria for any psychiatric disorder as adults. Furthermore, 50% of people with a lifetime history of complex SAD did not view themselves as very shy as young people (Cox, MacPherson, & Enns, 2005). These authors' findings were consistent with those of Heiser, Turner, and Beidel (2003), who found only modest support, at best, for a direct relationship between even extreme childhood shyness and SAD later in life.

We believe that final definitions await descriptions of the emotional states and self-reported traits of those who refer themselves to shyness treatment in comparison with those who refer themselves to SAD treatment, particularly given that a somewhat different pattern of comorbidity was revealed in our shyness clinic sample from the pattern found in SAD treatment samples (St. Lorant, Henderson, & Zimbardo, 2000). We continue to search for qualitative differences between these categories in both normative and clinical samples.

We define chronic shyness almost entirely in terms of the person's self-report, in order to avoid an external performance standard according to which observers assign individuals to diagnostic categories. Research in personality psychology suggests that self-reports are more valid for personality traits than observer ratings, particularly among those who openly report their traits (Lamiell, 1997; St. Lorant et al., 2000). We believe that SAD definitions imply that significant impairment in functioning is comparable across groups. Assessment of impairment is, at best, imperfect among clinical evaluators, particularly across settings and instruments, in spite of suggested guidelines for the global assessment of functioning in the DSM-IV (American Psychiatric Association, 1994). For instance, socioeconomic status and cultural influences often constrain what shy people are able to do. Those who are not performing well in school may be constrained by extraverted teachers who value active and competitive verbal exchanges over written expression and more collaborative verbal interaction with an emphasis on listening skills (Aronson, Blaney, Stephan, Sikes, & Snapp, 1978; Henderson, 2006). Those who appear higher functioning in some settings, by virtue of social class and privilege, may be under-achieving in relation to their peer group (Henderson, Martinez, & Zimbardo, 1999).

In summary, definitions of clinical samples of shy and socially phobic individuals are similar, but show differences as well. The emotional states of both shyness and social anxiety are probably nearly universal in normative samples, and people who are shy, socially anxious, or socially phobic in only one or two situations likely never present to clinicians. Such individuals may construe their distress as an intransigent temperamental factor, or simply a natural part of life. Furthermore, they may not be motivated to change if highly verbal participation or dominant assertive behavior is infrequently required in significant areas of their daily lives. Notably, adding to the literature concerning the heterogeneity of shyness, recent research has revealed a substantial proportion of highly shy people who report no social fears in diagnostic interviews (Heiser, Turner, Beidel, & Roberson-Nay, 2009).

PREVALENCE

Over the past 30 years, estimates of the prevalence of SAD in the general population have increased from 2% to over 12%, with 26% of women and 19% of men reporting they were "very shy" growing up (Cox et al., 2005; Kessler, Chiu, Demler, & Walters, 2005). Estimates of self-reported dispositional shyness have also increased during this time frame, from 40 to 58% (Carducci et al., 2007; Carducci & Zimbardo, 1995; Zimbardo, 1977). Sixty-four percent of those who label themselves as shy said they do not like being shy, and 65% considered it to be a personal problem for them. Among children, 38% of a sample of fifth graders said they were shy (Lazarus, 1982) and 32% of girls and 28% of boys were said to be shy by parents in a sample of 8–10-year-olds in the early studies (Caspi, Glen, Elder, & Bem, 1988). More recent adolescent self-reports include rates as high as 61% (Henderson & Zimbardo, 1993). In cross-cultural comparisons of shyness among 18–21-year-olds in the mid-1970s, the range of shyness prevalence in eight countries varied from a low of about 30% in Israel to a high of nearly 60% in Japan and Taiwan, with Mexico, Germany, India, Newfoundland, and the United States in between these extremes (Zimbardo, 1977). The highest levels of shyness in the US samples were also found among Asian Americans, while Jewish Americans were typically least shy. Remarkably, the current levels of shyness in the United States now approximate those reported earlier in Japan and Taiwan. We are not aware of evidence regarding the current prevalence of shyness in those Asian countries.

CULTURAL INFLUENCES

Cultural factors affect social anxiety and shyness. Culturally based self-definitions mediate social anxiety, and particular self-construals are related to particular types of social anxiety (Zimbardo & Zoppel, 1984). For example, in Japan the focus is on not offending others with one's behavior or appearance, while in the United States the focus is a concern for public scrutiny of oneself, or embarrassment.

Among the Japanese, shyness is promoted by a host of cultural conditions, among them training in emotional control and inhibition of emotional expression, as well as a focus on fine details of social rituals in order to avoid the shame of violating social protocol. *Amae* is a uniquely Japanese construct of passive dependence on and unquestioning loyalty and obedience to authority and superiors. *Amae* is practiced and experienced at every level of Japanese society and is a central determinant of the control of social, political, and personal actions (Zimbardo & Zoppel, 1984).

In Israel, by contrast, the societal focus is on rewarding risk-taking by giving full credit to the actor for succeeding, or for even trying, while attributing blame for failure on external circumstances rather than on dispositional inadequacies.

Such a culturally sanctioned orientation leads to tendencies to take social and intellectual risks since the individual has nothing to lose by trying: You get the credit for a hit; they get the blame for a miss. Not only does this action orientation reduce shyness, it leads to the development of the Yiddish concept of *chutzpa*, a sense of self-sufficiency that helps to propel one's self to initiate actions toward desired goals – regardless of talent, merit, seniority, or traditional constraints on risky actions (Pines & Zimbardo, 1977).

The consequences of shyness are also affected by one's culture. Swedish boys' careers are not negatively affected by shyness as they are in the United States (where shy men enter careers later than the nonshy, while they show no psychopathological problems). However, Swedish girls attain lower levels of education than nonshy girls, in contrast to American girls, who do not differ from their peers (Kerr, Lambert, & Bem, 1996). In both countries shy women assume more traditional roles. A study of shy children in China revealed that shy-inhibited children were more accepted than their peers and more likely to be considered for leadership positions, in contrast to studies of Western children (Xinyin, Rubin, & Boshu, 1995). Teachers also regarded them as more competent. Collectivistic countries in general appear more accepting toward socially reticent and withdrawn behaviors than individualistic countries, but personal norms do not differ and social anxiety and fear of blushing is higher in collectivist cultures, perhaps due to strict social norms (Beidel, Turner, & Dancu, 1985). However, China was not included in the sample, and recent results reveal self-reported shyness as lower in a Sri Lankan sample than in a British sample (Abeysinghe, 2009).

Stockli (2002), in a study of teacher-ratings of shy versus nonshy children, raises the question of whether the negative connotations attributed to shyness in the West disadvantage shy children scholastically. Interestingly, as well, a review of the literature on giftedness in children revealed that the majority of gifted children are introverted and many are quite sensitive due to heightened interpersonal awareness (Henderson, 2006). One wonders to what degree these children are labeled as shy. While no differences have been found in levels of intelligence between the shy and the nonshy, shy children in Switzerland have been found to underestimate their mathematical abilities. Cultural values and belief systems, coupled with societal practices and social norms, influence shy behavior, as well as how such behavior is viewed by others (Zimbardo & Zoppel, 1984).

COMORBIDITY IN A SHYNESS TREATMENT SAMPLE

A high degree of comorbidity in chronic shyness is consistent with comorbidity in SAD studies, according to our recent study of 114 patients between 1991 and 1997 (St. Lorant et al., 2000). Ninety-seven percent of our sample received a diagnosis of GSAD, according to the ADIS, a structured interview with good inter-rater reliability designed specifically to assess anxiety and related disorders (Di Nardo & Barlow, 1988). The most common additional disorders were dysthymia (29%) and GAD (27%).

A striking percentage (94%) received a coexisting personality disorder diagnosis, according to the Millon Clinical Multiaxial Inventory-II (MCMI-II), an instrument designed specifically to assess the criteria for personality disorders as specified in DSM-III-R (American Psychiatric Association, 1987; Millon, 1987). APD was the most frequent (67%), followed by schizoid (35%) and dependent (23%) personality disorders. Less frequently found were obsessive-compulsive (7.3%) and schizotypal (8.5%) personality disorders. The Minnesota Multiphasic Personality Inventory (MMPI), the most frequently researched objective personality assessment tool (Greene, 1991), further suggested compulsive (21%) and passive aggressive personality disorders (15%). In our treatment sample, we appear to have a larger percentage of schizoid personality disorder diagnoses and a lower incidence of PD than many samples of individuals with SAD (St. Lorant et al., 2000). Although method variance (the use of different measures and methods of evaluation) needs to be taken into account, these findings suggest that clients who present to the shyness clinic may have a somewhat different overall profile than clients who present to anxiety disorders clinics.

Alcohol abuse/dependence was suggested in less than 2% of Shyness Clinic clients according to the MMPI, in contrast to some samples of individuals with SAD, where abuse appears to be higher (Schneier, Martin, Liebowitz, Gorman, & Fyer, 1989). Some of our clients use alcohol to reduce social anxiety but tend to restrict intake, and many do not drink. Many clients also report fearing a loss of control if they "drink too much," consistent with earlier studies of shy college students in which shyness was negatively associated with alcohol use, except when positive expectancies existed (Bruch et al., 1992).

DEVELOPMENT OF CHRONIC SHYNESS

A number of factors are seen as instrumental in the development of problematic shyness, including parental and peer rejection, and parental over-protection, leading to a lack of self-efficacy. Specific conditioning events play a role; for example, being teased or shamed by teachers or other children in front of others, performance failures, traumatic events, and emotional or physical abuse or neglect (Zimbardo, 1982). Observational learning may also contribute to shyness; for example, viewing siblings or classmates who are humiliated or harshly treated, and thus imagining similar negative consequences to oneself.

Previous investigations of the relationship of shyness and SAD suggested that the onset of SAD was characterized by negative conditioning experiences while the onset of shyness was not (Turner et al., 1990). This suggestion was challenged by Zimbardo's findings because many negative conditioning experiences were reported by shy individuals on the Stanford Shyness Survey (Zimbardo, 1977). Another important possibility to be considered in light of current research is to what degree the negative stereotyping of shyness in Western countries is leading to the rise in cases of SAD.

Our current theory of the development of shyness is based on the work of previous researchers who studied the associations of private self-consciousness, attribution style, and negative emotional states (see Ingram, 1990 for a review). Because negative affective states draw attention inward, they are likely to lead to the trait of private self-consciousness, which is simply the tendency to focus inward on one's thoughts and emotions. It is frequently associated with seeing the self as responsible for external events.

We have demonstrated that self-blame and shame are exacerbated by private self-consciousness in shy adolescents and young adults (Henderson, 1992; Henderson & Zimbardo, 1993). We argue that children who experience rejection, and negative emotions in response to that rejection, will focus inward more frequently and become more attentive to these painful states. They begin to believe that they cause or contribute disproportionately to the negative or undesirable events occurring around them. This process generates further negative thinking, which in turn contributes to negative emotion in a dynamic, reciprocal downward spiral. Thinking patterns and maladaptive attributions of responsibility may be influenced by whatever emotion is present, whether fear, shyness, shame, or anger. If one is afraid, others look dangerous and the self appears vulnerable. If one is shy, others look attractive, but potentially critical and rejecting. If one does not measure up in one's own eyes and is ashamed, others appear contemptuous and the self abased. If one is angry, other people appear untrustworthy and hurtful. These vicious attribution cycles are likely to develop at relatively young ages, some evidence for which has been provided by Rubin and Krasnor (1986). We also believe that these ruminative cycles lead to negative beliefs about the self, others, and potential social transactions. In line with our theory, Trew and Alden (2009) have recently shown that rumination linked social anxiety to trait anger and also to outward anger expression.

Consistent with our research, social phobics who attribute their condition to genetic or somatic factors have been shown to demonstrate more severe symptomatology before and after cognitive behavioral treatment (Heimberg, Liebowitz, Hope, & Schneier, 1995). Are these findings evidence of the influence of genetic or temperament factors in SAD? Alternatively, as we believe, are they evidence of lower self-efficacy expectations and less motivation for change than if the person believes the cause of their problem has been learned and thus can be unlearned by retraining? In support of this notion, a study of implicit self-theories of shyness revealed that college students who believed that their shyness was biologically based were less likely to engage in new social learning opportunities than those who believed it was learned (Beer, 2002).

Empirical findings call into question the idea that inherent temperament components on the part of the shy inevitably must prevent adequate social behavior or social acceptance. Skilled social behavior by the shy has been demonstrated when their socially based shyness arousal is misattributed to an external source, such as a neutral noise source (Brodt & Zimbardo, 1981). Furthermore, a study of shy and nonshy college students involved in social interaction suggested that the actual experience of the two groups was not different. What differed was the belief on the part of the shy group that their feelings and thoughts were abnormal (Maddux, Norton, & Leary, 1988). Whatever the origins of shyness, social anxiety, and SAD, there appears to be a good deal of room to modify social perception and social behavior, whether early or later in the lifespan.

Areas of Overlap

Somatic symptoms tend to be similar for shy, socially anxious, and socially phobic adults, as are frequent negative cognitions (Leary & Kowalski, 1995; Turner et al., 1990; Zimbardo, 1977). Adolescent shy clients report frequent negative thoughts, including self-blame for negative social outcomes. Interestingly, children with SAD do not report negative cognitions with the same frequency as adults (Beidel & Morris, 1995). However, spontaneous thoughts about self-presentational issues occur in children by age eight, which suggests the presence of negative thoughts in socially anxious children (Banerjee & Yuill, 1998). Whether they are reported may be due to differences in expressive behavior tendencies rather than to differences in the actual frequency of their occurrence.

Deficits or biases in children's social cognition have been suggested as playing a role in social anxiety, and perhaps shyness as well (Crick & Ladd, 1993). We found that socially anxious children had poorer recognition of self-presentational motives and less appreciation of the links between beliefs, intentions, and emotions in faux pas situations, particularly when they were high in negative affect (Banerjee & Henderson, 2001).

Situations that present some form of perceived social difficulty are also similar across the three constructs. Children with SAD say that the most common upsetting event for them is an "unstructured peer encounter" (Beidel & Morris, 1995). This is also among the challenging situations that are most frequently reported retrospectively by Shyness Clinic clients and normative samples of shy adults (Henderson, 1992; Zimbardo, 1977). Specific upsetting events in childhood that have led to or exacerbated social distress are also common to all three phenomena (Heimberg, Dodge, & Becker, 1987; Leary & Kowalski, 1995; Zimbardo, 1977).

Age of Onset

Social anxiety is reported in elementary school (Beidel & Morris, 1995), and shy college students in treatment report a mean age of onset of 10 years for problematic shyness (Henderson et al., 1999). Forty percent of a sample of shy college students reported an onset in early childhood (Bruch, Giordano, & Pearl, 1986). Interestingly, males with an early onset reported the most behavioral problems. Social withdrawal becomes noticeable in early childhood and may or may not be a precursor to later shyness or SAD (Rubin, Coplan, & Bowker, 2008).

SAD usually begins in early to mid adolescence, with an average age of onset of around 16, and generally has a chronic, unremitting course (Turner et al., 1990). The second most frequent onset is elementary school, and it tends to be earlier for generalized than nongeneralized social phobics (Beidel & Morris, 1995).

SAD researchers have understandably reasoned that shyness stars much earlier than SAD, given the results of infant studies in which evidence of "behavioral inhibition" was seen as early as 21 months (Kagan & Reznick, 1986; Kagan & Snidman, 1991; Turner et al., 1990). Kagan has referred to this 10–15% of infants who reveal a variety of signs of inhibition as illustrating a "push from nature" in that negative direction. An equivalent percentage is pushed in the opposite direction toward being "bold," while the majority fall between these extremes. Jonathan Cheek was one of the first researchers to point out that a significant portion of a sample of inhibited infants were not shy at age seven. He also distinguished shyness from BI, in that shyness involves a cognitive concern about evaluation (Cheek & Briggs, 1982). Most researchers agree that shyness is a separate phenomenon and that BI is a precursor to shyness in some children but is demonstrably not so in a significant proportion of them, and nor is it a stable trait.

Adolescent Onset

Adolescence appears to be the age of onset for many kinds of social anxiety, phobic avoidance, and chronic shyness. Perspective-taking ability has been seen as one of the major reasons, in that awareness of discrepancies between the perspectives of others and the view of the self can promote painful negative social comparisons. The accuracy of perspective-taking in relation to the self, however, appears to vary both in shy children and adults (Alden & Wallace, 1991; Rubin & Asendorpf, 1993).

Self-blaming tendencies may lead to misperceptions of others' views of the self (Henderson & Zimbardo, 1993). Increased interpersonal avoidance also limits opportunities for feedback that can counter negative self-perceptions and provide occasions for receiving constructive feedback.

The awareness of a discrepancy between how one sees oneself and how one would ideally like to be seen by others or by the self creates many kinds of discomfort and negative behavior, according to a large body of both clinical and empirical literature (Carver & Scheier, 1986; Henderson & Zimbardo, 1993; Higgins, Klein & Strauman, 1987). These discrepancies may exert considerable influence on the development of chronic shyness and SAD in adolescence.

It will be important to continue to differentiate shyness, social anxiety, and SAD in children and adolescents, because the phenomenology and precursors may differ in systematic ways.

Zimbardo identified two additional primary contributors to the elevation of shyness levels in this adolescent age group. One was a newfound concern about one's attractiveness to the opposite sex. A second contributor appeared to be the onset of sexual desire and sexual thoughts, which adolescents felt had to be concealed and actively suppressed (see Zimbardo & Radl, 1981). Among adolescent girls another factor to consider, which is related to these two, is the dramatic changes in their body shape as they begin to look more sexually mature. In some cases, the men in their lives – fathers, brothers, uncles, and friends – may modify earlier patterns of holding or touching them as they move from being a girl to a woman.

INDIVIDUAL DIFFERENCES IN SHY AND SOCIALLY PHOBIC INDIVIDUALS

Shyness has been conceptualized as more heterogeneous than SAD (Turner et al., 1990). The heterogeneous appearance of shyness may reflect not only the continuum of mild defensive caution to extreme fears and social inhibition, but also the different domains of difficulty found in shyness. Some people report few negative thoughts, but are inhibited and avoidant; others report physiological responses that interfere with cognitive processing; still others report a great deal of worry, but display little overt behavioral difficulty (Pilkonis, 1977). Some report the presence of negative emotions such as shame and resentment, but little physiological arousal (Henderson, 1992). Clinical observation also reveals many socially anxious individuals (SAIs) who attribute their anxiety to more general feelings of insecurity, denying both shyness and phobic tendencies.

More recent research with individuals with SAD, however, has also revealed considerable heterogeneity in levels of social anxiety, social skill, degree of avoidance, and physiological arousal (Beidel & Morris, 1995; Heimberg et al., 1995; Hofmann & Roth, 1996). Heterogeneity in SAD may be related to degree of social anxiety, transient states of shyness versus trait-shyness, and degree of phobic avoidance or BI.

The behavior genetics concept of "niche picking" – that is, selecting the environment most suited to one's traits – may be the factor that separates problematic shyness, social anxiety, and SAD from adaptive shyness, transient social anxiety, and transient social avoidance (Rowe, 1997; Scarr & McCartney, 1983; Xinyin et al., 1995). Communal and collaborative environments, rather than highly competitive or authoritarian environments, which place a strong value on personal dominance, may provide more and better opportunities for the contributions of the shy.

Subgroups

These observations have led to several attempts to define subgroups. For example, Buss classified fearful shy individuals versus self-conscious shys (Buss, 1986). In the former group, fear of novelty and autonomic reactivity is hypothesized to be the major component; in the latter group, it is excessive awareness of public aspects of one's self. Pilkonis (1977) distinguished the privately shy from the publicly shy using cluster analysis. The privately shy were socially skilled but self-doubting and uncomfortable; the publicly shy were more visibly uncomfortable and less skilled.

Zimbardo (1977) divided shy individuals into two groups, shy introverts and shy extraverts. Shy introverts often preferred to be alone, liking ideas and inanimate objects. They were less socially skilled than shy extraverts, were reluctant to approach others, and dated infrequently. Turner and colleagues (1990) speculated that this group in the extreme resembled schizoid personality disorder and indeed this diagnostic group may comprise a proportion of our clinic sample. These individuals do, however, report desiring at least some connection with others.

The second group Zimbardo (1977) identified was socially skilled, but suffered internally. They were constrained by social expectations and concerned about social rules. Turner et al. (1990) speculated that these were the most likely candidates for SAD, being both sociable and shy. Shy extraverts appeared to function best in highly structured situations where everyone knew and played their roles as expected. Many talk show hosts, standup comedians, and professors in large lecture courses rather than seminars report being shy.

CHARACTERISTICS OF SHY AND SOCIALLY PHOBIC INDIVIDUALS

Somatic Symptoms

Heart palpitations, shakiness, blushing, muscle twitching, sweating, and urinary urgency are reported by social phobics and are also common physiological responses in shy and socially anxious college students and in our clinic patients (Beidel, Turner, & Dancu, 1985; Henderson, 1992; Zimbardo, 1977). However, there are fewer reports of nausea and chills among adult social phobics than for socially phobic children (Beidel, Christ, & Long, 1991). Shyness clinic clients also infrequently report these symptoms. Parental ratings of shyness and higher heart rates in a stressful task have been modestly correlated in children. There are, however, some contradictory findings. When heart rate was continuously monitored, by a portable microcomputer, there was no association between shyness and heart rate reactivity (Asendorpf & Meier, 1993).

Reports of higher cardiac rates also vary across studies of adults with SAD, with increased heart rates shown in socially challenging situations in some studies, but not others. Interestingly, individuals with SAD limited to one specific domain demonstrate the highest cardiac rates (Levin et al., 1993; Turner, Beidel, & Larkin, 1986). Pilkonis's description of the privately shy mentioned previously – i.e., those who reported more internal discomfort but less behavioral difficulty – may be similar to this specific SAD group (Pilkonis, 1977). No differences between individuals with SAD versus shy and nonshy individuals were shown on physiological measures in other studies, although individuals who were shy or diagnosed with SAD perceived more arousal (Edelmann & Baker, 2002; Heiser, et al., 2009). Socially anxious college students showed the same pattern during a public speaking task (Mauss, Wilhelm, & Gross, 2004). In our clinic sample, cardiac rates have not been measured directly, but most of our clients report high subjective anxiety ratings when engaging in simulations of feared social situations.

The exception is a small group of clients who report little somatic distress and low subjective anxiety ratings during simulated exposures. These clients tend to be behaviorally passive in interaction and often initiate little social contact outside the context of the group. We wonder whether these individuals resemble the adult version of passive isolation in familiar situations (Rubin & Asendorpf, 1993). This pattern may be related to the reciprocal effect of biological differences interacting with growing psychological inhibition in the face of rejection and negative experiences.

Cognitive Features and Perception

The cognitive components of shyness, social anxiety, and SAD have been the subject of considerable interest over the past 30 years. Early clinical observation and empirical studies revealed a plethora of findings regarding the tendencies to (1) worry; (2) regard normal experiences of shyness as shameful and unacceptable; (3) be preoccupied to the point of interference with performance and empathic behavior; (4) appraise interpersonal situations in threatening ways; and (5) make maladaptive attributions for social behavior (Beidel et al., 1985; Carducci & Zimbardo, 1995; Cheek & Briggs, 1982; Zimbardo, 1977). Our clients demonstrate a double standard in that they do not judge others, including other group members, for responses such as blushing, for which they expect negative judgment for their reactions. Recent research has also revealed a double standard wherein socially anxious women expect to be judged for acknowledging anxiety more than others would be judged, while simultaneously understanding the likelihood of negative social outcomes for hiding anxiety, which emotion-suppression research confirms (Voncken, Alden, & Bogels, 2006).

Self-blaming attributions are common in our shyness clinic clients, as are entrenched negative beliefs about the self. There are also frequent negative thoughts and beliefs about others. We have developed a new scale called the Estimations of Others Scale (EOS) to assess these negative thoughts and beliefs (Henderson & Horowitz, 1998). The scale has high internal reliability (0.91 alpha) in a college student sample. Shy students score significantly higher on this scale than the nonshy and clinic clients score significantly higher than the students.

Our research on perceptions of facial expressions of emotions has revealed that shy college students and Asian American students are slower to recognize disgusted facial expressions than the nonshy, being *less*, not more, sensitive to social threat emotions, as we had originally predicted. Asian Americans were slower to recognize facial expressions of anger than the nonshy, and the shy group did not differ from Asian Americans or the nonshy. Groups did not differ in sensitivity to fear, surprise, or sadness, and the shy and the Asian Americans were slower to recognize happiness. Earlier research had shown that shy and Asian Americans tend to value harmony and are higher in interdependent self-construals. In addition, they have a more reflective intellectual style that may make them less willing to acknowledge social threat emotions until they are obvious and the context is considered, particularly if they are not directed at them. We also suggest that less sensitivity to happiness expressions may be related to valuing pleasant versus high-intensity positive emotion (Henderson, Kurita, & Zimbardo, 2006).

Affective Features

Compared to normative samples, shy clients report considerably higher levels of social anxiety, shame, guilt, depression, and resentment, with higher levels of shame and anger predicting passive aggression (Henderson & Zimbardo, 1998). However, embarrassment is correlated with shyness in normative samples (Crozier & Russell, 1992). In contrast, one-third of an extremely shy group without SAD reported no social fears during a diagnostic interview (Heiser et al., 2009). Social anxiety, depression-related emotions, and embarrassment are frequently reported in the SAD treatment literature (Turner et al., 1990). The study of negative emotionality in socially anxious children is a growing area of research (Banerjee & Henderson, 2001).

Behavior

Behaviors associated with chronic shyness are similar to those associated with social anxiety and GSAD; that is, shy people speak less in social settings, less often initiate new topics of conversation, avert their gazes, exhibit nervous mannerisms, and show fewer facial expressions (Leary & Kowalski, 1995; Turner et al., 1990; Zimbardo, 1977). Shy behaviors are usually described by shy individuals and observers alike as reticent, quiet, awkward, or overactive (Cheek & Busch, 1981; Zimbardo, 1982). Shy college students are less visible and less assertive in the workplace, and are less likely to use career-planning resources (Cheek & Busch, 1981). They display less verbal fluency and fewer leadership skills. They also show less verbal creativity when faced with evaluation (Cheek & Stahl, 1986), but are equally creative when not under evaluative threat.

Conversations between the shy are dominated by talk about the immediate physical/social setting rather than about themselves, and leave ambiguous who is to speak next (Manning & Ray, 1993). The exception to this is "favored" topics, which are discussed extensively. Although most strangers seek "common ground" topics when starting conversations, it may become a dominant strategy for the shy because it offsets the painful silence when neither party talks. Shy individuals are less self-disclosing, even to the point of telling physicians and psychologists too little about problem areas to obtain adequate help (Zimbardo & Piccione, 1985). Genuine self-disclosure may also involve the risk of communicating negative thoughts and feelings about the self, which increases inhibition (Henderson, 1992).

When we consider nonverbal behavior, shy people keep others at a greater physical distance than those who are less shy (about 12 inches further away). The difference is greater with an opposite-sex stranger than with a same-sex stranger, and when a stranger is coming toward them than when they are moving toward the stranger (Carducci & Webber, 1979; Zimbardo, 1977). They maintain minimal eye contact and little smiling, and have a closed, "defensive" posture, low speaking voice, and constrained bodily movements, with minimal hand and arm gesturing (Zimbardo, 1977).

However, a recent study of socially anxious college students conducted by Alden and Bieling (1998) revealed that negative behaviors can be readily changed when negative appraisals of social situations are altered by an experimental manipulation. When told that their personality profiles were similar to those of their conversational partners, indicating that they would easily relate well to each other, anxious individuals were indistinguishable from nonanxious individuals in likeableness, appropriateness, and similarity.

Moreover, clinical observation has suggested that, when shy clients are not self-focused, their behavior is indistinguishable from nonshys and is often highly skilled. These observations lend at least clinical credence to the idea that behavioral deficits may disappear when critical self-consciousness is reduced and shy clients are focused on a cooperative task with others.

Family Characteristics

Parenting characteristics that may promote shyness are controlling, insensitive, or overprotective styles that involve frequent correction and shaming (Bruch, 1989). The important issue is when and how much parents should encourage or refuse to protect inhibited children so that they receive adequate socialization experiences. Individuals with SAD who report parental overprotection are less responsive to the behavior of a conversation partner, and their failure to respond to friendly overtures leads to rejection (Alden & Taylor, 2006). Many patients report minimal social interaction with peers and a lack of family support for such interaction. Some also report little interaction with family friends or relatives. Because extended family socializing predicts less shyness in young adults (Bruch, 1989), parental sociability in itself appears conducive to preventing shyness in children. Engfer (1993) found that parents of shy children were less sensitive to children's expressed needs and more prone to use strongly assertive strategies.

The self-critical tendencies of shy adults may be the result of restrictiveness and rejection by parents because these parental behaviors have been shown to be related to the development of self-criticism in adolescents more generally, particularly when received from the same-sex parent (Koestner, Zuroff, & Powers, 1991). Self-criticism remains stable into young adulthood for women, but not for men. However, men exhibit a relationship between self-criticism and inhibited aggressive impulses.

TREATMENT

Treatments for shyness, social anxiety, and SAD generally include cognitive restructuring, social skills training, and role-plays of threatening situations. A meta-analysis of SAD treatment suggested that both cognitive and behavior therapy treatments were effective for SAD, and some researchers suggest that exposure appears to be the most powerful mechanism for producing ameliorative change (Feske & Chambless, 1995; Turner & Beidel, 1992). Two studies of social anxiety treatment concluded that treatment is useful and that response to treatment is not significantly differentiated by approach or modality (DiGiuseppe, McGowan, Simon, & Gardner, 1990; Leary & Kowalski, 1995). A recent treatment update revealed no differences between exposures only and exposures with cognitive restructuring. Type of treatment, mode of delivery, number of hours, or length of treatment so far do not appear to effect outcome (Jorstad-Stein & Heimberg, 2009). However, one carefully controlled study demonstrated that exposures with cognitive restructuring were superior to exposures without cognitive restructuring for severe SAD (Mattick, Peters, & Clarke, 1989).

An important treatment consideration involves assessing the degree to which shyness or SAD is a consequence of inadequate social skills, or symptomatology related to other disorders. Skill deficiencies need to be differentiated from inhibition or anxious behavior and addressed in treatment. We agree with Caballo and Turner (1994), for example, who indicated that physical self-care may need to be addressed, particularly among those who fear dating. In contrast, high-functioning individuals with Asperger's syndrome will exhibit shy behavior but primarily need very concrete social skills training.

Butler and Wells (1995) noted that social phobics in treatment enter feared situations but disengage using subtle strategies such as avoiding eye contact. Some clients achieve more effective desensitization when simply asked to "stay in the moment" during conversation role-plays (Henderson, 2007). Wallace and Alden (1997) suggest that self-protective motivation accounts for continued avoidance of feared situations in spite of successful exposures.

Cognitive restructuring may fail to demonstrate impressive response rates in many studies because treatment may often neglect negative attributions and beliefs about the self and others that accompany severe shyness and SAD (Henderson, 2002). We believe that the frequent relapse seen in studies of SAD is at least partially due to inadequately addressed maladaptive attribution styles and negative beliefs. Consequently, since the early 1990s we have included a specific focus in our treatment on negative attributions and negative beliefs about the self and others. We also focus on the negative emotions that these attributions and beliefs engender: shame if the beliefs are about the self, and resentment and hurt if they are about others. Therapists also help clients link thoughts and emotions to early experiences in order to help clients develop insight into their anxiety and motives for interpersonal avoidance.

Addressing Attribution Style in Treatment and Assessing Results

We addressed self-blame and shame in social fitness training, as well as how the presence of private self-awareness exacerbates painful emotion and unsupportive thinking. We developed specific challenges to negative attributions and beliefs about the self and applied such challenges concomitantly with the usual cognitive restructuring techniques during exposures to feared situations, and have gathered data regarding the results of attribution retraining.

Pre- and post-testing of shyness clinic clients in 26-week groups has revealed that internal, global, stable, and self-blaming attributions in clients' three most challenging situations were significantly and substantially reduced in treatment, as was shame. Interestingly, shy students who were in an eight-week treatment at Stanford, who were also higher in general fearfulness according to the fear scale of Buss and Plomin's EAS Temperament Survey for Adults (Buss & Plomin, 1984), were the most self-blaming at pre-test. These results are sufficiently interesting to warrant more extensive investigation in relation to subgroups of shy clients.

A telephone follow-up study of clients treated between 1994 and 1999 also revealed that, on average, they were maintaining treatment gains in the form of reduced distress and avoidance, but with considerable variability. It is that variability that motivates our efforts to identify subgroups and to develop more specific treatment strategies for particular individuals, as well as new methods for enhancing treatment generalizability.

Naturalistic investigations of Shyness Clinic samples have also revealed that a coping style that is primarily internalizing predicts better outcomes in social fitness training. In addition, a flexible coping style – that is, being able to use both internalizing and externalizing coping strategies flexibly – is an additive predictor in reducing shyness as measured by our clinically sensitive shyness questionnaire, the ShyQ (Clinton, 2009; Henderson & Zimbardo, 2002; Kimpara, Henderson, & Beutler, 2008).

We also think that the approach of Beutler (2009) is better for assessing treatment outcome than relying solely on the results of randomized control treatment comparisons of different structured treatments. Beutler found few differences in benefits to patients after reviewing meta-analytic studies and a large mega-analysis comparing ESTs and treatment as usual conditions (TAUs). Effect sizes associated with comparisons between and among structured treatments also approximated zero (Beutler, 2009). He argues, therefore, that not all research questions are effectively addressed with randomized controlled trial designs, and has demonstrated that several patient moderating variables increase the power of treatments to produce benefits. Thus, social fitness training was found to produce a strong effect size ($d = 0.85$) among internalizing patients. Beutler integrates multiple research and statistical methods to study variables that include not only treatment variables but also client and therapist variables, the treatment alliance, and treatment compatibility.

Shyness Clinic Treatment

The Shyness Clinic has been a freestanding fee-for-service organization that functioned on a private practice model until recently, when the clinic was moved to the Pacific Graduate School of Psychology in CA, renamed Palo Alto University in 2009. This move has enabled us to train graduate students as well as postgraduates and practicing psychologists. Students also have access to our clinic database for research studies. Research findings from personality theory, social psychology, and clinical psychology are used to inform the techniques we use with clients. Although the major therapeutic work is done in small groups, prior to group assignment there is an initial evaluation of three to seven individual sessions depending on the degree of comorbidity.

Groups are mixed-gender and include six to eight participants, who meet weekly for two hours over 26 sessions. The first 13 weeks consist primarily of simulated exposures to feared situations, and include reports of behavioral homework and goal-setting for the following week. Clients also conduct homework assignments together, in pairs or small groups, such as telephoning each other, challenging each other's negative thoughts, and attending events together. In-group exposures involve other clients, research assistants, and volunteers who play the roles of conversational partners, employers, dating partners, and others. Group members and confederates provide feedback in the form of indicating which specific behaviors could be changed or eliminated in order to make them feel more comfortable. Specific skills for providing and receiving helpful versus nonhelpful feedback are taught throughout this period. Another strong emphasis of the educative component is that the quality of social interactions are negotiated and relative: the goal is for clients to learn to see themselves as one of the definers and initiators of social interactions, rather than attempting to follow perceived performance "rules" that "everyone else knows" and will be imposed upon them.

The second 13 weeks is directed toward specific skill training to address the areas of difficulty experienced by extremely shy clients. Self-disclosure, listening skills, expressing feelings verbally and nonverbally, trust-building, handling criticism, negotiation, anger management, and assertiveness training are among the topics included. Clients role-play various situations in small groups in order to practice these skills with treatment "partners" with whom they are becoming more intimate. This serves as a model for deepening friendships and developing intimacy as well as navigating relationships in particular contexts, such as on the job, meeting new people, and dating. Videotaping is provided for some group exercises and interactions, if clients are open to it. As clients self-disclose earlier experiences that led to their shyness to group members, therapists help clients link these experiences to current fear and avoidance.

In addition to the focus on behavioral skill training, we try to create a safe place: a large "sandbox" where clients can experiment, practice, and play. Playing includes nonverbal exercises taken from theater improvisation and sensitivity-training groups in order for clients to learn to "live in their bodies," creating a greater sense of physical and emotional freedom. Attention is given to how clients hold themselves and to their posture and walk, in order to help them understand what they are communicating nonverbally to others and to themselves, and to facilitate the making of deliberate choices regarding their nonverbal communication.

Shy clients tend to be over-ideational; they ruminate at great length about their performance in social situations, which not only perpetuates painful emotional states but also interferes with taking action. These exercises help them to trust themselves more at a "gut" level. We also help them to experiment with deliberately altering attentional focus. They practice interactions in which they are focused on paying attention to how they are doing in the conversation. They practice focusing on internal states and they practice focusing on the other person by looking for interesting things about the other and areas they have in common. These exercises afford clients the opportunity to experience for themselves what is most pleasurable about social interactions and to discuss the differences in these experiences. Learning how to give and how to receive compliments is also a vital skill we promote in sessions. For example, the response to a compliment is a simple "Thanks," as soon after it is received. It can be reciprocated by adding some phrase such as, "Coming from you, that makes me feel good, because you dress so well; write so well; have such a good sense of …"

The exposures and skill-building components of the group are based on social cognitive theory, which stresses both the development of competency and cognitive-emotional self-regulation (Bandura, 1997). Rules and strategies guide action though observational learning, exploration, instruction, and original cognitive syntheses of information, and skill execution varies with changing situations and purposes (p. 34). While reinforcement, nonreward, and modeling have been demonstrated to lead to the learning of social norms and behavior (Bandura, 2008), social cognitive theory presupposes a more complex and reciprocal causality among people and between people and the environment. Perceived self-efficacy is pivotal because it influences motivation and choice of activities. Self-efficacy plays an essential role in behavioral persistence in the face of challenging social tasks. If clients can increase their sense of personal self-efficacy in the form of taking responsibility for their behavior, but not for social outcomes over which they have no control, they are more likely to maintain the cognitive, emotional, and behavioral gains that accrue in treatment.

Interpersonal process theory provides an additional theoretical framework during the second 13 weeks (Leary, 1957). Harry Stack Sullivan (1953) suggested that peer relationships were the foundation of respect, interpersonal sensitivity, and cooperation. He emphasized special close relationships in particular as places where mutuality and reciprocity develop. We also use interpersonal motives theory to inform therapists' responses to clients' bids to be led or dominated (Horowitz et al., 2006). Therapists take care to gently counter bids to be led or dominated with egalitarian behavior and invitations to collaborate and lead in learning together.

Because extremely shy adults are often withdrawing by adolescence, providing a place to experiment socially in the safety of the group is likely to enable clients to utilize their own cognitive and emotional resources more effectively. They also have the opportunity to experience some emotional security through the process of interaction in the group, helping to provide a model of mutuality and reciprocity on which they can continue to build. Clients use the model to guide their practice in current homework exercises, and can continue to use it in future nontherapeutic settings and relationships. We are also working to develop a more systematic focus on mindfulness and compassion, based on the current research and clinical work of Paul Gilbert (2009).

SOCIAL FITNESS MODEL

We have chosen social fitness as our model of helping people deal with shyness, social anxiety, and SAD because it best fits our goal to transfer research and theory from social and personality psychology into behavioral, cognitive, and emotional regulation strategies that help individuals to thrive in social interaction. As individuals learn about the strategies and the theory behind them, practice new behaviors that are informed by them, and then practice those behaviors in their own lives outside the clinic, we believe they will become increasingly "socially fit." Perhaps more importantly, they will, in a sense, become practicing social researchers in terms not only of developing an understanding of their own social fitness, as we have understood it, but also to contributing further to theory and new practices themselves. Continuing homework exercises contribute to the generalizability of treatment effects, such as meeting with other graduates for coffee and goal setting, telephoning/texting/twittering each other, or meeting for support and consultation.

The concept of social fitness provides an umbrella term within an evolutionary framework that is continuous and dynamic, including many levels of social competence and incompetence, social comfort, and discomfort. Nevertheless, it contains categories that are phenomenologically discrete, such as personality types. Moreover, finding one's social "sport" or niche may involve matching discrete differences in personality to situations in which these characteristics are seen as strengths. We have noted previously that shyness, social anxiety, and SAD appear to be, at least to a certain extent, discrete. They are phenomenologically different from each other, according to the differing self-reports of people who endorse one, but not the others, as appropriate to their self-construals. It is also apparent that there is considerable variability in stimulus situations that trigger these reactions, as well as the nature and features of the reactions.

Using our physical fitness analogy as an example, both a long-distance runner and a tennis player may be highly coordinated and athletic along a continuum of genetic capabilities and a state of physical fitness earned through considerable effort, disciplined practice, and persistence. However, a tennis player is not a long-distance runner, and the two sports require some differing capabilities, different types of conditioning and practice, and perhaps temperamental differences. Furthermore, there are many ways in which to be physically fit and to enjoy one's own physical health and well-being – by jogging, hiking, surfing, playing soccer, volleyball, or football. Analogously, social fitness implies some measure of learned skill and a belief that one is "fit" enough to slip and fall, lose a surfboard, miss a goal, bungle a shot, make an error, or even be tackled with someone's full weight, and not only recover but learn from the experience, trusting that one can still play, individually and on the team.

Whether socially anxious, shy, or phobic regarding social situations, people can achieve some measure of social fitness and social success, both by "working out" and by choosing activities and situations to pursue that are suited to their individual temperaments. They can also understand that "temperament" is sometimes a word for well-ingrained habit patterns developed adaptively in situations that were traumatic or nonrewarding but that no longer serve a useful purpose. As behavior change in social fitness training occurs, along with new emotions and revised emotional and cognitive understandings, new "temperament" variables may appear.

In working with shyness groups over the years, LH has been sufficiently impressed with certain personality traits, such as ethical and caring behavior toward others, that incoming group members already possess that she has undertaken an interview study of "shy leaders." People are interviewed who are known to be outstanding leaders, either locally or in larger contexts, and who report that they are shy. Interviews are also conducted with at least one associate. Using independent ratings of transcribed interviews by the author and two researchers according to personality questionnaires, we are attempting to delineate the particular strengths of shy leaders. Pilot results suggest they tend to lead from behind and let others take the spotlight, are careful observers of people, are attentive listeners, are empathic, and feel strongly about their values in relation to their work. They are motivated, strategic, genuine, and somewhat androgynous (showing both masculine and feminine traits). They are also determinedly persevering, overpreparing for public speaking tasks and pushing past shyness to get the job done. They may be more likely than others to be recruited into leadership roles, rather than to seek them, and some report cultivating certain kinds of self-assertion.

Consistent with our observations, Kurtz and Tiegreen (2005) have shown that the "big five" personality variables of agreeableness and openness to experience as measured by the revised Neuroticism–Extroversion–Openness Personality Inventory (NEO-PI-R) are significantly correlated with ego development. Interestingly, the facet scale scores that were most predictive of ego development were aesthetics and modesty. Both are qualities we see consistently in our shyness clients, and qualities that are associated with shyness in the research literature (Ziller & Rorer, 1985). Shy leaders who are effective in achieving their goals and those of their association, while also modest, may allow others to share credit for success and thus build better team morale.

In conclusion, we believe that the pursuit of social fitness is an idealized quest in support of the overall health of individuals, cultures, and the planet as a whole. We know that social support networks are the best prophylactics against the negative effects on the body, mind, and spirit associated with social isolation. Social fitness should contribute to increasing the vitality of these networks. Personal social fitness in a healthy social ecology is essential for enhancing meaningful social support and, thereby, strengthening the bonds of the human connection.

REFERENCES

Abeysinghe, N. (2009). Shyness: A cross-cultural study. Unpublished MSc, University of Worcester, UK.

Alden, L. E., & Bieling, P. J. (1998). Interpersonal consequences of the pursuit of safety. *Behaviour Research and Therapy*, *36*, 53–64.

Alden, L. E., & Taylor, C. T. (2006). Parental overprotection and interpersonal behavior in generalized social phobia. *Behavior Therapy*, *37*, 14–24.

Alden, L. E., & Wallace, S. T. (1991). Social standards and social withdrawal. *Cognitive Therapy and Research*, *15*, 85–100.

American Psychiatric Association. (1987). *Diagnostic and statistical manual of mental disorders* (3rd ed., rev.) (DSM-III-R). Washington, DC: Author.

American Psychiatric Association. (1994). *Diagnostic and statistical manual of mental disorders* (4th ed.) (DSM-IV). Washington, DC: Author.

Aronson, E., Blaney, N., Stephan, C., Sikes, J., & Snapp, M. (1978). *The jigsaw classroom.* Beverly Hills, CA: Sage.

Asendorpf, J. B., & Meier, G. H. (1993). Personality effects on children's speech in everyday life: Sociability-mediated exposure and shyness-mediated reactivity to social situations. *Journal of Personality and Social Psychology*, *64*, 1072–1083.

Bandura, A. (1997). *Self-efficacy, the exercise of control.* New York: W. H. Freeman.

Bandura, A. (2008). Toward an agentic theory of the self. In H. Marsh, R. G. Craven, & D. M. McInerney, (Eds.), *Self-processes, learning, and enabling human potential: Dynamic new approaches: Vol. 2* (pp. 15–49). Charlotte, NC: Information Age Publishing.

Banerjee, R., & Henderson, L. (2001). Social-cognitive factors in childhood social anxiety: A preliminary investigation. *Social Development*, *10*, 558–572.

Banerjee, R., & Yuill, N. (1998). Children's explanations for self-presentational behavior. *European Journal of Social Psychology*, *29*, 105–111.

Beer, J. S. (2002). Implicit self-theories of shyness. *Journal of Personality and Social Psychology*, *80*, 1009–1024.

Beidel, D. C., Christ, M. A. G., & Long, P. J. (1991). Somatic complaints in anxious children. *Journal of Abnormal Child Psychology*, *19*, 659–670.

Beidel, D. C., & Morris, T. L. (1995). Social phobia. In J. S. March (Ed.), *Anxiety disorders in children and adolescents* (pp. 181–211). New York: Guilford Press.

Beidel, D. C., Turner, S. M., & Dancu, C. V. (1985). Physiological, cognitive and behavioral aspects of social anxiety. *Behavioral Research and Therapy*, *23*, 109–117.

Beutler, L. E. (2009). Making science matter in clinical practice: Redefining psychotherapy. *Clinical Psychology: Science and Practice*, *16*, 301–317.

Brodt, S. E., & Zimbardo, P. G. (1981). Modifying shyness-related social behavior through symptom misattribution. *Journal of Personality and Social Psychology*, *41*, 437–449.

Bruch, M. A. (1989). Familial and developmental antecedents of social phobia: Issues and findings. *Clinical Psychology Review*, *9*, 37–47.

Bruch, M. A., Giordano, S., & Pearl, L. (1986). Differences between fearful and self-conscious shy subtypes in background and current adjustment. *Journal of Research in Personality*. *20*, 172–186.

Bruch, M. A., Heimberg, R. G., Harvey, C., McCann, M., Mahone, M., & Slavkin, S. L. (1992). Shyness, alcohol expectancies, and alcohol use: Discovery of a suppressor effect. *Journal of Research in Personality*, *26*, 137–149.

Buss, A. H. (1986). Two kinds of shyness. In R. Schwarzer (Ed.), *Self-related cognition in anxiety and motivation* (pp. 65–75). Hillsdale, NJ: Erlbaum.

Buss, A. H., & Plomin, R. (1984). *Temperament: Early developing personality traits.* Hillsdale, NJ: Erlbaum.

Butler, G., & Wells, A. (1995). Cognitive-behavioral treatments: Clinical applications. In R. Heimberg, M. Liebowitz, D. Hope, & F. Schneier (Eds.), *Social phobia: Diagnosis, assessment and treatment* (pp. 310–333). New York: Guilford Press.

Caballo, V. E., & Turner, R. M. (1994). *Behavioral, cognitive and emotional differences between social phobic and non-phobic people.* Paper presented at the AABT 28th Annual Convention, San Diego, CA.

Carducci, B. J., Stubbins, Q. A., & Bryant, M. R. (2007). Still shy after all these (30) years, Poster presented at the American Psychological Association, 115th National Conference, Boston, MA.

Carducci, B. J., & Webber, A. W. (1979). Shyness as a determinant of interpersonal distance. *Psychological Reports*, *44*, 1075–1078.

Carducci, B. J., & Zimbardo, P. G. (1995). Are you shy? *Psychology Today*, 34–40, 64, 66, 68.

Carver, C. S., & Scheier, M. F. (1986). Analyzing shyness: A specific application of broader self-regulatory principles. In W. H. Jones, J. M. Cheek, & S. R. Briggs (Eds.), *Shyness: Perspectives on research and treatment* (pp. 173–185). New York: Plenum Press.

Caspi, A., Glen, H., Elder, J., & Bem, D. J. (1988). Moving away from the world: Life-course patterns of shy children. *Developmental Psychology*, *24*, 824–831.

Cheek, J. M., & Briggs, S. R. (1982). Self-consciousness and aspects of identity. *Journal of Research in Personality*, *16*, 401–408.

Cheek, J. M., & Busch, C. M. (1981). The influence of shyness on loneliness in a new situation. *Personality and Social Psychology Bulletin*, *7*, 572–577.

Cheek, J. M., & Stahl, S. S. (1986). Shyness and verbal creativity. *Journal of Research in Personality*, *20*, 51–61.

Clinton, D. (2009). *An Archival Study Examining the Effects and Interactions of Coping and Attributional Styles upon Treatment with a Chronically Shy Population*. Pacific Graduate School of Psychology.

Cox, B. J., MacPherson, P. S. R., & Enns, M. W. (2005). Psychiatric correlates of childhood shyness in a nationally representative sample. *Behaviour Research and Therapy*, *43*, 1019–1027.

Crick, N. R., & Ladd, G. W. (1993). Children's perceptions of their peer experience: Attributions, loneliness, social anxiety, and social avoidance. *Developmental Psychology*, *29*(2), 244–254.

Crozier, W. R., & Russell, D. (1992). Blushing, embarrassability and self-consciousness. *British Journal of Social Psychology*, *31*(4), 343–349.

Davies, P. G., Spencer, S. J., & Steele, C. M. (2005). Clearing the air: Identity safety moderates the effects of stereotype threat on women's leadership aspirations. *Journal of Personality and Social Psychology*, *88*, 276–287.

DiGiuseppe, R., McGowan, L., Simon, K., & Gardner, F. (1990). A comparative outcome study of four cognitive therapies in the treatment of social anxiety. *Journal of Rational-Emotive and Cognitive-Behavior Therapy*, *8*, 129–146.

Di Nardo, P. A., & Barlow, D. H. (1988). *Anxiety Disorders Interview Schedule-Revised (ADIS-R)*. Albany, NY: Phobia and Anxiety Disorders Clinic, State University of New York.

Eagly, A. H., & Karau, S. J. (2002). Role congruity theory of prejudice toward female leaders. *Psychological Review*, *109*, 573–598.

Edelmann, R. J., & Baker, S. R. (2002). Self-reported and actual physiological responses in social phobia. *British Journal of Clinical Psychology*, *41*, 1–14.

Engfer, A. (1993). Antecedents and consequences of shyness in boys and girls: A 6-year longitudinal study. In K. H. Rubin & J. B. Asendorpf (Eds.), *Social withdrawal, inhibition and shyness in childhood* (pp. 49–79). Hillsdale, NJ: Erlbaum.

Feske, U., & Chambless, D. L. (1995). Cognitive behavioral versus exposure only treatment for social phobia: A meta analysis. *Behavior Therapy*, *26*, 695–720.

Gilbert, P. (2009). *The compassionate mind*. London: Constable.

Greene, R. L. (1991). *MMPI-2/MMPI: An Interpretive Manual*. Needham Heights, MA: Allyn & Bacon.

Heimberg, R. G., Dodge, C. S., & Becker, R. E. (Eds.), (1987). *Social phobia*. New York: Guilford Press.

Heimberg, R. G., Liebowitz, M., Hope, D., & Schneier, F. (Eds.), (1995). *Social phobia: Diagnosis, assessment and treatment*. New York: Guilford Press.

Heiser, N. A., Turner, S. M., & Beidel, D. C. (2003). Syness: Relationship to social phobia and other psychiatric disorders. *Behaviour Research and Therapy*, *41*, 209–221.

Heiser, N. A., Turner, S. M., Beidel, D. C., & Roberson-Nay, R. (2009). Differentiating social phobia from shyness. *Journal of Anxiety Disorders*, *23*, 469–476.

Henderson, L. (1992). Shyness groups. In M. McKay & K. Paleg (Eds.), *Focal group psychotherapy*. Oakland, CA: New Harbinger Press.

Henderson, L. (2002). Fearfulness predicts self-blame and shame in shyness. *Personality and Individual Differences*, *32*, 79–93.

Henderson, L. (2006). Gifted and shy. *Duke Gifted Letter*, *6*, 5, 10.

Henderson, L. (2007). *Social Fitness Training: A cognitive behavioral protocol for the treatment of shyness and social anxiety disorder*. Palo Alto, CA: Shyness Institute.

Henderson, L., & Horowitz, L. M. (1998). The Estimations of Others Scale (EOS). Palo Alto, CA: Shyness Institute.

Henderson, L., Kurita, K., & Zimbardo, P. (2006). Shyness and communal vs. individualistic orientations: Sensitivity to emotion, Poster presented at the Association for Cognitive and Behavioral Therapies. Chicago, IL.

Henderson, L., Martinez, A., & Zimbardo, P. (1999). Social fitness training with attribution and self-concept restructuring; preliminary data with a college student population. Unpublished manuscript, Department of Psychology, Stanford University, www.shyness.com.

Henderson, L., & Zimbardo, P. (1993). *Self-blame attributions in shys vs. non-shys in a high-school sample*. Paper presented at the annual conference of the Anxiety Disorders Association of America, Charleston, SC.

Henderson, L., & Zimbardo, P. (1998). *Trouble in river city: Shame and anger in chronic shyness*. Paper presented at the American Psychological Association, 106th National Conference, San Francisco, CA.

Henderson, L., & Zimbardo, P. (2002). *Dimensions of shyness: The ShyQ*. Paper presented at the 82nd Annual Convention of the Western Psychological Association, Irvine, CA.

Higgins, E. T., Klein, R. L., & Strauman, T. J. (1987). Self-discrepancies: Distinguishing among self-states, self-state conflicts, and emotional vulnerabilities. In K. Yardley & T. Honess (Eds.), *Self and Identity: Psychosocial Perspectives* (pp. 173–186). New York: John Wiley & Sons Ltd.

Hofmann, S. G., & Roth, W. T. (1996). Issues related to social anxiety among controls in social phobia research. *Behavior Therapy*, *27*, 79–91.

Horowitz, L., Wilson, K., Turan, B., Zolotsev, P., Constantino, M., & Henderson, L. (2006). How interpersonal motives help clarify the meaning of an interpersonal behavior: A revised circumplex model. *Personality and Social Psychology Review*, *10*, 67–86.

Ingram, R. E. (1990). Self-focused attention in clinical disorders: Review and a conceptual model. *Psychological Bulletin*, *107*(2), 156–176.

Izard, C. E. (1972). *Patterns of emotions*. New York: Academic Press.

James, W. (1890). *The principles of psychology: Vol. 2*. New York: Holt.

Jorstad-Stein, E. C., & Heimberg, R. G. (2009). Social Phobia: An Update on Treatment. *Psychiatric Clinics of North America*, *32*, 641–663.

Kagan, J., & Reznick, J. S. (1986). Shyness and temperament. In W. H. Jones, J. M. Cheek, & S. R. Briggs (Eds.), *Shyness: Perspectives on research and treatment* (pp. 81–90). New York: Plenum.

Kagan, J., & Snidman, N. (1991). Infant predictors of inhibited and uninhibited profiles. *Psychological Science*, *2*(1), 40–44.

Kerr, M., Lambert, W. W., & Bem, D. J. (1996). Life course sequelae of chldhood shyness in Sweden: Comparison with the United States. *Developmental Psychology*, *32*, 1100–1105.

Kessler, R. C., Chiu, W. T., Demler, O., & Walters, E. E. (2005). Prevalence, severity, and comorbidity of 12-month DSM-IV disorders in the national comorbidity survey replication. *Archives of General Psychiatry*, *62*, 617–627.

Kimpara, S., Henderson, L., & Beutler, L. (2008). [A naturalistic study of the effectiveness of a treatment for chronic shyness and social phobia]. Unpublished data.

Koestner, R., Zuroff, D. C., & Powers, T. A. (1991). Family origins of adolescent self-criticism and its continuity into adulthood. *Journal of Abnormal Psychology*, *100*(2), 191–197.

Kurtz, J. E., & Tiegreen, S. B. (2005). Matters of conscience and conscientiousness: The place of ego development in the Five Factor Model. *Journal of Personality Assessment*, *85*, 312–317.

Lamiell, J. T. (1997). Individuals and the differences between them. In R. Hogan, J. Johnson, & S. Briggs (Eds.), *Handbook of personality psychology* (pp. 117–141). San Diego, CA: Academic Press.

Lane, C. (2007). *Shyness: How normal behavior became a sickness*. New Haven, CT: Yale University Press.

Lazarus, P. J. (1982). Incidence of shyness in elementary-school age children. *Psychological Reports*, *51*, 904–906.

Leary, M., & Kowalski, R. (1995). *Social Anxiety*. New York: Guilford Press.

Leary, T. F. (1957). *Interpersonal diagnosis of personality*. New York: Ronald Press.

Levin, A. P., Saoud, J. B., Strauman, T., Gorman, J. M., Fyer, A. J., Crawford, R., et al. (1993). Responses of "generalized" and "discrete" social phobics during public speaking. *Journal of Anxiety Disorders*, *7*, 207–222.

Maddux, J. E., Norton, L. W., & Leary, M. R. (1988). Cognitive components of social anxiety: An investigation of the integration of self-presentation theory and self-efficacy theory. *Journal of Social and Clinical Psychology*, *6*, 180–190.

Manning, P., & Ray, G. (1993). Shyness, self-confidence, and social interaction. *Social Psychology Quarterly*, *56*, 178–192.

Mattick, R. P., Peters, L., & Clarke, J. C. (1989). Exposure and cognitive restructuring for social phobia: A controlled study. *Behavior Therapy*, *20*, 3–23.

Mauss, I. B., Wilhelm, F. H., & Gross, J. J. (2004). Is there less to social anxiety than meets the eye? Emotion experience, expression, and bodily responding. *Cognition and Emotion*, *18*, 631–662.

Millon, T. (1987). *Manual for the Millon Clinical Multiaxial Inventory-II (MCMI-II)*. Minneapolis, MN: National Computer Systems.

Mosher, D. L., & White, B. B. (1981). On differentiating shame and shyness. *Motivation and Emotion*, *5*, 61–74.

Pilkonis, P. A. (1977). Shyness, public and private, and its relationship to other measures of social behavior. *Journal of Personality*, *45*, 585–595.

Pines, A., & Zimbardo, P. G. (1977). The personal and cultural dynamics of shyness: A comparison between Israelis, American Jews and Americans. *Mada (Israeli Science Magazine)*, *21*, 273–278.

Rowe, D. C. (1997). Genetics, temperament, and personality. In R. Hogan, J. Johnson, & S. Briggs (Eds.), *Handbook of personality psychology*. San Diego, CA: Academic Press.

Rubin, K. H., & Asendorpf, J. B. (1993). *Social withdrawal, inhibition and shyness in childhood*. Hillsdale, NJ: Lawrence Erlbaum.

Rubin, K. H., Coplan, R. J., & Bowker, J. C. (2008). Social withdrawal in childhood. *Annual Review of Psychology*, *60*, 141–171.

Rubin, K. H., & Krasnor, L. R. (1986). Social-cognitive and social-behavioral perspectives on problem solving. In M. Perlmutter (Ed.), *Cognitive perspectives on children's social and behavioral development. The Minnesota Symposia on Child Psychology: Vol. 18* (pp. 1–68). Hillsdale, NJ: Lawrence Erlbaum.

Scarr, S., & McCartney, K. (1983). How people make their own environments: A theory of genotype–environmental effects. *Child Development*, *54*, 424–435.

Schlenker, B. R., & Leary, M. R. (1982). Social anxiety and self-presentation: A conceptualization and model. *Psychological Bulletin*, *92*, 641–669.

Schneier, F. R., Martin, L. Y., Liebowitz, M. R., Gorman, J. M., & Fyer, A. J. (1989). Alcohol abuse in social phobia. *Journal of Anxiety Disorders*, *3*, 15–23.

Scott, S. (2006). The medicalisation of shyness: From social misfits to social fitness. *Sociology of Health and Illness*, *28*, 133–153.

St. Lorant, T., Henderson, L., & Zimbardo, P. (2000). Co-morbidity in chronic shyness. *Depression and Anxiety*, *12*, 232–237.

Steele, C. (1997). A threat in the air. *American Psychologist*, *52*, 613–629.

Stockli, G. (2002). Shyness in cultural context: A comparative study of correlates of shyness in school children in Switzerland and China. *Psychologie in Erziehung und Unterricht*, *49*, 151–159.

Sullivan, H. S. (1953). *The interpersonal theory of psychiatry*. New York: Norton.

Trew, J. L., & Alden, L. (2009). Predicting anger in social anxiety: The mediating role of rumination. *Behaviour Research and Therapy*, *47*(12), 1079–1084.

Turner, S., & Beidel, D. C. (1992). Reduction of fear in social phobics: An examination of extinction patterns. *Behavior Therapy*, *23*, 389–403.

Turner, S. M., Beidel, D. C., & Larkin, K. T. (1986). Situational determinants of social anxiety in clinic and nonclinic samples: Physiological and cognitive correlates. *Journal of Consulting and Clinical Psychology*, *54*, 523–527.

Turner, S. M., Beidel, D. C., & Townsley, R. M. (1990). Social phobia: Relationship to shyness. *Behaviour Research and Therapy*, *28*, 497–505.

Voncken, M. J., Alden, L. E., & Bogels, S. M. (2006). Hiding anxiety versus acknowledgment of anxiety in social interaction: Relationship with social anxiety. *Behaviour Research and Therapy*, *44*, 1673–1679.

Wallace, S. T., & Alden, L. E. (1997). Social phobia and positive social events: The price of success. *Journal of Abnormal Psychology*, *106*, 416–424.

Xinyin, C., Rubin, K. H., & Boshu, L. (1995). Social and school adjustment of shy and aggressive children in China. *Development and Psychopathology*, *7*, 337–349.

Ziller, R., & Rorer, B. (1985). Shyness-environment interaction: A view from the shy side through auto-photography. *Journal of Personality*, *53*, 626–639.

Zimbardo, P. G. (1977). *Shyness: What it is, what to do about it*. Reading, MA: Addison–Wesley.

Zimbardo, P. G. (1982). Shyness and the stresses of the human connection. In L. Goldberger & S. Breznitz (Eds.), *Handbook of stress: Theoretical and clinical aspects* (pp. 466–481). New York: Free Press.

Zimbardo, P. G., & Piccione, C. (1985). Can shyness affect your health? *Healthline*, *4*, 12, 13.

Zimbardo, P. G., & Radl, S. L. (1981). *The Shy Child*. New York: McGraw–Hill.

Zimbardo, P. G., & Zoppel, T. (1984). *The emic and etic of shyness*. Paper presented at the VII International Conference of Cross-Cultural Psychology, Acapulco, Mexico.

Chapter 4

Are Embarrassment and Social Anxiety Disorder Merely Distant Cousins, or Are They Closer Kin?

Rowland S. Miller
Department of Psychology and Philosophy, Sam Houston State University, Huntsville, TX 77341

If you're reading these words, you have almost certainly been embarrassed (Miller, 1996), but it is unlikely that you have experienced Social Anxiety Disorder (SAD). A remarkable number of people – as many as 13% of us – do experience SAD during their lifetimes (Furmark, 2002), so it is a common psychological problem. Still, most of us never slip into its grasp, while, in contrast, almost *all* of us have been embarrassed. Unlike SAD, a capacity for embarrassment seems to be ordinary and normal: A person who is genuinely immune to embarrassment, who cannot be embarrassed by anything he or she or others do, is odd, and possibly dangerous.

Indeed, the prevalence of embarrassment may result from its desirable functions in social life. Embarrassment may be commonplace because, unlike SAD, it is adaptive. In this chapter I suggest that, despite its unpleasantness, embarrassment is a useful social emotion that serves valuable interactive functions: It alerts one to unbecoming behavior, forestalls further transgressions, mollifies one's critics, and motivates desirable remedial responses. Embarrassment typically provides an efficient, efficacious way to overcome the minor mishaps that inevitably occur in our dealings with others. People who cannot be embarrassed may predictably be less proper and trustworthy than the rest of us, and they may seem implacable and remorseless; they are certainly less well-liked when they misbehave (Semin & Manstead, 1982). In short, embarrassment may be a beneficial component of social life.

In contrast, SAD impairs social life. Those with phobic fears of social situations experience excessive, irrational tension and distress that may interfere with – or entirely preclude – many typical public behaviors (Heiser, Turner, Beidel, & Roberson-Nay, 2009). Unlike embarrassment, SAD does not seem to serve any useful purpose. At best it is inconvenient and at worst it is debilitating. To add insult to injury (and, again, unlike embarrassment), SAD often

Social Anxiety: Clinical, Developmental, and Social Perspectives. DOI: 10.1016/B978-0-12-375096-9.00004-3

occurs in combination with other maladies such as depression, substance abuse, and obsessive-compulsive disorder (OCD) (Wenzel, Chapter 7, this volume).

What, then, may be the relationship – if any – that links embarrassment to SAD? Obviously, if one is desirable and the other detrimental, they do not seem to be siblings that spring from the same stock. On the other hand, despite their dissimilarities, they probably do not come from entirely different families. They have a key ingredient in common: neither would likely exist if people did not care what others thought of them. Embarrassment and SAD are notably different but they share a common ancestor – a grandparent – that places them on the same family tree without making them immediate kin. They are clearly related, but each has defining features that are not shared by the other. Call them first cousins.

This chapter addresses that assertion. It first considers embarrassment, surveying its nature, possible origins, and interactive effects. It then turns to social anxiety and SAD, delineating the differences between them and embarrassment.

THE NATURE OF EMBARRASSMENT

Embarrassment is an acute state of surprised, awkward abashment and chagrin that results from events that confound our expectations and increase the threat of unwanted evaluations from real or imagined audiences (Miller, 1996). It causes people to feel exposed and conspicuous, flustered and foolish, and inept and maladroit (Parrott & Smith, 1991; Tangney, Miller, Flicker, & Barlow, 1996). These are uncomfortable feelings, and, although embarrassing circumstances are often humorous, embarrassment is – at its core – an unpleasant experience.

Feelings

Accounts of embarrassment (Miller, 1992; Miller & Tangney, 1994; Parrott & Smith, 1991) routinely find that most embarrassments are startling; the predicaments that cause them are unanticipated, often resulting from abrupt and accidental changes in fortune. Thereafter, when embarrassment strikes, sufferers ordinarily feel unhappily noticeable and conspicuous; they believe that they are salient objects of others' attention and they often wish that they could escape or hide. Routinely accompanying this sense of exposure are feelings of awkwardness and nervous discomfort. People may feel ungainly and clumsy, incapable of any appropriate and graceful response to their predicament. Finally, underlying all of this is sheepish regret and chagrin. People are typically concerned about others' evaluations of them when they are embarrassed, and they usually suspect that they have made an unwanted impression. They rue this, are usually abashed, and are sometimes mortified.

Altogether, then, prototypical embarrassment involves startled, awkward sheepishness. These feelings ordinarily strike without warning, washing over people suddenly. Happily, however, they also tend to be short-lived (Miller & Tangney, 1994). Embarrassment does not persist for long periods of time, lasting only a few minutes instead of hours or days – a point nicely illustrated by the unique physiological marker of embarrassment, the blush.

Physiology

The visible reddening of the skin that typifies embarrassment (Edelmann, 2001) – blushing – occurs only in the upper chest, neck, and face, and it can be distinguished from the flushing that follows exercise or intoxication (Leary, Britt, Cutlip, & Templeton, 1992). In fact, facial veins are equipped with β-adrenergic receptors that are not commonly found in venous tissue and that cause them to behave differently from other capillaries in the skin (Mellander, Andersson, Afzelius, & Hellstrand, 1982); while other epidermal blood vessels are constricting in response to the activation of the sympathetic nervous system that underlies embarrassment (Hofmann, Moscovitch, & Kim, 2006), facial veins can dilate, bringing more blood near the surface of the cheeks (Drummond, 1989). All of this is entirely involuntary and cannot be consciously controlled – in fact, a sensation of warmth as one's cheeks grow red is ordinarily one's only clue that blushing has occurred (Shearn, Bergman, Hill, Abel, & Hinds, 1990) – but these reactions are short-lived; normal blushing lasts just a few minutes, fading gradually as one's embarrassment wanes (Shields, Mallory, & Simon, 1990).

Blushing and embarrassment do not readily occur in patients with damage to (Beer, Heerey, Keltner, Scabini, & Knight, 2003), or degeneration in (Sturm, Ascher, Miller, & Levenson, 2008), the medial regions of the prefrontal cortex. Children with damage in these areas never fully learn the norms of gentility and politesse the rest of us observe (Anderson, Bechara, Damasio, Tranel, & Damasio, 1999), and deterioration of these areas leaves previously well-mannered adults oddly heedless of potential social peril; they can behave flagrantly and indiscreetly with placid equanimity, even when others clearly disapprove. Notably, normal functioning in these regions also appears to be necessary if one is to have a normal "theory of mind" (that is, an ordinary recognition of the likely content of others' thoughts) (Stuss, Gallup, & Alexander, 2001). Thus, a capacity for embarrassment is linked to the ability to comprehend what others are thinking of us. Absent the capability to recognize and to care about others' evaluations of us, embarrassment is unlikely to occur.

This is a key point that speaks to the fundamental nature of embarrassment, and we will return to it later. Theorists also find it remarkable that, in being able to blush, our species is endowed with a distinctive physiological capacity that is a reasonably reliable marker of embarrassment and that occurs only in the areas of the body that are most likely to be visible to others (Miller, 2004). Why should such a response exist? One provocative possibility is that it is advantageous for others to know that we are embarrassed, so that blushing may have evolved as an interpersonal signal designed to communicate that fact (Castelfranchi & Poggi, 1990; Dijk, de Jong, & Peters, 2009). We will return to that argument later, as well; for now, we should note that blushing is not the only way we can tell whether or not someone is embarrassed.

Nonverbal Behavior

Embarrassment can be obvious in static photographs (Tracy, Robins, & Schriber, 2009), but in live interactions it unfolds in a dynamic *sequence* of facial and body movements that distinguish it from other states. When embarrassment strikes, people ordinarily avert their gaze (usually looking down and to the left) and then restlessly shift their gaze from place to place while continuing to avoid eye contact with others (Keltner, 1995). Then, a split-second later, they typically begin trying to prevent emerging smiles – biting their lips or pulling down the corners of their mouths – but ultimately fail, breaking into ambivalent, self-conscious grins that are less intense than their usual smiles of genuine amusement (Ambadar, Cohn, & Reed, 2009). They then tend to lower their heads and bring a hand to their faces to cover their eyes or mouths (Keltner, 1995); they also exhibit exaggerated body movements, shifting posture and gesturing broadly (Edelmann & Hampson, 1981). Finally, they make more speech errors, stammering and stuttering more than they do when they are poised and calm (Edelmann & Hampson, 1979).

This entire sequence ordinarily takes about five seconds from start to finish (Keltner, 1995), and it makes a person's embarrassment plain to anyone who is watching. Indeed, when someone in their midst becomes embarrassed, people usually know it; in general, observers can accurately gauge how embarrassed someone else is (Marcus & Miller, 1999). Moreover, when gaze aversion, smile controls, head movements, and face touches are all apparent, observers can reliably distinguish embarrassment from related states such as amusement, shame, and guilt (Keltner, 1995; Keltner & Buswell, 1996). Add a noticeable blush to these cues and embarrassment may be hard to miss, no matter where one travels (Consedine, Strongman, & Magai, 2003).

Altogether, then, embarrassment is characterized by particular feelings, physiological responses, and nonverbal behavior that make it unique. It shares some physical and phenomenological elements with other self-conscious moods and emotions (Hofmann et al., 2006), but careful analysis can differentiate it from related states (such as shame; see Miller & Tangney, 1994; Tangney et al., 1996).

Antecedent Events

Important distinctions also emerge from the events that elicit embarrassment. Embarrassment is, first and foremost, a *social* experience that almost never occurs when people are completely alone. Surveys of embarrassing incidents (e.g., Miller, 1992; Tangney et al., 1996) demonstrate that embarrassment always involves some form of (real or imagined) unwanted attention from others. People do report occasionally becoming embarrassed when no one else is present, but those episodes inevitably involve a threat of imminent discovery (when a person realizes, for instance, that he or she has entered the wrong restroom) or conscious recognition of what others would think if they knew (see Schlenker, 1980). If a person vividly imagines how others would react if they were present, solitary embarrassment is possible. This does not happen often, however: Only 2% of the embarrassments we encounter occur when we are alone, whereas almost a fifth of the shame we feel troubles us in private (Tangney et al., 1996).

Diverse events can cause us chagrin. Most embarrassments result from some mishap or misbehavior in which someone violates a norm of deportment, civility, self-control, or grace (Miller, 1992). There are many specific ways this may occur, ranging from physical pratfalls and other clumsiness to more subtle cognitive errors involving forgetfulness, temporary stupidity, and mistakes in judgment. Our possessions may also fail us, as pants rip or cars stall in busy intersections, or we may be abashed by doing others some minor inconvenience or harm. In such cases, embarrassment results from the sole actions of the embarrassed individual, and episodes like these account for almost two-thirds of all embarrassing circumstances (Miller, 1996). However, various other predicaments include other people and are more complex.

In particular, people need not misbehave in any way to become embarrassed. Abashed disquiet can result from interactions that take awkward turns even though no participant is maladroit. Innocent victims may be targeted for teasing or practical jokes by others who are either playful or malicious (Sharkey, Kim, & Diggs, 2001). Even more often (in 1 of every 10 embarrassments), people become embarrassed even when their own behavior is unremarkable because they are associated in others' eyes with someone else who does something embarrassing (Fortune & Newby-Clark, 2008; Miller, 1992). (These are events with which most parents of small children will be familiar!) Obviously, embarrassment does not emerge only from personal transgressions; it can be thrust upon us by the actions of others and may occur when we are merely hapless bystanders to others' misdeeds.

Still, in all of the instances mentioned above, whether through personal misconduct or the actions of others, circumstances conspire to make people look bad. In all these situations, embarrassment follows some discrete event that communicates a negative image of the embarrassed person to others. The adverse image may be ambiguous and undeserved – as when a companion misbehaves despite our efforts and we appear "guilty by association" – but an unappealing image is conveyed, nonetheless. Such damage is done in nearly all embarrassing events, allowing the possibility that embarrassment results from undesirable public image. There are, however, a few types of embarrassing circumstances that do not tidily fit this pattern.

For one thing, people can be embarrassed by excessive public attention even when desirable, praiseworthy images are in play. Simply being conspicuous and noticeable can cause embarrassment when there is nothing else at all to be embarrassed about (Crozier, 2004); for instance, selecting a member of an audience at random and asking everyone else to gaze steadily at him or her invariably causes the hapless target some embarrassment although nothing is really wrong (Lewis, 1995). People may even become embarrassed when they receive too many compliments and too much acclaim; being singled out for excessive public praise is sometimes embarrassing (Miller, 1992). Relatively few embarrassments result from simple conspicuousness and effusive praise; together they account for only 3% of the embarrassments people experience (Miller, 1996). Nevertheless, the embarrassing potential of such events demonstrates that actual harm to a person's public image need not be done for genuine embarrassment to occur.

Furthermore, people may even be embarrassed by exposure to social predicaments that do not actually involve them at all. Merely witnessing from afar a stranger's humiliating plight may engender a state of *empathic embarrassment* if observers envision how they would feel in such straits (Miller, 1987). Empathic embarrassment tends to be mild, but it is recognizably real embarrassment and accounts for another 3% of the embarrassing circumstances people encounter (Miller, 1987, 1992).

In sum, then, embarrassment usually follows events that do actual damage (whether justified or undeserved) to a person's image in the eyes of others. Occasionally, however, merely being the salient object of others' attention, or just envisioning another's predicament, can cause embarrassed chagrin. Theoretical efforts to explain the origins of embarrassment must encompass all of these antecedent events. Such efforts also need to explain why these antecedents do not trigger embarrassment until we are several years old.

The Development of Embarrassment

Experts differ in their estimates of when openness to embarrassment begins (see Lewis, 1995; Miller, 1996). Most, but not all (Barrett, 2005), studies find little evidence of rudimentary embarrassment in toddlers until they become self-conscious (usually around 1.5 years of age) and are able to recognize themselves in a mirror (DiBiase & Lewis, 1997). When this developmental milestone is reached, one-quarter of the children who are confronted with their own reflections display gaze aversion, smiling, and nervous hand movements that resemble embarrassed behavior in adults (Lewis, Sullivan, Stanger, & Weiss, 1989). Thereafter, slightly more than half of all 3-year-olds look embarrassed when they are asked to dance for an experimenter (Lewis, Stanger, Sullivan, & Barone, 1991). Behavior that resembles adult sheepishness and abashment thus occurs in rather young children.

What is indisputable, however, is that the sophistication and complexity of children's capacity for embarrassment continues to change and develop until they reach adolescence. Five-year-olds become embarrassed only when they are "caught in the act" and are actively rebuked by a disapproving audience (Bennett & Gillingham, 1991). Eight-year-olds react with embarrassment to any response – either derisive or supportive – to their predicaments from bystanders, but they remain unperturbed if their audiences watch silently. Only 11- and 13-year-olds are embarrassed (as adults are) by the mere knowledge that others are aware of their misbehavior, regardless of how those others react (Bennett, 1989). What makes this pattern compelling are studies of cognitive development and perspective-taking (e.g., Selman, 1976) that demonstrate that children's understanding of others' thoughts and feelings emerges in a manner that seamlessly complements the embarrassment data. Preschoolers have no idea what other people may be thinking of them, and, until they receive overt correction from others, they will blithely do things in public that would mortify an adult. Only in the face of unequivocal disapproval do they become embarrassed. By the time they are 11 or 13, however, they are capable of adult perspective-taking and can fully grasp what others may be thinking even when those others do nothing. Only then are they embarrassed by the assumed evaluations of others in the fashion of adults.

Thus, developmental studies suggest that embarrassment is rooted both in the self-conscious ability to hold oneself as the object of one's attention and in the complex cognitive ability to see oneself as others do. A third fundamental influence on the adult shape of embarrassment is socialization, the processes that teach children the social norms that will govern their public behavior (Saarni, 2008). Through painful experience, youngsters learn that certain behavior is likely to be met with teasing and ridicule. (Indeed, laughter at another person's embarrassing predicament is far more likely among fifth-graders, occurring more than half the time, than it is among adults (Miller, 1996)). In particular, children may come to dread excessive attention from others because it more often leads to disapproval and reproach than to acceptance and approbation. In this fashion, mere conspicuousness may gradually become embarrassing: "After hundreds of repetitions, conspicuousness becomes so closely associated with embarrassment that close scrutiny by others can cause embarrassment" (Buss, 1980, p. 233). Through modeling and social referencing, children can learn important lessons from others' predicaments, as well. As they come to apprehend others' feelings and watch the rough treatment others receive for misbehavior, classically conditioned empathic responses and stimulus generalization may slowly make them susceptible to empathic embarrassment (Hatfield, Cacioppo, & Rapson, 1994).

Ultimately, when they have already undergone thorough social seasoning and can finally intuit what passive audiences may be thinking of them, youngsters enter adolescence. Teenagers face provocative new social dilemmas (Buss, 1980). Puberty brings extraordinary physical and social changes, and teens enter unfamiliar and challenging new roles just as social acceptance becomes especially valuable to them. Certainly, "if God wanted to create a perfect recipe for embarrassment, the teen years might be it" (Miller, 1996, p. 87). In fact, teenagers do experience more intense embarrassments than adults do (Miller, 1992) and, as we will later see, most cases of SAD begin then, too (Schneier, Johnson, Hornig, Liebowitz, & Weissman, 1992; Stein, Walker, & Forde, 1996).

Individual Differences

Of course, by the time we are adults, some of us are more embarrassable than others. Individual differences in susceptibility to embarrassment, or *embarrassability*, can be readily assessed with a variety of measures (e.g., Kelly & Jones, 1997). The best-known of these, Modigliani's (1968) Embarrassability Scale, contains one-sentence items describing a variety of potentially embarrassing situations; respondents rate how embarrassed they would be in each of these predicaments, and the resulting global score reliably predicts how strongly they will react to the real embarrassments they encounter (Marcus & Miller, 1999; Miller, 1996). Highly embarrassable people do not experience different types of embarrassing predicaments from the rest of us, but they do become embarrassed more frequently and react more intensely than other people (Miller, 1992). Women also tend to be more embarrassable than men (Miller, 1995; Withers & Vernon, 2006).

Embarrassability is related to public self-consciousness, so that people who are routinely attuned to what others are thinking of them are more susceptible to embarrassment than are people who tend not to monitor their public images (Miller, 1995). Importantly, however, embarrassability is even more closely related to fear of negative evaluation (Miller, 2009). Highly embarrassable people dread disparagement from others. They fret about potential disapproval and worriedly anticipate unfavorable judgments when they come to others' attention. Obviously, this is one reason they react more strongly to a given predicament – their fear of negative evaluation ups the evaluative ante, making the potential damage done by an unwanted social image appear greater than the harm that seems to await people of lower embarrassability.

Interestingly, embarrassable people do not clumsily blunder their way into more awkward social situations than the rest of us; I found there to be no connection between embarrassability and one's global level of social skill (Miller, 1995). Although people with inhibited social skills tend to be shy and apprehensive (and relatively prone to SAD; Beidel & Turner, 2007) before anything goes wrong in an interaction, they do not manifest more embarrassment after some predicament occurs. Conversely, people with excellent social skills are evidently not immune to embarrassment; the various accidents and provocations from others that can cause embarrassment often entrap them, too.

On the other hand, if we break global skill into its constituent components (see Riggio, 1986), there is a noteworthy link between embarrassability and a certain specific skill, a sensitivity to social norms. Highly embarrassable people are especially aware of and concerned about the normative appropriateness of their behavior (Miller, 1995). They attend to social rules and dread violations of them, expecting more severe consequences to result. By comparison, people who are less susceptible to embarrassment are more easygoing; they are less attentive to norms and more placid if any are breached. This characteristic, combined with their higher fear of negative evaluation, places highly embarrassable people between a rock and a hard place: "They (1) hold themselves to stricter, less forgiving codes of conduct; and (2) chronically worry about what others are thinking of them, more than the rest of us do" (Miller, 1996, p. 101). In fact, embarrassability has less to do with a person's self-esteem than with his or her concern about social evaluation; highly embarrassable people tend to have low self-esteem, but the correlation between embarrassability and self-esteem disappears completely when fear of negative evaluation – which is also higher among people of low self-esteem – is taken into account (Miller, 1995).

The Fundamental Cause of Embarrassment

Contemplation of embarrassment's antecedents, development, and individual differences informs consideration of the central cause from which it springs. Two main contenders vie for the honor. Silver, Sabini, and Parrott (1987) persuasively argued that, at bottom, embarrassment occurs when people find themselves bewildered and uncertain of what to do and say next in social interactions (also see Sabini, Siepmann, Stein, & Meyerowitz, 2000). Silver et al. allowed that concerns over image often occurred during embarrassing predicaments, but they asserted that the only necessary stimulus for embarrassment was dramaturgical disarray that left "no character that one can coherently perform" (p. 51). The essential element of embarrassment, in this view, is the flustered awkwardness that results when unanticipated events disrupt one's expectations in social life.

An opposing perspective, held by me and others (e.g., Edelmann, 1987; Miller, 2009), counters that – although awkward uncertainty is certainly characteristic of embarrassing situations – the only indispensable catalyst for embarrassment is acute concern for what others may be thinking of us. Absent the acute threat of unwanted social evaluations that (almost) always underlies embarrassing predicaments, embarrassment would not occur.

Both of these models are valuable, heuristic perspectives rooted in prototypical, central features of embarrassment; after all, when people are asked to describe a "typical" episode of embarrassment, awkward indecision and social-evaluative concern are the two descriptors most likely to come to mind (Parrott & Smith, 1991). However, I favor the social evaluation model over the dramaturgic view for several reasons.

First, embarrassment springs from activity in regions of the brain that allow us to intuit what others are thinking of us. In particular, embarrassment is less intense or wholly absent in people who do not possess a normal theory of mind.

Second, as a mature capacity for embarrassment slowly develops during childhood, youngsters' reactions to embarrassing predicaments are more closely tied to their knowledge of others' evaluations of them than to the intrinsic awkwardness or silliness of the situation they are in. Young children may be completely unruffled by bizarre circumstances until they learn that others are critical of them; they get embarrassed only when others' disapproval is plain.

Third, susceptibility to embarrassment covaries with fear of negative evaluation but is uncorrelated with global social skill. If flustered uncertainty is the fundamental cause of embarrassment, we should expect people possessed of superior social skills to be rather less embarrassable than those who are more inept. Instead, the specific skill that best predicts embarrassability is a sensitivity to normative appropriateness that supports a social evaluation position.

Finally, I think the social evaluation model can account more flexibly and parsimoniously for the wide variety of events that can elicit embarrassment. As we have seen, the vast majority of such events entail actual, imminent, or potential damage to one's desired social identity. Almost all embarrassing circumstances create a real threat that others are about to form (if they have not already) unwanted judgments of the unfortunate target. In my view, fewer embarrassing predicaments easily fit a dramaturgic approach. For example, envision yourself slipping on an icy patch in a parking lot and going down hard, spilling some groceries; further assume that a witness is visible some distance across the lot. This pratfall would readily embarrass most of us, but it is difficult to argue that our distress is rooted in interactive uncertainty: Clearly, we should get up and pick up the groceries. Instead, I think the active ingredient in this embarrassing event is our awareness of the unattractive, ungainly image broadcast to the watching stranger. The same fall would be much less – or not at all – embarrassing if we were certain that no one else was present, not because our dramaturgic uncertainty would be reduced, but because there would be no unwanted social evaluations to dread.

But why should we care what random, distant strangers think of us? The social evaluation model suggests an evolutionary basis for the very existence of embarrassment that, although speculative, is another intriguing reason to prefer it to a dramaturgic perspective. Consider that, because they lived as members of small tribal groups, early humans would have been keenly motivated to maintain positive relations with others and to be accepted by their group (Baumeister & Leary, 1995). In that early era, social rejection may have literally been an evolutionary death sentence, with solitary humans being much less likely to survive and reproduce. Selective pressures would have favored advantageous psychological mechanisms that (1) alerted early humans to worrisome events that could lead to abandonment by others and (2) provided helpful means to forestall or prevent such ostracism or exclusion. Embarrassment may be such a mechanism (Miller, 2004): Despite its aversive character, embarrassment is an adaptive, propitious process in social life.

Behavioral Sequelae

They may feel discombobulated, but embarrassed people usually manage to respond to their predicaments in a conciliatory manner that helps them regain the acceptance of others. On occasion, they are so overwhelmed that they simply flee the scene without explanation. In rare instances, when they believe that others have intentionally caused their indignity, they counterattack with hostility and anger. Most of the time, however, people behave in humble, conciliatory, or jocular manners that are reassuring and pleasing to their audiences (Cupach & Metts, 1992; Miller, 1996).

For instance, the most common responses to an embarrassing event are efforts either to apologize, expressing regret and offering assurances of better behavior in the future, or to make restitution, actually repairing any damage or inconvenience that was caused. Together, these attempts at verbal or behavioral reparation occur in one of every three embarrassing situations (Miller, 1996). Another frequent response is humor, which is especially likely after physical pratfalls or failures of self-control (Cupach & Metts, 1992); people may acknowledge their transgressions – and perhaps show that they are uninjured – by lightheartedly making jokes at their own expense.

In general, then, embarrassed people are usually contrite, friendly, helpful, and eager to please (see Apsler, 1975). Unlike (for example) shame, which can generate surly, self-serving behavior (Tangney & Dearing, 2002), embarrassment appears to motivate polite, accommodating, and amicable behavior.

Others' Reactions

Significantly, the agreeable conduct of embarrassed people usually succeeds in impressing others favorably. This is a key point that is constantly misunderstood: After some public blunder, people routinely believe that observers are judging them more harshly than those others really are (Savitsky, Epley, & Gilovich, 2001). In fact, however, displays of appropriate embarrassment do not rouse rejection and make matters worse; instead, they ordinarily elicit acceptance and support from others. If a predicament has occurred, "*others will like us and treat us better if we do become embarrassed* than they will if we remain unruffled, cool, and calm" (Miller, 1996, p. 152; emphasis in original).

In one of the earliest demonstrations of this effect, Semin and Manstead (1982) showed research participants videotapes of a clumsy shopper whose cart knocks over a large stack of toilet paper rolls. In different versions of the tape, the shopper reacted with either evident embarrassment or unruffled poise and then either picked up the rolls or left them lying on the floor. Audiences liked the fellow better when he was abashed by his mishap than when he remained composed. He received the most favorable evaluations when he seemed obviously chagrined and picked up his mess, but, notably, he was even liked better when he got embarrassed and simply fled than when he stayed cool and calm and picked up the rolls. After a blunder, when it fit the situation, embarrassment engendered kinder judgments from others than did implacable aplomb.

Subsequent investigations have shown that blushing has similar effects. Even when they otherwise seem nonchalant, people who are apparently blushing after some clumsy mishap are judged more favorably than are those who seem unaffected by their actions (Dijk et al., 2009). In particular, blushing makes people seem more trustworthy, moral, sympathetic, and likeable when social predicaments occur (de Jong, 1999). Moreover, people behave as if they understand that blushing has interactive benefits; after inept performances, they become *less* distressed when they learn that their audiences have noticed their blushes and their evident chagrin (Leary, Landel, & Patton, 1996).

These data all support the intriguing possibility that embarrassment and blushing function as reliable gestures of appeasement – involuntary (and thereby sincere) nonverbal apologies – that palliate public predicaments (Castelfranchi & Poggi, 1990; Miller, 2004). Embarrassment demonstrates that someone is aware of his or her misbehavior. It also communicates the person's authentic alarm and regret and thereby signals his or her eagerness to do better in the future. Thus reassured of the person's good intentions, audiences can afford to remain tolerant of behavior that would otherwise be worrisome.

Importantly, however, embarrassment does not make a good impression when it does not fit the situation and is disproportional to one's predicament. Overstated, extreme reactions to trivial mistakes do not elicit sympathy from onlookers (Levin & Arluke, 1982), and blushing in the absence of any apparent predicament can be suspicious, signifying that one has a guilty conscience (de Jong, Peters, & De Cremer, 2003). Excessive embarrassability does not endear one to others, a point to which we will shortly return.

Nevertheless, when their chagrin is calibrated to its context, abashed actors usually receive supportive and kindly reactions from observers of their predicaments (Metts & Cupach, 1989). This was typically not so when we were children and our embarrassments were often met with heartless ridicule (Miller, 1996), and it is not always so now that we are adults. Still, more often than not, adult audiences respond to others' embarrassment with empathy, explicit reassurance, or friendly humor (Metts & Cupach, 1989). Even when audiences do or say something that makes someone's embarrassment worse, they frequently have friendly intentions (Sharkey, 1993). Only rarely do adults respond to a person's obvious embarrassment with criticism, rebuke, or malicious laughter. What is more, this seems to be true all over the world.

Embarrassment Across Cultures

Embarrassment has been studied in diverse cultures across the globe (e.g., Edelmann et al., 1989; Hashimoto & Shimizu, 1988), and it appears to operate similarly in all of them. The same sorts of circumstances elicit embarrassment, the feelings produced are the same, and the interactive consequences of the episodes are similar. When they describe embarrassed behavior from memory, denizens of different cultures do report small differences in their nonverbal displays (Edelmann et al., 1989), but these variations may be due more to their local stereotypes than to real differences in actual behavior. Certainly, blushing is characteristic of embarrassment in all peoples of the world.

One cultural contrast may be meaningful: Embarrassment may be a somewhat more serious event in collectivist cultures such as Japan than it is in individualistic cultures such as the United States (Singelis & Sharkey, 1995). Members of collectivist cultures stress their interdependence and family ties, so a person's misbehavior may seem to have more wide-ranging consequences, involving others' images to a greater extent than is the case in cultures that emphasize independence and autonomy. As a result, compared to North Americans, people in collectivist cultures may less often use humor to respond to embarrassment (e.g., Cupach & Imahori, 1993). Still, on the whole, people's responses to embarrassment – like the events that elicit it – are quite similar from culture to culture. Embarrassment appears to have reasonably consistent form and function around the world.

Reprise: The Nature of Embarrassment

Embarrassment takes years to develop, and its emergence coincides with the self-conscious ability to understand what others may be thinking of us. People also vary in their susceptibility to embarrassment, with those who are attentive to social norms and who dread social disapproval being more embarrassable. In a prototypical episode, unanticipated events that broadcast undesired images of us elicit involuntary, distinctive physiological and behavioral changes that make our abashment plain to observers. Awash with these feelings, we typically seek reassurance and are met with empathy and friendly support from others. Various aspects of embarrassment converge in suggesting that, if people genuinely did not care at all what others thought of them, they would not be embarrassable. People *do* care about social evaluation, however, and embarrassment may be an adaptive psychological mechanism that evolved to help us manage and overcome our inevitable small failures of grace and poise.

Two final prominent points about embarrassment remain to be made. First, embarrassment is unquestionably an *emotion*, not a mood. Emotions evidence (1) quick onset, (2) brief duration, and (3) unbidden occurrence, and appear to be the result of (4) relatively nonconscious, automatic appraisal (Ekman, 1992); that is, they emerge suddenly and spontaneously, without conscious consideration, but last only seconds or minutes, not hours or days. They are also characterized by coherent, particular patterns of feelings and behavior that distinguish them from other affective states (Roseman, Wiest, & Swartz, 1994). Embarrassment possesses each of these characteristics and thus is not simply a more diffuse and lasting mood.

Second, embarrassment is probably one of a small number of especially important, or basic, emotions that evolved to help people cope with fundamental tasks (Ekman, 1992). Such emotions – plausibly including happiness, sadness, fear, surprise, disgust, shame, and anger (Tracy, Robins & Schriber, 2009) – are presumed to have (1) singular physiological signatures that result from (2) antecedent events that are universal across cultures and are accompanied by (3) distinctive, and universal, expressions and behavior (Ekman, 1992). As we have seen, embarrassment possesses each of these features, as well (Keltner & Anderson, 2000).

Embarrassment is thus a distinct, discrete emotion – perhaps of particular importance – that is elicited by specific events and that engenders idiosyncratic and distinctive patterns of behavior. Arguably, it exists because it has functional value, helping us cope with recurring predicaments that all humans inevitably face.

EMBARRASSMENT AND SOCIAL ANXIETY DISORDER

As a patient reader, you may now know more about embarrassment than you ever intended to know! All of these varied facts and assertions will serve us well, however, as we now attempt to delineate the similarities and differences between embarrassment and its relative, SAD. I will examine five differences emerging from the phenomenology, timing, development, behavioral sequelae, and normality of the two states before concluding with a look at the common ground they share. I share the popular presumption (e.g., Beidel & Turner, 2007; McNeil, Chapter 1, this volume; Schneier, Blanco, Antia, & Liebowitz, 2002) that social anxiety and SAD differ mainly in intensity, not in their qualities, so most of my assertions about SAD will pertain to social anxiety as well. Nevertheless, we will need to distinguish social anxiety from SAD when we address the normality of these states.

Phenomenology

Embarrassment and SAD *feel* different. As we have seen, embarrassment is primarily composed of surprise, awkwardness, and chagrin. In contrast, the predominant feature of SAD is fear (American Psychiatric Association, 2000; Moscovitch, 2009). At bottom, phobic people are scared by the situations that cause them distress. Important distinctions among subtypes of SAD lie in the specific threats that make one miserable (Moscovitch, 2009) and the particular physiological reactions that result (McTeague et al., 2009), but uneasy, exaggerated dread of potential peril in public places is always present.

Indeed, the mental lives of those who suffer from social anxiety differ from those who are not anxious in several notable ways (Amir & Bomyea, Chapter 14, this volume; Miller, 2009). When they enter social situations, they are burdened with intrusive thoughts of past failures and worst-case outcomes that lead them to anticipate unhappy results before they occur (Vassilopoulos, 2005). Then, they scan their environments and monitor their own internal reactions in a state of high alert; they are unduly vigilant for signs of rejection and overly sensitive to their own unease (Bögels & Mansell, 2004; Schultz & Heimberg, 2008), and both forms of preoccupation make their anxiety worse (Zou, Hudson, & Rapee, 2007). Furthermore, they perceive disapproval where it does not exist (Huppert, Pasupuleti, Foa, & Mathews, 2007) and find fault even in positive events (Alden, Taylor, Mellings, & Laposa, 2008). Finally, when they are again alone, they ruminate, replaying past encounters in their minds and brooding over their perceived imperfections (Brozovich & Heimberg, 2008).

Thus, whereas embarrassment is comprised of startled chagrin, social anxiety is characterized by pervasive nervousness and trepidation. Importantly, social anxiety is longer-lasting, too.

Timing

Embarrassed emotion washes over people *after* they find themselves in a threatening situation; embarrassment is a reaction to presumed damage to one's social image that has already occurred (Schlenker & Leary, 1982). Surprised, flustered feelings characterize embarrassment because the reaction arises from unexpected events that often leave people at a loss for what to do. (For dramaturgic theorists, you may recall, bewildered uncertainty defines the emotion.) Embarrassing circumstances ambush people; in most cases, they are completely unanticipated.

In contrast, the situations that engender SAD are rarely surprising. Indeed, because they are such ordinary occurrences, they are often entirely foreseeable. Eating in a restaurant, using a public restroom, or signing a charge receipt while a cashier watches may all cause considerable distress to people with SAD (Beidel & Turner, 2007); clearly, such events are not painful because they are unexpected. On the contrary, SAD is often troubling long *before* a person encounters a frightening situation. The fear and apprehension that plague socially anxious people are typically anticipatory responses that occur in advance of any actual harm (Schlenker & Leary, 1982). SAD is a disruptive disorder not just because sufferers exaggerate the harm that may befall them, but because they are usually scared of harm that has not happened and never will.

This issue of the timing of embarrassment and SAD is meaningful because it speaks to the basic natures of the two states. Because it can occur long before one encounters a threatening situation and then persist in post-event processing (PEP) after the peril is past, SAD may result in acute anxiety that lasts for some time. The duration of these episodes argues that they should properly be considered moods, not emotions. The distinction matters because moods usually have more lasting influence on cognition and behavior than emotions such as embarrassment do (Isen, 1984). Embarrassment may often be consequential, but it is unlikely to have the pervading influence on a person's life that SAD can have.

Behavioral Sequelae

As a mood, social anxiety is less likely to be represented by coherent, unique nonverbal behavior than embarrassed emotion is, and, indeed, there are no distinguishing signals that a person is experiencing social anxiety *per se*. In fact, the behaviors that do tend to accompany SAD are often mistaken by observers for something else. When they experience intense social anxiety, people's interactive behavior is impoverished (Heerey & Kring, 2007); they either avoid troubling social situations altogether or behave in an inhibited, tentative fashion that is characterized by submissive withdrawal (Weeks, Rodebaugh, Heimberg, Norton, & Jakatdar, 2009). They avoid eye contact, keep their distance, nod, gesture, smile infrequently, and speak less fluently (Miller, 2009), and, instead of eliciting sympathy, their behavior often just seems unfriendly (Leary & Buckley, 2000). Ironically, then, by behaving in an aloof, guarded fashion, socially anxious people may elicit from others the very disapproval they dreaded in the first place (Alden & Taylor, 2004; Rodebaugh, 2009).

In contrast, embarrassed people are more likely to try to maintain and repair their current interactions than they are to run and hide from them. On occasion, in 1 of every 11 embarrassing situations, people are so overwhelmed by their predicaments that they simply flee them, exiting abruptly with no explanation (Miller, 1996). Far more often, however, embarrassed people stay put and try to regain the regard of their audiences with apologetic conciliation or humor. Once it occurs, embarrassment usually has a constructive effect on its social situations, but SAD is almost always destructive.

Development

Our mature capacities for embarrassment emerge hand-in-hand with our perspective-taking skills and appear to be complete by the time we are 11 years old (Bennett, 1989). The social experiences that accompany this growth probably help determine how conscientiously and/or fearfully we adhere to social norms, but the socialization of embarrassment seems to take place on a broad, and even cultural, scale (Buss, 1980). Embarrassment thus arises from developmental processes that do not vary much from person to person; all normal people are biologically and psychologically prepared to experience embarrassment, and individual differences in embarrassability seem to be more closely tied to ordinary variability in personality than to atypical physiology or unique personal experience.

By comparison, the sources of SAD seem to be more idiosyncratic, being present in some people and not at all in others. This may be true even of social anxiety, which, being milder than SAD, is considerably more widespread.

Although most people occasionally experience at least some social anxiety, predispositions to be especially socially anxious appear to be inherited (Stein & Gelernter, Chapter 11, this volume). There appear to be organismic differences involving noradrenergic, serotonergic, and dopaminergic neurotransmissions (Phan & Klumpp, Chapter 10, this volume) between those who are prone to social anxiety and those who are not, and inhibited temperaments that distinguish such children are present from birth (Kagan, Chapter 12, this volume).

However, theorists generally agree that biological predispositions like these interact with the family and social experiences people encounter to produce and shape SAD (e.g., Beidel & Turner, 2007; Kagan, Chapter 12, this volume). The parenting children receive can be influential (Rapee, 1997; Rapee & Heimberg, 1997), and specific traumatic social experiences may be formative as well. About half of those with SAD can recall a particular adverse event that coincided with the onset of their disorder (Stemberger, Turner, Beidel, & Calhoun, 1995), and, even when no single catastrophe is at fault, a variety of smaller setbacks can conceivably have cumulative deleterious effects (Mineka & Zinbarg, 1996). The role of such experiences may be one reason specific social anxiety disorders usually take longer to develop than embarrassment does; whereas 11-year-olds are fully susceptible to embarrassment, half of those who develop specific social fears do so after the age of 13 (Schneier et al., 1992; Stein et al., 1996).

Fuller discussion of these possibilities is beyond the scope of this chapter. Here, it is sufficient to reiterate that the factors that contribute to SAD seem to be more variable and less pervasive than are the influences that produce embarrassment. Of course, some influences on the two states are similar. For instance, both SAD and embarrassment are shaped by socialization, and its particular aspects can differ from culture to culture. Japanese people, for example, can experience a type of SAD that does not ordinarily occur in the United States: *taijin kyofusho* (TKS), a fear of causing others distress or harm through ineptitude or physical defect. TKS appears to emerge from norms regarding physical propriety that are more exacting than those in Western cultures (Kirmayer, 1991). Still, within a particular culture, individual differences in social anxiety and SAD seem to result from relatively idiosyncratic developmental processes involving types of genetic endowments, neurobiology, parenting, and traumas that – fortunately – do not affect everyone.

Thus, embarrassment appears to be a natural, ordinary product of human development, but SAD is rarer and arguably results from influences that are not ordinary at all. It should be no surprise, then, that one of these states is normal and the other is not (see Table 4.1).

Normality and Abnormality

People with SAD differ from the rest of us in several respects. They perceive social situations in pejorative, self-defeating ways that make those situations

TABLE 4.1 Distinguishing Embarrassment and Social Anxiety

Characteristic	Embarrassment	Social Anxiety
Phenomenology	Startled chagrin	Nervous trepidation
Nature of state	Emotion	Mood
Timing	Abrupt and reactive, after predicaments occur	Gradual and anticipatory, before predicaments occur
Duration	Short-lived	Long-lived
Onset of mature form	Early adolescence	Middle adolescence
Behavioral sequelae	Apologetic conciliation	Inhibited disaffiliation
Interactive result (in moderation)	Sympathy and acceptance	Mild disapproval
Proximal cause	Social-evaluative concern	Social-evaluative concern

seem more risky and less rewarding than they really are (Miller, 2009). They are at increased risk for a variety of damaging comorbid disorders, and the more generalized their SAD, the worse their related pathologies tend to be (Wenzel, Chapter 7, this volume). Finally, there is SAD itself: Sufferers cannot perform without impairment or extreme distress public actions the rest of us find unremarkable. Clearly, by any standard, SAD is an unwelcome, undesirable, abnormal condition.

Embarrassment is none of those things. Embarrassment is unpleasant, but it seems to fulfill useful interactive functions, and we would likely be worse off without it.

Of course, my assertions in these past two paragraphs are overly simplistic. Comparing embarrassment directly to SAD is a bit like comparing gentle summer rain to a tropical storm; to say the one is more desirable than the other is to belabor the obvious. A more sophisticated analysis must acknowledge that social anxiety has its benefits and embarrassment some potential drawbacks.

Collectively, people exhibit concerns over social evaluation that range from nearly nonexistent to the paralyzing incapacitation of SAD. Low, manageable levels of social anxiety are, of course, customary and commonplace in many situations; after all, anxiety is a normal response to intimidating challenges, and it (like embarrassment) probably evolved because it motivated beneficial behavior (Stein & Bouwer, 1997). Early humans who were roused by the prospect of negative evaluation from their fellows were probably more able to head off disapproval that could be dangerous (Baumeister & Tice, 1990). However, social anxiety is adaptive only within a delimited range and, outside those levels, abnormality results.

This volume focuses on the irrational, excessive, debilitating levels of social anxiety that we label as SAD, but we should not forget that *too little* social anxiety is dysfunctional, too. People without social anxiety – who are either always certain that they are being judged in a desired fashion or who care not at all what others think (Leary & Kowalski, 1995) – have a disability that is relatively unlikely to come to the notice of clinicians and researchers, but they are handicapped, nonetheless. They lack a feedback mechanism that would help them avoid social disapproval, and they may seem narcissistic, ruthless, or arrogant to others (Hofmann, Korte, & Suvak, 2009). Their relationships are likely less fulfilling than they otherwise could be.

In short, there is probably a curvilinear, inverted U relation between social anxiety and personal adjustment. Low-to-moderate social anxiety is presumably both normal and adaptive, but, as one's worries about others' judgments either become excessive or vanish completely, difficulty follows.

In my view, embarrassment is similar to social anxiety in this regard, but it is adaptive over a wider range of intensity. Even high embarrassability that increases one's reactions to existing predicaments does not inhibit or impair normal behavior to the extent that high social anxiety in advance of any evaluation does. There are limits even to embarrassment's usefulness, however, and outside the broad normal range it is disadvantageous to be either too little or too highly susceptible to embarrassment (Miller, 2007). At the low end, people who cannot be embarrassed may seem to lack a conscience (de Jong, 1999). At the high end, people overreact to trivial events, becoming discombobulated by situations that would not faze the rest of us. This is problematic because – whereas appropriate, measured embarrassment in response to a predicament makes good impressions on observers – excessive fluster and agitation make bad impressions (Levin & Arluke, 1982). By remaining unperturbed by compelling predicaments, people risk seeming crass and unfeeling, but by responding with exaggerated embarrassment they risk appearing inept (Miller, 1996).

Excessive embarrassability is also associated with *chronic blushing* that occurs in public settings in the absence of any overt predicament. Chronic blushers frequently find themselves blushing in ordinary situations that involve innocent contact with others, and they may come to dread their blushing episodes so much, and avoid interaction with others so thoroughly, that they meet the diagnostic criteria for SAD (Edelmann, 1990). Their maladaptive blushing appears to be a "pathological triggering" of appeasement behavior that is unwarranted (Stein & Bouwer, 1997), and it illustrates how the normal mechanisms associated with embarrassment can go awry.

Still, chronic blushing is not really an example of embarrassment run amok. Sufferers are typically socially anxious but are not embarrassed until their blushing starts, and only after their public loss of control makes them feel conspicuous do they ordinarily begin to feel abashed (Edelmann, 1990). Nevertheless, the trait of embarrassability is a good predictor of a person's tendency to be a chronic blusher (Leary & Meadows, 1991), and the fact that a miscalibrated signal of embarrassment can contribute to SAD is telling. Embarrassment and SAD are notably different but, at bottom, they serve the same master.

Similarities of the States

Underlying all the particular facts and specifics of SAD and embarrassment, a single foundation exists: If people were genuinely heedless of the judgments of others, they would experience neither state. Both kinds of affect presumably evolved because of their interpersonal functions: It was adaptive for people to be concerned about acceptance and approval from others, and useful to have alarm mechanisms that motivated both preventive and remedial behavior (Leary, Chapter 18, this volume; Miller, 2004). Hence, respectively, social anxiety and embarrassment are states experienced by all the peoples of the world (Horwath & Weissman, 1997).

Perhaps as a result of these shared evolutionary roots, social anxiety and embarrassment are also influenced by similar personality traits. The hallmark of both is fear of negative evaluation (Johnson, Turner, Beidel, & Lydiard, 1995; Miller, 1995). From that core constituent, embarrassment is shaped more by sensitivity to social norms, whereas social anxiety is more highly correlated with poor social skill, low self-esteem, and neuroticism (Baker & Edelmann, 2002; Leary & Kowalski, 1995; Norton, Cox, Hewitt, & McLeod, 1997). Still, the most important active ingredient is identical in the two states.

The situations that elicit the two states are similar to some extent, as well. Many circumstances that cause social anxiety are not embarrassing at all, but all events that cause embarrassment will also arouse social anxiety if they can be foreseen. Indeed, a defining characteristic of SAD is exaggerated fear of embarrassment (American Psychiatric Association, 2000). Almost everybody avoids embarrassment when they can, but some people go to extraordinary lengths to steer clear of situations that hold any potential for embarrassment (Miller, 2007). If they are able to do this without undue inconvenience, their extreme fear may go mostly unnoticed by others; however, if their avoidant behavior interferes with too many ordinary activities, their fear is judged to be SAD (Heckelman & Schneier, 1995). Thus, social anxiety and SAD have a longer reach than embarrassment does, but embarrassing situations can also be anxiety-arousing and the dread of such situations is one of the characteristics that make SAD so dreadful.

CONCLUSIONS

Our species is clearly equipped with psychological mechanisms that prepare us to monitor and react to social evaluation. Sensitivity to such stimuli, like other human characteristics, is probably normally distributed throughout the population, and embarrassability and social anxiousness may vary considerably from person to person (Leary & Kowalski, 1995; Miller, 2009). Susceptibilities to both states are completely normal in moderation. However, in some unfortunate people, presumably through the interactive influences of biological (e.g., neurotransmitter), psychological (e.g., perceptual), and social (e.g., family) factors, irrational fears of ordinary situations develop and interfere with social life (Beidel & Turner, 2007). These are undesirable mutations of normal processes, so they differ from embarrassment, which is typically a profitable, adaptive reaction to the inevitable predicaments of social life.

However, even when it is moderate, social anxiety differs from embarrassment. Social anxiety is an anticipatory mood state, whereas embarrassment is an emotion elicited by events that have already occurred. The two states feel different and engender different types of behavior: Social anxiety is characterized by inhibition and avoidance whereas embarrassment is typified by conciliation and remediation.

Nevertheless, they are recognizably kin to one another, born of the same fundamental human motivation to be accepted by others. One is benevolent and often light-hearted, the other less so, but they belong to the same extended family. Consider them cousins at work in the same family business.

REFERENCES

Alden, L. E., & Taylor, C. T. (2004). Interpersonal processes in social anxiety disorder. *Clinical Psychology Review*, *24*, 857–882.

Alden, L. E., Taylor, C. T., Mellings, T. M. J. B., & Laposa, J. M. (2008). Social anxiety and the interpretation of positive social events. *Journal of Anxiety Disorders*, *22*, 577–590.

Ambadar, Z., Cohn, J. F., & Reed, L. I. (2009). All smiles are not created equal: Morphology and timing of smiles perceived as amused, polite, and embarrassed/nervous. *Journal of Nonverbal Behavior*, *33*, 17–34.

American Psychiatric Association. (2000). *Diagnostic and statistical manual of mental disorders* (4th ed., text rev.) (DSM-IV-TR). Washington, DC: Author.

Anderson, S. W., Bechara, A., Damasio, H., Tranel, D., & Damasio, A. R. (1999). Impairment of social and moral behavior related to early damage in human prefrontal cortex. *Nature Neuroscience*, *2*, 1032–1037.

Apsler, R. (1975). Effects of embarrassment on behavior toward others. *Journal of Personality and Social Psychology*, *32*, 145–153.

Baker, S. R., & Edelmann, R. J. (2002). Is social anxiety disorder related to lack of social skills? Duration of skill-related behaviours and ratings of behavioral adequacy. *British Journal of Clinical Psychology*, *41*, 243–257.

Barrett, K. C. (2005). The origins of social emotions and self-regulation in toddlerhood: New evidence. *Cognition and Emotion*, *19*, 953–979.

Baumeister, R. F., & Leary, M. R. (1995). The need to belong: Desire for interpersonal attachments as a fundamental human motivation. *Psychological Bulletin*, *117*, 497–529.

Baumeister, R. F., & Tice, D. M. (1990). Anxiety and social exclusion. *Journal of Social and Clinical Psychology*, *9*, 165–195.

Beer, J. S., Heerey, E. A., Keltner, D., Scabini, D., & Knight, R. T. (2003). The regulatory function of self-conscious emotion: Insights from patients with orbitofrontal damage. *Journal of Personality and Social Psychology*, *85*, 594–604.

Beidel, D. C., & Turner, S. M. (2007). *Shy children, phobic adults: Nature and treatment of social anxiety disorder* (2nd ed.). Washington, DC: American Psychological Association.

Bennett, M. (1989). Children's self-attribution of embarrassment. *British Journal of Developmental Psychology*, *7*, 207–217.

Bennett, M., & Gillingham, K. (1991). The role of self-focused attention in children's attributions of social emotions to the self. *Journal of Genetic Psychology*, *152*, 303–309.

Bögels, S. M., & Mansell, W. (2004). Attention processes in the maintenance and treatment of social anxiety disorder: Hypervigilance, avoidance and self-focused attention. *Clinical Psychology Review*, *24*, 827–856.

Brozovich, F., & Heimberg, R. G. (2008). An analysis of post-event processing in social anxiety disorder. *Clinical Psychology Review*, *28*, 891–903.

Buss, A. H. (1980). *Self-consciousness and social anxiety*. San Francisco: W. H. Freeman.

Castelfranchi, C., & Poggi, I. (1990). Blushing as a discourse: Was Darwin wrong? In W. R. Crozier (Ed.), *Shyness and embarrassment: Perspectives from social psychology* (pp. 230–251). Cambridge: Cambridge University Press.

Consedine, N. A., Strongman, K. T., & Magai, C. (2003). Emotions and behaviour: Data from a cross-cultural recognition study. *Cognition and Emotion*, *17*, 881–902.

Crozier, W. R. (2004). Self-consciousness, exposure, and the blush. *Journal for the Theory of Social Behaviour*, *34*, 1–17.

Cupach, W. R., & Imahori, T. T. (1993). Managing social predicaments created by others: A comparison of Japanese and American facework. *Western Journal of Communication*, *57*, 431–444.

Cupach, W. R., & Metts, S. (1992). The effects of type of predicament and embarrassability on remedial responses to embarrassing situations. *Communication Quarterly*, *40*, 149–161.

de Jong, P. J. (1999). Communicative and remedial effects of social blushing. *Journal of Nonverbal Behavior*, *23*, 197–217.

de Jong, P. J., Peters, M. L., & De Cremer, D. (2003). Blushing may signify guilt: Revealing effects of blushing in ambiguous social situations. *Motivation and Emotion*, *27*, 225–249.

DiBiase, R., & Lewis, M. (1997). The relation between temperament and embarrassment. *Cognition and Emotion*, *11*, 259–271.

Dijk, C., de Jong, P. J., & Peters, M. L. (2009). The remedial value of blushing in the context of transgressions and mishaps. *Emotion*, *9*, 287–291.

Drummond, P. D. (1989). Mechanism of social blushing. In N. W. Bond & D. A. T. Siddle (Eds.), *Psychobiology: Issues and applications* (pp. 363–370). Amsterdam: Elsevier Science.

Edelmann, R. J. (1987). *The psychology of embarrassment*. Chichester, UK: Wiley.

Edelmann, R. J. (1990). *Coping with blushing*. London: Sheldon Press.

Edelmann, R. J. (2001). Blushing. In W. R. Crozier & L. E. Alden (Eds.), *International handbook of social anxiety: Concepts, research and interventions relating to the self and shyness* (pp. 301–323). Chichester, UK: Wiley.

Edelmann, R. J., Asendorpf, J., Contarello, A., Zammuner, V., Georgas, J., & Villanueva, C. (1989). Self-reported expression of embarrassment in five European countries. *Journal of Cross-Cultural Psychology*, *20*, 357–371.

Edelmann, R. J., & Hampson, R. J. (1979). Changes in non-verbal behaviour during embarrassment. *British Journal of Social and Clinical Psychology*, *18*, 385–390.

Edelmann, R. J., & Hampson, R. J. (1981). The recognition of embarrassment. *Personality and Social Psychology Bulletin*, *7*, 109–116.

Ekman, P. (1992). An argument for basic emotions. *Cognition and Emotion*, *6*, 169–200.

Fortune, J. L., & Newby-Clark, I. A. (2008). My friend is embarrassing me: Exploring the guilty by association effect. *Journal of Personality and Social Psychology*, *95*, 1440–1449.

Furmark, T. (2002). Social anxiety disorder: Overview of community surveys. *Acta Psychiatrica Scandinavica*, *105*, 84–93.

Hashimoto, E., & Shimizu, T. (1988). A cross-cultural study of the emotion of shame/embarrassment: Iranian and Japanese children. *Psychologia*, *31*, 1–6.

Hatfield, E., Cacioppo, J. T., & Rapson, R. L. (1994). *Emotional contagion*. New York: Cambridge University Press.

Heckelman, L. R., & Schneier, F. R. (1995). Diagnostic issues. In R. G. Heimberg, M. R. Liebowitz, D. A. Hope, & F. R. Schneier (Eds.), *Social anxiety disorder: Diagnosis, assessment, and treatment* (pp. 3–20). New York: Guilford Press.

Heerey, E. A., & Kring, A. M. (2007). Interpersonal consequences of social anxiety. *Journal of Abnormal Psychology*, *116*, 125–134.

Heiser, N. A., Turner, S. M., Beidel, D. C., & Roberson-Nay, R. (2009). Differentiating social anxiety disorder from shyness. *Journal of Anxiety Disorders*, *23*, 469–476.

Hofmann, S. G., Korte, K. J., & Suvak, M. K. (2009). The upside of being socially anxious: Psychopathic attributes and social anxiety are negatively associated. *Journal of Social and Clinical Psychology*, *28*, 714–727.

Hofmann, S. G., Moscovitch, D. A., & Kim, H. (2006). Autonomic correlates of social anxiety and embarrassment in shy and non-shy individuals. *International Journal of Psychophysiology*, *61*, 134–142.

Horwath, E., & Weissman, M. M. (1997). Epidemiology of anxiety disorders across cultural groups. In S. Friedman (Ed.), *Cultural issues in the treatment of anxiety* (pp. 21–39). New York: Guilford Press.

Huppert, J. D., Pasupuleti, R. V., Foa, E. B., & Matthews, A. (2007). Interpretation biases in social anxiety: Response generation, response selection, and self-appraisals. *Behaviour Research and Therapy*, *45*, 1505–1515.

Isen, A. M. (1984). Toward understanding the role of affect in cognition. In R. S. Wyer., Jr., & T. K. Srull (Eds.), *Handbook of social cognition: Vol. 3* (pp. 179–236). Hillsdale, NJ: Erlbaum.

Johnson, M. R., Turner, S. M., Beidel, D. C., & Lydiard, R. B. (1995). Personality function. In M. B. Stein (Ed.), *Social anxiety disorder: Clinical and research perspectives* (pp. 77–117). Washington, DC: American Psychiatric Press.

Kelly, K. M., & Jones, W. H. (1997). Assessment of dispositional embarrassability. *Anxiety, Stress & Coping: An International Journal*, *10*, 307–333.

Keltner, D. (1995). Signs of appeasement: Evidence for the distinct displays of embarrassment, amusement, and shame. *Journal of Personality and Social Psychology*, *68*, 441–454.

Keltner, D., & Anderson, C. (2000). Saving face for Darwin: The functions and uses of embarrassment. *Current Directions in Psychological Science*, *9*, 187–192.

Keltner, D., & Buswell, B. N. (1996). Evidence for the distinctness of embarrassment, shame, and guilt: A study of recalled antecedents and facial expressions of emotion. *Cognition and Emotion*, *10*, 155–171.

Kirmayer, L. J. (1991). The place of culture in psychiatric nosology: *Taijin kyofusho* and DSM-III-R. *Journal of Nervous and Mental Disease*, *179*, 19–28.

Leary, M. R., Britt, T. W., Cutlip, W. D., II, & Templeton, J. L. (1992). Social blushing. *Psychological Bulletin, 112*, 446–460.

Leary, M. R., & Buckley, K. E. (2000). Shyness and the pursuit of social acceptance. In W. R. Crozier (Ed.), *Shyness: Development, consolidation and change* (pp. 139–153). New York: Routledge.

Leary, M. R., & Kowalski, R. M. (1995). *Social anxiety*. New York: Guilford Press.

Leary, M. R., Landel, J. L., & Patton, K. M. (1996). The motivated expression of embarrassment following a self-presentational predicament. *Journal of Personality, 64*, 619–636.

Leary, M. R., & Meadows, S. (1991). Predictors, elicitors, and concomitants of social blushing. *Journal of Personality and Social Psychology, 60*, 254–262.

Levin, J., & Arluke, A. (1982). Embarrassment and helping behavior. *Psychological Reports, 51*, 999–1002.

Lewis, M. (1995). Embarrassment: The emotion of self-exposure and evaluation. In J. P. Tangney & K. W. Fischer (Eds.), *Self-conscious emotions: The psychology of shame, guilt, embarrassment and pride* (pp. 198–218). New York: Guilford Press.

Lewis, M., Stanger, C., Sullivan, M. W., & Barone, P. (1991). Changes in embarrassment as a function of age, sex and situation. *British Journal of Developmental Psychology, 9*, 485–492.

Lewis, M., Sullivan, M. W., Stanger, C., & Weiss, M. (1989). Self development and self-conscious emotions. *Child Development, 60*, 146–156.

Marcus, D. K., & Miller, R. S. (1999). The perception of "live" embarrassment: A social relations analysis of class presentations. *Cognition and Emotion, 13*, 105–117.

McTeague, L. M., Lang, P. J., Laplante, M. C., Cuthbert, B. N., Strauss, C. C., & Bradley, M. M. (2009). Fearful imagery in social anxiety disorder: Generalization, comorbidity, and physiological reactivity. *Biological Psychiatry, 65*, 374–382.

Mellander, S., Andersson, P., Afzelius, L., & Hellstrand, P. (1982). Neural beta-adrenergic dilatation of the facial vein in man: Possible mechanism in emotional blushing. *Acta Physiologica Scandinavia, 114*, 393–399.

Metts, S., & Cupach, W. R. (1989). Situational influence on the use of remedial strategies in embarrassing predicaments. *Communication Monographs, 56*, 151–162.

Miller, R. S. (1987). Empathic embarrassment: Situational and personal determinants of reactions to the embarrassment of another. *Journal of Personality and Social Psychology, 53*, 1061–1069.

Miller, R. S. (1992). The nature and severity of self-reported embarrassing circumstances. *Personality and Social Psychology Bulletin, 18*, 190–198.

Miller, R. S. (1995). On the nature of embarrassability: Shyness, social evaluation, and social skill. *Journal of Personality, 63*, 315–339.

Miller, R. S. (1996). *Embarrassment: Poise and peril in everyday life*. New York: Guilford Press.

Miller, R. S. (2004). Emotion as adaptive interpersonal communication: The case of embarrassment. In L. Z. Tiedens & C. W. Leach (Eds.), *The social life of emotions* (pp. 87–104). Cambridge, UK: Cambridge University Press.

Miller, R. S. (2007). Is embarrassment a blessing or a curse? In J. L. Tracy, R. W. Robins, & J. P. Tangney (Eds.), *The self-conscious emotions: Theory and research* (pp. 245–262). New York: Oxford University Press.

Miller, R. S. (2009). Social anxiousness, shyness, and embarrassability. In M. R. Leary & R. H. Hoyle (Eds.), *Handbook of individual differences in social behavior* (pp. 176–191). New York: Guilford Press.

Miller, R. S., & Tangney, J. P. (1994). Differentiating embarrassment and shame. *Journal of Social and Clinical Psychology, 13*, 273–287.

Mineka, S., & Zinbarg, R. (1996). Conditioning and ethological models of anxiety disorders: Stress-in-dynamic-context anxiety models. In D. A. Hope (Ed.), *Perspectives on anxiety, panic, and fear* (pp. 135–210). Lincoln, NE: University of Nebraska Press.

Modigliani, A. (1968). Embarrassment and embarrassability. *Sociometry, 31*, 313–326.

Moscovitch, D. A. (2009). What is the core fear in social anxiety disorder? A new model to facilitate individualized case conceptualization and treatment. *Cognitive and Behavioral Practice, 16*, 123–134.

Norton, G. R., Cox, B. J., Hewitt, P. L., & McLeod, L. (1997). Personality factors associated with generalized and non-generalized social anxiety. *Personality and Individual Differences, 22*, 655–660.

Parrott, W. G., & Smith, S. F. (1991). Embarrassment: Actual vs. typical cases, classical vs. prototypical representations. *Cognition and Emotion, 5*, 467–488.

Rapee, R. M. (1997). Potential role of childrearing practices in the development of anxiety and depression. *Clinical Psychology Review, 17*, 47–67.

Rapee, R. M., & Heimberg, R. G. (1997). A cognitive-behavioral model of anxiety in social anxiety disorder. *Behaviour Research and Therapy, 35*, 741–756.

Riggio, R. E. (1986). Assessment of basic social skills. *Journal of Personality and Social Psychology, 51*, 649–660.

Rodebaugh, T. L. (2009). Social anxiety disorder and perceived friendship quality. *Journal of Anxiety Disorders, 23*, 872–878.

Roseman, I. J., Wiest, C., & Swartz, T. S. (1994). Phenomenology, behaviors, and goals differentiate discrete emotions. *Journal of Personality and Social Psychology, 67*, 206–221.

Saarni, C. (2008). The interface of emotional development with social context. In M. Lewis, J. Haviland-Jones, & L. F. Barrett (Eds.), *Handbook of emotions* (3rd ed.) (pp. 332–347). New York: Guilford Press.

Sabini, J., Siepmann, M., Stein, J., & Meyerowitz, M. (2000). Who is embarrassed by what? *Cognition and Emotion, 14*, 213–240.

Savitsky, K., Epley, N., & Gilovich, T. (2001). Do others judge us as harshly as we think? Overestimating the impact of our failures, shortcomings, and mishaps. *Journal of Personality and Social Psychology, 81*, 44–56.

Schlenker, B. R. (1980). *Impression management: The self-concept, social identity, and interpersonal relations*. Monterey, CA: Brooks/Cole.

Schlenker, B. R., & Leary, M. R. (1982). Social anxiety and self-presentation: A conceptualization and model. *Psychological Bulletin, 92*, 641–669.

Schneier, F. R., Blanco, C., Antia, S. X., & Liebowitz, M. R. (2002). The social anxiety spectrum. *Psychiatric Clinics of North America, 25*, 757–774.

Schneier, F. R., Johnson, J., Hornig, C. D., Liebowitz, M. R., & Weissman, M. M. (1992). Social anxiety disorder: Comorbidity and morbidity in an epidemiologic sample. *Archives of General Psychiatry, 49*, 282–288.

Schultz, L. T., & Heimberg, R. G. (2008). Attentional focus in social anxiety disorder: Potential for interactive processes. *Clinical Psychology Review, 28*, 1206–1221.

Selman, R. L. (1976). Social-cognitive understanding: A guide to educational and clinical practice. In T. Lickona (Ed.), *Moral development and behavior* (pp. 299–316). New York: Holt, Rinehart and Winston.

Semin, G. R., & Manstead, A. S. R. (1982). The social implications of embarrassment displays and restitution behavior. *European Journal of Social Psychology, 12*, 367–377.

Sharkey, W. F. (1993). Who embarrasses whom? Relational and sex differences in the use of intentional embarrassment. In P. J. Kalbfleisch (Ed.), *Interpersonal communication: Evolving interpersonal relationships* (pp. 147–168). Hillsdale, NJ: Erlbaum.

Sharkey, W. F., Kim, M., & Diggs, R. C. (2001). Intentional embarrassment: A look at embarrassors' and targets' perspectives. *Personality and Individual Differences*, *31*, 1261–1272.

Shearn, D., Bergman, E., Hill, K., Abel, A., & Hinds, L. (1990). Facial coloration and temperature responses in blushing. *Psychophysiology*, *27*, 687–693.

Shields, S. A., Mallory, M. E., & Simon, A. (1990). The experience and symptoms of blushing as a function of age and reported frequency of blushing. *Journal of Nonverbal Behavior*, *14*, 171–187.

Silver, M., Sabini, J., & Parrott, W. G. (1987). Embarrassment: A dramaturgic account. *Journal for the Theory of Social Behavior*, *17*, 47–61.

Singelis, T. M., & Sharkey, W. F. (1995). Culture, self-construal, and embarrassability. *Journal of Cross-Cultural Psychology*, *26*, 622–644.

Stein, D. J., & Bouwer, C. (1997). A neuro-evolutionary approach to the anxiety disorders. *Journal of Anxiety Disorders*, *11*, 409–429.

Stein, M. B., Walker, J. R., & Forde, D. R. (1996). Public speaking fears in a community sample: Prevalence, impact on functioning, and diagnostic classification. *Archives of General Psychiatry*, *53*, 169–174.

Stemberger, R. T., Turner, S. M., Beidel, D. C., & Calhoun, K. S. (1995). Social anxiety disorder: An analysis of possible developmental factors. *Journal of Abnormal Psychology*, *104*, 526–531.

Sturm, V. E., Ascher, E. A., Miller, B. L., & Levenson, R. W. (2008). Diminished self-conscious emotional responding in frontotemporal lobar degeneration patients. *Emotion*, *8*, 861–869.

Stuss, D. T., Gallup, G. G., Jr., & Alexander, M. P. (2001). The frontal lobes are necessary for 'theory of mind.' *Brain*, *124*, 279–286.

Tangney, J. P., & Dearing, R. L. (2002). *Shame and guilt*. New York: Guilford Press.

Tangney, J. P., Miller, R. S., Flicker, L., & Barlow, D. H. (1996). Are shame, guilt, and embarrassment distinct emotions? *Journal of Personality and Social Psychology*, *70*, 1256–1264.

Tracy, J. L., Robins, R. W., & Schriber, R. A. (2009). Development of a FACS-verified set of basic and self-conscious emotion expressions. *Emotion*, *9*, 554–559.

Vassilopoulos, S. P. (2005). Anticipatory processing plays a role in maintaining social anxiety. *Anxiety, Stress, and Coping*, *18*, 321–332.

Weeks, J. W., Rodebaugh, T. L., Heimberg, R. G., Norton, P. J., & Jakatdar, T. A. (2009). "To avoid evaluation, withdraw": Fears of evaluation and depressive cognitions lead to social anxiety and submissive withdrawal. *Cognitive Therapy and Research*, *33*, 375–389.

Withers, L. A., & Vernon, L. L. (2006). To err is human: Embarrassment, attachment, and communication apprehension. *Personality and Individual Differences*, *40*, 99–110.

Zou, J. B., Hudson, J. L., & Rapee, R. M. (2007). The effect of attentional focus on social anxiety. *Behaviour Research and Therapy*, *45*, 2326–2333.

Chapter 5

Social Anxiety Disorder and Its Relationship to Perfectionism

Randy O. Frost, Katharine Glossner, and Sarah Maxner
Department of Psychology, Clark Science Center, Smith College, Northampton, MA 01060

Social evaluation and scrutiny by others are core features of social anxiety disorder (DSM-IV, American Psychiatric Association, 1994). According to Rapee and Heimberg (1997), individuals with social anxiety disorder perceive themselves as not meeting the expectations of others, and they believe others will evaluate them negatively as a result. Earlier cognitive behavioral models of social anxiety disorder contain similar elements (Beck & Emery, 1985; Clark & Wells, 1995; Schlenker & Leary, 1982). These features of social anxiety disorder have been central concepts in theorizing about perfectionism as well. Burns (1980) emphasizes the fear of being seen as foolish or inadequate in conceptualizing perfectionism. He suggests perfectionists are excessively sensitive to negative feedback (perceived or real), a theme echoed by later researchers (Flett, Hewitt, & DeRosa, 1996). Hamachek (1978) suggests that perfectionists overvalue performance and approval from others. Being perfect is a way of gaining such approval. If perfect performance is not possible, perfectionists employ strategies to avoid evaluation. Hollender (1965) also describes perfectionists as overly sensitive to rejection and excessively concerned with approval from others. In addition, because perfectionists lack a sense of self-competence, they depend on other people's evaluations to feel secure. Pacht (1984) echoes a similar theme.

Developments in the conceptualization and measurement of perfectionism make it possible to gain a much clearer picture of its role in various forms of psychopathology, including social anxiety disorder. This chapter will review the evidence linking perfectionism with social anxiety and social anxiety disorder, examining studies linking measures of social anxiety and perfectionism in nonclinical and social anxiety disorder samples, and studies of the role of perfectionism in social anxiety contexts. The implications of these findings for avoidance of social-evaluative situations will also be discussed. First, however, a brief overview of conceptualizations of perfectionism is warranted.

Multidimensional models have focused on specific components of perfectionism. Hewitt and Flett (1991a, 1991b) suggest three dimensions based on

Social Anxiety: Clinical, Developmental, and Social Perspectives. DOI: 10.1016/B978-0-12-375096-9.00005-5

the origin or target of excessively high standards. Self-oriented perfectionism reflects the tendency to set high standards for oneself and stress the importance of meeting those standards. Socially prescribed perfectionism involves the tendency to believe that other people set excessively high standards and are overly critical when these standards are not met. Other-oriented perfectionism involves the tendency to set excessively high standards for others. A considerable amount of research supports the reliability and validity of these dimensions.

Frost, Marten, Lahart, and Rosenblate (1990) define perfectionism as the setting of excessively high standards for performance accompanied by overly critical self-evaluations. Five perfectionistic dimensions and one related dimension constitute this conceptualization. Two dimensions involve the nature of perfectionistic thought and evaluations. Concern over mistakes reflects negative reactions to mistakes, the interpretation of mistakes as equivalent to failure, and the belief that one will lose the respect of others after failure. This dimension relates to a wide variety of psychological disorders, and it most clearly distinguishes perfectionists from those people who set high standards for themselves because they are highly competent and successful (Frost et al., 1990). Doubts about actions involves the tendency to doubt the quality of one's actions. It is closely associated with obsession-like doubting, but it relates to early theorizing about perfectionists' doubts about their competence (Hamachek, 1978; Hollender, 1965). Two other dimensions in this model concern beliefs about expectations and evaluation by parents. Parental expectations and parental criticism reflect the perception that parents set extremely high standards and are overly critical of attempts to meet them. Each of the early theorists (Burns, 1980; Hamachek, 1978; Hollender, 1965; Pacht, 1984) emphasized the role of parental expectations and criticism in the development of perfectionism. One dimension – personal standards – reflects the setting of excessively high standards for performance and the basing of one's self-evaluation on achieving them. This dimension has been emphasized by most theorists on perfectionism, but it is least likely to be related to psychopathology and most likely to be related to striving for positive achievement (Frost, Heimberg, Holt, Mattia & Neubauer, 1993; Lundh, 2004; Stoeber & Otto, 2006). The sixth dimension – organization – is somewhat distinct from the rest. It concerns the tendency to be orderly and organized. Hollender (1965) refers to this as the tendency to be "fussy or exacting" (p. 96).

The Hewitt and Flett and the Frost et al. conceptualizations overlap in significant ways. Frost et al. (1993) factor-analyzed the subscales from both multidimensional perfectionism scales and found two predominant features of perfectionism: positive achievement striving (PAS) and maladaptive evaluation concerns (MEC). Personal standards and organization from the Frost MPS, and self-oriented perfectionism and other-oriented perfectionism from the Hewitt and Flett measure, combined to make up PAS. The concern over mistakes, doubts about actions, parental expectations, parental criticism, and socially prescribed perfectionism scales combined to form the second factor, MEC. Data from this sample indicated that PAS was positively correlated with positive affect, but not negative affect, whereas MEC was positively correlated with depression and negative affect. Subsequent research has indicated close associations between concern over mistakes, doubts about actions, and socially prescribed perfectionism as well (Flett, Sawatzky, & Hewitt, 1995). A considerable amount of research has supported the two-dimensional structure of perfectionism, with varying labels for each (Bieling, Israeli, & Antony, 2004; Dunkley, Blankstein, Masheb, & Grilo, 2006; Stumpf & Parker, 2000; Terry-Short, Glynn Owens, Slade, & Dewey, 1995). Alden, Ryder, and Mellings (2002) proposed a similar two-component model of perfectionism specifically related to social anxiety composed of performance expectations and maladaptive self-appraisal. Like Frost et al.'s (1990) personal standards and Hewitt and Flett's (1991a, 1991b) self-oriented perfectionism, the performance expectations component captures the tendency to hold oneself to high standards. The maladaptive self-appraisal component is characterized by excessive criticism of oneself and one's abilities that results in feelings of anxiety and personal inadequacy and is similar to the maladaptive dimensions of perfectionism proposed by Frost et al. (1990) and Hewitt and Flett (1991a, 1991b). For the purposes of this chapter we will refer to these as perfectionism dimensions using the MEC and terminology PAS.

While much of the research on perfectionism has focused on the independent contribution of these dimensions of perfectionism, early definitions emphasized the combination of high personal standards and overly critical self-evaluations (Frost et al., 1990). A number of investigators have similarly suggested that high personal standards or PAS will be pathological or not, depending on the existence of MEC (Alden et al., 2002; Lundh, 2004; Lundh, Saboonchi, & Wångby, 2008; Stoeber & Otto, 2006).

PERFECTIONISM AND MEASURES OF SOCIAL ANXIETY IN NONCLINICAL SAMPLES

A number of studies involving nonclinical populations have reported relationships between perfectionism and measures of social anxiety, fear of negative evaluation, social skills, and social problem-solving. Flett, Hewitt, & DeRosa (1996) administered a series of questionnaires concerning social anxiety and social skills to undergraduates. Self-oriented and other-oriented perfectionism were not correlated with any of the social anxiety measures. However, socially prescribed perfectionism was significantly correlated with all of them. Subjects high in socially prescribed perfectionism were more shy and lonely, and had lower self-esteem and greater fear of negative evaluation. These findings replicated other studies linking socially prescribed perfectionism and social anxiety (Blankstein, Flett, Hewitt, & Eng, 1993; Hewitt & Flett, 1991b; Laurenti, Bruch, & Haase, 2008). The picture regarding social skills was more complex.

Self-oriented and other-oriented perfectionism were both positively correlated with the emotional sensitivity subscale and the social expressiveness subscale of the Social Skill Inventory. The emotional sensitivity subscale is thought to reflect the tendency to be sensitive to the emotional state of others, whereas the social expressiveness subscale reflects outgoing social behaviors (e.g., being the first to introduce oneself in a social encounter). Positive correlations with these measures argue against an association with social anxiety for these dimensions of perfectionism. Other-oriented perfectionism was also correlated with emotional expressiveness, which reflects gregariousness and behaviors drawing attention to oneself. Socially prescribed perfectionism, on the other hand, was negatively correlated with emotional control, which involved success at concealing true feelings and maintaining a calm exterior when upset. Socially prescribed perfectionism was also positively correlated with social sensitivity, the tendency to fear that one is being misunderstood or criticized.

The authors suggest that people high in socially prescribed perfectionism respond to perceived criticism with withdrawal and isolation, leading to more feelings of loneliness. The absence of association between self-oriented perfectionism and social anxiety indicates that PAS shows little or no association with social anxiety, which is consistent with other similar findings (Alden, Bieling, & Wallace, 1994; Wallace & Alden, 1991). In general, both self-oriented perfectionism and other-oriented perfectionism were associated with adaptive social skills, whereas socially prescribed perfectionism was associated with negative social skills.

Saboonchi and Lundh (1997) found the MEC perfectionism to be correlated with multiple measures of social anxiety, while the PAS subscales showed little or no association with these measures. Although it was possible that the association between MEC and social anxiety in this study might have been due to increased public self-consciousness, when the variance attributable to public self-consciousness was removed in a partial correlation, the correlations between MEC subscales and social anxiety remained significant. Furthermore, when MEC subscales were controlled in a partial correlation, the correlations between public self-consciousness and social anxiety were no longer significant. The authors conclude that "perfectionism is a more relevant construct in the study of anxiety than is public self-consciousness" (p. 927). Similarly, Ferrari (1992) found positive correlations between the Burns Perfectionism Scale (a unidimensional measure of MEC) and public and private self-consciousness, as well as social anxiety.

Shumaker and Rodebaugh (2009) examined the relative contribution of high personal standards (PAS) and MEC among speech-anxious college students using two different perfectionism measures. MEC predicted both state and trait social anxiety, while PAS predicted only state social anxiety. Higher levels of PAS were associated with lower social anxiety. Shumaker and Rodebaugh failed to find interaction effects between PAS and MEC, contradicting the theory that the combination of high PAS and high MEC would be associated with more psychopathology (Alden et al., 2002; Lundh, 2004; Stoeber & Otto, 2006).

DiBartolo, Li, and Frost (2008) found that both MEC and PAS dimensions of perfectionism were correlated with social anxiety in female undergraduates. However, partial correlations indicated that the MEC–social anxiety correlation remained significant when controlling for PAS, but the PAS–social anxiety correlation did not when MEC was controlled.

Flett, Hewitt, Blankstein, Solnik, and Van Brunschot (1996) examined the relationship between perfectionism and social problem-solving among two samples of undergraduates. They found that self-oriented and other-oriented perfectionism were positively correlated with problem-solving skills, social problem-solving, and positive cognitive orientation to problem-solving. They were also correlated with the tendency to solve problems in an adaptive way by breaking down the problem into manageable components, looking for alternate solutions, and systematic decision-making. In their second sample, however, a number of these associations did not replicate. Only other-oriented perfectionism was correlated with social problem-solving skills, problem definition, and seeking alternate solutions. Although weakened somewhat by the failure to replicate, these findings are consistent with the notion that parts of the construct of perfectionism are related to PAS and adaptation in certain contexts (Frost et al., 1993).

In contrast to these findings, socially prescribed perfectionism was negatively correlated with cognitive, emotional, and behavioral problem-solving orientations. These findings suggest that, when faced with a social problem, people high in socially prescribed perfectionism believe they do not have the ability to solve it. They are less likely to remain "cool, calm, and collected," and they are more likely to avoid the problem instead of dealing with it directly. Not only did these findings replicate in a second study, but they remained significant after controlling for both anxiety and depression. The study was correlational, so it is not clear what the direction of causality would be. The trait of socially prescribed perfectionism may lead people to develop negative orientations to problem-solving situations. If a person believes that others expect more from them than they are able to produce, or that others are judging them harshly for what they have produced, they may develop a belief that they cannot effectively solve problems. It is better to avoid them and it is awful when problems arise. On the other hand, it is possible that having such an orientation would lead someone to become perfectionistic. The mechanism by which having negative problem-solving reactions would lead to the development of high perceived expectations from others is unclear, however.

Interestingly, although socially prescribed perfectionism was associated with more negative problem orientations, it was not associated with any measures of social problem-solving skill (Flett, Hewitt, Blankstein, et al., 1996). Perfectionists appear to suffer no skill deficit, but instead they suffer from a problem in the interpretation of and reaction to social situations. This is consistent with our research on mistake monitoring and reactions to mistakes (Frost, Trepanier, Brown, & Heimberg, 1997; Frost et al., 1995). Perfectionists do not make mistakes more frequently, nor do they make more serious mistakes; however, they do engage in maladaptive patterns of self-evaluation, which, based on the findings just described, seem to include maladaptive coping orientations. One question that might be asked is: if perfectionists have such a bad orientation in their coping, why don't they develop poor problem-solving skills as a result? One answer might be that their perfectionism leads them to work much harder at coping, despite feeling bad about it. A more careful analysis of coping patterns of perfectionists and nonperfectionists might answer this question.

One conclusion to be drawn from this research is that MEC perfectionism is associated with social anxiety in normal populations, and PAS is *not* associated with social anxiety in normal populations, or at least not independently associated. An important question is whether this association is specific to social anxiety or whether it reflects a more global association between MEC and general anxiety. There are a number of studies showing correlations between MEC perfectionism and other types of anxiety (Christensen, Danko, & Johnson, 1993; Deffenbacher, Zwemer, Whisman, Hill, & Sloan, 1986; Flett, Hewitt, Endler, & Tassone, 1995; Flett, Hewitt, & Dyck, 1989; Hankin, Roberts, & Gotlib, 1997). In addition to anxiety, other studies have reported the MEC dimensions of perfectionism to be correlated with worry (Meyer, Miller, Metzeger, & Borkovec, 1990), life stress (Dean, Range, & Goggin, 1996; Flett, Hewitt & Hallett, 1995; Fry, 1995; Hewitt, Flett, & Ediger, 1996), and obsessive-compulsive symptoms (Frost et al., 1990; Rhéaume, Freeston, Dugas, Letarte, & Ladouceur, 1995). Perfectionism, especially the MEC dimensions, seems to be related to most forms of anxiety, including social anxiety, in nonclinical populations.

A related issue concerns the extent to which the association overlaps with general psychopathology. The negative evaluative concern dimensions of perfectionism have been found to correlate with the more general constructs of negative affect (Frost et al., 1993; Minarik & Ahrens, 1996), as well as depression (Frost et al., 1990; Minarik & Ahrens, 1996) in nonclinical populations. In an attempt to determine the uniqueness of these relationships, Minarik and Ahrens (1996) measured both anxiety and depression, as well as the Frost MPS, in a small undergraduate sample. Although MEC subscales were correlated with both anxiety and depression, when depression was controlled in a regression analysis, MEC no longer predicted anxiety. However, when anxiety was controlled, MEC perfectionism dimensions still predicted significant variance in depression. Although this measure of anxiety was not social anxiety, it raises the possibility that the variance social anxiety shares with MEC is in common with variance shared with depression. In order to answer this question, Kawamura, Hunt, Frost, and DiBartolo (2001) measured a number of specific types of anxiety, including social anxiety, and depression. A multiple regression analysis using the perfectionism dimensions as predictor variables and the social anxiety measures as dependent variables was conducted. Depression scores were forced into the regression in the first step followed by the subscales from the Frost MPS. For the FNE, concerns over mistakes, doubts about actions, and personal standards predicted a significant amount of variance in social anxiety (17%) after the contribution of depression was removed. Concern over mistakes and doubts about actions were positively related to social anxiety, whereas personal standards was negatively related. For a second measure of social anxiety, concerns over mistakes and personal standards combined to predict a significant amount of variance (5%) after controlling for depression. Again, concern over mistakes was positively correlated with social anxiety, and personal standards was negatively related. In a similar vein, Flett, Hewitt, Blankstein, et al. (1996) controlled for depression (as well as anxiety) when examining the relationship between perfectionism and social problem-solving orientation. Socially prescribed perfectionism remained significantly associated with poor problem-solving orientation when the influence of depression was controlled. Their data suggest that the relationship between these dimensions of perfectionism and social anxiety among nonclinical subjects is not accounted for by shared variance with depression. They also indicate, that despite the absence of a zero-order correlation between personal standards and measures of social anxiety, personal standards accounts for a significant amount of variance in social anxiety after the shared variance with depression is removed.

In summary, the findings from nonclinical populations indicate that the MEC perfectionism is associated with social anxiety and related constructs (social problem-solving orientation). There are some data indicating that these relationships are not accounted for by general levels of anxiety (Flett et al., 1996) or depression (Flett et al., 1996; Kawamura et al., 2001). There is considerable evidence that MEC is related to other forms of anxiety in addition to social anxiety and general anxiety (Frost et al., 1990; Meyer et al., 1990; Rhéaume et al., 1995). The relationship between PAS and social anxiety is less consistent. In some cases, PAS has been positively correlated with social anxiety, in some cases it has been negatively correlated, and in others it has not been related at all. There is little evidence that PAS is positively correlated with social anxiety when MEC is controlled. However, this does not rule out the possibility that PAS may be a vulnerability or interacting factor (Besser, Flett, & Hewitt, 2004).

PERFECTIONISM IN PATIENTS WITH SOCIAL ANXIETY DISORDER

A number of studies have examined the relationship between perfectionism and social anxiety disorder (previously known as social phobia) using patient samples. Juster et al. (1996) compared 61 patients who requested treatment for, and were diagnosed with, social phobia to a group of 39 nondisordered community volunteers. All subjects completed the Frost MPS as well as multiple measures of social anxiety. Three interview-based measures of social anxiety were included in the study.

Comparison of social phobia and community control groups revealed significant differences on four of the six subscales of the Frost MPS. Participants with social phobia scored higher on concern over mistakes, doubts about actions, and parental criticism than the community controls. The community controls scored higher on the organization subscale. High concern over mistakes may set the stage for the cycle of fear and avoidance of social situations that is typical of social anxiety disorder (social phobia). High scores on the doubts about actions subscale are consistent with the self-presentation model of social anxiety (Schlenker & Leary, 1982) that hypothesizes that individuals with social anxiety disorder doubt their ability to create the desired effect in a social encounter. The association of parental criticism with social anxiety disorder is consistent with some research on family background and parental influence. The research suggests that the parents of patients with social anxiety disorder place greater emphasis on the opinions of others (Bruch, Heimberg, Berger, & Collins, 1989) and rely more on the use of shame to discipline (Bruch & Heimberg, 1994). In addition, the Juster et al. findings suggest that these parents are more critical.

Correlations between perfectionism subscales and measures of social anxiety, general anxiety, and depression were calculated using the group of individuals diagnosed with social phobia. Concern over mistakes and doubts about actions were the only subscales with significant correlations. Concern over mistakes was significantly correlated with two of the four self-report measures of social anxiety and one of the interview measures. Doubts about actions was correlated with three of the four self-report measures of social anxiety and all three of the interview measures. Thus, even in a sample with a restricted range, concern over mistakes and doubts about actions were associated with measures of social anxiety.

Consistent with other research indicating that perfectionism is associated with a wide variety of psychopathology (Antony, Purdon, Huta, & Swinson, 1998), in the Juster et al. study both concern over mistakes and doubts about actions were correlated with measures of general psychopathology as well. This suggests the possibility that the relationship between concern over mistakes, doubts about actions, and social anxiety observed in the Juster et al. study could be accounted for by the shared variance with general psychopathology. However, the analysis revealed that concern over mistakes, doubts about actions, and personal standards accounted for a significant amount of variance in social anxiety beyond that accounted for by depression and general psychopathology. While concern over mistakes and doubts about actions were positively associated with social anxiety, personal standards was negatively associated. These findings using a sample of individuals diagnosed with social phobia (social anxiety disorder) mirror those of Kawamura et al.

(2001). The relationship between perfectionism subscales and social anxiety appears to be independent of the relationship between perfectionism and general psychopathology.

Lundh and Öst (1996) compared patients diagnosed with social phobia and age-, sex-, and education-matched controls. Consistent with the findings of Juster et al., the patients scored higher on concern over mistakes, doubts about actions, and parental criticism than the control subjects. Patients also had higher scores on parental expectations than controls. In addition, the concern over mistakes subscale correlated significantly with the interference produced by socially threatening words on the modified Stroop task.

Saboonchi, Lundh, and Öst (1999) replicated the Saboonchi and Lundh (1997) findings by comparing patients diagnosed with social phobia and panic disorder to community controls. Patients with social phobia had higher scores on concern over mistakes, doubts about actions, and parental criticism than community controls. These differences remained after controlling for public self-consciousness. Although social phobia patients had higher scores on concern over mistakes and doubts about actions than panic disorder patients, these differences disappeared when variance in common with public self-consciousness was controlled.

Bieling and Alden (1997) also compared individuals with diagnosed social phobia (social anxiety disorder) with nonanxious community controls, this time using Hewitt and Flett's MPS. Consistent with other studies, patients with social phobia scored higher on socially prescribed perfectionism, but not on self-oriented perfectionism. Subjects met and talked to someone of the opposite sex and rated their standards for themselves on this task, their guesses about what the other people would expect of them in the task, and their "social self-efficacy," or how well they thought they would handle the social situation. Patients in this study also had significantly lower levels of social self-efficacy than community controls. Although socially prescribed perfectionism was not related to social self-efficacy, it was related to the perception of what other people would expect of them on the task, particularly among social phobics. Among the participants diagnosed with social phobia, socially prescribed perfectionism was positively associated with ratings of other people's standards. No such relationship was observed among control subjects.

This study reveals more specific information about the relationship between perfectionism and social anxiety disorder. Social anxiety disorder is characterized by reduced perception of social self-efficacy, but MEC perfectionism is not. MEC perfectionism was associated with the perception of other people's standards among social phobics but not among controls. It would appear that only a subset of people with social anxiety disorder, those high in socially prescribed perfectionism, perceive others as setting high standards for them. It is surprising that ratings of others' expectations were not related to perfectionism among control subjects. Socially prescribed perfectionism is thought to be a measure of the perception of other people's expectations and has been found to be valid in numerous investigations involving nonclinical populations (Hewitt & Flett, 1991a, 1991b).

There is a consistency across these studies in the suggestion that, compared to nonanxious controls, individuals with social anxiety disorder are more perfectionistic, especially in their excessive concern over mistakes, their doubts about the quality of their performance, their view of their parents as hypercritical, and their tendency to believe that others are overly demanding in setting high standards for them. However, other studies have found similar differences in perfectionism dimensions when comparing other anxiety-disordered patients to community controls. For instance, Frost and Steketee (1997) found both obsessive-compulsive disorder (OCD) and panic disorder patients to score higher on concern over mistakes than community controls. Doubts about actions scores were higher for OCD subjects than panic subjects and community controls, who did not differ from each other. Hewitt and Flett (1991b) found that a group of mixed anxiety disorder patients differed from community controls on socially prescribed perfectionism but not self-oriented perfectionism.

There are a few studies examining differences among the anxiety disorders. Boivin, Todorov, and Marchand (1996) compared 82 agoraphobics and 40 OCD patients with 34 individuals diagnosed with social phobia (social anxiety disorder) on levels of perfectionism using both the Frost MPS and the Hewitt and Flett MPS. Participants with social phobia had higher concern over mistakes and parental criticism scores than agoraphobic subjects, whereas the OCD subjects had higher doubts about actions scores and self-oriented perfectionism than the other two groups. There were no differences among these groups on personal standards, parental expectations, and organization. Concern over mistakes, doubts about actions, and parental criticism scores for participants with social phobia were comparable to or higher than the data for this group reported by Juster et al. and Lundh and Öst. These scores also were considerably higher that the control subjects in either of these studies.

Antony et al. (1998) compared individuals with social phobia (social anxiety disorder), panic disorder, OCD, and specific phobia to nonclinical control participants. Subjects completed both the Frost MPS and the Hewitt and Flett MPS. Comparisons among these groups supported other findings that selected dimensions of perfectionism were elevated across most of the anxiety disorders. Specifically, concern over mistakes, doubts about actions, and socially prescribed perfectionism were elevated among individuals with OCD, panic disorder, and social phobia compared to community controls. Parental criticism was also elevated among the patients with social phobia. There was no elevation among patients with specific phobias. Comparisons among the anxiety disorder patient groups revealed that individuals diagnosed with social phobia scored higher on concern over mistakes than the panic disorder patients and the OCD patients. The patients with social phobia were also significantly higher in parental criticism and socially prescribed perfectionism than the OCD patients, and they were higher than the panic disorder patients on doubts about actions.

Lundh et al. (2008) used the FMPS to conduct cluster analyses of patients with social phobia (social anxiety disorder), panic disorder, and nonclinical controls. They found three high perfectionism clusters characterized by high MEC as well as high PAS, all of which were over-represented in the group with social anxiety disorder compared to the nonclinical group. One cluster characterized by high PAS and low MEC was found to be under-represented in the group with social anxiety disorder and over-represented in the nonclinical group. These findings support the Alden et al. (1994) and Lundh (2004) hypothesis that high PAS is adaptive when MEC is low (i.e., nonperfectionism is accepted), but maladaptive when combined with high MEC.

The findings comparing levels of perfectionism of social anxiety disorder patients to nonclinical samples are quite consistent. Individuals with social anxiety disorder have higher levels of MEC, specifically concern over mistakes, doubts about actions, parental criticism, and socially prescribed perfectionism. The PAS dimension of perfectionism (personal standards, parental expectations, and self-oriented perfectionism) do not appear to characterize individuals with social anxiety disorder, except when they are accompanied by high MEC. When the variance associated with depression and general psychopathology is controlled, there is some indication that PAS is negatively correlated with social anxiety (Juster et al., 1996). Finally, at least some data suggest that patients with social anxiety disorder score significantly higher on concern over mistakes and doubts about actions than other anxiety disorder patients.

PERFECTIONISM IN SOCIAL/EVALUATIVE CONTEXTS

The studies reviewed thus far clearly show a strong association between MEC perfectionism and social anxiety. Many of these studies rely on retrospective self-reports of social anxiety, however. Such accounts may be subject to distortion, or they may inaccurately reflect the processes that occur during socially threatening episodes. Important information about perfectionism and social anxiety can be gained by examining social-evaluative contexts. The following studies have examined perfectionism under conditions of social-evaluative threat. They provide a clearer idea of how perfectionism operates in everyday social contexts.

In one of the first studies of this sort, subjects high or low in overall perfectionism using the Frost MPS were assigned to a high or low threat condition by Frost and Marten (1990). The threat involved a writing task in which the evaluative nature of the task was emphasized. Under low evaluative threat, participants high in concern over mistakes did not differ from those low in concern over mistakes in their level of negative affect. However, under high evaluative threat, they reported significantly more negative affect. High-concern-over-mistakes participants' writing was judged to be of poorer quality than that of participants low in concern over mistakes, and the quality difference could not be accounted for by differences in negative affect. Frost and Marten hypothesize that high-MEC perfectionists' fear of evaluation may set in place a chain of events that leads to poorer performance on tasks that involve skills that require practice and feedback to develop. Specifically, they suggest that MEC perfectionists avoid most evaluative contexts, including those involving writing. That is, they are so afraid of having others think badly of their abilities that they avoid situations in which other people would review and criticize their writing. This results in less practice at writing and fewer opportunities to learn from feedback provided by others. Consequently, writing skills do not develop as they should. This leads to a host of other hypotheses about the role of social/evaluative threat and avoidance behavior. If true, other tasks requiring practice and feedback in which other people observe performance should be similarly affected. Although the writing task in this study was not a social task, the evaluative threat manipulation was presumed to be a social one in that other people would be evaluating and criticizing one's writing. Other studies examine social contexts more directly.

A prominent feature of social phobia is a fear of performing in front of others. There are a number of studies examining the influence of perfectionism on cognition, affect, and behavior during some kind of performance. The kinds of performance range from everyday mistakes to athletic competition. Most of these studies focus on thoughts, anxiety, and behavior during a public performance.

Athletics is one arena in which performance anxiety can play a dramatic role. Investigators have hypothesized that perfectionistic athletes fear mistakes and failure to such an extent that their enjoyment of a sport and their performance in it are diminished (Bunker & Williams, 1986; Burns, 1980). Frost and Henderson (1991) measured perfectionism and several features of athletic competition among female college athletes. Perfectionistic concern over mistakes and doubts about actions were highly correlated with a failure orientation toward sports. This orientation reflects a tendency to focus on failure and mistakes in performance. Items on this measure include "When I play poorly, I feel ashamed," and "I worry about choking in a big game." In contrast, personal standards from the Frost MPS was highly correlated with a success orientation. This orientation is reflected in items such as "I strive for perfection in my game" and "I have dreams of being the best in my sport." Although concern over mistakes was correlated with success orientation and personal standards with failure orientation, the magnitudes of these correlations were much smaller.

Concern over mistakes and doubts about actions were also highly correlated with a number of negative reactions to mistakes made during competition; specifically, social concerns (e.g., "I let the team down"), personal disappointment ("I feel I let myself down"), attentional focus ("I feel pressure to overcome my mistake"), forgetting ("I have a difficult time forgetting about my mistake"), and images ("Images of my mistake control my mind for the rest of the competition"). None of the other FMPS subscales were related to any of the reactions to mistakes in any consistent way. Corroborating these relationships were coaches' ratings of the athletes' ability to react to mistakes, pressure, and competition. Athletes high in concern over mistakes and doubts about actions were rated by their coaches as not recovering well from mistakes, as being less able to adapt quickly, as performing more poorly under pressure, and as not accepting criticism well compared with subjects with lower scores on these scales.

In addition to the general orientation to sports, the reaction to mistakes during competition, and the coaches' ratings, subjects indicated the frequency with which they had each set of thoughts or feelings in the 24-hour period before a competition. Each of the thoughts or feelings was examined separately. Concern over mistakes was highly correlated ($r = 0.61$) with the item "I worry about how the audience will perceive me." Concern over mistakes was also correlated with fears of making a mistake, lack of self-confidence, images of mistakes clogging the mind, and difficulty concentrating on other things. Personal standards, on the other hand, was correlated with dreams of perfection and thoughts about competition.

It is worth nothing here that the General Sports Orientation Questionnaire was originally designed with three subscales – success orientation, failure orientation, and focus on others. The focus on others subscale was designed to measure the tendency to focus on what other important people think about one's performance. Specifically, the items reflected a focus on worries about the evaluative thoughts of coaches, parents, and teammates. Unfortunately, this measure was so highly correlated with failure orientation that it was redundant. It is clear that, in the athletic context, failure orientation is basically a social phenomenon.

A number of subsequent studies have also found the PAS dimensions of perfectionism to be associated with success orientation that may improve performance, whereas MEC is associated with a failure orientation and self-deprecating attributions (Stoeber & Becker, 2008; Stoeber, Uphill, & Hotham, 2009). Stoeber and Becker (2008) reported that PAS was positively correlated with internal attributions for success in athletics but negatively correlated with internal attributions for failure. The opposite pattern was observed for MEC. High levels of MEC were associated with more internal attributions for failure and less internal attribution for success. The MEC dimension of perfectionism has also been found to be associated with burnout in elite athletes, whereas PAS negatively predicts burnout (Appleton, Hall, & Hill, 2009; Chen, Kee, Chen, & Tsai, 2008; Hill, Hall, Appleton, & Kozub, 2008).

In a similar type of study, Mor, Day, Flett, and Hewitt (1995) examined Hewitt and Flett's dimensions of perfectionism among a sample of professional performing artists. Both socially prescribed and self-oriented perfectionism were associated with higher debilitating performance anxiety and lower facilitating performance anxiety. Both of these dimensions were also associated with higher levels of somatic anxiety while performing, less happiness while performing, and lower goal satisfaction. As has been the case in other investigations, socially prescribed perfectionism was more highly correlated with these indices of social anxiety than self-oriented perfectionism.

Mor et al. (1995) suggest that the role of perfectionism in performance anxiety may be moderated by the extent to which performers believe they have the ability to control events. Regression analyses revealed significant interactions between self-oriented perfectionism and personal control on facilitating anxiety, debilitating anxiety, and goal satisfaction. There was only one significant interaction between socially prescribed perfectionism and personal control on goal satisfaction. In each of these interactions, there were no differences between subjects low in perfectionism who perceived themselves to have little control and subjects low in perfectionism who perceived themselves to have more control. Among subjects high in perfectionism, however, those experiencing low levels of personal control had more debilitating anxiety, less facilitating anxiety, and lower levels of goal satisfaction.

These findings are consistent with self-regulatory models (Bandura, 1986; Kowal & Pritchard, 1990), suggesting that low levels of perceived control lead self-oriented perfectionists to experience more negative affect and less goal satisfaction. It is interesting to note that the observed interactions with personal control were primarily for self-oriented perfectionism, even though it has been shown to be less directly related to anxiety generally (Frost & DiBartolo, 2002) and social phobia specifically (see earlier section). Perhaps the absence of observed correlations between self-oriented perfectionism and anxiety are misleading, and the relationship only becomes apparent when moderating variables are considered (Besser et al., 2004).

To examine another evaluative context, Alden et al. (1994) asked college students high or low in social anxiety to engage in a dyadic social interaction. After the interaction, subjects rated their own personal standards for success on the task, their perception of others' standards for them, their perceived social ability (self-efficacy), the frequency with which they evaluated their behavior during the task, and how important it was for them to meet their own and others' standards. Consistent with the other studies reviewed here, the socially anxious subjects scored higher on socially prescribed perfectionism but not on self-oriented perfectionism. They also rated themselves as having less social ability, but they did not differ on their perceptions of others' standards for them or on the importance of their own or other people's standards. The socially anxious subjects actually had lower personal standards than the nonanxious subjects.

Although social anxiety has been assumed to be associated with the perception of overly stringent expectations on the part of others, this study and that of Bieling and Alden (1997) failed to find that socially anxious people actually perceive others to set higher standards for them. If perfectionism is defined solely on the basis of the perception of others' standards for success, then social anxiety would seem not to be related to it. However, although many studies have described socially prescribed perfectionism as measuring the perception of overly demanding expectations from others, it is likely to encompass a somewhat broader construct such as MEC.

In examining what features of the self-regulatory process were related to perfectionism, Alden et al. (1994) found that only frequency of self-appraisal was associated with socially prescribed perfectionism. For self-oriented perfectionism the associations were more complex. Self-oriented perfectionism was related to the discrepancy between their own personal standards for success and their perceived abilities, as well as how important meeting their personal standards was to them. Although self-oriented perfectionism was associated with personal goals that exceeded their perceived social abilities, it was not associated with social anxiety.

More recently, Laurenti et al. (2008) found that socially prescribed perfectionism among college students was associated with a larger discrepancy between their ratings of other people's performance standards and their own self-efficacy ratings about an upcoming social encounter. Socially prescribed perfectionism was not related to the discrepancy or the frequency of negative self-statements at low levels of social anxiety. However, at high levels of social anxiety, high socially prescribed perfectionism was associated with a greater discrepancy between their beliefs about others' standards and their own self-efficacy, and it was also associated with a greater frequency of negative self-statements.

In a study examining reactions to mistakes, Frost et al. (1995) divided subjects into groups of high or low MEC (defined by the concern over mistakes subscale) and assigned them to perform a task characterized by frequent or infrequent mistakes. In the low-mistake-frequency condition, there was no difference between subjects with high MEC and those with low MEC on negative moods, confidence, or ratings of their beliefs that others would view them as less intelligent based on their performance. However, in the high-mistake-frequency condition, high-MEC participants reported significantly greater negative moods, lower confidence, and beliefs that others would view them as less intelligent based on their performance than low-MEC participants. Those with high MEC in both the low- and high-mistake-frequency conditions were less willing to share their results with others than those with low MEC. Interestingly, the mistake frequency manipulation did not change the willingness of those with low MEC to share their results. They were as willing to share the results of their performance with others after the high-mistake-frequency task as after the low-mistake-frequency task. Among those with high MEC, however, the high-mistake-frequency task significantly decreased subjects' willingness to share their results compared with the low-mistake-frequency task. These findings suggest that mistake-filled social contexts prime MEC perfectionistic reactions.

Several other features of this study are noteworthy. Those with high perfectionistic concern did not report making any more mistakes than those with low perfectionistic concern. This suggests that the definition of what is and is not a mistake is not affected by perfectionism and that concern over mistakes pertains to the evaluation of mistakes, not the threshold for detecting them.

Another finding of note was that high-MEC participants endorsed more personal imperatives (i.e., "should" statements) than those with low MEC. This have been important in theorizing about perfectionism (Burns, 1980; Hamachek, 1978; Pacht, 1984) and psychopathology (Beck, 1976; Ellis, 1962). The "tyranny of the should" was first described by Horney (1950) as a way to achieve perfection by generating a list of rigid dictates. Noncompliance with these dictates leads to self-blame, negative affect, and increased rigidity.

In a follow-up study, Frost et al. (1997) asked subjects high and low in MEC (concern over mistakes) to monitor their mistakes over a five-day period and to complete a brief evaluation sheet regarding each mistake. Consistent with the earlier study, those with high MEC did not record any more mistakes than those with low MEC. Also, independent ratings of each mistake by raters blind to subjects' levels of MEC failed to reveal any differences in the quality or severity of reported mistakes. However, the reactions of those with high and low MEC to their mistakes were quite different. Those with high concerns were more bothered by their mistakes, experienced more negative affect, and endorsed significantly more personal imperatives regarding their mistakes (e.g., "I should not have allowed this to happen"). They judged their mistakes to be more important and morally reprehensible than did those with low perfectionistic concerns. They were more worried about other people's reactions to their mistakes and wanted to keep them secret if possible. Interestingly, those with high MEC did not believe their mistakes caused more harm to others, but they believed their mistakes caused more harm to themselves than did the other group. This is interesting in the light of ratings by the high-MEC participants of the moral reprehensibility of their mistakes. The threat produced by their mistakes was to themselves and not to others.

Although both groups recalled similar numbers of mistakes at a two-week follow-up, those with high MEC thought more about and were more bothered by their mistakes during the two weeks than their counterparts were. It appears that the high-MEC participants ruminated more about their mistakes during the two weeks after the study. Perhaps, over time, people high in MEC ruminate over their mistakes and alter their assessments of their performance to conform to their negative self-evaluation.

PERFECTIONISM AND SOCIAL/EVALUATIVE AVOIDANCE

It is clear from the research reviewed so far that the central features of perfectionism related to social phobia are high-MEC dimensions such as excessive concern over mistakes, doubts about the quality of one's actions, and the perception that other people have excessively high expectations. These dimensions of perfectionism are not only related to measures of social anxiety in nonclinical populations; they also distinguish individuals with social anxiety disorder from other anxiety disorder patients and they predict negative affect (as well as other related variables) in social evaluative contexts. The PAS features of perfectionism (i.e., personal standards), although not directly related to social anxiety, have aspects that are inversely related when its association with MEC is partialled out. Beyond these effects, it is likely that these dimensions of perfectionism have an important impact on other social or self-evaluative behaviors. Hamachek (1978) suggests that perfectionists define themselves and their identity based on how others think of them. The only way to ensure acceptance is by being perfect. However, because this is impossible, perfectionists develop strategies to avoid rejection. Hamachek lists three such strategies: self-deprecation, shyness, and procrastination. The strategies for avoiding negative evaluation by others are, in all likelihood, not limited to these three. Any strategy that removes or avoids the threat of negative evaluation may be employed. The effects of such avoidance can be widespread. For instance, Frost and Marten (1990) hypothesized that MEC perfectionists avoid subjecting samples of their writing to scrutiny by others, thereby limiting their opportunities to benefit from feedback and practice. Several evaluation-avoidance strategies have been studied within the context of perfectionism.

Although Hamachek (1978) hypothesized that shyness would be an avoidance strategy of perfectionists, the relationship between shyness and perfectionism has yet to be established. Flett et al. (1996) found socially prescribed perfectionists scored higher on a measure of shyness, but Jackson, Towson, and Narduzzi (1997) failed to find self-oriented or socially prescribed perfectionism to predict shyness. However, in the Jackson et al. study, measures of the expectation of rejection and doubts about interpersonal competence were entered into the regression equation before the perfectionism measures. These constructs may have substantial overlap with certain features of perfectionism, such as concern over mistakes and doubts about actions.

In an early description of perfectionism, Burns (1980) suggested that perfectionists have a "disclosure phobia" based on their feelings that their personal flaws will be unacceptable to others and cause for rejection. Flett, Hewitt, and DeRosa (1996) further suggested that the loneliness and social anxiety they observed may result in perfectionists being less likely to disclose in personal situations. Both loneliness and social anxiety have been found to be associated with lower levels of self-disclosure (Meleshko & Alden, 1993). Based on the findings reviewed earlier, it could be expected that MEC perfectionists develop a set of behaviors that are meant to hide or mask potential mistakes. People possessing MEC tendencies fear negative evaluation so intensely that they will go to great lengths to avoid it, including avoidance of self-disclosure as well as active attempts to conceal.

Several studies have found evidence of a tendency to avoid disclosure among highly perfectionistic individuals. After their performance in a task characterized by a high number of mistakes, people high in MEC were less willing to share the results of their performance with others than people low in MEC (Frost et al., 1995). Even in a low-mistake-frequency task, those with high MEC were less willing to disclose, though the difference was considerably smaller. In a study of self-monitored mistakes (Frost et al., 1997), those with high MEC were more likely to keep their mistakes secret if possible. In another naturalistic study, those with high MEC were less likely to disclose their final exam score in a college class than those with low MEC (Brown et al., 1999). Interestingly, in this study, the combination of high PAS (personal standards) and meeting or exceeding present standards of performance were associated with greater willingness to disclose exam scores.

In a more recent study, Kawamura and Frost (2004) reported that MEC perfectionism was significantly correlated with self-concealment, general psychopathology, and distress. Self-concealment was significantly positively correlated with general psychopathology and distress; self-concealment also predicted distress. Self-concealment was associated with distress even after controlling for MEC, whereas MEC was not correlated with distress independent of self-concealment. Therefore, the findings suggest that self-concealment mediates the relationship between maladaptive perfectionism and distress. In a follow-up, DiBartolo et al. (2008) found that self-concealment and contingent self-worth partially mediated the relationship between MEC and social anxiety. Contingent self-worth fully mediated the relationship between PAS and social anxiety.

Self-concealment and lack of self-disclosure may have a host of negative consequences for MEC perfectionists. Frost and Marten (1990) have suggested one such consequence: the failure to develop important skills as a function of avoiding evaluative feedback. Extensive research has shown that the concealment of emotions has physical consequences (Pennebaker, 1985; Pennebaker, Kiecolt-Glaster, & Glaser, 1988). The loneliness findings of Flett et al. (1996) suggest that perfectionists may not develop social networks and intimate relationships as effectively, which may be related to disclosure and concealment. Furthermore, there are some findings of an association between sexual dysfunction and perfectionism, which may be related as well (DiBartolo & Barlow, 1996).

Another avoidance strategy related to concealment involves attempts to manage the impressions of others. Hewitt et al. (2003) suggest the existence of a perfectionistic self-presentation style that reflects underlying perfectionistic traits and is composed of three dimensions: perfectionistic self-promotion, the nondisplay of imperfection, and nondisclosure of imperfection. The nondisplay and nondisclosure of imperfection are very similar to self-concealment. They are associated with avoiding and concealing actions that are less than perfect (nondisplay) and verbal statements admitting imperfection (nondisclosure). In a series of studies on college students, Hewitt et al. (2003) found that these two perfectionistic self-presentation subscales accounted for significant variance in social phobia, but not general anxiety symptoms, after controlling for trait measures of perfectionism. Furthermore, both also predicted social interaction and social performance anxiety after controlling for self-presentation strategies (e.g., defensive, assertive).

Hewitt, Habke, Lee-Baggley, Sherry, & Flett (2008) examined reactions to a clinical interview among psychological/psychiatric clinic patients. Consistent with the notion that perfectionistic self-presentation is closely associated with social anxiety, nondisclosure of imperfection uniquely predicted ratings of the interviewer as threatening, post-interview dissatisfaction, overall negative self-evaluation of performance, and increases in heart rate when asked about mistakes.

A related type of impression-management strategy is self-handicapping, the purposeful undermining of performance when uncertain of one's ability to succeed. In doing so, the individual protects self-esteem by reinterpreting failure as a function of something other than lack of ability. Ferrari (1992) reported a significant correlation between the Burns Perfectionism Scale and a measure of self-handicapping. Similarly, Hobden and Pliner (1995) found that subjects high in socially prescribed perfectionism engaged in more self-handicapping behavior following noncontingent rather than contingent success, but only in public. Consistent with the conceptualization of this construct, this suggests they are more concerned with what others think than with their own view. Hobden and Pliner suggest this indicates a need to "self-present" rather than "self-protect." Self-oriented perfectionists self-handicapped in both public and private conditions, suggesting a need to do both.

The growing research on the relationship self-concealment has with social anxiety suggests that it is an important link between perfectionism and social anxiety. Although the direction of causality in this relationship is not clear, one possible implication of this research is that changing presentation style may be an effective therapeutic strategy for reducing social anxiety.

Other constructs related to both perfectionism and social anxiety may be important as well. Judgments about the probability and negative consequences of potential events have been found to be related to perfectionism. DiBartolo et al. (2007) reported that MEC predicted perceived probability and psychological costs associated with negative events. Furthermore, perceived probability significantly mediated the relationships between MEC and social anxiety, depression, anxiety, and stress, whereas psychological costs only mediated the relationship between MEC and social anxiety. Neither mediated the relationship between PAS and social anxiety.

Yet another evaluation-avoidance strategy is procrastination. By procrastinating, the perfectionist can avoid negative evaluation as long as possible. Indeed, Horney (1950) suggested that perfectionists dread starting any project or working toward a goal because of the potential negative consequences. A number of studies support the hypothesis that perfectionism leads to procrastination. Frost et al. (1990) found the severity of procrastination correlated with concern over mistakes, doubts about actions, and parental criticism. Frequency of procrastination was positively correlated with parental criticism and negatively correlated with parental expectations and organization. All the Frost et al. MPS dimensions were correlated with fear of failure as a reason for procrastination. Concern over mistakes, doubts about actions, and both parental dimensions were also positively correlated with task aversiveness. Stoeber (1998) also found concern over mistakes and doubts about actions to be positively correlated with procrastination, whereas organization was negatively correlated with it.

Using the Hewitt and Flett MPS, Saddler and Sacks (1993) found socially prescribed perfectionism, but not self-oriented perfectionism, to be correlated with procrastination. Flett, Blankstein, Hewitt, and Koledin (1992) found socially prescribed perfectionism to be correlated with generalized procrastination, frequency of academic procrastination, the extent to which procrastination is a problem, and fear of failure. Self-oriented and other-oriented perfectionism had only one small correlation with fear of failure. Using a multiple regression strategy, Martin, Flett, Hewitt, Krames, and Szanto (1996) found the Hewitt and Flett MPS accounted for 13% of the variance in procrastination scores. Socially prescribed perfectionism was positively associated with procrastination, whereas self-oriented perfectionism was negatively associated with it. Ferrari (1992) factor-analyzed measures of social anxiety, perfectionism, self-handicapping, and self-presentation among samples of procrastinators and nonprocrastinators. Among the procrastinators, perfectionism loaded with measures of social anxiety, acquisitive and protective self-presentation, and self-handicapping. Among the nonprocrastinators, perfectionism loaded with measures of acquisitive self-presentation. Ferrari concludes that, for procrastinators, "perfect behavior may be a strategic act of self-presentation aimed at 'getting along' with others," but among nonprocrastinators "it is a striving for excellence motivated by 'getting ahead' of others" (p. 75).

A little-studied aspect of social interactions in social phobia concerns the evaluation of social events. Laposa, Cassin, and Rector (2010) found that, among social phobics, perfectionism was associated with the negative interpretation of positive social events. Perhaps perfectionism contributes both to the avoidance of potentially negative social events and the absence of reward from positive social events.

THE EFFECT OF TREATMENT FOR SOCIAL PHOBIA ON PERFECTIONISM

Only a small number of studies have examined the role of perfectionism in the treatment of social anxiety disorder. Two issues have been addressed: whether perfectionism changes with treatment of social anxiety disorder and whether perfectionism predicts treatment outcomes. Lundh and Öst (2001) examined the effect of CBT on perfectionism in a sample of 24 social anxiety disorder patients. Subjects were assigned to one of three different treatments: individual

CBT, group CBT, or self-help. Patients showed significant reductions in doubts about actions, concern over mistakes, personal standards, and parental criticism subscales of the Frost MPS. At post-treatment, those classified as treatment responders (75% of the sample) reduced their Frost MPS subscale scores to nonclinical levels, but only because their pretreatment scores were lower than those of nonresponders. Treatment nonresponders showed reductions in perfectionism subscales comparable to those of treatment responders. The results of the Lundh and Öst study indicate that CBT for social anxiety disorder reduces both MEC and PAS perfectionism as measured by the Frost MPS, even when the treatment does not impact social anxiety.

Rosser, Issakidis, and Peters (2003) compared 61 outpatients enrolled in group CBT for social anxiety disorder on pre- and post-treatment measures of perfectionism (Frost MPS). Concern over mistakes (Frost MPS) decreased significantly from pre- to post-treatment, but pretreatment concern over mistakes did not predict outcome on social anxiety measures as would be expected based on Lundh and Öst (2001).

Ashbaugh et al. (2007) expanded upon the findings of Rosser et al. (2003) and Lundh and Öst (2001) to further examine the role perfectionism plays in predicting treatment outcome. One hundred and seven outpatients with a principle diagnosis of social anxiety disorder participated in 12 sessions of CBT for social anxiety disorder. In addition, participants completed a battery of questionnaires that included the Frost MPS and measures of social anxiety and general psychopathology at pre- and post-treatment. Participants' social anxiety decreased significantly from pre- to post-treatment. Depression, anxiety, and stress were also significantly decreased from pre- to post-treatment. Post-treatment scores on the Frost MPS concern over mistakes and doubts about actions subscales significantly decreased from pretreatment levels.

To determine whether perfectionism predicted changes in social anxiety, residual change scores were calculated for FMPS total and subscales. Doubts about actions residual change scores predicted change in social anxiety post-treatment even after controlling for pretreatment social anxiety and general psychopathology. None of the dimensions of perfectionism mediated changes in social anxiety.

In summary, the results from the treatment outcome studies indicate that CBT designed for social anxiety disorder is effective in reducing both MEC and PAS, but there is limited evidence that high MEC interferes with treatment for social phobia.

SUMMARY AND CONCLUSIONS

A review of the evidence suggests that concern about social evaluation and scrutiny are concepts closely related to both social anxiety disorder and MEC perfectionism. Specifically, there is ample evidence that certain domains of perfectionism, those characterized by MEC, are related to social anxiety in normals, social anxiety disorder in patients, and reactions to social-evaluative threat. These relationships cannot be accounted for by depression or negative affect. In fact, there is evidence that PAS is negatively associated with social anxiety when the influence of depression is controlled. Although more research is needed, there is some reason to suspect that MEC leads to an avoidant style of coping with social threat that involves attempts at self-concealment, procrastination, and self-handicapping. These can be seen as attempts to avoid scrutiny and negative evaluation by others. They may lead to a myriad of negative consequences, including inhibition of skill development (i.e., writing, athletic performance), problems in developing interpersonal relationships (i.e., due to disclosure phobia), anxiety, and depression. A more detailed study of avoidance behavior among perfectionists would clarify the scope and consequences of such behavior, and it may be necessary for the development of treatment strategies for MEC perfectionism.

REFERENCES

Alden, L., Bieling, P., & Wallace, S. (1994). Perfectionism in an interpersonal context: A self-regulation analysis of dysphoria and social anxiety. *Cognitive Therapy and Research*, *18*(4), 297–316. doi:10.1007/BF02357507.

Alden, L., Ryder, A., & Mellings, T. (2002). Perfectionism in the context of social fears: Toward a two-component model. *Perfectionism: Theory, research, and treatment* (pp. 373–391). Washington, DC: American Psychological Association. doi:10.1037/10458–015.

American Psychiatric Association. (1994). *Diagnostic and statistical manual of mental disorders* (4th ed.) (DSM-IV). Washington, DC: Author.

Antony, M., Purdon, C., Huta, V., & Swinson, R. (1998). Dimensions of perfectionism across the anxiety disorders. *Behaviour Research and Therapy*, *36*(12), 1143–1154. doi:10.1016/S0005-7967(98)00083-7.

Appleton, P., Hall, H., & Hill, A. (2009). Relations between multidimensional perfectionism and burnout in junior-elite male athletes. *Psychology of Sport and Exercise*, *10*(4), 457–465. doi:10.1016/j.psychsport.2008.12.006.

Ashbaugh, A., Antony, M., Liss, A., Summerfeldt, L., McCabe, R., & Swinson, R. (2007). Changes in perfectionism following cognitive-behavioral treatment for social phobia. *Depression and Anxiety*, *24*(3), 169–177. doi:10.1002/da.20219.

Bandura, A. (1986). *Social foundations of thought and action: A social cognitive theory*. Englewood Cliffs, NJ: Prentice Hall.

Beck, A. T. (1976). *Cognitive therapy and the emotional disorders*. New York: International Universities Press.

Beck, A. T., & Emery, G. (1985). *Anxiety disorders and phobias: A cognitive perspective*. New York: Basic Books.

Besser, A., Flett, G., & Hewitt, P. (2004). Perfectionism, cognition, and affect in response to performance failure vs success. *Journal of Rational-Emotive & Cognitive Behavior Therapy*, *22*(4), 301–328. doi:10.1023/B:JORE.0000047313.35872.5c.

Bieling, P., & Alden, L. (1997). The consequences of perfectionism for patients with social phobia. *British Journal of Clinical Psychology*, *36*(3), 387–395.

Bieling, P., Israeli, A., & Antony, M. (2004). Is perfectionism good, bad, or both? Examining models of the perfectionism construct. *Personality and Individual Differences, 36*(6), 1373–1385. doi:10.1016/S0191-8869(03)00235-6.

Blankstein, K., Flett, G., Hewitt, P., & Eng, A. (1993). Dimensions of perfectionism and irrational fears: An examination with the fear survey schedule. *Personality and Individual Differences, 15*(3), 323–328. doi:10.1016/0191-8869(93)90223-P.

Boivin, I., Todorov, C., & Marchand, A. (1996). *Perfectionism in three anxiety disorders.* Paper presented at the 10th World Congress of Psychiatry, Madrid, Spain.

Brown, E., Heimberg, R., Frost, R., Makris, G., Juster, H., & Leung, A. (1999). Relationship of perfectionism to affect, expectations, attributions and performance in the classroom. *Journal of Social & Clinical Psychology, 18*(1), 98–120.

Bruch, M., & Heimberg, R. (1994). Differences in perceptions of parental and personal characteristics between generalized and nongeneralized social phobics. *Journal of Anxiety Disorders, 8*(2), 155–168. doi:10.1016/0887-6185(94)90013-2.

Bruch, M., Heimberg, R., Berger, P., & Collins, T. (1989). Social phobia and perceptions of early parental and personal characteristics. *Anxiety Research, 2*(1), 57–65.

Bunker, L., & Williams, J. M. (1986). Cognitive techniques for improving performance. In J. M. Williams (Ed.), *Applied sport psychology* (pp. 225–242). Mountainview, CA: Mayfield.

Burns, D. (1980). The perfectionist's script for self-defeat. *Psychology Today, November*, 34–52.

Chen, L., Kee, Y., Chen, M., & Tsai, Y. (2008). Relation of perfectionism with athletes' burnout: Further examination. *Perceptual and Motor Skills, 106*(3), 811–820. doi:10.2466/PMS.106.3.811-820.

Christensen, B., Danko, G., & Johnson, R. (1993). Neuroticism and the belief that one is being scrutinized and evaluated by others. *Personality and Individual Differences, 15*(3), 349–350. doi:10.1016/0191-8869(93)90228-U.

Clark, D., & Wells, A. (1995). A cognitive model of social phobia. *Social phobia: Diagnosis, assessment, and treatment.* New York: Guilford Press, pp. 69–93.

Dean, P., Range, L., & Goggin, W. (1996). The escape theory of suicide in college students: Testing a model that includes perfectionism. *Suicide and Life-Threatening Behavior, 26*(2), 181–186.

Deffenbacher, J., Zwemer, W., Whisman, M., Hill, R., & Sloan, R. (1986). Irrational beliefs and anxiety. *Cognitive Therapy and Research, 10*, 281–292. doi:10.1007/BF01173466.

DiBartolo, P., & Barlow, D. (1996). Perfectionism, marital satisfaction, and contributing factors to sexual dysfunction in men with erectile disorder and their spouses. *Archives of Sexual Behavior, 25*(6), 581–588. doi:10.1007/BF02437840.

DiBartolo, P., Li, C., Averett, S., Skotheim, S., Smith, L., Raney, C., et al. (2007). The relationship of perfectionism to judgmental bias and psychopathology. *Cognitive Therapy and Research, 31*(5), 573–587. doi:10.1007/s10608-006-9112-z.

DiBartolo, P., Li, C., & Frost, R. (2008). How do the dimensions of perfectionism relate to mental health? *Cognitive Therapy and Research, 32*(3), 401–417. doi:10.1007/s10608-007-9157-7.

Dunkley, D., Blankstein, K., Masheb, R., & Grilo, C. (2006). Personal standards and evaluative concerns dimensions of 'clinical' perfectionism: A reply to Shafran et al. (2002, 2003) and Hewitt et al. (2003). *Behaviour Research and Therapy, 44*(1), 63–84. doi:10.1016/j.brat.2004.12.004.

Ellis, A. (1962). *Reason and emotion in psychotherapy.* New York: Lyle Stuart.

Ferrari, J. (1992). Procrastinators and perfect behavior: An exploratory factor analysis of self-presentation, self-awareness, and self-handicapping components. *Journal of Research in Personality, 26*(1), 75–84. doi:10.1016/0092-6566(92)90060-H.

Flett, G., Blankstein, K., Hewitt, P., & Koledin, S. (1992). Components of perfectionism and procrastination in college students. *Social Behavior and Personality*, *20*(2), 85–94. doi:10.2224/sbp.1992.20.2.85.

Flett, G., Hewitt, P., Blankstein, K., Solnik, M., & Van Brunschot, M. (1996). Perfectionism, social problem-solving ability, and psychological distress. *Journal of Rational-Emotive & Cognitive Behavior Therapy*, *14*(4), 245–275. doi:10.1007/BF02238139.

Flett, G., Hewitt, P., & Dyck, D. (1989). Self-oriented perfectionism, neuroticism and anxiety. *Personality and Individual Differences*, *10*(7), 731–735. doi:10.1016/0191-8869(89)90119-0.

Flett, G., Hewitt, P., Endler, N., & Tassone, C. (1995). Perfectionism and components of state and trait anxiety. *Current Psychology*, *13*(4), 326–350.

Flett, G., Hewitt, P., & Hallett, C. (1995). Perfectionism and job stress in teachers. *Canadian Journal of School Psychology*, *11*(1), 32–42.

Flett, G., Sawatzky, D., & Hewitt, P. (1995). Dimensions of perfectionism and goal commitment: A further comparison of two perfectionism measures. *Journal of Psychopathology and Behavioral Assessment*, *17*(2), 111–124. doi:10.1007/BF02229013.

Flett, G. L., Hewitt, P. L., & DeRosa, T. (1996). Dimensions of perfectionism, psychosocial adjustment, and social skills. *Personality and Individual Differences*, *20*(2), 143–150.

Frost, R., & DiBartolo, P. (2002). Perfectionism, anxiety, and obsessive-compulsive disorder. In *Perfectionism: Theory, research, and treatment* (pp. 373–391). Washington, DC: American Psychological Association. doi:10.1037/10458-015.

Frost, R., & Henderson, K. (1991). Perfectionism and reactions to athletic competition. *Journal of Sport & Exercise Psychology*, *13*(4), 323–335.

Frost, R., Heimberg, R., Holt, C., Mattia, J., & Neubauer, A. (1993). A comparison of two measures of perfectionism. *Personality and Individual Differences*, *14*(1), 119–126. doi:10.1016/0191-8869(93)90181-2.

Frost, R., & Marten, P. (1990). Perfectionism and evaluative threat. *Cognitive Therapy and Research*, *14*(6), 559–572. doi:10.1007/BF01173364.

Frost, R., & Steketee, G. (1997). Perfectionism in obsessive-compulsive disorder patients. *Behaviour Research and Therapy*, *35*(4), 291–296. doi:10.1016/S0005-7967(96)00108-8.

Frost, R., Marten, P., Lahart, C., & Rosenblate, R. (1990). The dimensions of perfectionism. *Cognitive Therapy and Research*, *14*(5), 449–468.

Frost, R., Trepanier, K., Brown, E., & Heimberg, R. (1997). Self-monitoring of mistakes among subjects high and low in perfectionistic concern over mistakes. *Cognitive Therapy and Research*, *21*(2), 209–222. doi:10.1023/A:1021884713550.

Frost, R., Turcotte, T. A., Heimberg, R. G., Mattia, J. I., Holt, C. S., & Hope, D. A. (1995). Reactions to mistakes among subjects high and low in perfectionistic concern over mistakes. *Cognitive Therapy and Research*, *19*(2), 195–205.

Fry, P. (1995). Perfectionism, humor, and optimism as moderators of health outcomes and determinants of coping styles of women executives. *Genetic, Social, and General Psychology Monographs*, *121*(2), 211–245.

Hamachek, D. E. (1978). Psychodynamics of normal and neurotic perfectionism. *Psychology*, *15*(1), 27–33.

Hankin, B., Roberts, J., & Gotlib, I. (1997). Elevated self-standards and emotional distress during adolescence: Emotional specificity and gender differences. *Cognitive Therapy and Research*, *21*(6), 663–680.

Hewitt, P. L., & Flett, G. L. (1991a). Dimensions of perfectionism in unipolar depression. *Journal of Abnormal Psychology*, *100*(1), 98–101.

Hewitt, P. L., & Flett, G. L. (1991b). Perfectionism in the self and social contexts: conceptualization, assessment, and association with psychopathology. *Journal of Personality and Social Psychology*, *60*(3), 456–470.

Hewitt, P. L., Flett, G. L., & Ediger, E. (1996). Perfectionism and depression: Longitudinal assessment of a specific vulnerability hypothesis. *Journal of Abnormal Psychology*, *105*(2), 276–280.

Hewitt, P., Flett, G., Sherry, S., Habke, M., Parkin, M., Lam, R. W., et al. (2003). The interpersonal expression of perfection: Perfectionistic self-presentation and psychological distress. *Journal of Personality and Social Psychology*, *84*(6), 1303–1325. doi:10.1037/0022-3514.84.6.1303.

Hewitt, P., Habke, A., Lee-Baggley, D., Sherry, S., & Flett, G. (2008). The impact of perfectionistic self-presentation on the cognitive, affective, and physiological experience of a clinical interview. *Psychiatry: Interpersonal and Biological Processes*, *71*(2), 93–122. doi:10.1521/psyc.2008.71.2.93.

Hill, A., Hall, H., Appleton, P., & Kozub, S. (2008). Perfectionism and burnout in junior elite soccer players: The mediating influence of unconditional self-acceptance. *Psychology of Sport and Exercise*, *9*(5), 630–644. doi:10.1016/j.psychsport.2007.09.004.

Hobden, K., & Pliner, P. (1995). Self-handicapping and dimensions of perfectionism: Self-presentation vs self-protection. *Journal of Research in Personality*, *29*(4), 461–474. doi:10.1006/jrpe.1995.1027.

Hollender, M. (1965). Perfectionism. *Comprehensive Psychiatry*, *6*(2), 94–103. doi:10.1016/S0010-440X(65)80016-5.

Horney, K. (1950). *Neurosis and human growth; The struggle toward self-realization*. Oxford: W. W. Norton.

Jackson, T., Towson, S., & Narduzzi, K. (1997). Predictors of shyness: A test of variables associated with self-presentational models. *Social Behavior and Personality*, *25*(2), 149–154. doi:10.2224/sbp.1997.25.2.149.

Juster, H. R., Heimberg, R. G., Frost, R. O., Holt, C. S., Mattia, J. I., & Faccenda, K. (1996). Social phobia and perfectionism. *Personality and Individual Differences*, *21*(3), 403–410.

Kawamura, K., & Frost, R. (2004). Self-concealment as a mediator in the relationship between perfectionism and psychological distress. *Cognitive Therapy and Research*, *28*(2), 183–191.

Kawamura, K. Y., Hunt, S. L., Frost, R. O., & DiBartolo, P. M. (2001). Perfectionism, anxiety, and depression: Are the relationships independent? *Cognitive Therapy and Research*, *25*(3), 291–301.

Kowal, A., & Pritchard, D. (1990). Psychological characteristics of children who suffer from headache: A research note. *Journal of Child Psychology and Psychiatry*, *31*(4), 637–649. doi:10.1111/j.1469-7610.1990.tb00803.x.

Laposa, J., Cassin, S., & Rector, N. (2010). Interpretation of positive social events in social phobia: An examination of cognitive correlates and diagnostic distinction. *Journal of Anxiety Disorders*, *24*, 203–210. doi:10.1016/j.janxdis.2009.10.009.

Laurenti, H., Bruch, M., & Haase, R. (2008). Social anxiety and socially prescribed perfectionism: Unique and interactive relationships with maladaptive appraisal of interpersonal situations. *Personality and Individual Differences*, *45*(1), 55–61. doi:10.1016/j.paid.2008.02.018.

Lundh, L., & Öst, L. (1996). Stroop interference, self-focus and perfectionism in social phobics. *Personality and Individual Differences*, *20*(6), 725–731. doi:10.1016/0191-8869(96)00008-6.

Lundh, L., & Öst, L. (2001). Attentional bias, self-consciousness and perfectionism in social phobia before and after cognitive-behaviour therapy. *Scandinavian Journal of Behaviour Therapy*, *30*(1), 4–16. doi:10.1080/02845710130014042[8].

Lundh, L. (2004). Perfectionism and acceptance. *Journal of Rational-Emotive & Cognitive Behavior Therapy*, *22*(4), 255–269. doi:10.1023/B:JORE.0000047311.12864.27.

Lundh, L., Saboonchi, F., & Wångby, M. (2008). The role of personal standards in clinically significant perfectionism. A person-oriented approach to the study of patterns of perfectionism. *Cognitive Therapy and Research, 32*(3), 333–350. doi:10.1007/s10608-006-9109-7.

Martin, T., Flett, G., Hewitt, P., Krames, L., & Szanto, G. (1996). Personality correlates of depression and health symptoms: A test of a self-regulation model. *Journal of Research in Personality, 30*(2), 264–277. doi:10.1006/jrpe.1996.0017.

Meleshko, K., & Alden, L. (1993). Anxiety and self-disclosure: Toward a motivational model. *Journal of Personality and Social Psychology, 64*(6), 1000–1009. doi:10.1037/0022-3514.64.6.1000.

Meyer, T., Miller, M., Metzger, R., & Borkovec, T. (1990). Development and validation of the Penn State Worry Questionnaire. *Behaviour Research and Therapy, 28*(6), 487–495. doi:10.1016/0005-7967(90)90135-6.

Minarik, M., & Ahrens, A. (1996). Relations of eating and symptoms of depression and anxiety to the dimensions of perfectionism among undergraduate women. *Cognitive Therapy and Research, 20*(2), 155–169. doi:10.1007/BF02228032.

Mor, S., Day, H., Flett, G., & Hewitt, P. (1995). Perfectionism, control, and components of performance anxiety in professional artists. *Cognitive Therapy and Research, 19*(2), 207–225. doi:10.1007/BF02229695.

Pacht, A. (1984). Reflections on perfection. *American Psychologist, 39*(4), 386–390. doi:10.1037/0003-066X.39.4.386.

Pennebaker, J. (1985). Traumatic experience and psychosomatic disease: Exploring the roles of behavioural inhibition, obsession, and confiding. *Canadian Psychology/Psychologie canadienne, 26*(2), 82–95. doi:10.1037/h0080025.

Pennebaker, J., Kiecolt-Glaser, J., & Glaser, R. (1988). Disclosure of traumas and immune function: Health implications for psychotherapy. *Journal of Consulting and Clinical Psychology, 56*(2), 239–245. doi:10.1037/0022-006X.56.2.239.

Rapee, R. M., & Heimberg, R. G. (1997). A cognitive-behavioral model of anxiety in Social Anxiety Disorder. *Behaviour Research and Therapy, 35*, 741–756.

Rhéaume, J., Freeston, M., Dugas, M., Letarte, H., & Ladouceur, R. (1995). Perfectionism, responsibility and obsessive-compulsive symptoms. *Behaviour Research and Therapy, 33*(7), 785–794. doi:10.1016/0005-7967(95)00017-R.

Rosser, S., Issakidis, C., & Peters, L. (2003). Perfectionism and social phobia: Relationship between the constructs and impact on cognitive behavior therapy. *Cognitive Therapy and Research, 27*(2), 143–151. doi:10.1023/A:1023505108426.

Saboonchi, F., & Lundh, L. (1997). Perfectionism, self-consciousness and anxiety. *Personality and Individual Differences, 22*(6), 921–928. doi:10.1016/S0191-8869(96)00274-7.

Saboonchi, F., Lundh, L., & Öst, L. (1999). Perfectionism and self-consciousness in social phobia and panic disorder with agoraphobia. *Behaviour Research and Therapy, 37*(9), 799–808. doi:10.1016/S0005-7967(98)00183-1.

Saddler, C., & Sacks, L. (1993). Multidimensional perfectionism and academic procrastination: Relationships with depression in university students. *Psychological Reports, 73*(3, Pt 1), 863–871.

Schlenker, B., & Leary, M. (1982). Social anxiety and self-presentation: A conceptualization model. *Psychological Bulletin, 92*(3), 641–669. doi:10.1037/0033-2909.92.3.641.

Shumaker, E., & Rodebaugh, T. (2009). Perfectionism and social anxiety: Rethinking the role of high standards. *Journal of Behavior Therapy and Experimental Psychiatry, 40*(3), 423–433. doi:10.1016/j.jbtep.2009.04.002.

Stoeber, J. (1998). The Frost Multidimensional Perfectionism Scale revisited: More perfect with four (instead of six) dimensions. *Personality and Individual Differences, 24*(4), 481–491.

Stoeber, J., & Becker, C. (2008). Perfectionism, achievement motives, and attribution of success and failure in female soccer players. *International Journal of Psychology, 43*(6), 980–987. doi:10.1080/00207590701403850.

Stoeber, J., & Otto, K. (2006). Positive conceptions of perfectionism: Approaches, evidence, challenges. *Personality and Social Psychology Review, 10*(4), 295–319. doi:10.1207/s15327957pspr1004.

Stoeber, J., Uphill, M., & Hotham, S. (2009). Predicting race performance in triathlon: The role of perfectionism, achievement goals, and personal goal setting Retrieved from PsycINFO database. *Journal of Sport & Exercise Psychology, 31*(2), 211–245.

Stumpf, H., & Parker, W. (2000). A hierarchical structural analysis of perfectionism and its relation to other personality characteristics. *Personality and Individual Differences, 28*(5), 837–852. doi:10.1016/S0191-8869(99)00141-5.

Terry-Short, L., Glynn Owens, R., Slade, P., & Dewey, M. (1995). Positive and negative perfectionism. *Personality and Individual Differences, 18*(5), 663–668. doi:10.1016/0191-8869(94)00192-U.

Wallace, S., & Alden, L. (1991). A comparison of social standards and perceived ability in anxious and nonanxious men. *Cognitive Therapy and Research, 15*(3), 237–254. doi:10.1007/BF01173016.

Chapter 6

Social Phobia as a Deficit in Social Skills

Ariel Stravynski, Angela Kyparissis, and Danielle Amado
Department of Psychology, University of Montreal, QC, Canada

INTRODUCTION

When considering SP as a presumably unique pattern of behaviors, one is struck by its elusive and mostly negative quality as well as by the extent to which the interpersonal, social, and occupational spheres of life of those who complain of it are perturbed (Schneier et al., 1994).

Social phobic conduct is strongly characterized by evasions, withdrawals, and absences. In short, from an observer's point of view, to a large extent by what the patient does not do.

Some activities and situations vital to participation in social life are seldom engaged in or entered into. Opportunities for advancement and the enrichment of social or personal life are often forgone. In the relatively circumscribed social interactions these patients engage in, little is said and feelings or opinions are walled in and remain mostly unexpressed. These individuals' very suffering is concealed as well. Their anxious distress – a constant feature of their lives – is typically dissimulated and kept secret.

What Could Account for This Peculiar Pattern of Conduct?

One of the various envisageable explanations for this wide-ranging reticence is that social phobic individuals in general, or especially those presenting the generalized pattern (the majority), lack the requisite social skills in order to perform proficiently in various social (and anxiety-evoking) situations (Curran, 1979, p. 319; Marks, 1985, p. 615; Stravynski & Greenberg, 1989, p. 208).

The anxious distress reported by patients would appear in such scheme of things to be a byproduct of the inability to act effectively, although conceivably one could claim just as plausibly that performance is undermined by an unmanageable and therefore disorganizing degree of anxiety (Eysenck & Calvo, 1992).

Social Anxiety: Clinical, Developmental, and Social Perspectives. DOI: 10.1016/B978-0-12-375096-9.00006-7

Whether currently unskilled social phobic individuals have ever been socially skilled and, if so, how these skills have been lost is an additional theoretical puzzle awaiting resolution.

The hypothesis of skills deficits has also important therapeutic implications. As a putative causal factor of SP, it is viewed as calling for and indeed being amenable to treatment by, social skills training.

Aim and Method

Our main goal in this chapter is to assess the evidence having a bearing on the "skill deficits" account of SP. Before reaching that stage, however, several intermediate steps need to be taken.

We must first clarify the concept of "social skills" generally and then inquire into its soundness in regards to SP specifically. Subsequently, as psychological constructs cannot have an existence apart from the way in which they are measured, we shall have to investigate the validity of the corresponding tests devised to identify and to quantify social skills deficits generally and their extent in SP in particular.

The theoretical construct (if it is that) of skills deficits, as well as the psychometric measures assessing it, are indispensable to the practical testing of the hypothesis. Once the matter of their validity is dealt with, we should be able to proceed and tackle the more precise questions of whether subgroups of social phobic individuals differ from one another in this respect and whether social phobic patients differ in their social skills from normal and/or other contrast populations. The demonstration of such differences is a necessary (but not sufficient) condition for the ultimate query: do skills deficits play a causal role in the social phobic pattern of behavior?

Finally, we shall gauge the value of the concept of skills deficits indirectly, through the perspective of treatment by means of social skills training.

THE NOTION OF SOCIAL SKILLS

The notion of social skills originates in attempts to make sense of normal social conduct. One possible perspective on social behavior is to consider it in analogy (first put forward by Argyle & Kendon, 1967) to a motor skill; i.e., an individual acting according to pre-established rules in pursuit of certain goals (e.g., dancing, skating, writing). This perspective stresses both the rule-bound aspect of social behavior as well as its dynamism; i.e., as undergoing constant changes in light of various signals emanating from the social environment. A failure to perform proficiently – as in a sporting activity – is accounted for (by analogy) in terms of a lack of requisite skills (Trower, Bryant, & Argyle, 1978).

This outlook of problematic or deficient "social skills" is an attempt to account for the commonplace observation that certain individuals are socially inept, are forgoing socializing, or have failed to realize a certain normative potential; e.g., to find a mate or hold a position commensurate with their level of education.

Heuristically, this explanatory hypothesis had caught the imagination of numerous theoreticians and has had a wide influence not least among practicing clinicians. In consequence, it has been applied to various patterns of abnormal behavior: depression (Lewinsohn, 1974), sexual dysfunctions in men (Lobitz & LoPiccolo, 1972), and of course SP (see Stravynski & Greenberg, 1989), among others.

Such an account ties problems in social skills with membership of certain categories of psychopathology (e.g. Hersen, 1979). However, the very breadth of application of this concept may paradoxically beg the question: does it have any specific content?

What Are Social Skills?

Before delving into the meaning of social skills, it may be useful to clarify the concept of skill. The notion of skill in itself, despite its frequent use and wide-ranging application, has proved exceedingly difficult to define (see Adams, 1987). One definition puts it as: "clearly a learned ability which involves co-ordination of different elements in a goal-directed manner . . . Skilled behavior may be viewed as an active self-assembled coalition of diverse resources in the service of a unitary goal. This relational aspect of skill includes not only the interactive relations among different segments of the act in question but the interaction between this act and the external environment"

O'Connor, 1989, p. 219

This rather abstract definition is in stark contrast with the fact that a very appealing feature of the "skills deficits" hypothesis is that it involves a seemingly sensible and down-to-earth reasoning unburdened by abstract concepts. The impression of clarity and concreteness, unfortunately, is somewhat deceptive. As remarked by Curran (1979), "everyone seems to know what good and poor social skills are . . . [but] no one can define them adequately" (p. 321).

One of the first and oft-quoted definitions of social skills (Libet & Lewinsohn, 1973) regarded it as "the complex ability to maximize the rate of positive reinforcement and to minimize the strength of punishment from others" (p. 311). This functional definition does not pinpoint specific behaviors, but relies on their success in generating rewards and minimizing punishment as an indication of skill.

This is so ambiguous as to leave, for example, the less than socially successful individuals without any guidance as to what they could do to improve their lot. Furthermore, this definition doubtlessly also encompasses behaviors that are usually considered less than adequate; e.g., temper tantrums, illness behavior, or moraliness unsavor (e.g. hypocrisy, manipulativeness, deceit).

Another functional (and rather sweeping) definition (albeit a negative one in terms of social inadequacy) emphasizes control over others: "a person can be regarded as socially inadequate if he is unable to affect the behavior and feelings of others in the way he intends and society accepts"

Trower et al., 1978, p. 2

A different sort of definition (see Curran, 1979 and McFall, 1982 for overviews) goes to the other extreme by providing details of what are deemed essential elements of skillful performance. Eye contact, appropriate content of speech, and reciprocity (among others) are put forward as such. Lists of elements, however concrete or comprehensive, do not make a definition. Nor is it clear why the listed elements are given prominence while many others that come to mind remain languishing in obscurity.

Other definitions still (e.g. Bellack, 1979) further argue for the integration of an amalgam of cognitive processes (e.g., social perception) to the behavioral elements of social skills (p. 98). Although this splitting of constituting elements must be ultimately judged by its validity and utility, this may also pose a risk of weakening the construct of social skills through its expansion to the extent of it becoming a metaphor for all behavior.

Although no satisfactory definition of social skills (and by implication their absence or inadequacy) is available today, the term has wide currency in clinic-lore and seems to be endowed with a certain concrete obviousness in the eyes of its users. Embedded in this face validity seems to be the sense that "it" is a set of behaviors or characteristics and, therefore, palpably recognizable.

In Wlazlo, Schroeder-Hartig, Hand, Kaiser, and Münchau (1990), for example, clinicians had little trouble identifying skill-deficient patients from the clinical notes. Conversely, Juster, Heimberg, and Holt (1996) argue that "in our clinic most social phobic persons are found to possess adequate social skills but are inhibited when it comes to applying their skills in social situations" (p. 84). The conceptual and empirical basis for both sets of observations remains unclear. By using the same term of "skill," are all referring to the same construct encompassing the same set of activities?

Perhaps greater clarity in this respect might be profitably gained from considering the way the notion of social skills has been used in research.

Two Views of Social Skills

The notion of social skills has been thoroughly analyzed by McFall (1982, pp. 1–12) and Curran (1979, pp. 319–354) and our discussion relies on both.

The construct of social skills may be said to have been construed in two different ways. One might be termed intrapersonal and the other interpersonal. The intrapersonal considers social skills a mental construct or trait, while the interpersonal defines it behaviorally as a pattern of activities. In some studies, the two approaches are confusingly mixed; while the design and measurement follow a behavioral perspective, the conclusions are compatible with a mental trait perspective.

The Intrapersonal View of Social Skills

Regarding social skills as a psychological process "within" the individual – or, in short, a trait – is the most common use of the term. A trait is a hypothetical mental construct; it is a shorthand for certain mental processes that predispose an individual to act in a particular way. Being "socially skilled" in the intrapersonal sense is not an observable performance, but, rather, an underlying quality that manifests itself in or may be inferred from actual behavior. Trower (1995), for example, distinguishes between the components of social skills – i.e., behaviors or repertoires of actions (the components) – and social skill – i.e., the process of generating skilled behavior (p. 55). The value of such a view is in the explanation it offers; i.e., the mental construct (or process) is the driving force within that gives rise to the action without. As a trait, social skills are something that one has, an attribute of the person.

As with all traits, so with social skills – such an analysis runs the risk of resorting to what amounts to a tautology. Initially, inadequate social skills are inferred from an inept performance. Yet the very same lackluster performance is subsequently seen as *resulting* from the deficient skills. Such an account is untenable, however, as the inferred trait cannot be used simultaneously as a causal explanation for the same behavior. For a hypothetical structure to be endowed with explanatory power, it must be shown to be valid in a series of independent studies; i.e., that it makes a difference and that it has a myriad of predictable consequences. Such independent demonstrations are lacking.

An advantage of the trait approach to social skills is that it does not require a specific definition of such skills, for such a definition, as we have seen earlier, is clearly unavailable. As it is an abstraction, it is sufficient that such a construct meets certain psychometric criteria to be considered useful, even if not entirely valid. The practical question we shall be considering later is whether it does. The omens in this respect are not good.

As with all trait conceptions (e.g., intelligence), social skills are seen as inherent to an individual; ploddingly stable over time and fairly consistent over situations. These assumptions are central to and embedded in the assessment of social skills as a trait; these methods would be incoherent otherwise. Whether this is actually the case remains to be seen.

The Interpersonal View of Social Skills

Within this approach, social skills are construed as specific features of behavior deemed the "building blocks of the individual's overall performance in each interpersonal situation" (McFall, 1982, p. 7). The specific appropriate social skills are a function of given situations and the ensuing interactions with the persons involved. Thus, "social skills are an attribute of a person's situation-specific behavior, not of the person per se" (p. 7). It follows that "no particular behavior can be considered intrinsically skillful, independent of its context" (p. 7). Although clear at a theoretical level (and especially as an incisive critique of the trait approach), the interpersonal perspective has its own short-comings and ambiguities.

It is not clear for example what units of behavior (constituent structures of behavior) it is important to consider, nor how to measure their effects (function of behavior) on the environment. Nor is it obvious what makes a performance satisfactory.

The implication of this approach for assessment is that situations must be taken into account so that behaviors are set in context. Its most far-reaching consequence, however, is that, ultimately, social skills are idiosyncratic and context-dependent. Consequently, these cannot be measured by some general test.

This, then, is the backdrop against which the intricate issue of how to assess and quantify social skills or their deficits, to put it negatively, has to be addressed.

ASSESSMENT OF THE SOCIAL SKILLS OF SOCIAL PHOBIC INDIVIDUALS

Given the theoretical ambiguity of the fundamental notion of "social skills," the task of developing precise and valid measurement methods has to be carried out on rather shaky foundations. Undaunted, researchers have constructed a number of such devices.

The various proposed methods for the assessment of social skills have been comprehensively reviewed in McNeil, Ries, and Turk (1995) and earlier in Hersen and Bellack (1977). These may be divided roughly in two: self-report inventories of behavior and simulations of behavior observed by assessors.

In what follows, the psychometric characteristics of the measurement devices we have selected will be summarized in their application to social phobic subjects whenever available. It must be borne in mind that most instruments have been developed with student or other subjects. Schematically, these characteristics are typically designated as reliability and validity. Reliability refers to the accuracy of the measurement, conceived of as agreement between assessors, occasions of testing, or different items of the test and the overall score.

Whereas numerous types of validity studies can be imagined, commonly two kinds have been reported. Convergent validity concerns the degree of correspondence between the measurement of aspects of social skills and other measures of related phenomena. Discriminant validity denotes a negative relationship. Occasionally, two types of criterion validity have been reported. Concurrent validity concerns the degree to which the measurement of social behavior goes hand in hand with related features of psychopathology at the present or – as in predictive validity – that might occur in the future.

As carrying out a comprehensive review is not our purpose, we shall consider only several instruments with sufficient background research to document some of their psychometric characteristics with social phobic subjects. These are of the most direct relevance to our inquiry.

Self-reports

Scale for Interpersonal Behavior (SIB; Arrindell & van der Ende, 1985)

This is a multidimensional self-report scale (originally devised in Dutch) of assertiveness measuring four domains rated each for performance and related distress. The domains are: (1) display of negative feelings (15 items); (2) expression of personal shortcomings (14 items); (3) display of assertion (9 items); (4) expression of positive feelings (8 items).

Distress is rated on a 5-point dimension ranging from 1 = "not at all" to 5 = "extremely." Performance is quantified in terms of categories of frequency ranging from 1 = "never do" to 5 = "always do."

Each domain has a score; a general score (separate for distress and performance) is the summation of the scores of all domains. We summarize in Table 6.1 the evidence regarding the soundness of the test.

In summary, the accuracy of this instrument is rather impressive. However, it is not altogether certain what it ultimately measures as its validity rests on moderate correlations with other instruments. The relationship of the SIB with the social behavior of social phobic individuals in their own lives remains for the time being unexplored.

The Social Performance Survey Schedule (SPSS; Lowe & Cautela, 1978)

This is a 100-item self-report questionnaire of "social performance" listing social behaviors rated on a 4-point scale of categories of frequency ranging from 0 = "never" to 4 = "very much." The social behaviors were generated from lists supplied by undergraduate students with some additions by the investigators.

Fifty items describe positive and an additional 50 describe negative behaviors. The scale rests on the assumption that "the more often positive social behaviors are emitted, and the less often negative social behaviors are emitted, the better one's social performance" (1978, pp. 537–538).

The raw score is a straightforward summation of ratings on positive items, and negative ones for which the ratings are inversed (e.g., "never" = 4 and "very much" = 0) to reflect their negative valuation in a positive way. The adjusted scores are meant to be the absolute difference between a normative rating on each item minus an actual score. To create the norms, 12 students were asked to rate the scale in an "ideal way." We summarize in Table 6.2 the evidence regarding the soundness of the test.

In summary, although the test shows reasonable accuracy, evidence that it measures the actual social behavior that we are interested in is rather weak.

TABLE 6.1 Psychometric Characteristics of the Scale for Interpersonal Behavior (SIB)[1,2]

Reliability		Validity			
			Internal		External
Test–retest	**Internal Consistency**	**Concurrent**	**Convergent**	**Discriminant**	**Generalizability**
Interval = 22–40 days: *r* (dis.) = 0.85 *r* (per.) = 0.73	α (dis.) = 0.95–0.97 (**) α (per.) = 0.91–0.97 (**)	*r* (SIB dis./FQ) = 0.53–0.73 (**) *r* (SIB per./FQ) = −0.15 (ns) – −0.38 (**)	*r* (SIB dis./SIB per.) = −0.53 (**) *r* (SIB dis./FSS) = 0.65 (**) *r* (SIB dis./SCL-90) = 0.62 (**) *r* (SIB dis./STAI-s) = 0.27 (**) *r* (SIB dis./STAI-t) = 0.36 (**) *r* (SIB per./SCL-90) = −0.13 (ns) *r* (SIB per./STAI-s) = −0.07 (ns) *r* (SIB per./STAI-t) = −0.18 (*)		
Interval = 41–93 days: *r* (dis.) = 0.70 *r* (per.) = 0.80	Similar results for the English version (α = 0.92–0.95)				
Interval = 48.3 days: *r* (per.) = 0.91	α (per.) = 0.70–0.87				Swedish version
Interval = 47.8 days: *r* (per.) = 0.71	α (per.) = 0.70–0.90		*r* (SIB per./PSS-Fa) = 0.35 (*) *r* (SIB per./PSS-Fr) = 0.23 (ns) *r* (SIB per./SPS) (ns)		Turkish version
Interval = 15–30 days: *r* (dis.) = 0.66 *r* (per.) = 0.70	α (dis.) = 0.82–0.96 α (per.) = 0.68–0.93	*r* (SIB dis./FQ) = 0.50–0.54 (***) *r* (SIB per./FQ) = −0.33 – −0.43 (***)	*r* (SIB dis./SIB per.) = −0.37– − 0.63 (***) *r* (SIB dis./RAS) = 0.64 (***) *r* (SIB dis./SSEI) = −0.49 (ns) – −0.57 (***) *r* (SIB per./RAS) = −0.59 (***) *r* (SIB per./SSEI) = −0.58 – −0.63 (***)	APD > SP > N (dis.) (****) APD < SP < N (per.) (****)	French version

	α (dis.) = 0.83–0.95 α (per.) = 0.77–0.93	*r* (SIB dis./SIB per.) = –0.36 (***)	English – Dutch students, Netherlands
	α (dis.) = 0.83–0.95 α (per.) = 0.78–0.93	*r* (SIB dis./SIB per.) = −0.34 (****) *r* (SIB dis./FSS) = 0.42 (***) *r* (SIB dis./s-EPQ-R) = −0.15 (***) *r* (SIB dis./s-EPQ-R) = −0.33 (***) *r* (SIB dis./s-EPQ-R) = −0.30 (***) *r* (SIB per./FSS) = −0.22 (***) *r* (SIB per./s-EPQ-R-p) = 0.10 (***) *r* (SIB per./s-EPQ-R-e) = 0.37 (***) *r* (SIB per./s-EPQ-R-n) = −0.16 (***)	English – US students

Note: There are no p values given for test–retest correlations.
[1]*Based on the following studies: Arrindell et al. (2001); Arrindell et al. (1990); Arrindell, Sanderman, van der Molen, van der Ende, and Mersch (1988); Arrindell and van der Ende (1985); Arrindell et al. (1999); Bouvard et al. (1999); Bridges, Sanderman, Breukers, Ranchor, and Arrindell (1991); Eskin (1992, 1993); Mersch, Breukers, and Emmelkamp (1992).*
[2]*Abbreviations, acronyms, and symbols: dis. = distress; FQ = Fear Questionnaire (social phobia subscale); FSS = Fear Survey Schedule (social fear items); ns = non-significant; per. = performance; p = psychoticism scale); PSS = Perceived Social Support (Fa = from family; Fr = from friends); RAS = Rathus Assertiveness Scale; SCL-90 = Symptom Checklist (social inadequacy subscale); s-EPQ-R = short-scale Eysenck Personality Questionnaire-Revised (e = extraversion scale; n = neuroticism scale; SPS = Suicide Probability Scale; SSEI = Social Self-Esteem Inventory; STAI = State–Trait Anxiety Inventory (s = state; t = trait); (*) =* $p < 0.05$*; (**) =* $p < 0.01$*; (***) =* $p < 0.001$*; (****) =* $p < 0.0001$*.*

TABLE 6.2 Psychometric Characteristics of the Social Performance Survey Schedule[1,2]

Reliability		Validity		
Test–retest	**Internal Consistency**	**Predictive**	**Convergent**	**Discriminant**
Unadjusted scores: $r = 0.87$ r (SPSS-P) = 0.88 r (SPSS-N) = 0.85	Unadjusted scores: $\alpha = 0.94$		Unadjusted scores: r (SPSS/SADS) = −0.42 (***)	Unadjusted scores: F > M
Adjusted scores: $r = 0.86$ r (SPSS-P) = 0.76 r (SPSS-N) = 0.87	Adjusted scores: $\alpha = 0.88$		Adjusted scores: r (SPSS/SADS) = −0.38 (***)	Adjusted scores: F > M
		r (SPSS-P/SPRS) = 0.29 (ns) r (SPSS-N/SPRS) = 0.35 (*)	r (SPSS-P/KAS-R1) = −0.12 (ns) r (SPSS-P/KAS-R1-P) = 0.52 (*) r (SPSS-P/KAS-R1-N) = −0.19 (ns) r (SPSS-N/KAS-R1) = −0.73 (**) r (SPSS-N/KAS-R1-P) = 0.38 (**) r (SPSS-N/KAS-R1-N) = −0.74 (**)	TBI < N (SPSS, SPSS-P) TBI = N (SPSS-N) TBI < N (SPSS-P, SPSS-N)

Note: There are no p values given for test–retest correlations.
[1]Based on the following studies: Long, McDonald, Tate, Togher, and Bornhofen (2008); Lowe and Cautela (1978).
[2]Abbreviations, acronyms, and symbols: F = females; KAS_R1 = Katz Adjustment Scale (P = positive scale; N = negative scale); M = males; N = negative social behaviors; N = normal control subjects; ns = non-significant; SPRS = Sydney Psychosocial Reintegration Scale; SPSS = Social Performance Survey Schedule (P = positive social behaviors); TBI = Traumatic Brain Injury Patients; (*) = $p < 0.05$; (**) = $p < 0.01$; (***) = $p < 0.001$.

Overall, then, although on the face of it self-report measures show satisfactory accuracy, ultimately it remains unclear to what extent what is being reported actually corresponds to the subject's actions in real life. Furthermore, although in principle social performance is usually considered as considerably influenced by context, the measures are in fact treating social performance as a trait.

Role-Play Tests

The construction of most RPTs is guided by the interpersonal view of social skills, namely as being situation-specific and rather individual. As such, most RPTs were ad hoc creations. Additionally, most departed from a straightforward behavioral focus on active conduct in combining role-play with a rating of subjective anxiety experienced during the simulations. This theoretical hybrid usually goes by the name of the Behavioral Assessment Test. A major complication in RPTs is how to analyze and make sense of the performance they elicit from the subjects. To resolve this dilemma, there is no help but to seek guidance from theory. This brings us back to the definition of "social skills." In this respect, the definitions are of high practical importance, not simply a matter of logical tidiness. In practice, two approaches have been taken.

The first, the "molecular" approach, focuses on various verbal – i.e., speech content and paralinguistic dimensions (e.g., intonation, length of speech, pauses) – and nonverbal (e.g., gaze, posture, hand-movement) elements of social performance. These are sought across behaviors. Such elements were in all likelihood chosen because they have an intuitive appeal (as seeming building blocks) and are easy to "make sense" of as there is no theoretical (operational) definition grounding to this practice.

The second, the "molar" approach, focuses on global behaviors in key domains, e.g., assertion, courtship, etc., deemed to be essential to social performance. These are typically rated (on Likert-type scales) by assessors on the strength of their intuitive judgment of what constitutes a skillful performance of a specific activity. Although it is reassuring to know that there seems to be evidence of good reliability in such practice, "it is not clear precisely what these ratings actually reflect" (Bellack, 1979, p. 168).

These two levels of assessment are not mutually exclusive and have been combined in some studies. As such, they make for a certain confusion, as the results cannot be compared. For the sake of our survey, we chose the most psychometrically elaborate and sophisticated RPT, as follows.

The Simulated Social Interaction Test (SSIT; Curran, 1982)

The SSIT provides descriptions of eight short situations described by a narrator. A confederate is present and gives the prompt to which the subject is meant to respond. All the proceedings are videotaped.

The situations include criticism, being the focus of attention, anger, meeting someone of the opposite sex, expression of warmth, conflict with a close relative, interpersonal loss, and receiving compliments. These themes were drawn from factor-analytic investigations identifying the most common difficulties (e.g., Goldsmith & McFall, 1975; Richardson & Tasto, 1976). At the end of each description, the subject is prompted to respond. Although the role-plays are intended to be short, no specific duration is suggested.

The simulated performance is rated on two dimensions with an 11-point Likert-type scale ranging from "not at all skillful" (1) to "extremely skillful" (11) for performance and ranging from "extremely anxious" (1) to "not at all anxious" (11) for anxiety.

Two key features of the test may give rise to some concern even at this point. First, it adopted a global ("molar") approach to the rating of social skills because the authors "have not yet empirically determined the components of social skills for our criterion situation" (Curran, 1982, p. 363). It is troubling that such an important choice was determined by nothing better than the lack of a better option.

Second, aspects of the training of the judges of social skill raise questions. Initially, six senior clinicians had reached agreements on ratings of bogus patients' performance. Subsequently, these ratings become the criterion ratings (i.e., the proper normative response that the assessors must rate). Thus, the process of training consisted in "recalibration" of the assessors' judgments (correlation coefficients had to be at least $r = 0.8$) to conform to those that the senior clinicians agreed upon.

Although this procedure forces agreement (i.e., reliability) among assessors, it may paradoxically, through pressure to conform, undermine the validity of what constitutes skillful behavior. We summarize in Table 6.3 the evidence regarding the soundness of the test.

In summary, the strengths of this test reside in it having a representative selection of difficult situations and a high rate of inter- and intra-assessor reliability. This assessment method differentiated psychiatric patients from normal control subjects. Its weaknesses consist in modest agreement (convergent validity) with independent ratings performed in other settings and with nontrained observers (nurses, research assistants) or even with those of the subjects themselves. Surprisingly, assessors' agreements varied despite the setting of a high threshold by the experimenters. However, perhaps the greatest shortcoming of this test is the absence of any support for its external (ecological) validity: that it provides information that may be considered as equivalent to observing what people do in actual life. Being on the ward can hardly be considered a representative sample of routine social life. The author of the test concedes: "we are still not content with the information yield from such ratings" (Curran, 1982, p. 371).

Overall then, this one device for measuring social skills has, accuracy aside, few confidence-inspiring psychometric characteristics.

Is the Use of Role-Play Tests as Behavioral Measures of Social Skills Warranted?

Our critique draws on thorough discussions by McNamara and Blumer (1982) and Bellack (1979).

Role-play tests are typically used as substitutes for the observation of real social conduct in its natural setting: "Role-play assessment is based on the assumption that actions displayed in the role-play reflect behavior of that person in a corresponding

TABLE 6.3 Psychometric Characteristics of the Simulated Social Interaction Test (SSIT)[1,2]

Reliability		Validity	
Inter-rater Agreement	**Internal Consistency**	**Convergent**	**Discriminant**
With mixed psychiatric patients: *r* (ski.) = −0.59–0.76 (*) *r* (anx.) = 0.45–0.68 (*) When raters are: Nurses: *r* (ski.) = 0.51 (**) RAs: *r* (ski.) = 0.64 (**) Interviewers: *r* (ski.) = 0.62 (**) Video judges: *r* (ski.) = 0.94 (**)	α (ski.) = 0.69 α (anx.) = 0.96 ICC (ski.) = 0.22 ICC (anx.) = 0.73	*r* (SSIT/beh. on the ward) = 0.51–0.94 (*) Men: *r* (SSIT ski./SIB per.) = 0.27 (ns) *r* (SSIT anx./SIB dis.) = −0.01 (ns) Women: *r* (SSIT ski./SIB per.) = 0.41 (*) *r* (SSIT anx./SIB dis.) = −0.48 (*)	National Guardsmen Psychiatric outpatients
With social phobic patients: *r* (ski.) = 0.91 (***) *r* (anx.) = 0.70 (***)			

Note: There are no p values given for test–retest correlations.
[1]Based on the following studies: Curran (1982); Curran et al. (1982); Curran, Wessberg, Monti, Corriveau, and Coyne (1980); Mersch, Breukers, and Emmelkamp (1992).
[2]Abbreviations, acronyms, and symbols: anx. = anxiety; beh. = behaviours; dis. = distress; ICC = inter-class correlation; ns = non-significant; per. = performance; RAs = research assistants; SIB = Scale for Interpersonal Behavior; ski. = skills; α = Cronbach's alpha, (*) = $p < 0.05$; (**) = $p < 0.01$; (***) = $p < 0.001$.

non-role play setting" (McNamara & Blumer, 1982, p. 520). This cardinal postulate is backed by little research in general and none in regard to SP. The paradigms in use for validation studies either compare role-plays to non-role-plays (usually observation of behavior during a waiting period before engaging in role-play) or having the role-play assessed by a significant person of the subject's as to its representativeness. Although appealing as economical substitutes for observation, each alternative is inadequate in some respect as neither is a proper reflection of real-life behavior.

Nevertheless, RPTs are typically used in the following ways:

1. To estimate treatment effects: differentiating the patients' post-treatment state from that at pretreatment;

2. To tell contrast-groups apart: distinguishing groups identified beforehand as socially skilled and nonskilled or of different degrees of skill; e.g., discrete versus generalized social phobia (GSP), SP with and without an additional APD.

Overall some studies that have used RPTs (or behavioral assessment tests) with social phobic individuals indeed reported the above-mentioned distinctions. However, the differences highlighted were usually in terms of severity of subjective anxiety ratings rather than in conduct. Behavior, moreover, was not always assessed. Such use of the role-play as a seemingly superior anxiety test is paradoxical as the impetus behind the use of role-plays is the possibility of observing behavior.

Although good reliability has been reported by Curran (1982) for the SSIT, it is not – as we have seen earlier – synonymous with validity. Construct validity is at this point not demonstrated, while there is little interest in what is perhaps the most important test of validity – a predictor of real-life behavior. This shortcoming calls into question the very foundation of the use of RPTs.

After searching reviews, both Bellack (1979, p. 167) and McNamara and Blumer (1982, p. 545) had suggested suspending the use of role-plays until better demonstrations of validity emerge. "Firm conclusions regarding role play's ultimate ecological validity must be therefore postponed until further research delimits how useful role playing is at representing real world behavior" (p. 167). These recommendations are probably as pertinent today.

Finally, a framework for analyzing the performance displayed in RPTs is sorely lacking. This is the upshot of the fact that no theoretical or operational definition of social skills is available. In practice, the analysis of performance is conducted in ways that generally preclude comparisons and paradoxically diminish the likelihood of outlining elements of convergent validity.

In sum, if we were very strict and narrowly purposeful, our survey might have come to a halt here. Lacking a clear theoretical vision of what social skills (and conversely their absence or deficiency) are, as well as meaningful means to identify and quantify them, we could have dismissed our quest out of hand and put an end to our inquiry at this stage. However, as our purpose is the exploration itself, we shall carry on regardless and attempt to answer several questions while ignoring the earlier-mentioned drawbacks but bearing them in mind.

SKILLS DEFICITS AND SOCIAL PHOBIA – DIRECT AND INDIRECT EVIDENCE

Are Highly Shy/Socially Anxious Individuals Less Skilled than Those Who Are Not?

Although they do not concern SP as described in diagnostic manuals, but rather shyness – a wider but related construct – the pioneering studies of

Twentyman and McFall (1975) and Pilkonis (1977) may nonetheless be useful in shedding some light on it. It is likely that some of the participants in these studies would fulfill the criteria for SP current today.

In Twentyman and McFall (1975), 31 shy (defined as having had less than one date a month) male students were compared to nine confident ones. Participants' behavior was measured in several ways: (1) weekly diaries of all their interactions with women; (2) role-play simulating a phone call proposing a date; (3) role-play of six social interactions involving 3-minute conversations with an unseen confederate (hidden behind a one-way mirror); and (4) a five-minute role-play of "asking out a classmate" face to face. These were recorded and analyzed.

The shy subjects reported greater levels of subjective anxiety in the simulation of a phone call and face to face but not in the other situations. Additionally, there were no differences in pulse rates during and in between the role-plays. The shy subjects, however, took less time to complete the role-play. Independent raters found the shy subjects globally less skillful and more anxious in two out of three role-plays (ratings on a 5-point Likert-type scale).

Most importantly, shy subjects – as gathered from their diaries – had fewer interactions with women in fewer situations and these were of shorter duration. In other words, shy individuals behaved differently in the domain most important to their lives. Whether this is due to lack of skill or the result of purposeful behavior (e.g., active avoidance) or some other reason cannot be ascertained from the study.

In Pilkonis (1977), 22 shy students (selected on the basis of scores on the Stanford Shyness Survey) were compared to 24 nonshy subjects on a number of social activities involving interacting with an individual of the opposite sex and giving a speech. Although the tasks were performed in the laboratory, these were not strictly speaking role-plays as the subjects were misled about the goals of the study.

The shy sat further away from the experimenter, were less able to initiate and structure conversations, and took longer before starting the conversation. During the exchange, they talked less and paused more. Shy individuals performed less well in an unstructured situation (e.g., conversation) as opposed to a well-defined one (e.g., making a speech), and tended to smile and nod more as well as engaging in "self-manipulation." There were no differences between the groups either in terms of the duration or the quality of speech. The author interpreted this to suggest that "a willingness to employ social skills may be at issue here, rather than a complete deficit of such skills" (p. 602).

Some differences between the sexes were found. Shy men had more difficulties than anyone did, whereas nonshy men did best. According to the author, men and women are anxious in different ways. This study, in addition to highlighting behavioral differences (a discriminant function allowed the correct reclassification of 91% of the shy subjects), strongly brought out the interaction between behavior and situation.

As in Twentyman and McFall (1975), Wessberg, Mariotto, Conger, Farrel, and Conger (1979) adopted "low-frequency dating" as an operational definition of social anxiety. In this study of male students, 9 low-frequency daters were compared to 19 medium and 17 high-frequency daters on two role-plays, each involving getting acquainted, punctuated by a waiting period. Subjects who dated frequently were rated as less anxious than those who dated least (but not the intermediate group). Furthermore, there were differences between the groups in term of ratings of skills (e.g., compliments, smiling). Subjects in all groups, however, exhibited greater skill in the role-plays than in the naturalistic waiting period, during which the subjects were unaware of being filmed. It is noteworthy that all subjects recognized this period as resembling most the way they were naturally.

In an additional study, Dow, Biglan, and Glaser (1985) compared 25 socially anxious women (scoring above 15 on the Social Avoidance and Distress; Watson & Friend, 1969) to eight nonanxious ones (scoring less than eight) on role-plays of "getting acquainted" with strangers of the same and the opposite sex. Additional role-plays to taped descriptions of situations and prompts were performed.

Highly anxious subjects were rated as having less social skills by peers, confederates, and observers. However, as in Pilkonis (1977), only one significant difference on specific behavioral variables was found: anxious women spoke less. This reoccurred in the taped situations test, in which anxious women differed only in giving fewer compliments and making fewer "positive statements."

In the self-monitoring of their own real-life social behavior, socially anxious women observed themselves as speaking to fewer people. When speaking to someone they tended to give fewer compliments, to share less personal experiences, and to agree more. The authors interpreted these differences as evidence of "skill deficits in specific conversational skills" (p. 280). However that may be, the study illustrates the fact that socially anxious women engage in real-life social situations differently, even if their performance in forced and imaginary circumstances cannot be easily distinguished from that of nonanxious individuals. These results recall those reported by Wessberg et al. (1979) described earlier. Because of the relatively small original sample size, made worse by seemingly catastrophic losses of data, these results must be viewed as tentative.

In a study inquiring into verbal communication skills (Lewin, McNeil, & Lipson, 1996), student subjects were divided in three groups according to their ratings of subjective anxiety: "circumscribed speech fear" ($n = 8$), "generalized social anxiety" ($n = 8$), and "low anxiety" individuals ($n = 16$), and compared. It is not clear whether the anxious subjects may be considered socially phobic.

All participants role-played a five-minute speech and filled out the State-Trait Anxiety Inventory-state form (STAI-S; Spielberger, 1970) before and after it. The verbal data were analyzed in four categories of speech dysfluency.

There were differences between the groups in terms of the number of subjects who finished their speech before the allotted five minutes. This was considered as escaping/avoiding the situation; escape behavior was highest in the speech fear group and lowest in the low anxiety group. This was not true, however, in terms of the number of words spoken: differences were detectable only between speech fear and low anxiety groups.

On the many variables quantifying the various speech dysfluencies, both anxious groups tended to differ from the less anxious one. Whether these features reflect skill or are features of a state of anxiety is difficult to say. However, there were no correlations between any verbal measures and the STAI-S score. If we do consider the measures as aspects of skill, their abstract nature does not allow us to reconstruct any meaningful behaviors that they could be related to.

In an attempt to approach the question more naturalistically, Segrin and Kinney (1995) divided 64 undergraduate students into the socially anxious (SA, $n = 31$) and the nonsocially-anxious (NSA, $n = 33$) by means of a cut-off point on the Social Reticence Scale (Jones & Briggs, 1986). All participants unwittingly took part in a five-minute unstructured interaction with a confederate while "waiting for the experiment to start." Subjects in the SA group were considered by the confederates (who were unaware of group membership) as having poorer social skills than those in the NSA group. In contrast, independent observers who rated tapes of the same interactions considered the groups equivalent in their social skills; similar results emerged in an analysis of the verbal content of subjects' responses. Overall, SA subjects – with one exception – were mostly like the NSA subjects.

In Strahan and Conger (1998), 333 undergraduate male students completed the SPS of the Social Phobia and Anxiety Inventory (Turner, Beidel, Dancu, & Stanley, 1989); the highest and lowest third of subjects in the distribution of social anxiety scores were selected (high SA, $n = 27$, and low SA, $n = 26$). Subsequently, all subjects underwent a simulated interview conducted by a female confederate; judges rated the taped interviews. Overall, no differences between the two groups were found in terms of either performance or verbal content.

In a study comparing a naturalistic and a contrived social exchange, Thompson and Rapee (2002) administered the Fear of Negative Evaluation (FNE; Watson & Friend, 1969) scale to 245 female students and selected the highest and the lowest 28 from the distribution. Fifty accepted to participate and were divided into low SA ($n = 24$) and high SA ($n = 26$).

All participants took part in unstructured (waiting in the company of a confederate for the experiment to begin) and structured (simulation of getting to know someone at a party) phase. In contrast to the two earlier studies, observers rated the SA participants as less skilled during the waiting period; the differences were less pronounced during the simulated conversation.

Wenzel, Graff-Dolezal, Macho, and Brendle (2005) investigated a narrowly defined population – romantically involved undergraduate couples. Those who scored one standard deviation above (SA, $n = 13$) and below (NSA, $n = 14$) the mean of the SAD and FNE (Watson & Friend, 1969) and had a "romantic partner" were selected.

All couples discussed three topics (neutral, problematic, and positive features of their relationship) and were rated on five types of communication skills. While no differences were found on three of the types of communication skills (e.g., asking questions, offering an opinion, paraphrasing the other's point of view), members of the SA group had greater difficulties in expressing themselves clearly during the problem discussion while fidgeting more and speaking more softly during all tasks. Additionally, they displayed less eye contact, smiled and initiated less (during conversation), and gave fewer compliments.

In summary, the available studies give a conflicting picture as to whether disparities in social skill may be said to distinguish groups of SAIs. However that may be, the relative and rather small differences between these subgroups, when found, are not foremost from the point of view of our inquiry, as these may be indicative of differences of degree. A plodding musician at home is but a pale reflection of the virtuoso concert pianist, yet both play the piano. It is the absolute level of social performance that is of most interest to us. Unfortunately, we have neither valid means nor norms of social skill that would allow us to determine the standing of the social phobic group on that dimension.

The Twentyman and McFall (1975) and Wenzel et al. (2005) studies then, although not of social phobic individuals in a formal sense, do suggest that SAIs behave differently at least as far as courtship of the opposite sex and communication among romantic partners is concerned. Whether this reflects deficits in skills is impossible to say.

Are the Social Phobics' Skills Different from Those of Normal Individuals?

Only a small number of studies allow us to pursue this question directly. The fact that they have used various definitions of social skill complicates matters even further. Rapee and Lim (1992) compared 28 social phobic (13 generalized, 15 specific) to 31 control participants. The RPT that all subjects underwent consisted of a brief speech given in front of a small audience. The performance was analyzed in terms of two broad categories: specific elements of behavior (e.g., eye contact, clarity of voice) and global aspects (e.g., subject's capacity to arouse interest), and rated on 5-point Likert-type scales by observers and the subjects themselves.

Significant differences were found on comparisons of the amalgamated scores of both specific and global aspects of performance. Most importantly, no differences in terms of specific behaviors were reported. For this reason, although statistically significant, the meaning of the association between lesser skill and social phobia remains obscure. Typically, subjects' self-ratings of performance tended to be lower than those of observers, especially for the social phobic subjects.

In Alden and Wallace (1995), 32 generalized social phobic participants were contrasted to 32 control community residents who simulated "getting acquainted" for five minutes. Half the subjects from both groups were assigned to a "positive" (e.g., the confederate was friendly and encouraging) and half to a "negative" (e.g., the confederate was cool and allowed silent pauses) condition.

Meaningfully, both groups performed better with an encouraging rather than with a distant confederate. Social phobic participants were more visibly anxious (nonverbal indices), had fewer "verbal behaviors," and were found to convey less warmth and to be less likeable than the controls, as rated on a variety of Likert-type scales. Theoretically, the meaning of these statistical differences is not entirely clear. Although the authors did conclude that "the social phobic patients in both conditions were less skillful than control subjects," what this statement relates to is ambiguous, as it ignores what constituent elements of skill were rated or how any of this relates to the subjects' conduct in real-life.

In Hofmann, Gerlach, Wender, and Roth (1997), 24 social phobic and 25 normal participants were compared. The role-plays included were: speaking with the interviewer, telling the interviewer what the participant did the day before, preparing a talk with the interviewer, sitting in front of two persons (all three minutes each), and a simulation of giving a speech prepared earlier (10 minutes). The participants' performance in all five situations was analyzed in terms of gaze while the first two minutes of the speech were also rated for speech disturbances (defined as silent pauses, errors, and dysfluencies).

No differences between the experimental groups were found in terms of gaze across situations – however calculated. As to speech disturbances, social phobic participants showed mostly less fluidity than the controls regardless of subgroup (the only difference was that the generalized subgroup had a longer overall time of pauses). These results, although suggesting that social phobic individuals experience difficulties in conversation, do not allow the drawing of general conclusions as to the state of their communication skills. Curiously, although differences in subjective anxiety ratings between subgroups were highlighted on some scales, these failed to show on the STAI-S (Spielberger, 1970). This would suggest that, while the subgroups are located on different points of a continuum of severity, it is not necessarily one of anxiety.

In a study testing hypotheses issued from Trower and Gilbert's (1989) model of social anxiety, Walters and Hope (1998) compared 22 social phobic subjects to 21 nonanxious controls in terms of a simulated impromptu speech and conversations with same and opposite sex confederates (not for all subjects). The videotaped role-plays were rated for behaviors assumed to reflect cooperation, dominance, submissiveness, and escape/avoidance.

Social phobic subjects faced their interlocutors less, expressed less praise (construed as cooperation), and engaged in less bragging and commanding (construed as dominance). It is noteworthy that in other respects, i.e., in terms of other descriptors of the constructs, no differences were observed. Unexpectedly and counterintuitively, the social phobic participants were neither found to be more submissive nor more avoidant than the nonanxious controls.

This study is important in showing that social phobic subjects behave somewhat differently from controls in simulated social interactions. Whether and to what extent these behaviors are indicators of the studied theoretical constructs remains an open question. How these constructs reflect adequate social behavior and what this might possibly be (optimally equidistant between dominant vs. submissive and cooperative vs. avoidant?) remains to be justified.

Fydrich, Chambless, Perry, Buergener, and Beazley (1998) asked 34 social phobic individuals, 28 normal individuals, and 14 individuals corresponding to criteria of various other anxiety disorders to simulate initiating and maintaining a conversation with a confederate of the opposite sex. Overall, observers rated the quality of the performance of the social phobic group as poorer than that of the normal and the other anxiety disorders groups.

In Norton and Hope (2001), 54 social phobic, 28 normal, and 23 dysthymic individuals simulated: (1) giving a brief speech, (2) engaging in a conversation (unstructured), and (3) engaging in conversation with a neighbor who had just moved in (structured). Observers rated the performance of the social phobic subjects as poorer than that of the dysthymic and the normal participants either on single tasks or all three pooled together.

In Baker and Edelmann (2002), 18 generalized social phobic individuals were compared to 18 normal individuals and 18 subjects characterized by other anxiety disorders in terms of a simulated interaction with a person they were meeting for the first time. Independent observers found the performance of social phobic individuals less adequate than that of normals; the differences in comparison with the other anxiety disorders group, although still significant, were less pronounced. Despite statistically significant differences between the groups on average, the authors emphasized the considerable overlap between them. For example, two social phobic individuals were rated as the most adequate normal subjects. At the other end of the spectrum, one normal participant was considered as barely more adequate than the least adequate of social phobic individuals.

In Stangier, Heidenreich, and Schermelleh-Engel (2006), 20 generalized social phobic participants, 17 normal participants, and 14 participants with other anxiety disorders simulated giving a short speech and engaging in conversation with a confederate. Observers rated the social phobic group as displaying greater nervousness (e.g., less eye contact) and less friendliness than subjects of the two control groups, who did not differ.

In Voncken and Bogels (2008), 48 generalized social phobic and 27 normal individuals simulated giving a short speech and engaged in conversation with two confederates. In contrast to previous studies, confederate ratings showed no statistically significant difference (at $p < 0.05$) between the groups in either speech making or the adequacy of engaging in conversation.

In summary, the studies available do not allow us to answer the question we have asked. First, on a global level of "performance," the results are contradictory. Second, on the level of specific skills, where differences have been identified, no convergence in deficits is in evidence. In most studies, social skill remains undefined and role-play performance, as its measure, is analyzed in ways that do not allow the integration of the fragmented bits into a meaningful whole; i.e., as a means to an end.

Are Any Social Phobic Individuals Deficient in Their Social Skills?

To our knowledge there are no studies that have attempted to put this question to a test directly; we shall, therefore, have to seek answers indirectly, through byways as it were. A number of studies lend themselves to such a purpose in that they have used role-plays as "behavioral assessments;" i.e., a measure of social skills or social anxiety, within a battery of other tests, with the original purpose being of investigating SP itself (e.g., in comparison to APD) or its putative subtypes (specific, generalized) as distinct entities. In what follows we shall proceed to review these studies.

In Turner, Beidel, and Townsley (1992), 88 social phobic participants were divided into specific ($n = 27$) and generalized ($n = 61$) subgroups. All subjects role-played (1) a 10-minute speech that had to last "at least 3 minutes" rated in terms of subjective anxiety; (2) a conversation on a first date; and (3) a conversation with a new neighbor of the same sex. These were rated for a number of molecular components of behavior (e.g., gaze, voice tone, number of verbal initiations, length of speech) and overall impression of skill. No differences between experimental groups were found on any dimension. Additionally, no differences were observed between the two subsets following a subsequent analysis of the subjects within the generalized group that met or did not meet criteria for APD.

In a similar study, Herbert, Hope, and Bellack (1992) compared two subsets of 23 "generalized" social phobic participants of which 14 also met criteria for APD. The subjects underwent a role-play consisting of three situations: making an impromptu speech of three minutes, initiating a conversation, and maintaining it. The subjects rated their subjective anxiety and the performance was analyzed in terms of overall skill, paralinguistic behavior, speech content, and nonverbal behavior. As in the earlier study, no differences in behavior were found between the two experimental groups although participants with APD were more anxious before simulating the speech (but not afterwards).

These results were further reanalyzed in light of a more stringent definition of the generalized subtype of SP originally proposed by Heimberg and

Holt (1989). After reclassification, it was found that this more severe group of generalized social phobic participants were rated as significantly less skilled on an overall composite score than their reclassified counterparts; no specific differences, however, in either behavior or thought were observed.

A study in similar vein was conducted by Tran and Chambless (1995), who had 16 specific, 13 generalized, and 16 generalized social phobic participants also meeting criteria for APD participate in three four-minute role-plays: impromptu speech and conversation with individuals of the same and the opposite sex. Assessors behind a one-way mirror rated performance for general impression of social skill. Simultaneously, the subjects rated their impression of their own skill as well as the subjective anxiety they had experienced.

Specific social phobic individuals were rated as giving a better impression of skill than did the generalized subject also meeting criteria for APD. These results were obtained consistently with both self-ratings and observer ratings across role-plays.

In summary, from the comparisons of several subcategories of SP, there is little evidence to suggest that, despite apparent differences in severity, these might differ in degree or quality of social skills – however measured.

Are Better Skills Acquired through Social Skills Training?

An indirect way of inquiring into the validity of the concept of social skills in SP would be to see whether it improves following a course of therapy designed to remedy it; e.g., social skills training.

Uncontrolled Studies

Chambless, Tran, and Glass (1997) describe a trial of cognitive behavior therapy with the sample described earlier in Tran and Chambless (1995). The outcomes measured by various behavioral assessment tests were as follows: self-ratings showed significant improvements across role-plays and remained at that level at six-month follow-ups. Observer ratings of social skills showed an improvement after treatment but this was not maintained at follow-up. Ostensibly, this study suggests that inadequate social skills may be changed in the course of therapy and perhaps maintained over time – the results are conflicting on this. As we were unable to answer the question of whether social phobic patients are deficient in their skills in an absolute sense, it is difficult to gauge the meaning of the changes documented in Chambless et al. (1997).

In Turner, Beidel, Cooley, Woody, and Messer (1994), 13 social phobic patients underwent 29 sessions (total of 54 hours) of "social effectiveness therapy." Among other tests, patients took part in role-plays requiring making a speech of 10 minutes and having a conversation with confederates of the same and the opposite sex. There was a significant improvement in "overall effectiveness" (as measured by the conversation role-play) after treatment that involved a spell of social skills training (eight sessions of two hours each) in addition to variants of exposure and practice in between sessions. Whether this improvement in performance implies an improvement in component social skills is not clearly established.

In van Dam-Baggen and Kraaimaat (2000a), 56 social phobic participants were divided into two equal groups (reticent and nonreticent) on the basis of their scores on the Inventory of Interpersonal Situations (van Dam-Baggen and Kraaimaat, 1999) and treated by a varying number of sessions of social skills training determined by demand. In both sets of patients, a significant and equivalent improvement in the frequency of social activities was reported. Whether the increased activity resulted from the deployment of better skills cannot be determined.

Herbert, Rheingold, and Goldstein (2002) treated 21 patients by six sessions of CBT combined with social skills training. Social skills were measured by means of three simulated activities: interactions with one and two strangers and an impromptu speech. An improvement in the performance observed during the role-plays after treatment was observed.

In summary, social skills training has been shown to result in improvement in performance in role-plays and increase in social activities of social phobic patients. Whether this occurred as a consequence of improved social skills remains uncertain. Moreover, it is unclear whether the improvement is specific to social skills training. Perhaps a more definitive answer to this question may be provided by controlled studies of social skills training.

Controlled Studies

In Wlazlo et al. (1990), 167 patients (corresponding to GSP/APD in DSM-III terms) were treated by either group social skills training or exposure *in vivo* – administered individually or in a group. Social skills training was administered over 25 sessions of 1.5 hours each. Group exposure involved a total of 34 hours of treatment, whereas the individual format involved 12 hours. One hundred and three patients completed treatment and 78 were followed up, for 2.5 years on average. At the end of treatment, the three regimens brought about significant and equivalent improvement in terms of social anxiety and tendency to avoid. These gains maintained and slightly strengthened over the follow-up period. For the sake of subsequent analysis, the sample was subdivided into two groups: those with primary "skills deficits" and those with primary "social anxiety." Overall, those classified as "skill deficient" did less well in treatment. Matching type of problem with kind of treatment (i.e., social skills training for patients identified as skill deficient) did not yield greater improvement. The internal validity of this study, however, is somewhat compromised by the fact that the exposure condition also included some training in social skills as well as in "social perception."

Skills deficits were said to be measured in this study by a self-report scale (Unsicherheitsfragebogen (UF) questionnaire – in German (Ullrich & Ullrich,

1998)). As the content of the measure seems to be a mixture of feelings (e.g., fear of failure and criticism, feeling of guilt) as well as abilities (e.g., making and refusing requests), it is doubtful that skills deficits, however defined, were actually assessed. Nonetheless, on the strength of improvements registered on this scale, patients in all treatment conditions (i.e., also in exposure) were said to have acquired social skills.

Subsequently, patients were divided into primarily "social phobic" (anxious) or "skill deficient" based on case records by experienced clinicians. It is not clear what the basis of this subdivision was as neither independent definition nor its anchoring points were provided. On the evidence of treatment outcome, one may surmise that the patients labeled "skill deficient" could be the most severely phobic.

In Mersch, Emmelkamp, Bogels, and Van der Sleen (1989) and Mersch, Emmelkamp, and Lips (1991), social skills training was compared to cognitive restructuring while also testing the value of matching treatment with patients' patterns of fear. On the basis of extreme responses to a role-play and a "rationality" test, 39 patients were classified as either predominantly behavioral (unskilled but rational) or cognitive (irrational but skillful). Half of each category of patients was assigned to the behavioral treatment (social skills training) and half to the cognitive treatment. Both treatment conditions resulted in significant and equivalent improvement on all measures. There was no support, however, for the notion that a match between predominant feature and treatment results in greater therapeutic gains. Nor did a significant lessening of social anxiety in this study lead to increased social activity.

Social skills were measured in this study by the SSIT described earlier (Curran, 1982). Patients' (classified as behavior reactors) skills improved following social skills training or a cognitive therapy (only on patients' self-ratings).

In van Dam-Baggen and Kraaimaat (2000b), 48 social phobic patients were assigned to 17 1.5-hour sessions on a weekly basis of either group social skills training or cognitive therapy. These were followed by three monthly sessions during a three-month follow-up. Self-reports of frequency of social activities were considered as measurement of social skills. Social skills training did result in a statistically greater frequency of social activities than did cognitive therapy, both at the end of treatment and at a three-month follow-up. Whether this is due to newly improved skills remains unknown.

In Stravynski, Ardel, Bounader et al. (2000), 60 social phobic patients were assigned to 14 sessions of an interpersonal approach to the treatment of SP with or without social skills training (conducted in groups). Both treatment conditions included the setting of interpersonal targets that constituted the content of treatment and had those targets assigned as homework to be performed in between sessions. Social functioning in both groups improved significantly and equivalently after treatment, remaining stable at 6- and 12-month follow-ups. Contrary to some of the previous results, social skills training in this study was not shown to result in or enhance distinct changes in social functioning.

In a related, as yet unpublished, study (Stravynski et al., 2010), 102 social phobic patients were randomly assigned to 14 sessions of either an interpersonal approach aiming at improving participation in individually relevant social encounters and including social skills training, a discussion group, or a brief individual supervision. All treatment conditions included interpersonal homework to be performed between sessions.

Seventy-six patients completed treatment. Patients in all treatment conditions improved significantly and equally in terms of reduced anxiety and avoidance, general psychopathology, and better social functioning that maintained over the 6- and 12-month follow-ups. As in Stravynski, Ardel, Bounader et al. (2000), social skills training had no unique or greater effect on social functioning.

Herbert and colleagues (2005) assigned 65 patients to 12 sessions of CBT either alone or combined with social skills training (both conducted in groups). Social skills were estimated by means of simulated interactions with one and two strangers, and an impromptu speech. The combined condition resulted in significantly better performance on all features of the three role-plays measured.

In summary, in Mersch et al. (1989) and Herbert et al. (2005), social skills training results in improved social skills as measured by role-plays. Paradoxically, in Mersch et al. (1989, 1991), a predicted superior improvement following a matching treatment failed to materialize, thereby weakening both the notion of skills deficits and the treatment – social skills training – meant to make them good.

As to the other studies surveyed in this section, which mostly used wider measures of social activity or social functioning, these did not show social skills training to result in unique improvements.

Is Improvement in Performance of Social Tasks Related to Skill-Acquisition?

Stravynski, Marks, and Yule (1982) assigned 27 outpatients (GSP/APD in today's terminology) to twelve 1.5 hour sessions of either social skills training alone or social skills training combined with cognitive restructuring. Twenty-two patients completed treatment. In each treatment condition patients improved significantly and equally on all measures of outcome, i.e., decrease in subjective anxiety, increase in social activities, and a corresponding improvement in social functioning with friends and at work. Only treated behaviors improved; little meaningful generalization to other behaviors occurred. During an initial no-treatment phase, no improvement was observed. At six-month follow-up, improvement remained stable.

Although changes in social skills were not measured in this study, it did document performance during interpersonal encounters in real-life through self-monitoring by the patients. A subsequent reanalysis of this data (Stravynski, Grey, & Elie, 1987) revealed that treatment had a sequentially diminishing impact on trained behavior. In other words, the greatest improvement in terms of frequency of performance was found in the first targeted interpersonal behavior; it gradually diminished with the introduction of treatment to each newly targeted interpersonal behavior. The sequentially diminishing impact of treatment did not seem to be compatible with "a skills-acquisition process that might be reasonably expected to take the form of gradual competence building and similarly gradual and steady improvement" (p. 228).

Discussion

Our inquiry into SP from the perspective of social skills deficits has been disappointing overall, not least because of the elusiveness of the master-concept and the inescapable attendant difficulties arising from practical attempts to measure it. Perhaps this is fitting, as the putative social phobic pattern of behavior itself is strongly characterized by reticence and evasion in pursuit of safety; we may need gentler methods to tease it out of its self-protective shell.

What appeared initially (admittedly at a casual glance) a potentially productive way of understanding SP (or some subtypes of it) and a guiding light for clinicians toward proper treatment has proven insubstantial. No evidence has emerged to link SP consistently with "deficits of social skills," let alone to suggest that they may play a causal role in its genesis. Nor has social skills training – the method presumed to improve deficiencies in social skills – been shown consistently to result in such outcomes in SP. At most, its results have been comparable to other methods, e.g., cognitive modification (Mersch et al., 1991), that have not aimed at improving social skills. Furthermore, when change in social behavior following social skills training was measured (Stravynski et al., 1987), improvement was not found to have followed a skills-acquisition pattern.

In sum, social skills and their putative deficiencies in SP seem to be metaphors; a manner of speaking of the ineffable as if it were something else. However sad for those attached to it, the demise of an idea – especially one of uncertain validity – need not be a destructive event. Conversely, it may set the stage for the surveying of familiar territory from new or different vantage points.

SOCIAL PHOBIA AS A PROBLEM IN SOCIAL FUNCTIONING

Although not much that is wrong with the social skills of social phobics has come to light, it is undeniable that something is very much the matter with the way these individuals live socially, be it in limited situations or generally. This we know at least indirectly, from the repercussions of this way of being; perturbed social and personal lives and lower economic and social attainments are typical (see Stravynski, 2007, pp. 114–115 for a summary). We know very little, however, about the particular social phobic pattern of social functioning – if such a pattern indeed exists in nature.

Most research on SP assumes such a pattern while attempting, for example, to explain its origins. In keeping with the diagnostic manuals (DSM, ICD), we conceive of SP in abstract terms, namely as a hypothetical entity characterized by additional hypothetical constructs such as anxiety – but not in terms of (observable) social activities.

The merit of the skills deficits hypothesis (as an outlook) was that it attempted to account for SP in its own terms, as a difficulty in social functioning. Its drawback – common to many other attempts – was to conceive of SP as a known and established entity requiring etiological explanation. Such a position, however, overlooks the fact that at the present we are uncertain to what extent SP is a distinct psychological pattern (see Stravynski, 2007, pp. 75–141 for a comprehensive engagement with the question). Rather more important – from our vantage point – is the question of whether there is an overall pattern of social behaviors characterizing SP and what this might be.

The social difficulties of social phobic individuals are usually seen as a consequence of some pathological process underlying it (e.g., anxiety), while this in turn is a consequence of a breakdown on a more fundamental level (e.g., neurotransmission, patterns of thought). Such a construal of SP in analogy to a medical view separates the disease (that the individual carries within) from the resulting social impairment displayed in the environment (the sickness – see Stravynski, 2007, p. 68). Whether a reified SP may be separated from its problematic social functioning must be considered doubtful. On an observed level (as opposed to a speculative one), SP is a short-hand for a psychopathological pattern of behavior; i.e., how individuals in that category act and live their lives.

Unfortunately, but not surprisingly in light of the above widely shared view, there are no published studies documenting social phobic behavior in real-life situations nor delineating a social phobic pattern of behavior in various spheres of life. To answer these necessary questions, a different kind of research is needed, more along the lines of ethnography, i.e., social phobic individuals as members of an exotic cult (Lillard, 1998), and ethology (Boice, 1982), i.e., social phobic individuals as organisms struggling to adjust to (and transform) their environments. These – rather than laboratory experiments – are more likely to tease out the purposeful nature of the overall social phobic pattern.

A first step in this direction was taken by Amado and Stravynski (2010) in a study based on field observations of four social phobic individuals going about their daily lives. The observations in real life situations were cross-validated with the participants themselves, diaries they kept, and clinical notes and interviews with close significant others. All social phobic participants, regardless of subtype, were characterized by a distinct and overarching self-protective pattern of interpersonal behavior. This was not observed in shy and nonshy normal individuals serving as control subjects. The social phobic self-protective pattern was found to come apart gradually and finally vanish after successful therapy (see Stravynski, Arbel, Lachance, & Todorov, 2000 for a description of individual cases), lending support to the previous findings.

THE TREATMENT OF SOCIAL PHOBIA AS AN ANTIDOTE TO ITS ETIOLOGY, OR, SOCIAL SKILLS TRAINING FOR SOCIAL SKILLS DEFICITS

Regardless of its scientific merits, an etiological hypothesis such as that of "skills deficits" often provides a powerful rationale or even a rationalization for a certain approach to treatment. Thus, social skills training is seen as building whatever is lacking in the individual patient's repertoire of social skills.

Such a construction of treatment (of SP) as an antidote to its etiology follows an older idealized pattern set by the medical model (of, say, infectious disease). In keeping with it, psychotropic medication is seen as setting right the dysregulation of neurotransmitters presumed to give rise to the problems or, to take another example, cognitive therapy is assumed to straighten the crooked thinking allegedly causing the anxious distress. It is interesting that the two notions – etiology and treatment – are frequently unveiled simultaneously although the relevant evidence for either is slight.

Although appealing to some, this ideal must remain unrealized, as the hypothetical etiology of SP (in terms of underlying defects within the person, be they skills deficits or otherwise) remains for the time being unidentified. The prospects of this happening in the future do not appear to be bright, as, in terms of underlying characteristics, social phobic patients are more like normal individuals than they are different from them (see Stravynski, 2007, pp. 90–95).

More importantly, there are few convincing demonstrations that social skills training results in improved skills (e.g., Mersch et al., 1991; Wlazlo et al., 1990). Moreover, the outcomes of social skills training and the two anxiety reduction methods it was compared with in the above studies were indistinguishable either in terms of anxiety reduction (to an equal degree) or social functioning (unchanged). This is in contrast with the outcome reported in Stravynski et al. (1982), in which social skills training resulted in less anxiety and improved social functioning.

What underlies the difference in outcome? Perhaps the better outcome (from the point of view of social functioning) in the latter approach was due to the fact that its content of treatment was not determined by the idea of building up generic hypothetical skills deemed necessary for social functioning, be they molecular (e.g., appropriate eye contact, timing, etc.) or not. Such an approach might be termed the structuralist perspective. Rather, in Stravynski et al. (1982) (an approach that might be termed interpersonal or functionalistic), individual patients were trained to develop personal ways of dealing with their real-life social/interpersonal circumstances and to use them in situations very much a part of their daily lives. Admitting to being clumsy, seeking people out, and being opinionated and provocative are examples of behaviors targeted in such treatment. Apart from the issue of what is the proper content of training (as dictated by the structuralistic or functionalistic perspectives), a further question arises. Is the framework of social skills training at all necessary for a beneficial improvement in social functioning to occur? The answer to this query is of considerable theoretical and practical interest.

An early study involving patients meeting criteria for APD (Stravynski, Lesage, Marcouiller, & Elie, 1989) queries the role of social skills training as an essential technique. In it, 28 subjects were assigned to two combined treatment conditions each consisting of five sessions of social skills training plus homework and five sessions of group discussion plus homework, administered in a different order in accordance with a latin-square (crossover) design.

Equivalent and significant improvements in social functioning and social skills were observed in both treatment conditions (combining each, both treatment modalities, in reverse order). Most importantly from our point of view, no differences in outcome were found between the treatment modalities; i.e., social skills training and discussion during the sessions and homework in between them.

In Stravynski, Ardel, Lachance et al. (2000), we put the same hypothesis to another test. In this study, we compared two treatments both aiming at the improvement of social phobic patients' social functioning, one including social skills training (modeling, role rehearsal, feedback) and the other without it. In both treatment conditions, the patients had predetermined individual behaviors aiming at better participation in various social encounters. The behaviors targeted for treatment came in for attention in the clinic as well as being assigned as homework tasks to be practiced in between sessions.

The regimen without social skills training promoted improvement in social functioning by means of the targeted behaviors being practiced during the session and being assigned as tasks to be performed in between sessions. In contrast to the condition using social skills training, however, no attempts were made to improve upon how the patient enacted the targeted behavior spontaneously; nor were the staple ingredients of social skills training (modeling, role-rehearsal, etc.) used. This condition was designed to assume the form of social skills training but without its essence.

We found that both treatment conditions (30 patients completed treatment in each) resulted in highly significant reductions in the level of subjective anxiety and in improvements in social functioning in most areas of social life (e.g., work, friends). Clinically however, the most meaningful result was that 60% of patients in each condition no longer met DSM-IV criteria for SP at one-year follow-ups.

These outstanding outcomes illustrate the promise of treating social phobics' difficulties of social functioning in their own right, unfettered by the intertwined notions of skills deficits put right by social skills training. It is to the problems of these patients in terms of social participation, fitting in, and assuming social roles that we ought presently to turn our attention.

CONCLUSION

In conclusion, social skills – as an idea – have not offered us a privileged vantage point from which to peer into SP. The main failing seems to be at a conceptual level; we do not know what social skills (or their deficits) are, and, unsurprisingly, we fail to measure them with any confidence. Specifically, there is an over-insistence in the RPTs on components of social behaviors while ignoring their functions in real-life (e.g., as elements in a pattern of self-protection; see Stravynski, 2007, pp. 3–15). In that sense, they seem to be abstracted from any social reality to a striking degree.

What needs to be done now? We believe it advisable to separate the tasks of understanding the maladjusted pattern of conduct we call SP from therapeutic attempts to change it; these pursuits may be simply unrelated. The social life of social phobics could be profitably studied in its own right, as a meaningful goal-directed activity and not as an expression of some underlying problem. The methods most likely to lend themselves to such studies are ones that do not seek to locate a "social phobic structure" within the individual. Rather, they would consider SP as a hypothetical and purposeful individual pattern of conduct (or way of being) within certain situations and life circumstances, to be documented through a combination of patiently gathered observations and the collection of individual life-stories documenting its development and vicissitudes.

REFERENCES

Adams, J. A. (1987). Historical review and appraisal of research on the learning retention and transfer of human motor skills. *Psychological Bulletin*, *101*, 41–74.

Alden, L. E., & Wallace, S. T. (1995). Social phobia and social appraisal in successful and unsuccessful social interactions. *Behaviour Research and Therapy*, *33*, 497–505.

Amado, D., & Stravynski, A. (2010). Is social phobia characterized by a distinct interpersonal pattern? An ethnographic study (in preparation).

Argyle, M., & Kendon, A. (1967). The experimental analysis of social performance. In L. Berkowitz (Ed.), *Advances in experimental social psychology: Vol. 3* (pp. 55–98). San Diego, CA: Academic Press.

Arrindell, W. A., Bridges, K. R., van der Ende, J., St. Lawrence, J. S., Gray-Shellberg, L., Harnish, R., et al. (2001). Normative studies with the Scale for Interpersonal Behaviour (SIB) II US students. A cross-cultural program with Dutch data. *Behaviour Research and Therapy*, *39*, 1461–1479.

Arrindell, W. A., Sanderman, B., Hageman, W. J., Pickersgill, M. J., Kwee, M. G. T., van der Molen, H. T., et al. (1990). Correlates of assertiveness in normal and clinical samples: A multidimensional approach. *Advances in Behaviour Research and Therapy*, *12*, 153–282.

Arrindell, W. A., Sanderman, R., van der Molen, H., van der Ende, J., & Mersch, P. P. (1988). The structure of assertiveness: A confirmatory approach. *Behaviour Research and Therapy*, *26*, 337–339.

Arrindell, W. A., & van der Ende, J. (1985). Cross-sample invariance of the structure of self-reported distress and difficulty in assertiveness. *Advances in Behaviour Research and Therapy*, *7*, 205–243.

Arrindell, W. A., van der Ende, J., Sanderman, R., Oosterhof, L., Stewart, R., & Lingsma, M. M. (1999). Normative studies with the Scale for Interpersonal Behaviour (SIB): I. Nonpsychiatric social skills trainees. *Personality and Individual Differences*, *27*, 417–431.

Baker, S. R., & Edelmann, R. J. (2002). Is social phobia related to lack of social skills? Duration of skill-related behaviours and ratings of behavioural adequacy. *British Journal of Clinical Psychology*, *41*, 243–257.

Bellack, A. S. (1979). A critical appraisal of strategies for assessing social skill. *Behavioral Assessment*, *1*, 157–176.

Boice, R. (1982). An ethological perspective on social skills research. In J. P. Curran & P. M. Monti (Eds.), *Social skills training: A practical handbook for assessment and treatment* (pp. 374–396). New York: Guilford.

Bouvard, M., Arrindell, W. A., Guérin, J., Bouchard, C., Rion, A. C., Ducottet, E., et al. (1999). Psychometric appraisal of the Scale for Interpersonal Behavior (SIB) in France. *Behaviour Research and Therapy*, *37*, 741–762.

Bridges, K. R., Sanderman, R., Breukers, P., Ranchor, A., & Arrindell, W. A. (1991). Sex differences in assertiveness on the U.S. version of the Scale for Interpersonal Behavior (SIB). *Personality and Individual Differences*, *12*, 1239–1243.

Chambless, D. L., Tran, G. Q., & Glass, C. R. (1997). Predictors of response to cognitive-behavioral group therapy for social phobia. *Journal of Anxiety Disorders*, *11*, 221–240.

Curran, J. P. (1979). Social skills: Methodological issues and future directions. In A. S. Bellack & M. Hersen (Eds.), *Research and practice in social skills training* (pp. 319–354). New York: Plenum Press.

Curran, J. P. (1982). A procedure for the assessment of social skills: The Simulated Social Interaction Test. In J. P. Curran & P. M. Monti (Eds.), *Social skills training: A practical handbook for assessment and treatment* (pp. 348–373). New York: Guilford.

Curran, J. P., Wessberg, H. W., Farrell, A. D., Monti, P. M., Corriveau, D. P., & Coyne, N. A. (1982). Social skills and social anxiety: Are different laboratories measuring the same construct? *Journal of Consulting and Clinical Psychology*, *50*, 396–406.

Curran, J. P., Wessberg, H. W., Monti, P. M., Corriveau, D. P., & Coyne, N. A. (1980). Patients versus controls on a social skill/anxiety role-play test. Paper presented at the 88th annual convention of the American Psychological Association, Montreal, Canada.

Dow, M. G., Biglan, A., & Glaser, S. R. (1985). Multimethod assessment of social anxious and socially nonanxious women. *Behavioral Assessment*, *7*, 273–282.

Eskin, M. (1992). Swedish translations of the Suicide Probability Scale, Perceived Social Support from Friends and Family Scales, and the Scale for Interpersonal Behavior: A reliability analysis. *Scandinavian Journal of Psychology*, *34*, 276–281.

Eskin, M. (1993). Reliability of the Turkish version of the Perceived Social Support from Friends and Family scales, Scale for Interpersonal Behavior, and Suicide Probability Scale. *Journal of Clinical Psychology*, *49*, 515–522.

Eysenck, M. W., & Calvo, M. G. (1992). Anxiety and performance: The processing efficiency theory. *Cognition and Emotion*, *6*, 409–434.

Fydrich, T., Chambless, D. L., Perry, K. J., Buergener, F., & Beazley, M. B. (1998). Behavioral assessment of social performance: A rating system for social phobia. *Behaviour Research and Therapy*, *36*, 995–1010.

Goldsmith, J. B., & McFall, R. (1975). Development and evaluation of an interpersonal skill-training program for psychiatric patients. *Journal of Abnormal Psychology*, *84*, 51–58.

Heimberg, R. G., & Holt, C. S. (1989). The issue of subtypes in the diagnosis of social phobia: A report to the social phobia subworkgroup for DSM-IV. Unpublished manuscript.

Herbert, J. D., Gaudiano, B. A., Rheingold, A. A., Myers, V. H., Dalrymple, K., & Nolan, M. (2005). Social skills training augments the effectiveness of cognitive behavioral group therapy for social anxiety disorder. *Behavior Therapy*, *36*, 125–138.

Herbert, J. D., Hope, D. A., & Bellack, A. S. (1992). Validity of the distinction between generalized social phobia and avoidant personality disorder. *Journal of Abnormal Psychology*, *101*, 332–339.

Herbert, J. D., Rheingold, A. A., & Goldstein, S. G. (2002). Brief cognitive behavioral group therapy for social anxiety disorder. *Cognitive and Behavioral Practice*, *9*, 1–8.

Hersen, M. (1979). Modification of skill deficits in psychiatric patients. In A. S. Bellack & M. Hersen (Eds.), *Research and practice in social skills training* (pp. 189–236). New York: Plenum Press.

Hersen, M., & Bellack, A. S. (1977). Assessment of social skills. In A. R. Ciminero, H. Adams, & K. Calhoun (Eds.), *Handbook of behavioral assessment* (pp. 509–554). New York/Chichester: Wiley.

Hofmann, S. G., Gerlach, A. L., Wender, A., & Roth, W. (1997). Speech disturbances and gaze behavior during speaking in subtypes of social phobia. *Journal of Anxiety Disorders*, *11*, 573–585.

Jones, W. H., & Briggs, S. R. (1986). Manual for the Social Reticence Scale: A measure of shyness. Palo Alto, CA: Consulting Psychologists Press.

Juster, H. R., Heimberg, R. G., & Holt, C. S. (1996). Social phobia: Diagnostic issues and review of cognitive behavioral treatment strategies. *Progress in Behavior Modification*, *30*, 74–98.

Lewin, M. R., McNeil, D. W., & Lipson, J. M. (1996). Enduring without avoiding: Pauses and verbal dysfluencies in public speaking fear. *Journal of Psychopathology and Behavioral Assessment*, *18*, 387–402.

Lewinsohn, P. M. (1974). Clinical and theoretical aspects of depression. In K. S. Calhoun, H. E. Adams, & K. M. Mitchell (Eds.), *Innovative treatment methods in psychopathology* (pp. 63–120). New York: Wiley.

Libet, J. M., & Lewinsohn, P. M. (1973). Concept of social skills with special reference to the behavior of depressed persons. *Journal of Consulting and Clinical Psychology*, *40*, 304–312.

Lillard, A. (1998). Ethnopsychologies: Cultural variations in theories of mind. *Psychological Bulletin*, *1*, 3–32.

Lobitz, W. C., & LoPiccolo, J. (1972). New methods in the behavioral treatment of sexual dysfunction. *Journal of Behavior Therapy and Experimental Psychiatry*, *3*, 275–281.

Long, E., McDonald, S., Tate, R., Togher, L., & Bornhofen, C. (2008). Assessing social skills in people with very severe traumatic brain injury: Validity of the Social Performance Survey Schedule (SPSS). *Brain Impairment*, *9*, 274–281.

Lowe, M. R., & Cautela, J. R. (1978). A self-report measure of social skill. *Behavior Therapy*, *9*, 535–544.

Marks, I. M. (1985). Behavioral treatment of social phobia. *Psychopharmacology*, *21*, 615–618.

McFall, R. M. (1982). A review and reformulation of the concept of social skills. *Behavioral Assessment*, *4*, 1–33.

McNamara, J. R., & Blumer, C. A. (1982). Role playing to assess social competence. Ecological validity considerations. *Behavior Modification*, *6*, 519–549.

McNeil, D. W., Ries, D. J., & Turk, C. L. (1995). Behavioral assessment: Self-report, physiology, and overt behavior. In R. G. Heimberg, M. R. Liebowitz, D. A. Hope, & F. R. Schneier (Eds.), *Social phobia: Diagnosis, assessment and treatment* (pp. 202–231). New York: Guilford Press.

Mersch, P. P., Breukers, P., & Emmelkamp, P. M. G. (1992). The Simulated Social Interaction Test: A psychometric evaluation with Dutch social phobic patients. *Behavioral Assessment*, *14*, 133–151.

Mersch, P. P. A., Emmelkamp, P.-M.-G., Bogels, S.-M., & Van der Sleen, J. (1989). Social phobia: Individual response patterns and the effects of behavioral and cognitive interventions. *Behaviour Research and Therapy*, *27*, 421–434.

Mersch, P. P. A, Emmelkamp, P.-M.-G., & Lips, C. (1991). Social phobia: Individual response patterns and the effects of behavioral and cognitive interventions. A follow-up study. *Behaviour Research and Therapy*, *29*, 357–362.

Norton, P. J., & Hope, D. A. (2001). Kernels of truth of distorted perceptions: Self and observer ratings of social anxiety and performance. *Behavior Therapy*, *32*, 765–786.

Pilkonis, P. A. (1977). The behavioral consequences of shyness. *Journal of Personality*, *45*, 596–611.

Rapee, R. M., & Lim, L. (1992). Discrepancy between self- and observer ratings of performance in social phobics. *Journal of Abnormal Psychology*, *101*, 728–731.

Richardson, F. C., & Tasto, D. L. (1976). Development and factor analysis of a social anxiety inventory. *Behavior Therapy*, *7*, 453–462.

Schneier, F. R., Heckelman, L. R., Garfinkel, R., Campeas, R., Fallon, B. A., Gitow, A., et al. (1994). Functional impairment in social phobia. *Journal of Clinical Psychiatry*, *55*, 322–331.

Segrin, C., & Kinney, T. (1995). Social skills deficits among the socially anxious: Rejection from others and loneliness. *Motivation and Emotion*, *19*, 1–24.

Spielberger, C. (1970). *Manual for state–trait anxiety inventory*. Palo Alto, CA: Consulting Psychologist.

Stangier, U., Heidenreich, T., & Schermelleh-Engel, K. (2006). Safety behaviors and social performance in patients with generalized social phobia. *Journal of Cognitive Psychotherapy: An International Quarterly*, *20*, 17–31.

Strahan, E., & Conger, A. J. (1998). Social anxiety and its effects on performance and perception. *Journal of Anxiety Disorders*, *12*, 293–305.

Stravynski, A. (2007). *Fearing others. The nature and treatment of social phobia*. New York: Cambridge University Press.

Stravynski, A., Arbel, N., Bounader, J., Gaudette, G., Lachance, L., Borgeat, F., et al. (2000). Social phobia treated as a problem in social functioning: A controlled comparison of two behavioural group approaches. *Acta Psychiatrica Scandinavica*, *102*, 188–198.

Stravynski, A., Arbel, N., Chenier, N., Lachance, L., Sidoun, P., & Todorov, C. (2010). Treating social phobia interpersonally: Dismantling the ingredients of a behavioural approach (in preparation).

Stravynski, A., Arbel, N., Lachance, L., & Todorov, C. (2000). Social phobia viewed as a problem in social functioning: A pilot study of group behavioral treatment. *Journal of Behavior Therapy*, *31*, 163–175.

Stravynski, A., & Greenberg, D. (1989). Behavioural psychotherapy for social phobia and dysfunction. *International Review of Psychiatry*, *1*, 207–218.

Stravynski, A., Grey, S., & Elie, R. (1987). Outline of the therapeutic process in social skills training with socially dysfunctional patients. *Journal of Consulting and Clinical Psychology*, *55*, 224–228.

Stravynski, A., Lesage, A., Marcouiller, M., & Elie, R. (1989). A test of the therapeutic mechanism in social skills training with avoidant personality disorder. *Journal of Nervous and Mental Disease*, *177*, 739–744.

Stravynski, A., Marks, I., & Yule, W. (1982). Social skills training with and without cognitive modification. *Archives of General Psychiatry*, *39*, 1378–1385.

Thompson, S., & Rapee, R. M. (2002). The effect of situational structure on the social performance of socially anxious and non-anxious participants. *Journal of Behavior Therapy and Experimental Psychiatry*, *33*, 91–102.

Tran, G. Q., & Chambless, D. L. (1995). Psychopathology of social phobia: Effects of subtype and avoidant personality disorder. *Journal of Anxiety Disorders*, *9*, 489–501.

Trower, P. (1995). Adult social skills: State of the art and future directions. In W. O'Donohue & L. Krasner (Eds.), *Handbook of psychological skills training: Clinical techniques and applications* (pp. 54–80). Boston, MA: Allyn & Bacon.

Trower, P., Bryant, B., & Argyle, M. (1978). *Social skills and mental health*. London: Methuen.

Trower, P., & Gilbert, P. (1989). New theoretical conceptions of social anxiety and social phobia. *Clinical Psychology Review*, *9*, 19–35.

Turner, S. M., Beidel, D. C., Cooley, M. R., Woody, S. R., & Messer, S. (1994). A multicomponent behavioral treatment for social phobia: Social effectiveness therapy. *Behaviour Research and Therapy*, *32*, 381–390.

Turner, S. M., Beidel, D. C., Dancu, C. V., & Stanley, M. A. (1989). An empirically derived inventory to measure social fears and anxiety: The Social Phobia and Anxiety Inventory. *Psychological Assessment*, *1*, 35–40.

Turner, S. M., Beidel, D. C., & Townsley, R. M. (1992). Social phobia: A comparison of specific and generalized subtypes and avoidant personality disorder. *Journal of Abnormal Psychology*, *101*, 326–331.

Twentyman, C. T., & McFall, R. M. (1975). Behavioral training of social skills in shy males. *Journal of Consulting and Clinical Psychology*, *43*, 384–395.

Ullrich, R., & Ullrich, R. (1998). Einuebung von Selbstvertra ven und Sozialer kompeteriz, Anleitung fuer den Therapeuten II. Der Ursicherheitsfrabogen (4th ed.). München, Germany: J. Pfeiffer Verlag.

van Dam-Baggen, R., & Kraaimaat, F. (1999). Assessing social anxiety: The Inventory of Interpersonal Situations, IIS. *European Journal of Psychological Assessment*, *15*, 25–36.

van Dam-Baggen, R., & Kraaimaat, F. W. (2000a). Social skills training in two subtypes of psychiatric inpatients with generalized social phobia. *Scandinavian Journal of Behaviour Therapy*, *29*, 14–21.

van Dam-Baggen, R., & Kraaimaat, F. (2000b). Group social skills training or cognitive group therapy as the clinical treatment of choice for generalized social phobia? *Journal of Anxiety Disorders*, *14*, 437–451.

Voncken, M. J., & Bogels, S. M. (2008). Social performance deficits in social anxiety disorder: Reality during conversation and biased perception during speech. *Journal of Anxiety Disorders*, *22*, 1384–1392.

Walters, K. S., & Hope, D. A. (1998). Analysis of social behavior in individuals with social phobia and nonanxious participants using a psychobiological model. *Behavior Therapy*, *29*, 387–407.

Watson, D., & Friend, R. (1969). Measurement of social-evaluative anxiety. *Journal of Consulting and Clinical Psychology*, *33*, 448–457.

Wenzel, A., Graff-Dolezal, J., Macho, M., & Brendle, J. R. (2005). Communication and social skills in socially anxious and nonanxious individuals in the context of romantic relationships. *Behaviour Research and Therapy*, *43*, 505–519.

Wessberg, H. W., Mariotto, M. J., Conger, A. J., Farrel, A. D., & Conger, J. C. (1979). Ecological validity of role plays for assessing heterosocial anxiety and skill of male college students. *Journal of Consulting and Clinical Psychology*, *47*, 525–535.

Wlazlo, Z., Schroeder-Hartig, K., Hand, I., Kaiser, G., & Münchau, N. (1990). Exposure in vivo vs. social skills training for social phobia: Long-term outcome and differential effects. *Behaviour Research and Therapy*, *28*, 181–193.

Chapter 7

Relation to Clinical Syndromes in Adulthood

Amy Wenzel
Department of Psychiatry, University of Pennsylvania, Philadelphia, PA 19104

SAD typically begins early in life and follows a chronic course, often resulting in comorbid presentations at some time in the lives of people who suffer from it. In many cases, comorbidity is associated with greater functional impairment and lower quality of life (e.g., Magee, Eaton, Wittchen, McGonagle, & Kessler, 1996). Research conducted over the past 30 years has indicated that there is substantial overlap between SAD and other anxiety and depressive disorders, and to a lesser extent between SAD and other conditions, such as alcohol and drug use disorders. This pattern of results emerges regardless of whether community or clinical samples are studied, of whether lifetime or current prevalence rates are calculated, and of whether DSM-III, DSM-III-R, or DSM-IV criteria are used to assign diagnoses.

In this chapter, I first summarize results from older research that established the high rate of comorbidity between SAD and several disorders, including other anxiety disorders, mood disorders, and alcohol and substance use disorders, according to DSM-III and DSM-III-R criteria. Next, I summarize the epidemiological research for the same instances of comorbidity that has been conducted on the basis of our current diagnostic system, DSM-IV. Subsequently, I highlight contemporary information on the comorbidity between SAD and other conditions that have received less systematic attention in the empirical research, such as eating disorders, BDD, bipolar disorder, psychosis, and suicidality. Finally, I compare comorbidity rates from a cross-cultural standpoint.

COMORBIDITY IN STUDIES USING DSM-III AND DSM-III-R CRITERIA

Table 7.1 provides a summary of major studies that were designed to identify rates of comorbidity in people with SAD diagnosed according to DSM-III or DSM-III-R criteria. Three studies included in this table document lifetime

Social Anxiety: Clinical, Developmental, and Social Perspectives. DOI: 10.1016/B978-0-12-375096-9.00007-9

TABLE 7.1 Comorbidity in Social Anxiety Disorder Diagnosed According to DSM-III or DSM-III-R Criteria

Comorbid Disorder	Community Sample: DSM-III Criteria; Lifetime Prev. (Three Studies)	Community Sample: DSM-III-R Criteria; Lifetime Prev. (One Study)	Clinical Sample: DSM-III-R Criteria; Lifetime Prev. (Three Studies)	Clinical Sample: DSM-III Criteria; Current Prev. (Two Studies)	Clinical Sample: DSM-III-R Criteria; Current Prev. (Four Studies)
Anxiety Disorders	n/a	56.9 (1)	n/a	n/a	n/a
AG	4.5–44.9 (2)	23.3 (1)	7.0–10.0 (2)	0.0–2.0 (2)	3.0–14.7 (2)
GAD	26.9 (1)	13.3 (1)	25.0–35.0 (3)	4.0–5.3 (2)	8.0–34.0 (4)
OCD	11.1–18.6 (2)	n/a	5.0–18.0 (3)	4.0–10.5 (2)	1.4–16.0 (3)
PD	4.7–26.9 (3)	10.9 (1)	0.0–49.1 (3)	0.0–2.0 (2)	2.8–9.0 (2)
PD with AG	n/a	n/a	25.0–42.0 (2)	n/a	17.0–36.0 (2)
PTSD	5.4 (1)	15.8 (1)	5.0–12.0 (2)	n/a	11.0 (1)
Simple Phobia	37.5–60.8 (3)	37.6 (1)	15.0–21.0 (3)	5.3–23.0 (2)	11.1–25.0 (3)
Mood Disorders	n/a	41.4 (1)	n/a	n/a	n/a

MDD	14.6–42.3 (3)	37.2 (1)	70.2 (1)	2.0–5.3 (2)	2.8 - 48.8 (3)
Dysthymic Disorder	11.5–12.5 (2)	14.6 (1)	31.6 (1)	15.8–23.0 (2)	5.6–21.0 (2)
Mania or Hypomania	1.5–11.5 (3)	5.1 (1)	3.5 (1)	n/a	n/a
Substance Use Disorder	n/a	39.6 (1)	n/a	n/a	n/a
Alcohol Abuse	15.4–18.8 (3)	10.9 (1)	28.1 (1)	5.3 (1)	n/a
Alcohol Dependence	n/a	23.9 (1)	n/a	n/a	n/a
Drug Abuse	13.0 (1)	5.3 (1)	15.8 (1)	n/a	n/a
Drug Dependence	n/a	14.8 (1)	n/a	n/a	n/a
No Comorbid Diagnosis	0.6–31.0 (2)	19.0 (1)	3.5–55.0 (3)	53.0–58.0 (2)	23.0–57.0 (3)

Values in columns represent the ranges of percentages of the people with social anxiety disorder who were diagnosed with the comorbid disorder specified. Values in parentheses are the number of studies that examined the particular disorder. Abbreviations are as follows: AG = agoraphobia; GAD = generalized anxiety disorder; MDD = major depressive disorder; n/a = disorder was not assessed in the study; OCD = obsessive-compulsive disorder; PD = panic disorder; prev. = prevalence; PTSD = post-traumatic stress disorder.

DSM-III SAD and Axis I comorbidity in large-scale epidemiological studies examining psychiatric disorders; that is, these studies identified people who met diagnostic criteria for SAD at any point in their lives and determined whether they met diagnostic criteria for other disorders at any point in their lives. I regard these studies as using community samples because participants were recruited to be representative of the general population from which they were drawn. These investigations included an analysis of the Epidemiologic Catchment Area (ECA) study data, drawn from four sites (Schneier, Johnson, Hornig, Liebowitz, & Weissman, 1992); an analysis of ECA data from the Duke University site (Davidson, Hughes, George, & Blazer, 1993); and the Zurich Study (Degonda & Angst, 1993). In most cases, there was a wide range of comorbidity estimates across studies; for example, rates of comorbid agoraphobia ranged from 4.5% at the Duke University ECA site (Davidson et al., 1993) to 44.9% at the remaining four ECA sites (Schneier et al., 1992). It is unclear why the rates between the Davidson et al. (1993) and Schneier et al. (1992) reports are so discrepant, as both used the same interview to achieve diagnoses (i.e., the Diagnostic Interview Schedule; Robins, Helzer, Croughan, & Ratcliff, 1981) and trained lay interviewers to administer this instrument. However, it is notable that there was potential unreliability in the diagnoses of SAD, as Schneier et al. (1992) achieved a kappa coefficient of only 0.40.

One large community epidemiological study in Table 7.1 was designed to identify rates of Axis I comorbidity in DSM-III-R lifetime SAD – the National Comorbidity Survey (NCS; Magee et al., 1996). It could be hypothesized that rates of comorbidity would be expected to increase in people diagnosed with DSM-III-R SAD as compared to people diagnosed with DSM-III SAD, as DSM-III-R diagnostic criteria were broadened from fear and avoidance of specific performance situations (e.g., public speaking, eating in public) to allow for a generalized type of SAD (McNeil, 2001). It is reasonable to speculate that a generalized form of SAD, consisting of fear and avoidance of a number of social and performance situations, would represent a more severe disorder and hence be associated with higher rates of comorbidity. However, results from Magee et al. (1996) did not support this prediction – the majority of the lifetime rates of comorbidity fell in between the low and high ends of rates of lifetime comorbidity diagnosed according to DSM-III criteria. Like the community epidemiological studies examining DSM-III-diagnosed disorders, Magee et al. (1996) found that only a minority had never been diagnosed with a comorbid disorder at any time in their lives.

Three additional studies in Table 7.1 examined lifetime rates of Axis I comorbidity in DSM-III-R-diagnosed SAD, but these studies used clinical samples rather than community samples (Goisman, Goldenberg, Vasile, & Keller, 1995; Schwalberg, Barlow, Alger, & Howard, 1992; van Ameringen, Mancini, Styani, & Donison, 1991). Clinical samples comprise people who are presenting for treatment at a clinic, either for SAD or for another psychiatric disorder. It would be expected that rates of comorbidity would be higher in these samples, as their psychiatric symptoms are severe enough to bring them in for treatment. This prediction was confirmed for a few specific disorders; for example, the rates of comorbid GAD, comorbid PD, comorbid major depressive disorder (MDD), comorbid dysthymic disorder, comorbid alcohol abuse, and comorbid drug abuse were higher in at least one of the studies using a clinical sample than in Magee et al. (1996). Curiously, rates of comorbid agoraphobia and comorbid simple phobia were substantially lower than the rates calculated by Magee et al. (1996).

Lifetime rates of comorbidity rates provide information about the degree to which psychiatric disorders cluster together, but they do not necessarily capture a person's clinical presentation at any one moment. Current rates of comorbidity, in contrast, illustrate the degree to which psychiatric disorders are present at the same time or are at least present within a discrete window that can last anywhere between 4 weeks and 12 months (Wittchen & Fehm, 2003). Regardless of whether community or clinical samples are considered, these rates are generally lower than rates of lifetime comorbidity because the co-occurrence of the two psychiatric disorders must take place at one particular point in time. Two studies included in Table 7.1 examined rates of current comorbidity in a clinical sample of people who were diagnosed with DSM-III SAD (Barlow, DiNardo, Vermilyea, Vermilyea, & Blanchard, 1986; DiNardo & Barlow, 1990), and four studies in this table examined rates of current comorbidity in clinical samples of people who were diagnosed with DSM-III-R SAD (Goisman et al., 1995; Lecrubier & Weiller, 1997; Sanderson, DiNardo, Rapee, & Barlow, 1990; Turner, Beidel, Borden, Stanley, & Jacob, 1991). The most common current psychiatric disorders were PD with agoraphobia, simple phobia, and dysthymic disorder.

In all, results from studies examining comorbidity in people with DSM-III and DSM-III-R SAD indicate that comorbidity is common. However, it is difficult to draw more specific conclusions beyond this general observation. Other than simple phobia, there were wide ranges in the estimates of other comorbid anxiety and mood disorders. In some cases, these wide ranges were observed in epidemiological studies that used identical methodologies (e.g., Davidson et al., 1993; Schneier et al., 1992). These discrepancies raise questions about the validity and the robustness of strategies that researchers have used to document comorbidity. Differences in operational definitions of particular disorders also may have accounted for discrepancies in the rates of comorbidity between studies. For example, Goisman et al. (1995) and Schwalberg et al. (1992) included categories of uncomplicated PD, agoraphobia without PD, and PD with agoraphobia. In contrast, all other studies except DiNardo and Barlow (1990) and Sanderson et al. (1990) presented rates for PD and agoraphobia, but not for PD with agoraphobia. Because operational definitions of particular Axis I disorders were not specified in the methodologies of these studies, it cannot be discerned whether individuals with these disorders in most of the studies were uncomplicated cases or were diagnosed with PD with agoraphobia. These caveats point to the fact that readers must have a detailed understanding of the designs of studies that examine comorbidity among psychiatric disorders and take into account methodological nuances in drawing conclusions.

COMORBIDITY IN STUDIES USING DSM-IV CRITERIA

Two main methodological differences stand out between most studies that examine Axis I comorbidity according to DSM-IV criteria and most studies that examine Axis I comorbidity according to DSM-III or III-R criteria. First, nearly all of the studies examining the prevalence and comorbidity of DSM-IV disorders use the Composite International Diagnostic Interview (CIDI; Kessler & Ustun, 2004), which was developed by the WHO and which corresponds to DSM-IV criteria. In contrast, only two of the studies reviewed in the previous edition of this chapter used the previous version of this instrument, which corresponded to DSM-III-R criteria (i.e., Lecrubier & Weiller, 1997; Magee et al., 1996). One advantage of the CIDI is that it assesses social anxiety across a broad range of social and performance situations, which decreases the likelihood that clinically significant cases of SAD are overlooked (Wittchen & Fehm, 2003). In addition, scholars have noted that there is less variability in the prevalence and comorbidity rates yielded by the CIDI (e.g., Chartier, Walker, & Stein, 2003), which could remedy the confusing pattern of results noted in the previous section. Although some research has found that the CIDI yields only a fair concordance with diagnoses achieved by another standard clinical interview, the SCID-IV Disorders (First, Spitzer, Gibbon, & Williams, 2002; Haro et al., 2006), researchers generally regard prevalence rates obtained by the CIDI as reliable but conservative.

A second methodological difference between studies examining comorbidity according to DSM-III and DSM-III-R criteria and studies examining comorbidity according to DSM-IV criteria is that odds ratios are reported in addition to simple percentages. Odds ratios indicate whether events occur with equal likelihood in two groups; an odds ratio of 1.0, for example, indicates that an event is equally likely to occur in both groups. For the purpose of this chapter, odds ratios tell us whether comorbidity is more likely to occur in people who are diagnosed with SAD as compared to people who are not diagnosed with SAD. Moreover, confidence intervals supplied along with odds ratios in individual studies give us information regarding the degree to which odds are truly different from 1.0 – if the upper and lower ranges of the confidence interval do not include 1.0, then it is safe to conclude that there is an effect. Advantages of considering odds ratios in the study of comorbidity include (1) that the reader can determine with greater precision whether rates of comorbidity in people with social anxiety are indeed elevated relative to people without SAD and (2) that confounding factors that could influence rates of comorbidity can be controlled, such as demographic variables.

Lifetime Comorbidity Rates

Table 7.2 summarizes rates of lifetime DSM-IV Axis I comorbidity in SAD from five studies. Wittchen, Stein, and Kessler (1999) calculated rates of DSM-IV lifetime comorbidity in the 3021 young adults between the ages of 14 and 24 who participated in Germany's Early Developmental Stages of Psychopathology Study. Although this chapter targets comorbidity in adults, the Wittchen et al. study is included here because most adult epidemiological studies recruit participants who are 18 years and older; thus, the age range of Wittchen et al.'s sample overlaps substantially with samples in other studies described in this chapter. Diagnoses were made using a computerized version of the CIDI. Grant et al. (2005) calculated rates of DSM-IV lifetime comorbidity in 43 093 adults aged 18 and older who participated in the National Epidemiologic Survey on Alcohol and Related Conditions. Diagnoses were made according to the National Institute on Alcohol Abuse and Alcoholism's Alcohol Use and Associated Disabilities Interview Schedule – DSM-IV edition (Grant, Dawson, & Hasin, 2001), which was administered by lay interviewers. The authors contrasted their instrument with the CIDI, noting that it ensures that diagnoses of SAD are not better accounted for by anxiety that is substance-induced or by a medical condition. Mohammadi, Ghanoizadeh, Mohammadi, and Mesgarour (2006) examined DSM-IV lifetime comorbidity rates in 25 180 Iranian people aged 18 and older using the Schedule for Affective Disorders and Schizophrenia (Endicott & Spitzer, 1978) translated to Farsi. Finally, Ruscio et al. (2008) calculated rates of DSM-IV lifetime comorbidity using data from the National Comorbidity Survey Replication (NCS-R; Kessler & Merikangas, 2004), in which the CIDI was administered by lay interviewers to 9282 adults aged 18 and older. Their odds ratios controlled for sociodemographic variables such as age, gender, and race/ethnicity.

The remaining study included in Table 7.2 (Brown, Campbell, Lehman, Grisham, & Mancill, 2001) calculated lifetime comorbidity rates in a clinical sample of 1127 patients seeking treatment at their anxiety disorders clinic. Diagnoses were assigned according to the ADIS-IV – Lifetime Version (DiNardo, Brown, & Barlow, 1994). Brown et al. (2001) reported two types of lifetime comorbidity – comorbidity in patients who had a principal diagnosis of various anxiety disorders and comorbidity in patients who had an anxiety disorder regardless of whether it was designated as principal. Values representing the latter designation are summarized in Table 7.2 in order to be comparable to other epidemiological studies, most of which identify comorbidity regardless of the severity of either disorder.

The values depicting the odds of having comorbid lifetime SAD and other lifetime psychiatric disorders in community epidemiological studies indicate that the presence of SAD increases the odds of having almost every other anxiety or mood disorder. Between 80 and 90% of people who were diagnosed with lifetime SAD in these samples had at least one other lifetime Axis I

TABLE 7.2 Lifetime Comorbidity in Social Anxiety Disorder Diagnosed According to DSM-IV Criteria

Comorbid Disorder	Wittchen, Stein, & Kessler (1999): Community Sample	Grant et al. (2005): Community Sample	Mohammadi et al. (2006): Community Sample	Ruscio et al. (2008): Community Sample	Brown et al. (2001): Clinical Sample
Anxiety Disorders	49.9 (3.71)*	54.1 (7.4)*	n/a	63.9 (5.9)*	67.0 (no OR)
AG	8.8 (5.45)*	n/a	n/a	6.8 (11.9)*	n/a
GAD	2.3 (2.42)*	23.3 (8.4)*	7.7 (9.41)*	24.1 (5.2)*	28.0 (1.26)*
OCD	2.3 (3.95)*	n/a	17.4 (12.40)*	n/a	16.0 (0.92)
Panic Disorder	6.2 (4.68)*	22.0 (5.7)*	12.1 (10.97)*	15.2 (4.9)*	30.0 (0.55)*
PD with AG	n/a	n/a	n/a	n/a	27.0 (0.55)*
PTSD	5.9 (6.23)*	n/a	4.8 (14.12)*	19.0 (3.9)*	8.0 (1.12)
Specific Phobia	43.6 (3.67)* (includes phobia NOS)	38.1 (6.6)*	66.7 (295.17)*	36.5 (5.4)*	21.0 (0.78)*
Mood Disorders	n/a	56.3 (5.5)*	n/a	51.8 (4.8)*	72.0 (no OR)

MDD	25.5 (2.69)*	34.1 (3.3)*	15.0 (5.76)*	47.2 (4.6)*	60.0 (1.18)*
Dysthymic Disorder	10.9 (5.03)*	11.5 (3.9)*	n/a	14.8 (6.2)*	20.0 (1.92)*
Mania or Hypomania	n/a	19.5 (3.9–6.1)*	4.8 (7.70–6.40)*	13.8 (4.6)*	n/a
Substance Use Disorder	41.3 (1.64)*	n/a	n/a	29.0 (2.8)*	n/a
Alcohol Abuse	19.4 (1.14)	20.9 (1.2)*	n/a	26.2 (2.8)*	17.0 (1.26)
Alcohol Dependence		22.3 (2.7)*	n/a		
Drug Abuse	7.5 (1.67)	12.5 (1.6)*	n/a	18.5 (3.0)*	11.0 (1.13)
Drug Dependence		9.8 (4.2)*	n/a		

*All values in columns are percentages of the people with social anxiety disorder who were diagnosed with the comorbid disorder specified. Values in parentheses are odds ratios. A * next to the odds ratio signifies that the 95% confidence interval did not include 1.0. Abbreviations are as follows: AG = agoraphobia; GAD = generalized anxiety disorder; MDD = major depressive disorder; NOS = not otherwise specified; OCD = obsessive-compulsive disorder; OR = odds ratio; PD = panic disorder; PTSD = post-traumatic stress disorder; n/a = disorder was not assessed in the study. Cells that combine alcohol abuse and dependence and drug abuse and dependence give percentages and odds ratios that combine the diagnoses. Two studies (i.e., Grant et al., 2005; Mohammadi et al., 2006) provided separate rates of bipolar I and bipolar II disorder; in these cases, the percentages were combined and the odds ratios for bipolar I and bipolar II disorders, respectively, are provided in parentheses.*

diagnosis (Grant et al., 2005; Ruscio et al., 2008). Specifically, between one-half and two-thirds of those with lifetime SAD had at least one other lifetime anxiety disorder, and over half of those with lifetime SAD had a lifetime mood disorder. There was a substantial range in the comorbidity rates of specific anxiety and mood disorders; for example, rates of comorbid lifetime GAD ranged from 2.3 to 24.1%. In general, rates of lifetime comorbidity ranged from approximately 5 to 20% for agoraphobia, OCD, PD, and post-traumatic stress disorder (PTSD); comorbidity rates extended to an upper limit of 25% for GAD and comorbidity rates for specific phobia reached as high as 67%. Between 25 and 50% of people with lifetime SAD endorsed lifetime MDD; approximately 10–15% of people with lifetime SAD endorsed lifetime dysthymic disorder; and between 5 and 20% of people with lifetime SAD endorsed bipolar I or bipolar II disorder. According to these community epidemiological studies, the odds of having a comorbid alcohol or substance use disorder were lower than most odds of having a comorbid anxiety or mood disorder, although the percentages indicated that up to 20–25% of people with SAD will be diagnosed with one of these disorders.

Contrary to expectation, rates of lifetime comorbidity were higher in Brown et al.'s (2001) clinical sample than in the community samples in only some instances. A higher percentage of this clinical sample was diagnosed with at least one other lifetime anxiety disorder or at least one lifetime mood disorder than the community samples. In addition, this clinical sample had higher rates of lifetime comorbidity with GAD, MDD, and dysthymic disorder than the community samples. Brown et al. reported higher rates of OCD and PTSD than some of the community studies, but lower rates than at least one other community study. Although their rate of 4.0% for diagnoses of lifetime PD is much lower than the rates obtained in the community studies, it must be considered that they included a separate category for PD with agoraphobia. It is likely that cases of PD only *and* PD with agoraphobia were included in the rates of PD reported in community studies. Moreover, Brown et al. reported lower rates of alcohol abuse than all of the community studies, although the odds ratio was similar to two of the community studies.

It is interesting to note in Brown et al.'s (2001) study that SAD was one of two anxiety disorders associated with the *lowest* rates of comorbidity with other anxiety and mood disorders – 72% for lifetime comorbid diagnoses and 46% for current comorbid diagnoses. Many of the odds ratios reflecting the likelihood of specific comorbid diagnoses are lower than 1.0 (see Tables 7.2 and 7.3). However, before concluding that SAD is associated with a lowered risk of comorbidity in treatment-seeking samples, it is important to consider the reference group, which consists of other people with any anxiety or mood disorder who were seeking treatment at a specialty clinic. Thus, a more accurate conclusion from this study is that SAD is associated with a lowered risk of comorbidity relative to other anxiety and mood disorders, but not necessarily relative to people representative of the general population who are not diagnosed with SAD. Nevertheless, the finding that 72% of their patients with SAD had at least one comorbid disorder is striking, given that higher rates were obtained in the community epidemiological studies (e.g., 80–90%; Grant et al., 2005; Ruscio et al., 2008). It is possible that higher rates were obtained in the community studies because they assessed some disorders not included in Table 7.2 and not assessed by Brown et al. (2001), such as impulse-control disorders.

All of the comorbidity rates presented in Table 7.2 are for SAD in general and do not differentiate between the generalized and nongeneralized subtype. GSAD describes people who report three or more social and evaluate fears, whereas non-generalized social anxiety disorder describes people who have one or two pre-dominant fears, usually those that involve public speaking or some sort of other public performance (Wittchen & Fehm, 2003). Wittchen et al. (1999) broke down comorbidity rates as a function of subtype. Results indicated that the nongeneralized subtype increased the odds of MDD, PD, and specific phobia. In contrast, the generalized subtype increased the odds of these disorders to an even greater degree, and it also increased the odds of dysthymic disorder, agoraphobia, GAD, OCD, and PTSD. Although they did not break down SAD into generalized and nongeneralized subtypes, Ruscio et al. (2008) found a lifetime comorbidity rate of 62.9% for people with SAD who reported 1–4 social fears, 75.2% for those who reported 5–7 social fears, 81.5% for those who reported 8–10 social fears, and 90.2% for those who reported 11 or more social fears. This pattern of results supports the notion that the generalized subtype is a more severe pathology than the nongeneralized subtype, at least when severity is defined by the presence of comorbid psychiatric disorders.

Current Comorbidity Rates

Table 7.3 summarizes rates of current DSM-IV Axis I comorbidity in SAD from five studies, three of which were conducted with community samples. Lampe, Slade, Issakisis, and Andrews (2003) examined rates of comorbidity in 10641 people aged 18 and older who participated in the Australian National Survey of Mental Health and Well-Being. Diagnoses were assigned through a computerized version of the CIDI when participants had met criteria for a particular disorder in the previous 12 months. Grant et al. (2005) calculated 12-month comorbidity rates in the National Epidemiologic Survey on Alcohol and Related Conditions using the Alcohol Use and Associated Disabilities Interview Schedule – DSM-IV edition, which was described in the previous section. Fehm, Beesdo, Jacobi, and Fiedler (2008) examined rates of comorbidity in 4174 people aged 18–65 who participated in the German National Health Interview and Examination Survey. Diagnoses were assigned through a computerized version of the Munich Composite Diagnostic Interview (M-CIDI), which is a modified version of the CIDI that accounts for a wider range of DSM-IV diagnoses than previous versions of the CIDI. Participants were regarded as having current diagnoses of psychiatric disorders if they met diagnostic criteria during the previous 12 months.

TABLE 7.3 Current Comorbidity in Social Anxiety Disorder Diagnosed According to DSM-IV Criteria

Comorbid Disorder	Lampe et al. (2003): Community Sample	Grant et al. (2005): Community Sample	Fehm et al. (2008): Community Sample	Brown et al. (2001): Clinical Sample	Kashdan et al. (2006): Clinical Sample
Anxiety Disorders	53.4 (6.3)*	48.8 (9.1)*	71.2 (22.2)*	59.0 (no OR)	n/a
AG	17.4 (7.8)*	n/a	17.0 (20.7)*	n/a	34.6 (9.28)*
GAD	33.9 (3.0)*	17.3 (10.6)*	22.2 (35.4)*	27.0 (1.23)	50.0 (8.39)*
OCD	7.7 (1.3)	n/a	11.5 (41.5)*	13.0 (0.90)	34.6 (74.01)*
PD	20.6 (4.9)*	15.3 (8.5)*	25.6 (26.4)*	26.0 (0.50)*	34.6 (7.94)*
PD with AG	(incorporated into above value)	n/a	n/a	23.0 (0.50)*	n/a
PTSD	14.6 (1.4)	n/a	n/a	5.0 (1.18)	73.1 (no OR)
Specific Phobia	n/a	37.3 (7.9)*	29.5 (6.6)*	16.0 (0.64)*	n/a
Mood Disorders	43.5 (2.9)*	38.3 (6.0)*	65.3 (19.7)*	48.0	n/a
MDD	40.5 (2.4)*	19.9 (4.1)*	50.5 (15.9)*	32.0 (1.29)*	69.2 (13.13)*

Dysthymic Disorder	12.0 (1.5)	6.6 (4.9)*	38.1 (20.2)*	17.0 (2.18)*	61.5 (12.48)*
Mania or Hypomania	n/a	16.2 (7.2–3.1)*	5.7 (12.6)*	n/a	n/a
Substance Use Disorder	22.1 (1.3)	n/a	n/a	n/a	n/a
Alcohol Abuse	16.7 (1.5)	4.4 (1.0)	n/a	n/a	3.8 (2.31)
Alcohol Dependence	n/a	8.6 (2.3)*	10.3 (3.9)*	n/a	15.4 (8.35)*
Drug Abuse	8.7 (0.9)	2.6 (1.7)*	n/a	n/a	n/a
Drug Dependence	n/a	2.9 (4.6)*	n/a	n/a	n/a

*All values in columns are percentages of the people with social anxiety disorder who were diagnosed with the comorbid disorder specified. Values in parentheses are odds ratios. A * next to the odds ratio signifies that the 95% confidence interval did not include 1.0. Abbreviations are as follows: AG = agoraphobia; GAD = generalized anxiety disorder; MDD = major depressive disorder; n/a = disorder was not assessed in the study; OCD = obsessive-compulsive disorder; OR = odds ratio; PD = panic disorder; PTSD = post-traumatic stress disorder. One study (i.e., Grant et al., 2005) provided separate rates of bipolar I and bipolar II disorder; in this case, the percentages were combined and the odds ratios for bipolar I and bipolar II disorders, respectively, are provided in parentheses.*

Two additional studies in Table 7.3 reported rates of current Axis I comorbidity in clinical samples. Brown et al. (2001) used the ADIS-IV to assess current psychiatric disorders in their sample of patients seeking treatment at their anxiety disorders clinic, which were assigned when participants met diagnostic criteria for the disorders at the time of the assessment. Kashdan, Frueh, Knapp, Herbert, and Magruder (2006) examined comorbidity in 733 veterans who were seen in four Veterans' Affairs primary care clinics, with 26 of these veterans being diagnosed at the time of the assessment. Comorbid psychiatric disorders were assigned during a telephone interview conducted by master's level clinicians, who used the Clinician-Administered PTSD Scale (Blake et al., 1990) to assess PTSD and the Mini International Neuropsychiatric Interview (Sheehan et al., 1997) to assess all other Axis I conditions.

Results from the three studies that used community samples indicate that between 50 and 70% of people with a current diagnosis of SAD were diagnosed with another current anxiety disorder and that between 30 and 60% were diagnosed with a current mood disorder. These rates are not appreciably different from the lifetime comorbidity rates described in the previous section. The range of comorbidity rates of specific anxiety and mood disorders was somewhat smaller than the ranges of lifetime comorbidity rates; for example, rates of comorbid current GAD ranged from 17.3 to 33.9%. In general, rates of current comorbidity range from approximately 5 to 20% for AG, OCD, and PD; comorbidity rates extended to 25–30% for PD and GAD; and one community study suggested that the rate of current comorbid specific phobia was as high as 37%. Between 38 and 65% of people with current SAD endorsed current MDD; between 6 and 38% of people with current SAD endorsed current dysthymic disorder; and 5–16% of people with current SAD endorsed bipolar I or bipolar II disorder. As seen with lifetime comorbidity rates, the odds of having a current comorbid alcohol or substance use disorder were lower than most odds of having a comorbid anxiety or mood disorder, although Lampe et al.'s (2003) study suggests that over 20% of people with current SAD are diagnosed with some form of current alcohol or drug use disorder.

The two studies that calculated current rates of comorbidity in clinical samples yielded discrepant results. The current comorbidity rates reported by Brown et al. (2001) were similar to, and at times lower than, current comorbidity rates reported by studies that used community samples. In contrast, Kashdan et al. (2006) identified high rates of comorbidity in their sample of veterans diagnosed with SAD who were seeking treatment at Veterans' Affairs primary care clinics. For example, over 70% of the veterans diagnosed with SAD also carried diagnoses of PTSD. The only diagnosis that was not elevated in this sample was alcohol abuse. It is likely that the high rate of comorbidity can be accounted for by the unique nature of the veteran sample, as less than a third of the respondents in the sample were employed and nearly half of them had been in a war zone at some point in their lives.

Like the studies summarized in Table 7.2, all of the comorbidity rates in Table 7.3 pertain to diagnoses of SAD in general, which includes both the generalized and nongeneralized subtypes. No epidemiological studies have broken down current comorbidity rates as a function of subtype. However, Fehm et al. (2008) identified rates of comorbidity among people who met full criteria for SAD, people who were subthreshold for SAD (i.e., those who met Criterion A for a diagnosis of SAD but were missing one criterion), and those who were symptomatic for SAD (i.e., those who reported social fears but who were missing two or more criteria). They identified a dose–response relation between the severity of SAD and the amount of comorbidity, such that the odds of being diagnosed with all of the other disorders considered were substantially elevated in people with SAD, whereas the odds were much lower (but in most cases still elevated) in those who were only symptomatic. This study was the first to demonstrate that subthreshold levels of social anxiety are associated with significant life interference and distress, in the form of comorbid psychiatric disorders.

COMORBIDITY BETWEEN SOCIAL ANXIETY DISORDER AND OTHER CONDITIONS

Eating Disorders

Over the past 10–15 years, much scholarly attention has been given to the overlap between eating disorders and anxiety disorders, especially SAD (e.g., Bulik, Sullivan, Fear, & Joyce, 1997). In their review of this topic, Swinbourne and Touyz (2007) concluded that SAD and OCD are the two most comorbid anxiety disorders in people who are diagnosed with eating disorders. Rates of DSM-IV SAD in people who are diagnosed with DSM-IV eating disorders in general range from 18 (Iwasaki, Matsunaga, Kiriike, Tanaka, & Matsui, 2000) to 23% (Kaye et al., 2004). DSM-IV comorbidity rates are even higher when specific eating disorder subgroups are considered; for example, rates of comorbid SAD up to 88 and 68% have been detected in patients with anorexia and bulimia, respectively (Hinrichson, Wright, Waller, & Meyer, 2003). Some scholars have proposed that SAD might constitute one pathway to the development of eating disorders because it is temporally primary in the majority of cases (Swinbourne & Touyz, 2007).

Body Dysmorphic Disorder

Empirical research has examined the overlap between SAD and BDD with the rationale that both share core features such as fear of embarrassment and rejection and avoidance of social situations (Coles et al., 2006). Rates of lifetime comorbidity between the two disorders according to DSM-III-R criteria range from 12 (Hollander, Cohen, & Simeon, 1993; Perugi et al., 1997) to

38% (Phillips & Diaz, 1997). Gunstad and Phillips (2003) calculated a 31% rate of current comorbidity between the two disorders, with SAD being diagnosed according to DSM-III-R criteria and BDD being diagnosed according to DSM-IV criteria. In the most extensive study to examine comorbidity between the two disorders using DSM-IV criteria, Coles et al. (2006) reported in a sample of 178 people with BDD that 39.3 met criteria for lifetime SAD and 34.3% met criteria for current SAD. Those with comorbid diagnoses were less likely to be employed and more likely to report suicide ideation and poor adjustment than those with BDD alone. BDD is also observed in between 8 (Zimmerman & Mattia, 1998) and 12% (Wilhelm, Otto, Zucker, & Pollack, 1997) of people with primary diagnoses of SAD, with SAD being temporally primary in nearly all cases.

Bipolar Disorder

Although the main focus of research on comorbid anxiety disorders in bipolar disorder has been on its comorbidity with PD and OCD, a few reports in the past decade have examined the overlap between bipolar spectrum disorders and SAD. Empirical research on this topic suggests that the lifetime comorbidity rate of SAD and bipolar I disorder ranges from 4.2 (Rihmer, Szádóczky, Füredi, Kiss, & Papp, 2001) to 20% (Tamam & Ozpoyraz, 2002). Rihmer et al. (2001) found that the rate of comorbid SAD and bipolar II disorder was almost triple the rate of its comorbidity with bipolar I disorder. One study (Pini et al., 2006) calculated a current (i.e., past month) comorbidity rate between SAD and bipolar I disorder of 10.1%. Patients with comorbid SAD and bipolar disorder report more severe psychiatric symptoms than patients with bipolar disorder alone (Pini et al., 2006; Tamam & Ozpoyraz, 2002) and are more likely to exhibit psychotic symptoms (Azorin et al., 2007).

The lifetime comorbidity rates indicate that the comorbidity between SAD and bipolar disorder is higher than would be expected by chance alone, but they say little about the clinical presentations of people who have carried both diagnoses at some point in their lifetime. Some scholars speculate that comorbid anxiety disorders, including SAD, are most likely to be present in mixed or dyphoric manic episodes (Freeman, Freeman, & McElroy, 2002), and there is some evidence that bipolar symptoms develop in the context of antidepressant treatment for SAD (Perugi et al, 1999).

Psychosis

Recent attention has also been given to the comorbidity between psychotic disorders and anxiety disorders, with the reasoning that comorbid anxiety has the potential to exacerbate the course of illness and hinder recovery. Empirical research demonstrates that DSM-IV SAD is especially comorbid with schizophrenia, with rates ranging from 11 (Mazeh et al., 2009) to 39.1% (Ciapparelli et al., 2007). In fact, empirical research indicates that SAD is the single anxiety disorder associated with the highest rate of comorbidity in psychotic individuals (Braga, Mendlowicz, Marrocos, & Figueira, 2005). Ciapparelli et al.'s (2007) work also demonstrated that rates of SAD are significantly higher in patients with schizophrenia than in patients who had psychotic episodes but were assigned other diagnoses. Research shows that symptoms of social anxiety correlate positively with an index of global severity of psychotic symptoms (Ciapparelli et al., 2007), lower quality of life, and lower social adjustment (Pallanti, Quercioli, & Hollander, 2004) in psychotic patients.

Suicidality

Although variables relevant to suicide (i.e., suicide ideation, suicide attempts) do not constitute a psychiatric diagnosis, they are often considered in investigations of comorbidity because they represent serious mental health problems. In both the NCS (Kessler et al., 1994) and the NCS-R (Kessler & Merikangas, 2004), lifetime history of suicide ideation was assessed via the question, "Have you ever seriously thought about committing suicide?", and lifetime history of suicide attempt was assessed via the question, "Have you ever attempted suicide?" In the NCS, lifetime suicide ideation and suicide attempt were not elevated in people who were diagnosed with lifetime DSM-III-R SAD (Sareen, Houlahan, Cox, & Asmundson, 2005). In contrast, in the NCS-R, lifetime DSM-IV SAD was associated with elevations in both of these variables, even while controlling for other anxiety disorders (Cougle, Keough, Riccardi, & Sachs-Ericsson, 2009). Specifically, almost 35% of the respondents with SAD endorsed a history of suicide ideation, and over 14% admitted that they had made a suicide attempt. An important difference between the two studies is that Sareen, Houlahan, et al. (2005) included a covariate that accounted for the presence of three or more diagnoses, which could have reduced the statistical significance of the anxiety disorders under consideration (Cougle et al., 2009).

The third study that examined suicidality associated with anxiety disorders used data from the Netherlands Mental Health and Incidence Survey (Bijl, van Zessen, & Ravelli, 1998), in which 7076 adults aged 18–65 were administered a computerized version of the CIDI in order to achieve DSM-III-R diagnoses (Sareen, Cox, et al., 2005). A lifetime history of suicide ideation was assessed via the question, "Have you ever felt so low that you thought about committing suicide?", and a lifetime history of suicide attempt was assessed via the question, "Have you ever attempted suicide?" SAD was associated with a lifetime history of suicide ideation, even after adjusting for demographic variables and an array of other psychiatric diagnoses. Exactly 25% of the sample endorsing suicide ideation met criteria for lifetime SAD. In contrast, over 27% of the sample endorsing a history of suicide attempt was diagnosed with SAD, relative to approximately 7% of those who did not endorse a history of suicide attempt. However, odds ratios for suicide attempt were not appreciably different from 1.0 when demographic and other psychiatric disorders were included in multi-variate analyses. In addition, a diagnosis of SAD increased the odds of new cases of suicide ideation during the three-year follow-up period after controlling for demographic variables and psychiatric diagnoses. Collectively, results from these studies suggest that there are higher rates of a lifetime history of suicide ideation in people diagnosed with SAD relative to people who do not carry this diagnosis, but that a history of suicide attempt is likely explained by the presence of comorbid psychiatric diagnoses.

CROSS-CULTURAL EXPRESSIONS OF COMORBIDITY

Nearly all of the studies described in this chapter were conducted in either the United States or Western Europe. In this section, I highlight results from the few studies that were conducted in non-Western countries. There is reason to believe that patterns of comorbidity might be different in non-Western countries than in Western countries. For example, the prevalence of SAD itself is much lower in some Asian countries than in Western countries (Wittchen & Fehm, 2003). If this pattern holds true for other disorders, then the likelihood of overlap would be especially low in these countries.

Two recent studies described the comorbidity between SAD and other psychiatric disorders in African countries. Bella and Omigbodun (2009) interviewed 413 Nigerian college students with the CIDI and determined that a current diagnosis of SAD was associated with a lifetime history of depression and depression during the past 12 months but not with current alcohol use or abuse. Kadri, Agoub, El Gnaoui, Berrada, and Moussaoui (2007) interviewed 800 adults aged 15 years or older with the Mini International Neuropsychiatric Interview in Moroccan Arabic language and found current (i.e., one month) rates of comorbidity that ranged from 13.8% between SAD and PD and between SAD and PTSD to 34.5% between SAD and OCD, and 41.4% between SAD and agoraphobia. The rates of comorbidity in the two latter instances were much higher than current rates of comorbidity found by researchers in Western countries.

As mentioned previously, rates of lifetime comorbidity between SAD and various psychiatric disorders in Iranian adults were reported by Mohammadi et al. (2006). Although many of the comorbidity percentages are similar to those found in studies conducted in Western countries, the odds ratios were much higher. This is likely due to the fact that psychiatric disorders were generally diagnosed much less frequently in this Iranian study than in the other studies; for example, the lifetime prevalence of SAD was only 0.83% in this sample – a far cry from the 12.2% detected by Ruscio et al. (2008) in the NCS-R, conducted in the United States. In fact, the authors remarked that their results were likely underestimates of psychiatric disorders in their country, as they speculated that respondents might not have been comfortable disclosing emotional distress to interviewers and that emotional distress is often expressed as somatization in their culture.

Clearly, much more epidemiological research must be conducted to identify prevalence and comorbidity rates of psychiatric disorders in non-Western countries. Researchers are encouraged to take into account not only the particular country under consideration but also the ethnic and religious composition of the participants. Such research has the potential to provide clues into the sociocultural mechanisms that affect the expression and course of psychiatric disorders such as SAD.

COMMENT AND FUTURE DIRECTIONS

Comorbidity is more the rule than the exception in SAD, particularly in the generalized subtype. Up to 90% of people who have SAD at some point in their lifetime will meet criteria for another Axis I disorder at some point in their lifetime. Although such a statistic has caused some to question whether SAD is a unique type of psychopathology, rather than a prodromal expression of another disorder, it should be noted that many studies find rates of comorbidity that are even higher in other anxiety and mood disorders (e.g., Grant et al., 2005). When SAD is accompanied by another Axis I disorder, symptom severity and functional impairment tend to increase (Acarturk, de Graaf, van Straten, ten Have, & Cuijpers, 2008).

Research on samples of respondents who are diagnosed according to DSM-IV criteria support results from older studies, which suggest that rates of comorbidity between SAD and other anxiety disorders and depressive disorders can reach as high as 50%, perhaps even higher. Although rates of comorbidity between SAD and substance use disorders are lower (i.e., 20–25%), people with SAD are still at elevated risk to develop problems with substance use, perhaps because they use substances to self-medicate (Carrigan & Randall, 2003). However, research conducted in the past 10 years suggests that comorbidity in SAD is not limited to overlap with other anxiety disorders, depressive disorders, and substance use disorders. Accumulating evidence suggests that there are elevated rates of SAD in people who are diagnosed with eating disorders, BDD, bipolar disorder, and psychosis. Moreover, people with SAD are at increased risk to experience suicide ideation. Clearly, SAD is a debilitating disorder in many instances, and it will be important for future research to identify the particular clinical presentations of SAD that are associated with the greatest amount of functional impairment and subjective distress.

Before long, a new edition of our diagnostic system will be in place (i.e., DSM-V; Reiger, Narrow, Kuhl, & Kupfer, 2009) and scholars undoubtedly will be vying for funding for epidemiological research that will yield the prevalence and comorbidity of psychiatric disorders, as defined by the revised criteria. This research is crucial in order to have accurate knowledge of the degree to which various disorders and their comorbid clinical presentations are found in community and clinical samples. However, such research is descriptive in nature and tells us little about the reasons why certain disorders co-occur.

Although it will be important to continue to establish rates of comorbidity in some understudied groups (e.g., people from non-Western countries), researchers are encouraged to move beyond the mere documentation of comorbidity and begin to identify empirically the path by which comorbidity between SAD and other psychiatric disorders emerges, the mechanism by which SAD puts people at risk for other psychiatric disorders, and the manner in which comorbidity affects patients' clinical course and response to treatment. Moreover, studies examining the psychopathology and treatment of SAD often exclude people with comorbid conditions from their samples. This practice runs the risk of yielding research findings that have limited relevance, at best, to the typical person who struggles with SAD. It is hoped that scholars will recognize that comorbidity is a central feature of SAD and recruit representative samples to enhance the external validity of research on this topic.

REFERENCES

Acarturk, C., de Graaf, R., van Straten, A., ten Have, M., & Cuijpers, P. (2008). Social phobia and number of social fears, and their association with comorbidity, health-related quality of life, and help seeking: A population-based study. *Social Psychiatry and Psychiatric Epidemiology*, *43*, 273–279.

Azorin, J-M., Akiskal, H., Akiskal, K., Hantouche, E., Châtenet-Duchêne, L., Gury, C., et al. (2007). Is psychosis in DSM-IV mania due to severity? The relevance of selected demographic and comorbid social phobia features. *Acta Psychiatrica Scandinavia*, *115*, 29–34.

Barlow, D. H., DiNardo, P. A., Vermilyea, B. B., Vermilyea, J., & Blanchard, E. B. (1986). Co-morbidity and depression among the anxiety disorders: Issues in diagnosis and classification. *Journal of Nervous and Mental Disease*, *174*, 63–72.

Bella, T. T., & Omigbodun, O. O. (2009). Social phobia in Nigerian university students: Prevalence, correlates, and co-morbidity. *Social Psychiatry and Psychiatric Epidemiology*, *44*, 458–463.

Bijl, R. V., van Zessen, G., & Ravelli, A. (1998). Prevalence of psychiatric disorder in the general population: Results of the Netherlands Mental Health Survey and Incidence Study (NEMESIS). *Social Psychiatry and Psychiatric Epidemiology*, *33*, 587–595.

Blake, D. D., Weathers, F. W., Nagy, L. N., Kaloupek, D. G., Klauminzer, G., Charney, D. S., et al. (1990). A clinician rating scale for assessing current and lifetime PTSD. *Behavior Therapist*, *18*, 187–188.

Braga, R., Mendlowicz, M. V., Marrocos, R. P., & Figueira, I. L. (2005). Anxiety disorders in outpatients with schizophrenia: Prevalence and impact on the subjective quality of life. *Journal of Psychiatric Research*, *39*, 409–414.

Brown, T. A., Campbell, L. A., Lehman, C. L., Grishman, J. R., & Mancill, R. B. (2001). Current and lifetime comorbidity of the DSM-IV anxiety and mood disorders in a large clinical sample. *Journal of Abnormal Psychology*, *110*, 585–599.

Bulik, C. M., Sullivan, P. F., Fear, J. L., & Joyce, P. R. (1997). Eating disorders and antecedent anxiety disorders: A controlled study. *Acta Psychiatrica Scandinavia*, *96*, 101–107.

Carrigan, M., & Randall, C. (2003). Self-medication in social phobia: A review of the alcohol literature. *Addictive Behaviors*, *28*, 269–284.

Chartier, M. J., Walker, J. R., & Stein, M. B. (2003). Considering comorbidity in social phobia. *Social Psychiatry and Psychiatric Epidemiology*, *38*, 728–734.

Ciapparelli, A., Paggini, R., Marazziti, D., Carmassi, C., Bianchi, M., Taponecco, C., et al. (2007). Comorbidity with Axis I anxiety disorders in remitted psychotic patients 1 year after hospitalization. *CNS Spectrums*, *12*, 913–919.

Coles, M. A., Phillips, K. A., Menard, W., Pagano, M. E., Fay, C., Weisberg, R. B., et al. (2006). Body dysmorphic disorder and social phobia: Cross-sectional and prospective data. *Depression and Anxiety*, *23*, 26–33.

Cougle, J. R., Keough, M. E., Riccardi, C. J., & Sachs-Ericcsson, N. (2009). Anxiety disorders and suicidality in the National Comorbidity Survey – Replication. *Journal of Psychiatric Research*, *43*, 825–829.

Davidson, J. R. T., Hughes, D. L., George, L. K., & Blazer, D. G. (1993). The epidemiology of social phobia: Findings from the Duke Epidemiologic Catchment Area Study. *Psychological Medicine*, *23*, 709–718.

Degonda, M., & Angst, J. (1993). The Zurich Study: XX. Social phobia and agoraphobia. *European Archives and Psychiatry and Clinical Neuroscience*, *243*, 95–102.

DiNardo, P. A., & Barlow, D. H. (1990). Syndrome and symptom co-occurrence in the anxiety disorders. In J. D. Maser & C. R. Cloninger (Eds.), *Comorbidity of mood and anxiety disorders* (pp. 205–230). Washington, DC: American Psychiatric Press.

DiNardo, P. A., Brown, T. A., & Barlow, D. H. (1994). *Anxiety Disorders Interview Schedule for DSM-IV: Lifetime version (ADIS-IV-L)*. San Antonio, TX: The Psychological Corporation.

Endicott, J., & Spitzer, R. L. (1978). A diagnostic interview: The schedule for affective disorders and schizophrenia. *Archives of General Psychiatry*, *35*, 837–844.

Fehm, L., Beesdo, K., Jacobi, F., & Fiedler, A. (2008). Social anxiety disorder above and below the diagnostic threshold: Prevalence, comorbidity, and impairment in the general population. *Social Psychiatry and Psychiatric Epidemiology*, *43*, 257–265.

First, M. B., Spitzer, R. L., Gibbon, M., & Williams, J. B. W. (2002). *Structured Clinical Interview for DSM-IV Disorders, Research Version, Non-Patient Edition (SCID-I/NP)*. New York: Biometrics Research, New York State Psychiatric Institute.

Freeman, M. P., Freeman, S. A., & McElroy, S. L. (2002). The comorbidity of bipolar and anxiety disorders: Prevalence, psychobiology, and treatment issues. *Journal of Affective Disorders*, *68*, 1–23.

Goisman, R. M., Goldenberg, I., Vasile, R. G., & Keller, M. B. (1995). Comorbidity of anxiety disorders in a multicenter anxiety study. *Comprehensive Psychiatry*, *36*, 303–311.

Grant, B. F., Dawson, D. A., & Hasin, D. S. (2001). *The Alcohol Use Disorders and Disabilities Interview Schedule – DSM-IV Version*. Bethesda, MD: National Institute on Alcohol Abuse and Alcoholism.

Grant, B. F., Hasin, D. S., Blanco, C., Stinson, F. S., Chou, P., Goldstein, R. B., et al. (2005). The epidemiology of social anxiety disorder in the United States: Results from the National Epidemiologic Survey on Alcohol and Related Conditions. *Journal of Clinical Psychiatry*, *66*, 1351–1361.

Gunstad, J., & Phillips, K. A. (2003). Axis I comorbidity in body dysmorphic disorder. *Comprehensive Psychiatry*, *44*, 270–276.

Haro, J. M., Arbabazadeh-Bouchez, S., Brugha, T. S., de Girolamo, G., Guyer, M. E., Jin, R., et al. (2006). Concordance of the Composite International Diagnostic Interview Version 3.0 (CIDI 3.0) with standardized clinical assessments in the WHO World Mental Health Surveys. *International Journal of Methods in Psychiatric Research*, *15*, 167–180.

Hinrichson, H., Wright, F., Waller, G., & Meyer, C. (2003). Social anxiety and coping strategies in eating disorders. *Eating Behaviors*, *4*, 117–126.

Hollander, E., Cohen, L., & Simeon, D. (1993). Body dysmorphic disorder. *Psychiatric Annals*, *23*, 359–364.

Iwasaki, Y., Matsunaga, H., Kiriike, N., Tanaka, H., & Matsui, T. (2000). Comorbidity of axis I disorders among eating-disordered subjects in Japan. *Comprehensive Psychiatry*, *41*, 454–460.

Kadri, N., Agoub, M., El Gnaoui, S., Berrada, S., & Moussaoui, D. (2007). Prevalence of anxiety disorders: A population-based epidemiological study in metropolitan area of Casablanca, Morocco. *Annals of General Psychiatry, 6,* np Retrieved November 1 2009, from www.annals-general-psychiatry.com/content/6/1/6.

Kashdan, T. B., Frueh, B. C.., Knapp, R. G., Herbert, R., & Magruder, K. M. (2006). Social anxiety disorder in Veterans' Affairs primary care clinics. *Behaviour Research and Therapy*, *44*, 233–247.

Kaye, W., Bulik, C. M., Thornton, L., Barbarich, N., Masters, K., & The Price Foundation Collaborative Group. (2004). Comorbidity of anxiety disorders with anorexia and bulimia nervosa. *American Journal of Psychiatry*, *161*, 2215–2221.

Kessler, R. C., McGonagle, K. A., Zhao, S., Nelson, C. B., Hughes, M., Eshleman, S., et al. (1994). Lifetime and 12-month prevalence of psychiatric disorders in the United States: Results from the National Comorbidity Survey. *Archives of General Psychiatry*, *51*, 8–19.

Kessler, R. C., & Merikangas, K. R. (2004). The National Comorbidity Survey Replicaton (NCS-R): Background and aims. *International Journal of Methods in Psychiatric Research*, *13*, 60–68.

Kessler, R. C., & Ustun, T. B. (2004). The World Mental Health (WMH) Survey Initiative version of the World Mental Health Organization (WHO) Composite International Diagnostic Interview (CIDI). *International Journal of Methods in Psychiatric Research*, *13*, 93–121.

Lampe, L., Slade, T., Issakidis, C., & Andrews, G. (2003). Social phobia in the Australian National Survey of Mental Health and Well-Being (NSMHWB). *Psychological Medicine*, *33*, 637–646.

Lecrubier, Y., & Weiller, E. (1997). Comorbidities in social phobia. *International Clinical Psychopharmacology*, *12*(Suppl 6), S17–S21.

Magee, W. J., Eaton, W. W., Wittchen, H. U., McGonagle, K. A., & Kessler, R. C. (1996). Agoraphobia, simple phobia, and social phobia in the National Comorbidity Survey. *Archives of General Psychiatry*, *53*, 159–168.

Mazeh, D., Bodner, E., Weizman, R., Delayahu, Y., Cholostoy, A., Martin, T., et al. (2009). Co-morbid social phobia in schizophrenia. *International Journal of Social Psychiatry*, *55*, 198–202.

McNeil, D. M. (2001). Terminology and evolution of constructs. In S. G. Hofmann & P. M. DiBartolo (Eds.), *From social anxiety to social phobia: Multiple perspectives* (pp. 8–19). Boston, MA: Allyn & Bacon.

Mohammadi, M-R., Ghanizadeh, A., Mohammadi, M., & Mesgarpour, B. (2006). Prevalence of social phobia and its comorbidity with psychiatric disorders in Iran. *Depression and Anxiety*, *23*, 405–411.

Pallanti, S., Quercioli, L., & Hollander, E. (2004). Social anxiety in outpatients with schizophrenia: A cause of relevant disability. *American Journal of Psychiatry*, *161*, 53–58.

Perugi, G., Akiskal, H., Giannotti, D., Frare, F., Di Vaio, S., & Cassano, G. (1997). Gender-related differences in body dysmorphic disorder (dysmorpho-phobia). *Journal of Nervous and Mental Disease*, *185*, 578–582.

Perugi, G., Akiskal, H. S., Ramacciotti, S., Nassini, S., Toni, C., Milanfranchi, A., et al. (1999). Depressive comorbidity of panic, social phobic, and obsessive compulsive disorders re-examined: Is there a bipolar connection? *Journal of Psychiatric Research*, *33*, 53–61.

Phillips, K. A., & Diaz, S. (1997). Gender differences in body dysmorphic disorder. *Journal of Nervous and Mental Disease*, *188*, 170–175.

Pini, S., Maser, J. D., Dell'Osso, L., Abelli, M., Muti, M., Gesi, C., et al. (2006). Social anxiety disorder comorbidity in patients with bipolar disorder: A clinical replication. *Journal of Anxiety Disorders*, *20*, 1148–1157.

Reiger, D. A., Narrow, W. E., Kuhl, E. A., & Kupfer, D. J. (2009). The conceptual development of DSM-V. *American Journal of Psychiatry*, *166*, 645–650.

Rihmer, Z., Szádóczky, E., Füredi, J., Kiss, K., & Papp, Z. (2001). Anxiety disorders comorbidity in bipolar I, bipolar II, and unipolar major depression: Results from a population-based study in Hungary. *Journal of Affective Disorders*, *67*, 175–179.

Robins, L. N., Helzer, J. E., Croughan, J., & Ratcliff, K. S. (1981). National Institute of Mental Health diagnostic interview schedule: Its history, characteristics, and validity. *Archives of General Psychiatry*, *38*, 381–389.

Ruscio, A. M., Brown, T. A., Chiu, W. T., Sareen, J., Stein, M. B., & Kessler, R. C. (2008). Social fears and social phobia in the USA: Results from the National Comorbidity Survey Replication. *Psychological Medicine*, *38*, 15–28.

Sanderson, W. C., DiNardo, P. A., Rapee, R. M., & Barlow, D. H. (1990). Syndrome comorbidity in patients diagnosed with a DSM-III-R anxiety disorder. *Journal of Abnormal Psychology*, *99*, 308–312.

Sareen, J., Cox, B. J., Afifi, T. O., de Graff, R., Asmundson, G. J. G., ten Have, M., et al. (2005). Anxiety disorders and risk for suicidal ideation and suicide attempts: A population-based longitudinal study of adults. *Archives of General Psychiatry*, *62*, 1249–1257.

Sareen, J., Houlahan, T., Cox, B. J., & Asmundson, G. J. G. (2005). Anxiety disorders associated with suicidal ideation and suicide attempts in the National Comorbidity Survey. *Journal of Nervous and Mental Disease*, *193*, 450–454.

Schneier, F. R., Johnson, J., Hornig, C. D., Liebowitz, M. R., & Weissman, M. M. (1992). Social phobia: Comorbidity and morbidity in an epidemiologic sample. *Archives of General Psychiatry*, *49*, 282–288.

Schwalberg, M. D., Barlow, D. H., Alger, S. A., & Howard, L. J. (1992). Comparison of bulimics, obese binge eaters, social phobics, and individuals with panic disorder on comorbidity across DSM-III-R anxiety disorders. *Journal of Abnormal Psychology*, *101*, 675–681.

Sheehan, D. V., Lecrubier, Y., Sheehan, K. H., Janavs, J., Weiller, E., Keskiner, A., et al. (1997). The validity of the Mini International Neuropsychiatric Interview (MINI) according to the SCID-P and its reliability. *European Psychiatry*, *12*, 232–241.

Swinbourne, J. M., & Touyz, S. W. (2007). The comorbidity of eating disorders and anxiety disorders: A review. *European Eating Disorders Review*, *15*, 253–274.

Tamam, L., & Ozpoyraz, N. (2002). Comorbidity of anxiety disorders among patients with bipolar I disorder in remission. *Psychopathology*, *35*, 203–209.

Turner, S. M., Beidel, D. C., Borden, J. W., Stanley, M. A., & Jacob, R. G. (1991). Social phobia: Axis I and II correlates. *Journal of Abnormal Psychology*, *100*, 102–106.

van Ameringen, M., Mancini, C., Styan, G., & Donison, D. (1991). Relationship of social phobia with other psychiatric illnesses. *Journal of Affective Disorders*, *21*, 93–99.

Wilhelm, S., Otto, M. W., Zucker, B., & Pollack, M. H. (1997). Prevalence of body dysmorphic disorder in patients with anxiety disorders. *Journal of Anxiety Disorders*, *11*, 499–502.

Wittchen, H-U., & Fehm, L. (2003). Epidemiology and natural course of social fears and social phobia. *Acta Psychiatrica Scandinavia*, *108*, 4–18.

Wittchen, H-U., Stein, M. B., & Kessler, R. C. (1999). Social fears and social phobia in a community sample of adolescents and young adults: Prevalence, risk factors, and comorbidity. *Psychological Medicine*, *29*, 309–323.

Zimmerman, M., & Mattia, J. I. (1998). Body dysmorphic disorder in psychiatric outpatients: Recognition, prevalence, comorbidity, demographic, and clinical correlates. *Comparative Psychiatry*, *39*, 265–270.

Chapter 8

Avoidant Personality Disorder and Its Relationship to Social Phobia

James Reich

Department of Psychiatry, UCSF Medical School, and Department of Psychiatry and Behavioral Health, Stanford Medical School; San Francisco, CA 94123

INTRODUCTION

In this chapter I will first summarize past findings and then update them with the findings of studies done in the past 10 years.

There has been a long-standing question as to how social fears relate to personality disorders. At one time anxiety was considered the hallmark of a personality disorder; e.g., the concept of neurosis. The development of the APD category in DSM-III stimulated interest in the relationship of social fears to personality disorders. By examining the relationship of SP to the personality disorders, clinicians and researchers could examine this question empirically in disorders defined by specific criteria.

The conceptualization of APD in DSM-III relied heavily on the work of Millon (1991). Millon felt that, although APD would overlap to some extent with schizoid, schizotypal, dependent, and paranoid personality disorders, it was a clear category in its own right. (Many DSM personality disorders overlap with each other to some extent.) For Millon the distinction between APD and SP was clear. As he put it, "Avoidant is essentially a problem of relating to persons; SP is largely a problem of performing in situations. The avoidant PD has a feeling of low self-esteem; SP implies no such self critical judgment" (1991, p. 356, emphasis added).

DIAGNOSTIC ISSUES USING THE DSM

The diagnosis of both SP and APD using the DSM system has been a moving target as the criteria change somewhat with each revision (see Table 8.1). The DSM-III criteria for APD emphasized low self-esteem, social withdrawal, and sensitivity to rejection. The criteria for SP emphasized social withdrawal but

Social Anxiety: Clinical, Developmental, and Social Perspectives. DOI: 10.1016/B978-0-12-375096-9.00008-0

TABLE 8.1 DSM Criteria for APD and for SP

	Social Phobia	Avoidant PD
DSM-III criteria	A persistent, irrational fear of and compelling desire to avoid a situation in which the individual is exposed to possible scrutiny by others and fears that he or she may act in a way that will be humiliating or embarrassing Causes significant distress Not due to APD or other mental disorder	Hypersensitivity to rejection Unwillingness to enter into relationships Social withdrawal Desire for affection and acceptance Low self-esteem
DSM-III-R criteria	A persistent fear of one or more social phobic situations in which the person is exposed to possible scrutiny by others and fears that he or she may do something or act in a way that will be humiliating or embarrassing Unrelated to other Axis I or III disorders Exposure to phobic stimulus causes anxiety response Situation is avoided or endured with anxiety Causes occupational or social dysfunction or subjective distress May be generalized	A pervasive pattern of social discomfort, fear of negative evaluation, and timidity, beginning in early adulthood and present in a variety of contexts as indicated by four of the following: • Easily hurt by criticism • No close friends • Unwilling to get involved with people • Avoids activities with significant interpersonal contact • Reticent in social situations • Fears being embarrassed • Exaggerates potential difficulties
DSM IV criteria	A marked and persistent fear of one or more social or performance situations Exposure to feared social situation invariably provokes anxiety Feared situations are avoided or endured with distress Significant occupational or social dysfunction may be generalized	A persistent pattern of social inhibition, feelings of inadequacy, and hypersensitivity to negative evaluation, as indicated by four of the following: • Avoids activities involving significant interpersonal contact • Unwilling to get involved with people • Shows restraint in intimate relationships • Preoccupied with being criticized or rejected • Inhibited in new interpersonal situations • Views self as socially inept, unappealing, or inferior • Is unusually reluctant to take personal risks

also listed fear of being humiliated, which could be seen as very similar to the APD criteria of low self-esteem. Already we have questions about the overlap of the two disorders. If someone is afraid of social situations due to fear of humiliation, would that not lead to low self-esteem? If someone avoided social situations due to low self-esteem but did not have performance difficulties, behavior theory would tell us that the low self-esteem would decondition as societal pressures brought the person into more and more social situations. At the DSM-III level there are two reasons the disorders would be diagnosed separately, one a matter of scope and the other arbitrary. The item of scope is the concept that the difficulty in SP is much more restricted (applies to fewer situations) than APD. The second reason for separate diagnosis is definitional, that SP can not be diagnosed in the presence of APD by definition in DSM-III.

At the DSM-III-R level there is still the same conceptual overlap, but several factors have now made the overlap stronger. The definitional exclusion of an SP diagnosis in the presence of APD has (appropriately) been dropped. Research in SP has now shown that it can appear in more than one setting and therefore can be generalized. The DSM-III-R has responded to this empirical data by creating a generalized version of SP. This again reduces the distance between the two disorders. The underlying theoretical concept that APD is social withdrawal without performance problems and SP is performance problems without self-esteem difficulties is more or less retained. The APD criteria of reticence in social situations and fears of being embarrassed do begin to sound like performance difficulties, however.

DSM-IV makes some changes but we are still basically left with the initial diagnostic question of whether we are cutting nature at the joint or at the bone by postulating one disorder (APD) of internal image (problems with self-esteem), but not performance anxiety, and another disorder (SP) of social performance problems without internal image problems (e.g., problems with self-esteem.) To further examine the relationship between the two we must turn to the empirical data.

REVIEW OF EARLY FINDINGS

I have reviewed the findings until 2000 elsewhere (Reich, 2000, 2009). I will summarize some of the earlier findings here.

Studies Comparing SP to APD

I will consider the older empirical literature comparing SP and APD. One aspect examined is the comorbidity of the two disorders. If the disorders were separate we would expect, at best, modest comorbidity. If they were highly related or identical disorders we would expect a much higher overlap. (We would not expect 100% overlap due to inherent measurement errors – especially for the personality disorders – and the different wording of the two sets of criteria.) If there was a high overlap we would want to examine differences between GSP and APD to determine whether, although highly overlapping and similar, there were distinct criteria or features that justified a distinction between the two.

Of the 13 studies reporting on overlap, the average comorbidity was 56% (range 22 to 89%; see Table 8.2). These figures were drawn from a wide range of populations using different measurement instruments in a wide range of settings. Different interview techniques were used in different settings and interviewers had different levels of training in diagnosing personality disorders. In addition, as disorders wax and wane, there is an additional source of variability. Given that this is about the same level of agreement that might be found comparing two different DSM personality measurement instruments on the same population and that subthreshold cases were usually not taken into account, this probably represents the highest level of overlap we could expect from these diverse settings and measurement techniques. It seemed clear that GSP highly, if not completely, overlapped with APD.

The Association of SP to Other Personality Disorders

Earlier studies that examined SP and other personality disorders showed some mild association with the DSM schizoid personality disorder cluster, but more strongly to the DSM anxious personality disorder cluster. It is quite possible that some of the association with the schizoid personality cluster (especially in the self-report instruments) may be due to measurement artifact. Overall, after APD, dependent personality disorder had the strongest association.

Treatment and Outcome Studies for SP and APD

Although treatment response is not part of the definition for SP or APD, these studies can give us valuable nosologic information. If the same treatments work for different disorders, or symptoms of one disorder get better as a second disorder is treated, this increases the possibility that these disorders are related or may even be the same disorder.

Psychopharmacological Treatment Studies

Although the early studies in this area vary in many respects, there was evidence that benzodiazepines, selective serotonin reuptake inhibitors (SSRIs), and various forms of MAOIs may be effective for APD or for avoidant traits associated with SP. Many of these studies had good sample size and careful measurements of avoidant personality traits, and they demonstrated that, as SP symptoms were treated, avoidant personality traits were also reduced (see Table 8.3).

Psychological Treatments

Eight psychological treatment studies of APD or SP associated with APD were reviewed previously (Reich, 2000). These studies used cognitive or behavioral

TABLE 8.2 Earlier Studies Comparing SP to APD

Study	Population	Instruments*	Procedure	Findings
Alpert et al. (1997)	Patients with major depression who also had SP or APD, $n = 92$	SCIDI, II (DSM-IIIR)	Cross-sectional examination	66% had both APD & SP. Of those with APD & SP, 55% had atypical depression
Alnaes and Torgersen (1988)	Consecutive psychiatric outpatients, $n = 289$	SCID1, SIDP (DSM-III)	Cross-sectional examination	84% of SP also had APD
Brown, Heimberg, & Juster (1995)	Patients from an Anxiety Disorder clinic who had SP, $n = 110$	ADIS-R, PDE (DSM-III-R)	Examine subtypes of SP and APD on outcome cog/beh tx	GSP plus APD had more depression
Emmanuel et al. (1993)	Outpatients with GSP, $n = 44$	SCID-II (DSM-III-R)	Cross-sectional comparison of overlap of personality disorders with GSP	73% of GSP had APD
Fahlen (1995a)	SP recruited for a drug trial, $n = 63$; SP $n = 58$ controls	SCID and clinical personality interview. 140-item avoidant personality questionnaire. (DSM-III-R)	Cross-sectional comparisons and factor analysis	60% had APD and 18% had subthreshold APD
Feske, Perry, Chambless, Renneberg, & Goldstein (1996)	Anxiety outpatients with generalized SP (GSP), $n = 48$	DSM-III-R criteria	Cross-sectional comparison	71% had APD. APD had more severe sx social fears and more depression
Hofmann, Newman, Becker, Taylor, & Roth (1995)	Patients recruited for study with SP, SP + AVD, controls, $n = 52$	SCIDI, II (DSM-III)	Comparison of SP & SP + APD in behavioral trial of public speaking	Differences in heart rate SP & SP-APD. 88% with APD also had GSP

(*Continued*)

TABLE 8-2 (*Continued*)

Study	Population	Instruments*	Procedure	Findings
Herbert, Hope, & Bellak (1992)	Patients recruited for a beh tx program. All had GSP, $n = 23$	SCID-R ADIS-R (DSM-III-R)	Comparison of GSP with and without APD	61% of GSP also met APD. APD had lower GAS and more comorbid dx
Holt, Heimberg, & Hope (1992)	Patients recruited from an anxiety disorders clinic, $n = 30$	ADIS-RPDE (DSM-III-R)	GSP with and without APD and SP without APD compared	APD appears to just identify a slightly more severe type of GSP
Hope, Herbert, & White (1995)	SP recruited for a beh tx study, $n = 23$	SCID-R, ADIS-R (DSM-III-R)	Examined subtypes of SP and APD	61% of SP had APD. No higher association of APD with GSP than specific SP
Jansen, Arntz, Merckelbach, & Mersch (1994)	Patients from a Netherlands outpatient psych clinic, $n = 117$	Axis I clinical interview, Axis II SCID-II (DSM-III-R)	Panic vs. SP for personality variables	Fear of being embarrassed discriminated best between panic and SP. 31% of SP had APD
Mersch, Marijke, Jansen, & Arntz (1995)	Patients recruited by Swedish newspaper for SP tx study, $n = 34$	Axis I, clinical interview, Axis II SCID-II (DSM-III-R)	SP with and without personality disorder	23% had APD. Those with APD were somewhat more disabled
Noyes, Woodman, Holt, Reich, & Zimmerman (1995)	Panic and SP patients recruited from news media, SP $n = 46$	SICD (DSM-III-R), PDQ (DSM-III)	Examined personality traits in panic and SP	GSP had 50% more personality traits from the anxious and schizoid clusters than SP
Reich, Noyes, & Yates, 1989	SP outpatients, $n = 14$	Axis I, SCIDI, SCIDII (DSM-III-R)	Pharm tx study	50% of SP also had APD

Sanderson, Wetzler, Beck, & Betz (1994)	SP, GSP outpatients, $n = 51$	SCID-II (DSM-III-R)	Cross-sectional comparison	61% had a personality disorder and 37% had APD
Schneier, Spitzer, Gibbon, Fyer, & Liebowitz (1991)	SP drawn from an anxiety disorders clinic, $n = 50$	Axis I, semi-structured interview Axis II, SCID-II (DSM-III-R)	Comparison of subtypes of SP and relationship to APD	APD in discrete SP = 21%. APD in GSP = 89%
Tran & Chambless (1995)	Outpatients with a primary dx of SP, $n = 45$	Axis I, SCID (DSM-III-R) Axis II, MCMI or MCMI-II	Comparison of subtypes of SP	GSP more socially disabled than SP. APD-GSP had more depression than GSP
Turner, Beidel, Borden, Stanley, & Jacob (1991)	Outpatients SP, GSP, $n = 71$	SCID (DSMII-R)	Cross-sectional, association with personality disorders	37% had a personality disorder; 22% prevalence of APD
Turner, Beidel, & Townsley (1992)	SP from an anxiety disorder clinic, $n = 89$	ADIS-R, SCID-II (DSM-III-R)	Comparison of specific SP, GSP, and APD	GSP is more similar to than different from APD, differing on only one of four dimensions (social anxiety); there was no difference in social skills between GSP and APD
Turner, Beidel, Dancu, & Keys (1986)	SP from an anxiety disorder clinic, $n = 21$	Axis I, ADIS Axis II, consensus (DSM-III)	Comparison of SP and APD	GAS and SP very similar, but indication that APD have poorer social skills

Abbreviations: PDE = Personality Disorder Examination (Loranger et al., Cornell University); SCID = Structured Clinical Interview for DSM Disorders (Spitzer et al., New York State Psychiatric Institute); ADIS-R = Anxiety Disorder Interview Schedule – Revised (Barlow et al., Boston University).

TABLE 8.3 Earlier Treatment Studies of Social Phobia and Avoidant Personality Disorder

Study (psycho-therapy)	Population	Instruments	Procedure	Findings
Alden and Capreol (1993)	76 outpatients with APD	MCMI and PDE (DSM-III)	Three active cognitive/behavioral tx and a control gp	APD patients responded to tx, although some tx better suited to specific subtypes
Brown, Heimberg, & Juster (1995)	Patients from an anxiety disorder clinic who had SP, $n = 110$	ADIS-R, PDE (DSM-III-R)	beh/cog tx on three gps: APD + GSP, GSP, SP	All groups improved from their baseline scores
Feske, Perry, Chambless, Renneberg, & Goldstein (1996)	Anxiety outpatients with generalized SP (GSP), $n = 48$	DSM-III-R criteria	Exposure-based tx of SP, SP + APD	Both groups improved from baseline
Hofmann, Newman, et al. (1995); Hofmann, Ehlers, Newman, & Roth (1995)	Outpatients, SP, SP + APD, $n = 16$	Axis I, SCID Axis II, unstructured interview (DSM-III-R)	gp beh tx speaking anxiety	Both groups improved equally
Hope, Herbert, White (1995)	SP recruited for a beh tx study, $n = 23$	SCID-R, ADIS-R (DSM-III-R)	cog/beh gp tx, SP, GSP, GSP + APD	The presence of APD in GSP did not affect tx response
Mersch, Marijke, Jansen, & Arntz (1995)	Patients recruited by Swedish newspaper for SP tx study, $n = 34$	Axis I, clinical interview Axis II SCID-II (DSM-III-R)	SP with and without personality disorder, beh tx	gps with and without a personality disorder benefited from tx
Renneberg, Goldstein, Phillips, & Chambless (1990)	Outpatients with APD from an anxiety disorder clinic, $n = 17$	SCID I and II (DSM-III-R)	Intensive gp tx APD	sx improved and some benefits maintained at one year

Stravynski, Belisle, Marcouiller, Lavalee, & Ellie (1994)	Psychiatric outpatients with APD, but "no significant" Axis I dx, $n = 28$	Clinical interview (DSM-III)	Eight sessions of social skills training	Clinical improvement maintained at 3 mth
Study (psycho-pharmacologic)				
Deltito & Perugi (1986)	Outpatient with SP + APD, $n = 1$	Clinical interview (DSM-III)	Treatment MAOI	Good clinical response
Deltito & Stam (1989)	Outpatients with APD, $n = 4$	Clinical interview (DSM-III-R)	tx MAOI or fluoxetine	Good clinical response
Fahlen (1995b)	SP outpatients, $n = 57$	Standardized interviews, personality trait questionnaire (DSM-III-R)	tx reversible MAOI	At endpoint sig reduction in APD in tx gp as compared to controls
Liebowitz et al. (1992)	SP outpatients 75% had GSP, $n = 74$	DSM-III criteria	Drug trial, atenolol, phenelzine, and placebo	64% response to phenelzine at 8 wk with sig reduction in APD traits
Reich, Noyes, & Yates (1989)	SP outpatients, $n = 14$	Axis I, SCIDI, SCIDII (DSM-III-R)	tx alprazolam	Significant reduction in avoidant personality traits over 8 wk
Versiani et al. (1992)	SP outpatients, $n = 78$	SCID-I (DSM-III-R)	Drug trial, MAOI vs. placebo	82–91% of the MAOI group reported being almost asymptomatic

treatments or both. Overall it appears that both APD and SP comorbid with APD do respond to treatment. The SP without GSP tends to be least disabled, followed by GSP followed by GSP comorbid with APD. Although all start at different baselines of morbidity, all seem to respond to treatment (see Table 8.3).

Course of SP

Early prospective studies on the course of SP generally find that SP tends to be chronic with low remission rates. This rate is the same for SP without GSP, and GSP. There are no studies of the course of GSP plus APD. This is most likely due to the high level of overlap of GSP and APD, making it hard to find pure samples of either GSP or APD to compare it to. For practical purposes we can assume that GSP and APD have a similar course.

APD and State Effects

Reich (2000) also reported empirical evidence that AVP symptoms could be affected by state anxiety and depression (see longer discussion below).

FINDINGS FROM MORE RECENT LITERATURE

Other Relevant Reviews

Alden, Laposa, Taylor, and Ryder (2002) focus on dimensional research on the question of the relationship of APD to SP. This approach is also present in the work of Taylor, Laposa, and Alden (2004). The findings here are that both APD and SP tend to have low levels of extraversion and higher neuroticism. It is possible that there also may be a mild decrease in novelty-seeking in APD.

Recent Empirical Evidence on the Construct of APD

Two reports focused on whether APD represented an internally consistent diagnosis (Baille & Lampe, 1998; Grillo et al., 2001). Both of these studies examined several hundred patients and examined whether APD appeared to be an internally consistent diagnosis. Both reports found that a single factor model seemed to fit the data best and that APD was internally consistent. A third report, which had over a thousand subjects, examined whether the APD criteria fit a prototype and whether there was a natural cut-off point to indicate transition into a disorder from a trait (Hummelen, Wilberg, Pedersen, & Karterud, 2006). The findings were that APD appeared to be a homogenous disorder and that there was no number of criteria to indicate where the pathology increased to indicate a personality disorder. APD appeared to be a dimensional construct. Basically these three studies are in agreement.

Recent Empirical Evidence on the Relationship of APD to SP

There are also a number of empirical reports on the relationship of APD to SP. One report examined over a thousand patients with standardized techniques (Hummelen, Wilberg, Pedersen, & Karterud, 2007). They found that the two disorders were highly related in symptoms but that APD had more disability and appeared to be a more severe disorder with more personality problems and a lower level of conscientiousness. An Australian epidemiologic study of over 10000 subjects compared SP to APD (Lampe, Slade, Issakidis, & Andrews, 2003). There was a high degree of overlap of symptoms. Those subjects severe enough to have the APD diagnosis had a greater burden of affective disorder. APD prevalence was 6.5% with no gender difference. Those with more significant APD and SP symptoms had deficits in the ability to form relationships and hold employment, and had increased comorbidity with anxiety and depressive disorders.

A longitudinal study of personality disorders ($n = 157$) found a significant association between APD and SP (McGlashan et al., 2000). Another report from the same group examined whether those subjects with APD who also had SP differed (Ralevski et al., 2005). They concluded that these two groups did not differ and felt that this was evidence that APD and SP might be alternate conceptualizations of the same disorder. A Swedish self-report epidemiological study with 581 subjects examined the overlap of APD and SP (Tillfors, Furmak, Ekselius, & Frederikson, 2004). They found that the disorders were similar, the major difference being a decrease in function in the APD group that appeared to be unrelated to the level of anxiety. A large clinical epidemiological study of 859 psychiatric outpatients and personality disorders found a 14.9% prevalence of APD (Zimmerman, Rothschild, & Chelminski, 2005). There was a high association with SP and the presence of major depression, GAD, PD, and PTSD significantly increased the probability of finding APD.

Basically, all the empirical findings in this section are similar and show that APD and SP do not have differentiating major features, although they show that APD has more dysfunction than SP. This would be expected if APD is the same disorder only with somewhat more severe symptoms.

State Personality Effects

Recently there has been an increased understanding of state effects, also referred to as state personality disorder (Reich, 2005, 2007). This is the phenomenon where personality traits appear under the stress of an Axis I disorder or other stress and remit when that stress is gone. It has become more and more recognized that many personality disorders have both state (transient, stress-induced symptoms) and trait (relatively enduring) components.

There are a number of reports that lend credence to the idea that APD has state components. One report indicates that the presence of APD in GSP can be predicted with 85% accuracy by a combination of introversion and depression (van Velzen, Emmerlkamp, & Scholing, 2000). It would appear that depression predicts state personality aspects. A two-year follow-up of 266 subjects with APD indicated both state and trait components (McGlashan et al., 2005). Two state components that were specified were (1) avoiding jobs that are interpersonal and (2) avoiding potentially embarrassing situations. In another report from the same group the finding was that APD tended not to remit if an underlying anxiety or depressive disorder had not remitted, which would be consistent with the state personality model (Shea et al., 2004). The findings cited above of increased prevalence of APD with the presence of certain Axis I disorders is also consistent with this finding. Overall, the empirical findings are consistent with a state personality component to APD.

Genetic Findings

There is one recent major report on the genetics of APD and its relationship to SP (Reichborn-Kjennerud et al., 2007). This study examined 1427 female twin pairs to examine similarities and differences in genetic predisposition. The results were rather striking – the genetic basis of the two disorders is identical, although environment may affect the nature of the development of symptoms.

DISCUSSION

Looking at both the old and new data moves us toward some fairly solid findings. First, we know that APD appears to be an internally consistent disorder that likely has no cut-off number of symptoms to indicate that it is a disorder rather than a dimensional symptom construct. It appears to have both state and trait personality components. With the exception of some increased disability in APD compared to SP, the two disorders share the same symptoms, respond to the same treatments, and are genetically identical and appear to be the same disorder.

What we have is a well-validated dimensional personality disorder with enough clinically significant symptoms to warrant clinical attention and treatment. The only real question is nosological – how to classify SP and APD, as they appear to be the same disorder.

One question is whether AVP belongs in the section of personality disorders. There is no cut-off number of criteria where pathology suddenly begins. The DSM approach has been to consider personality pathology disorders with an identifiable cut-off point. However, researchers have now come to understand that the disability caused by many personality disorders is related more to the number of criteria met and not to specific cut-off points. I believe that personality pathology of clinical significance, even though it is continuous, is worthy of inclusion in the DSM personality section and is consistent with evolving empirical evidence.

Another aspect worth discussing is treatability. Personality disorders have been considered a class that is relatively treatment-resistant. Our evidence is that a fair amount of APD pathology will respond to treatment. This again is consistent with our evolving knowledge of treatment of this and other personality disorders. We have come to understand that the courses of personality disorders are much more variable than we once thought and there is evidence of at least partial response to treatment. Once again, the evolving course of knowledge would make us accept amenability to treatment as an aspect of certain personality disorders.

The evidence indicates that APD and SP are different manifestations of one disorder. The question then becomes whether this single disorder belongs on Axis I or II. It would appear that the best route would be hierarchical, to merge the less severe form with the more severe. As APD is the more severe form, this would have us place both disorders in the personality category but with the understanding that the milder variant (SP) resembles an anxiety disorder.

CONCLUSIONS

AVP is an internally consistent personality disorder that can be reliably measured. As with many other personality disorders, it has both state and trait personality components. AVP causes morbidity through interfering with social interactions and may affect such important life parameters as dating, marriage, friendship, and employment. AVP is also relatively common in general and clinical populations. This prevalence and morbidity make it an appropriate focus of clinical treatment. AVP and SP share symptoms (differing only in severity), are responsive to the same pharmacological and psychotherapeutic interventions, and seem to be identical genetically. The best conceptualization is that SP is a milder variant of APD and that they are the same disease. APD's potential response to treatment engenders cautious clinical optimism about its treatment.

REFERENCES

Alden, L. E., & Capreol, M. J. (1993). Avoidant personality disorder, interpersonal problems as predictors of treatment response. *Behavior Therapy*, *24*, 357–376.

Alden, L. E., Laposa, J. M., Taylor, C. T., & Ryder, A. G. (2002). Avoidant personality disorder: current status and future directions. *Journal of Personality Disorders*, *16*(1), 1–29.

Alnaes, S., & Torgersen, S. (1988). The relationship between DSM-III symptom disorders (Axis I) and personality disorders (Axis II) in an outpatient population. *Acta Psychiatrica Scandinavica*, *78*, 485–492.

Alpert, J. E., Uebelacker, L. A., McLean, N. E., Nierenberg, A. A., Pava, J. A., Worthington, J. J., et al. (1997). Social phobia, avoidant personality disorder and atypical depression: Co-occurrence and clinical implications. *Psychological Medicine*, *27*, 627–633.

Baille, A. J., & Lampe, L. A. (1998). Avoidant personality disorder: Empirical support for DSM-IV revisions. *Journal of Personality Disorders*, *12*(1), 23–30.

Brown, E. J., Heimberg, R. G., & Juster, H. R. (1995). Social phobia subtype and avoidant personality disorder: Effect on severity of social phobia, impairment, and outcome of cognitive behavioral treatment. *Behavior Therapy*, *26*, 467–486.

Deltito, J. A., & Perugi, G. (1986). A case of social phobia with avoidant personality disorder treated with MAOI. *Comprehensive Psychiatry*, *27*, 255–258.

Deltito, J. A., & Stam, M. (1989). Psychopharmacological treatment of avoidant personality disorder. *Comprehensive Psychiatry*, *30*, 498–504.

Emmanuel, N., Brawman-Mintzer, O., Johnson, M., Morton, M., Lydiard, A., & Ballenger, J. (1993). Personality disorders in social phobia. Presented at the 13th Annual Meeting of the Anxiety Disorder Association of America, Charleston, SC.

Fahlen, T. (1995a). Personality traits in social phobia I: Comparisons with healthy controls. *Journal of Clinical Psychiatry*, *56*, 560–568.

Fahlen, T. (1995b). Personality traits in social phobia II: Changes during drug treatment. *Journal of Clinical Psychiatry*, *56*, 569–573.

Feske, U., Perry, K. J., Chambless, D. L., Renneberg, B., & Goldstein, A. J. (1996). Avoidant personality disorder as a predictor for treatment outcome among generalized social phobics. *Journal of Personality Disorders*, *10*, 174–184.

Grillo, C. M., McGlashan, T. H., Morey, L. C., Gunderson, J. G., Skodol, A. E., & Stout, R. L. (2001). Internal consistency, intercriterion overlap and diagnostic efficiency of criteria set for DSM-IV schizotypal, borderline, avoidant and obsessive-compulsive personality disorders. *Acta Psychiatrica Scandinavica*, *104*, 264–272.

Herbert, J. D., Hope, D. A., & Bellak, A. S. (1992). Validity of the distinction between generalized social phobia and avoidant personality disorder. *Journal of Abnormal Psychology*, *101*, 332–339.

Hofmann, S. G., Ehlers, A., Newman, M. G., & Roth, W. T. (1995). Psychophysiological differences between subgroups of social phobia. *Journal of Abnormal Psychology*, *104*, 224–231.

Hofmann, S. G., Newman, M. G., Becker, E., Taylor, C. B., & Roth, W. T. (1995). Social phobia with and without avoidant personality disorder: Preliminary behavior therapy outcome findings. *Journal of Anxiety Disorders*, *9*, 427–438.

Holt, C. S., Heimberg, G. H., & Hope, H. A. (1992). Avoidant personality disorder and the generalized subtype of social phobia. *Journal of Abnormal Psychology*, *2*, 318–325.

Hope, A. H., Herbert, J. D., & White, C. (1995). Diagnostic subtype, avoidant personality disorder, and efficacy of cognitive-behavioral group therapy for social phobia. *Cognitive Therapy and Research*, *19*, 399–417.

Hummelen, B., Wilberg, T., Pedersen, G., & Karterud, S. (2006). An investigation of the validity of the Diagnostic and Statistical Manual of Mental Disorders, Fourth Edition. Avoidant Personality Disorder construct as a prototype category and the psychometric properties of the diagnostic criteria. *Comprehensive Psychiatry*, *47*, 376–383.

Hummelen, B., Wilberg, T., Pedersen, G., & Karterud, S. (2007). The relationship between avoidant personality disorder and social phobia. *Comprehensive Psychiatry*, *48*, 348–356.

Jansen, M. A., Arntz, A., Merckelbach, H., & Mersch, P. P. A. (1994). Personality disorders and features in social phobia and panic disorder. *Journal of Abnormal Psychology*, *103*, 391–395.

Lampe, L., Slade, T., Issakidis, C., & Andrews, G. (2003). Social phobia in the Australian National Survey of Mental Health and Well-being (NSMHWB). *Psychological Medicine*, *33*, 637–646.

Liebowitz, M. R, Schneier, F., Campeas, R., Hollander, E., Hatterer, J., Fyer, A., et al. (1992). Phenelzine vs atenolol in social phobia: A placebo-controlled comparison. *Archives of General Psychiatry*, *49*, 290–300.

McGlashan, T. H., Grilo, C. M., Sanislow, C. A., Ralevski, E., Morey, L. C., Gunderson, J. G., et al. (2005). Two year prevalence and stability of individual DSM-IV criteria for schizotypal, borderline, avoidant and obsessive-compulsive disorders: Toward a hybrid model of Axis II disorders. *American Journal of Psychiatry*, *162*, 883–889.

McGlashan, T. H., Grilo, C. M., Skodol, A. E., Gunderson, J. G., Shea, M. T., Morey, L. C., et al. (2000). The collaborative longitudinal personality disorders study: baseline Axis I/II and II/II diagnostic co-occurrence. *Acta Psychiatrica Scandinavica*, *102*, 256–264.

Mersch, P. P., Marijke, A., Jansen, M. A., & Arntz, A. (1995). Social phobia and personality disorder: Severity of complaint and treatment effectiveness. *Journal of Personality Disorders*, *9*, 143–159.

Millon, T. (1991). Avoidant personality disorder: A brief review of issues and data. *Journal of Personality Disorders*, *5*, 353–362.

Noyes, R., Woodman, C. L., Holt, C. S., Reich, J. H., & Zimmerman, M. B. (1995). Avoidant personality traits distinguish social phobia and panic disorder subjects. *Journal of Nervous and Mental Disease*, *183*, 145–153.

Ralevski, E., Sanislow, C. A., Grilo, C. M., Skodol, A. E., Gunderson, J. G., Shea, T. M., et al. (2005). Avoidant personality disorder and social phobia: Distinct enough to be separate disorders? *Acta Psychiatrica Scandinavica*, *112*, 208–214.

Reich, J. (2000). The relationship of social phobia to avoidant personality disorder: A proposal to reclassify avoidant personality disorder based on clinical empirical findings. *European Psychiatry*, *15*, 151–159.

Reich, J. (2005). State and trait in personality disorders. In J. Reich (Ed.), *Personality disorders: Current research and treatments* (pp. 3–21). New York: Taylor & Francis.

Reich, J. (2007). State and trait in personality disorders. *Annals of Clinical Psychiatry*, *19*, 37–44.

Reich, J. (2009). Avoidant personality disorder and its relationship to social phobia. *Current Psychiatry Reports*, *11*, 89–93.

Reich, J. H., Noyes, R., & Yates, W. (1989). Alprazolam treatment of avoidant personality traits in social phobic patients. *Journal of Clinical Psychiatry*, *50*, 91–95.

Reichborn-Kjennerud, T., Czajkowski, N., Torgersen, S., Neale, M. C., Ørstavik, R. E., Tambs, K., et al. (2007). The relationship between avoidant personality disorder and social phobia: A population based twin study. *American Journal of Psychiatry*, *164*, 1722–1728.

Renneberg, B., Goldstein, A. J., Phillips, D., & Chambless, D. L. (1990). Intensive behavioral group treatment of avoidant personality disorder. *Behavior Therapy*, *21*, 363–377.

Sanderson, W., Wetzler, S., Beck, A., & Betz, F. (1994). Prevalence of personality disorders among patients with anxiety disorders. *Psychiatry Research*, *51*, 391–395.

Schneier, F. R., Spitzer, R. L., Gibbon, M., Fyer, A. B., & Liebowitz, M. R. (1991). The relationship of social phobia subtypes and avoidant personality disorder. *Comprehensive Psychiatry*, *32*, 496–502.

Shea, M. T., Stout, R. L., Yen, S., Pagano, M. E., Skodol, A. E., Morey, L. C., et al. (2004). Associations in the course of personality disorders and Axis I disorders over time. *Journal of Abnormal Psychology*, *4*, 499–508.

Stravynski, A., Belisle, M., Marcouiller, M., Lavalee, Y., & Ellie, R. (1994). The treatment of avoidant personality disorder by social skill training in the clinic or in real life settings. *Canadian Journal of Psychiatry*, *39*, 377–383.

Taylor, C. T., Laposa, J. M., & Alden, L. E. (2004). Is avoidant personality disorder more than just social avoidance? *Journal of Personality Disorders*, *18*(6), 571–594.

Tillfors, M., Furmark, T., Ekselius, L., & Fredrikson, M. (2004). Social phobia and avoidant personality disorder: One spectrum disorder? *Nordic Journal of Psychiatry*, *58*, 147–152.

Tran, G. Q., & Chambless, D. L. (1995). Psychopathology of social phobia: Effects of subtype and of avoidant personality disorder. *Journal of Anxiety Disorders*, *9*, 489–501.

Turner, S. M., Beidel, D. C., Borden, J. W., Stanley, M. A., & Jacob, R. G. (1991). Social phobia: Axis I and Axis II correlates. *Journal of Abnormal Psychology*, *100*, 102–106.

Turner, S. M., Beidel, D. C., Dancu, C. V., & Keys, D. J. (1986). Psychopathology of social phobia and comparison to avoidant personality disorder. *Journal of Abnormal Psychology*, *4*, 389–394.

Turner, S. M., Beidel, D. C., & Townsley, R. (1992). Social phobia: A comparison of specific and generalized subtypes and avoidant personality disorder. *Journal of Abnormal Psychology*, *101*, 326–331.

Van Velzen, C. J. M., Emmelkamp, P. M. G., & Scholing, A. S. (2000). Generalized social phobia versus avoidant personality disorder: Differences in psychopathology, personality traits, and social and occupational functioning. *Journal of Anxiety Disorders*, *14*, 395–411.

Versiani, M., Nardi, A. E., Mundim, F. D., Alves, A. B., Liebowitz, M. R., & Amrein, R. (1992). Pharmacotherapy of social phobia: A controlled study with moclobemide and phenelzine. *British Journal of Psychiatry*, *161*, 353–360.

Zimmerman, M., Rothschild, L., & Chelminski, I. (2005). The prevalence of DSM-IV personality disorders in psychiatric outpatients. *American Journal of Psychiatry*, *162*, 1911–1918.

Chapter 9

Social Anxiety in Children and Adolescents: Biological, Developmental, and Social Considerations

Michael F. Detweiler[1], Jonathan S. Comer[2], and Anne Marie Albano[2]
[1]USAF Educational, Developmental, and Intervention Services (EDIS) Program, RAF Lakenheath, UK, [2]NYS Psychiatric Institute, New York, NY 10032

During Victorian times, the clinical approach to psychology was often dominated by the concept of "precocity," in which children and adolescents were conceptualized as being merely miniature versions of adults. The implications of this conceptualization were both numerous and profound, not the least of which being a fostering of an ignorance of the relationship between ontogeny and pathology. Over time, this precocial view was eventually abandoned in favor of one with a greater appreciation for lifespan developmental processes. Most child and adolescent practitioners today receive clinical training steeped in a developmental perspective (Cicchetti & Cohen, 1995; Cicchetti & Toth, 2009; Ollendick & Hirshfeld-Becker, 2002). In this chapter, we discuss the phenomenon of social anxiety in children and adolescents. We adopt a biopsychosocial model of pathology where case formulation is approached with thorough appreciation for the various individual factors at play within the context of larger family: academic and cultural systems (Adler, 2009; Engel, 1977; Santrock, 2007). We propose that pediatric social anxiety is a product of the interaction among various biological, developmental, and social factors and begin with a thorough review of these systems. Next, we propose a model of social anxiety that outlines the reciprocal interaction between youth and these biopsychosocial systems. Finally, we describe an evidence-based therapeutic intervention for pediatric SP and conclude with recommendations for clinicians who work with this unique clinical population.

Social Anxiety: Clinical, Developmental, and Social Perspectives. DOI: 10.1016/B978-0-12-375096-9.00009-2

HISTORY AND MORPHOLOGY OF SOCIAL ANXIETY DISORDER (SOCIAL PHOBIA)

SP as a clinical diagnosis first appeared in the DSM-III (American Psychiatric Association, 1980) and has undergone considerable revision over the past thirty years. Initially, a distinction was made between adult and pediatric manifestations of the disorder, with minors diagnosed with AVD. This disorder was initially described only as a chronic and excessive withdrawal from others significant enough to interfere with peer relationships and failed to identify any subtypes of social fears other than this generalized form. Unfortunately, there was considerable overlap between the criteria of AVD and SP. The differential diagnosis was hampered further by the presence of a third diagnosis, overanxious disorder in childhood and adolescence (OAD), which allowed for social fears but itself overlapped considerably with GAD. The revised DSM-III-R (American Psychiatric Association, 1987) did not expressly forbid the diagnosis of SP in child and adolescent populations, but it did not specifically reference them in the criteria either, leading many clinicians to refrain from assigning this diagnosis to youth (Stein, Chavira, & Jang, 2001). With growing recognition that many cases of AVD and OAD overlapped with other disorders (Beidel, 1991; Francis, Last, & Strauss, 1992), DSM-IV (American Psychiatric Association, 1994) finally did away with the latter two diagnoses, improving the differential diagnosis. As evidence, Kendall and Warman (1997) reported that only 18% of their clinic sample met DSM-III-R criteria for SP, whereas 40% of that same sample met DSM-IV criteria thanks to this revision in diagnostic criteria (with the 40% roughly equivalent to the DSM-III-R SP plus AVD groups).

Under the current DSM-IV-TR (American Psychiatric Association, 2000), the criteria for SP (SAD) with children and adolescents are largely similar to those for adults, with certain exceptions. A marked and persistent social/performance fear of negative evaluation must be present. However, with children, there must be evidence of anxiety present in interactions with peers, as opposed to merely with adults. Exposure to the feared situation must result in an anxious behavioral response. However, in children, an emotional reaction such as freezing, crying, or acting out via tantruming also qualifies. Finally, children are permitted to display limited insight and it is not necessary for them to recognize the severity of their anxiety as being excessive or unreasonable to meet diagnostic criteria. With the exceptions of possibly expanding the list of specifiers and/or adding the requirement of a minimum duration of symptom presentation, the proposed changes to the SAD criteria for DSM-V appear to be largely cosmetic and should not prove to be a radical departure from the current criteria.

Both the prevalence and impact of anxiety disorders are profound. Comprising over one-third of the total, anxiety disorders are the most common psychiatric illnesses in the United States (Kessler, Berglund et al., 2005).

Greenberg and colleagues (1999) conducted an economic impact study and concluded that the annual cost of anxiety disorders in the United States during the 1990s was approximately $42 billion, or roughly one-third of the total health budget and representing over $1500 per individual. Anxiety disorders are also the most common disorders observed in child and adolescent populations (Beesdo, Knappe, & Pine, 2009; Bernstein & Borchardt, 1991; Costello, Egger, & Angold, 2004; Costello et al., 1996). It is well-established that SP most commonly begins in late childhood or adolescence, typically around 13 years of age, and rarely following age 25 (Beesdo et al., 2007; Kessler, Berglund et al., 2005; Wittchen & Fehm, 2003). Estimates of the prevalence rate for SP vary somewhat in the literature based upon the nature of assessment and geographic location of participant catchment. Also noteworthy of mention are the substantial diagnostic changes that occurred between DSM-III and DSM-IV limit the degree to which prevalence rates can be compared, and the reader is cautioned to be mindful of which diagnostic criteria were used when considering published estimations (for example, see Wittchen & Fehm, 2003).

Traditionally, the lifetime prevalence rate for SP has been estimated to be somewhere between 5 and 15% (Comer & Olfson, in press; Heimberg, Stein, Hiripi, & Kessler, 2000). Kessler, Chiu, Demler, and Walters (2005) reported the adult prevalence of SP to be about 6.8%. Cox, Pagura, Stein, and Sareen (2009) studied a data set of over forty thousand individuals from the National Epidemiologic Survey on Alcohol and Related Conditions and found the lifetime prevalence for GSP to be 2.8%. The pattern is similar for child and adolescent populations. Costello and colleagues (1996) reported a one-year prevalence of SP of 13% for children and adolescents aged 9 to 17. Estimates of the prevalence of pediatric SP in the United States range from 5 to 10%, with an average of around 7% (Fichter, Kohlboeck, Quadflieg, Wyschkon, & Esser, 2009; Schneier, 2006). Beesdo and colleagues (2009) conducted a comprehensive review of the reported prevalence rates of SP and other anxiety disorders in children and adolescents and concurred with a prevalence estimate of 7%. Common for most anxiety disorders, a gender difference is also clearly observed with SP by adolescence; the prevalence rate for females is nearly double that of males, although there is a developmental effect whereby the difference generally increases with increasing age (Beesdo et al., 2009; Craske, 2003; Pine, Cohen, Gurley, Brook, & Ma, 1998; Wittchen, Nelson, & Lachner, 1998).

BIOLOGICAL FACTORS

Youth, particularly adolescence, is a period marked by elevated activity across numerous biological processes (Holmbeck & Updegrove, 1995; Ojeda, Lomniczi, Sandau, & Matagne, 2010). Pediatric clinical syndromes are best approached with acknowledgment of those maturational changes under way for children at varying points of development. In-depth discussion of the biological basis for SAD is beyond the scope of this chapter and is available elsewhere in this volume (Phann & Klumpp, Chapter 10; Stein & Gelernter, Chapter 11; Kagan, Chapter 12). Therefore, we have restricted our discussion to those specific biological contributors to social anxiety that are most influential for youth.

Genetic Influence

Clinicians have long suspected that there is a genetic component to social anxiety, but the evidence has traditionally varied in breadth and scope. Differences in estimates are due to various factors, such as the nature of the dependent variable studied (e.g., clinical anxiety disorder vs. subclinical anxiety symptoms) or source of information (Gregory & Eley, 2007; Murray, Creswell, & Cooper, 2009), but the magnitude of genetic influence upon anxiety in general is believed to be moderate (Gregory & Eley, 2007). Evidence has clearly demonstrated a higher base rate of anxiety disorders in the children of parents who themselves have anxiety disorders, as well as vice versa (Biederman, Rosenbaum, Bolduc, Faraone, & Hirshfeld, 1991; Cooper, Fearn, Willetts, Seabrook, & Parkinson, 2006; Last, Hersen, Kazdin, Francis, & Grubb, 1987; Last, Hersen, Kazdin, Orvaschel, & Perrin, 1991; Turner, Biedel, & Costello, 1987; Warner, Mufson, & Weissman, 1995; Weissman, Leckman, Merikangas, Gammon, & Prusoff, 1984). Studies also have demonstrated the aggregation of SP specifically among family members, particularly the generalized subtype (Fyer, Mannuzza, Chapman, Liebowitz, & Klein, 1993; Fyer, Mannuzza, Chapman, Martin, & Klein, 1995; Mancini, van Ameringen, Szatmari, Fugere, & Boyle, 1996; Mannuzza et al., 1995; Reich & Yates, 1988; Stein et al., 1998).

Twin studies are helpful in teasing out the differential contribution of genetic and environmental influences upon social behavior and/or psychiatric disorders (Gregory & Eley, 2007). Unfortunately, however, there are few twin studies examining social anxiety specifically and more research is warranted. Kendler, Neale, Kessler, Heath, & Eaves, (1992) examined twins identified from the Virginia twin registry and found a 24.4% concordance rate of SP for monozygotic twins and a 15.3% concordance rate for dizygotic twins, yielding a heritability index (h^2) of about 30% for SP. However, this study has significant limitations in that it included only female twin pairs and utilized DSM-III diagnostic criteria. Ogliari et al. (2006) conducted a twin study focusing upon 378 Italian twin pairs ranging from late childhood through adolescence (ages 8–17) and reported an h^2 of around 0.6 for self-reported symptoms of social anxiety.

Behavioral genetic twin studies have classified three main influences upon behavior (Gregory & Eley, 2007) – genetic influences (inherited from family members), shared environmental influences (nongenetic environmental factors often shared with immediate family members such as parenting style, living environment, diet, etc.), and nonshared environmental influences (nongenetic environmental factors usually not shared with immediate family members, such as illness history, specific friendships, trauma history, etc.). Eley and colleagues (2003) employed both phenotypic and genetic approaches in an examination of over four thousand British preschool twin pairs. With regards to parental report of a subclinical shyness/inhibition temperamental trait, they found high levels of genetic influence accounting for around two-thirds of the variance, with one-third due to nonshared environmental factors. In a subsequent study, Eley, Rijsdijk, Perrin, O'Connor, and Bolton (2008) conducted a multivariate analysis of anxiety phenotypes in a sample of young people that included those who met diagnostic criteria for SP by age six (as assessed by semistructured clinical interview). They found nonshared environmental factors to be the only significant influence upon SP (79%), with only small nonsignificant influences from genetic (14%) and (10%) shared environmental factors.

Complicating matters, we now understand that genetic influence can be a dynamic process (Bird, 2007; Kendler, Gardner, & Lichtenstein, 2008). Even with a stable genetic "architecture," genetic "influence" can wax and wane over an individual's lifespan in response to environmental or developmental influences such as puberty (Eaves, Long, & Heath, 1986; Whitelaw & Whitelaw, 2006). In their seminal meta-analysis, Bergen, Gardner, and Kendler, (2007) alert us to the importance of maintaining a developmental perspective when considering heritability. For example, the heritability of a phenotype observed in early childhood may be different from the heritability of that same phenotype observed in adolescence or young adulthood. Consider for a moment that young children typically passively receive the genetic contribution and environmental control of their parents. Teens and young adults, however, take a more active approach and begin to seek out reinforcing environments based more upon their own unique genotypic expression, creating a stronger interaction between genetics and environment as they both shape and are shaped by the settings they encounter. Results of the Bergen et al. meta-analysis revealed an age-related increase in heritability (h^2 ranging from approximately 0.10 at age 10 to 0.60 by age 25) with anxiety symptoms demonstrating the highest effect size for per-year increase of any domain assessed ($+0.030$, $t = 4.22$, $p = 0.0056$).

Brain/Cognitive Development

One of the more exciting areas of research in recent years belongs to an emerging field attempting to integrate the findings of social cognitive neuroscience with those of clinical developmental psychopathology (Yeates et al., 2007). Where neuroscience is the interdisciplinary study of those underlying brain systems associated with human thoughts, emotions, and behaviors (Kandel, Schwartz, & Jessell, 2000), social cognitive neuroscience specifically focuses upon the brain–behavior relationship as it pertains to an individual's social functioning (Brothers, 1990; Moss & Damasio, 2001). Social cognitive neuroscience models drew heavily upon observations of children who suffered traumatic brain injuries. After it was observed that many of the interpersonal functioning deficits displayed following damage to the brain were similar to those characteristic of some clinical syndromes, the call came for greater integration between neuroscience and developmental psychopathology. For example, in much the same way that a neuropsychologist may capitalize upon an extensive knowledge of neural systems to help clarify a decline in school functioning into more specific terms of deficits in processing speed versus working memory versus attention (each with their own implications for intervention), the social cognitive neuroscience model may strive to clarify a decline in social functioning in terms of deficits of areas such as interpersonal problem-solving versus social communication versus emotion regulation. Today, there is a growing elucidatory research base identifying the development of brain structures and systems that play a part in the emergence of social competence during childhood and adolescence (see Adolphs, 2001). Further findings will undoubtedly provide insight into the role of neurobiological factors affecting social anxiety; however, progress is hindered to the extent that adaptive social functioning as a construct has proven difficult to define (c.f., Bukowski, Rubin, & Parker, 2001; Cavell, 1990; Rubin, Bukowski, & Parker, 2006).

Although a thorough discussion of all the brain systems involved in social competence is beyond the scope of this chapter, three warrant mentioning in terms of their relationship to both social development and social anxiety.

Amygdala

The amygdala is an almond-shaped structure located within the anterior portion of the temporal lobes, comprising a component of the limbic system and known to play a part in controlling emotion, motivation, and memory. It plays a clear role in the processing of both social cues and emotional expression and is involved with the sympathetic nervous system's response to anxiety, leading many to identify the amygdala as playing a role in social anxiety (Birbaumer et al., 1998; Etkin & Wager, 2007; Rosen & Schulkin, 1998; Shin & Liberzon, 2010). Normally, the amygdala responds to facial cues with an increase in activity as perceived social threat increases (Morris et al., 1996). Individuals with SP have been shown to demonstrate an attentional bias for negative social cues (e.g., Alden & Wallace, 1995). As would be expected, research has shown a correlation between the degree of amygdala activity and the severity of social anxiety when presented with social threat cues. This has been demonstrated both in individuals diagnosed with SP (Phan, Fitzgerald, Nathan, & Tancer, 2006) and in those not yet meeting diagnostic criteria but high in BI, a risk factor for a future SP diagnosis (Pérez-Edgar et al., 2007). Furthermore, individuals with increased social anxiety have been shown to display social skills deficits (Beidel & Turner, 1998) and damage to the amygdala typically leads to profound deficits in social functioning, such as difficulty with emotional processing, problem-solving, and the ability to discern the emotional nuance of facial expressions or body language (Ammerlaan, Hendriks, Colon, & Kessels, 2008; Cristinzio, N'Diaye, Seeck, Vuilleumier, & Sander, 2010; Scott et al., 1997; Shaw et al., 2004; see also Corden, Critchley, Skuse, & Dolan, 2006). Finally, individuals and nonhuman primates with damaged or surgically removed amygdalae often demonstrate restricted emotional expression in social contexts; decreased display of prosocial skills such as maintaining adequate eye contact; and occasionally (although not always) increased social withdrawal, escape, and avoidance behaviors in response to the presence of others (Mori & Yamadori, 1989; Ozmen, Erdogan, Duvenci, Ozyurt, & Ozkara, 2004; Spezio, Huang, Castelli, & Adolphs, 2007). Avoidance is viewed as a maintaining factor in social anxiety, with exposure-based interventions that limit avoidance shown to yield the largest effect sizes in studies examining different treatment approaches for social anxiety (Gould, Buckminster, Pollack, Otto, & Yap, 1997; Hope, Heimberg, & Bruch, 1995).

When specifically considering child populations, one must be mindful of the interaction between the amygdala's development and the emergence of social competence and social anxiety. Development of the amygdala continues for about two years following birth and this maturation both affects the social behavior of the infant and is affected by the reciprocal social stimulation the child receives in return (Joseph, 1999). Accordingly, infants demonstrate increasingly prosocial behavior (Hasselmo, Rolls, & Baylis, 1989; Yakovlev & Lecours, 1967) in the early stages of the amygdala's maturation. This not only demonstrates newly acquired social skills, but also serves to solicit additional adult social interaction, furthering the development of the amygdala and fine-tuning the child's emerging social competence. Infants raised in socially impoverished environments often display delays in neural development within the amygdala and subsequent deficits in social functioning later in life (Jacobson, 1986; Tranel & Hyman, 1990).

Developmentally speaking, it behooves infants to interact with as wide a social network as possible during the early stages of amygdala maturation in order to capitalize on the bidirectional influence of context upon development. We would not expect to see a volitional restriction of socialization until such time as maturation has progressed sufficiently so as to not be hindered by the lack of social stimuli. In fact, this is exactly what is observed. Stranger anxiety (i.e., a developmentally appropriate behavioral response to unfamiliar adults marked by distress and behavioral withdrawal) typically peaks around nine months of age (Ainsworth, Blehar, Waters, & Wall, 1978; Bronson, 1974; Schaffer, 1966; Waters, Matas, & Sroufe, 1975). This emergence corresponds directly with more advanced stages of amygdala development in which the infant has already developed an improved ability to discern between different faces, genders, emotions, and subtle social cues (see Caron, Caron, & Meyers, 1985). In fact, phases of infant social emotional development have been shown to correlate with differential maturation rates of the amygdala and supporting systems, in turn influencing infant approach-avoidant behavior and the formation of loving attachments with caregivers in corresponding fashion (Joseph, 1999).

Prefrontal cortex

Along with the amygdala, the prefrontal cortex is another key component of the neural circuit involved with the processing of social threat (Adolphs, 2001; Blair, Morris, Frith, Perrett, & Dolan, 1999; Gallagher & Frith, 2003; Gross & Hen, 2004; Hariri, Mattay, Tessitore, Fera, & Weinberger, 2003; Haxby, Hoffman, & Gobbini, 2002; Monk et al., 2003). In simplistic terms, the amygdala is believed to be involved with the identification of the emotional quality of a stimulus, whereas the prefrontal cortex is believed to be involved with activating the higher cognitive processes necessary for regulating emotion and choosing a subsequent course of reaction to the stimulus (Nelson, Leibenluft, McClure, & Pine, 2005). The prefrontal cortex is assumed to provide the cognitive resources to boost the efficiency of those behaviors commonly referred to as representing "executive functioning" (Amunts et al., 2004; Aron, Robbins, & Poldrack, 2004; Buchsbaum, Greer, Chang, & Berman, 2005; Curtis & D'Esposito, 2003; Duncan, 2001; Langenecker, Nielson, & Rao, 2004). As such, this area's role in the processing of social behavior becomes clear when you consider that social competence requires an adaptive management of attentional skills, problem-solving, and a host of additional executive functioning skills governed by the prefrontal cortex (White, Helfinstein, Reeb-Sutherland, Degnan, & Fox, 2009).

As with the amygdala, evidence of the relationship between the prefrontal cortex and anxiety comes in the form of data demonstrating differences in the activation patterns correlated with subjective social anxiety (Sripada et al., 2009; Tillfors et al., 2001; Tillfors, Furmark, Marteinsdottir, & Fredrikson, 2002). Monk et al. (2006) conducted an experiment in which functional magnetic resonance imaging (FMRI) captured the brain activity of adolescents as they completed a task measuring attention while presented with angry and neutral faces. Adolescents with GSP showed greater activation in the ventrolateral area of the prefrontal cortex compared to nonanxious adolescents as they were spontaneously demonstrating a significantly different degree of attentional avoidance of angry faces. Damage to the prefrontal cortex often results in disruptions in behavior required for competent social functioning. Mah, Arnold, and Grafman (2004) compared the ability of adults with prefrontal cortex lesions with control subjects on a social perception task and found an association between damage to this brain area and poorer social perception ability.

A distinguishing characteristic of the prefrontal cortex is its protracted developmental timeline. Many regions of the prefrontal cortex follow a nonlinear developmental trajectory and do not reach physical maturity until the early adulthood period of the late teens to early twenties (Casey, Giedd, & Thomas, 2000; Conklin, Luciana, Hooper, & Yarger, 2007; Giedd et al., 1999; Sowell et al., 2003; Sowell, Thompson, Holmes, Jernigan, & Toga; 1999; Toga, Thompson, & Sowell, 2006). In the frontal lobes, the peak in gray matter volume (the neural material comprising cell bodies and their dendrites) coincides with the onset of puberty and is, followed by an increase in the volume of white matter (WM) (the neural material comprising the myelinated connecting nerve fibers) in the prefrontal cortex thereafter and throughout the mid-twenties (Barnea-Goraly et al., 2005; Giedd et al., 1996; Giedd et al., 1999; Reiss, Abrams, Singer, Ross, & Denckla, 1996; Sowell, Thompson, Tessner, & Toga, 2001; Sowell et al., 2003; Toga et al., 2006). The period from late adolescence throughout the third decade of life is marked by synaptic fine-tuning within the prefrontal cortex through a process of increased axonal myelination and synaptic pruning to allow for improved communication between inter-related brain areas (Durston et al., 2001; Giedd, 2004; Huttenlocher, 1979; Huttenlocher, De Courten, Garey, & van Der Loos, 1983; Reiss et al., 1996; Sowell et al., 2001;Yakovlev & Lecours, 1967). This neurodevelopmental process of improving communication between inter-related brain areas in late adolescence and early adulthood has implications for the experience of social anxiety, as described below.

Amygdala-Prefrontal Cortex Connectivity

Rather than simply being two neural structures similar in function, there is evidence that the amygdala and prefrontal cortex work in conjunction as part of a more complex emotion-regulation circuit (Adolphs, 2003; Baxter, Parker, Lindner, Izquierdo, & Murray, 2000; Gross & Hen, 2004; Hariri et al., 2003; McClure et al., 2007) with implications for both social functioning in general and the development of affective disorders such as SAD (Drevets, 2003; Mayberg, 1997, 2007; Pezawas et al., 2005; Rauch, Shin, & Phelps, 2006). In simplistic terms, the prefrontal cortex is believed to develop into a top-down modulator of the amygdala's emotional reactivity to threat or fear-inducing stimuli (Casey, Getz, & Galvan, 2009; Hare et al., 2008; Tottenham et al., 2009). This executive control of amygdala activation by the prefrontal cortex in response to threatening situations facilitates the flexibility of attentional and behavioral processes presumed to be necessary for not only successful social functioning (Blair, 2004; Blair & Cipolotti 2000; Hariri et al., 2003; Kringelbach & Rolls, 2003) but also the process of habituation (Hugdahl & Nordby, 1994; Wright et al., 2001).

Recall that the prefrontal cortex has a protracted developmental timeline that continues well into the second or third decade of life. During adolescence, changes occur at the cellular level that involve the generation of new synapses and a subsequent synaptic pruning that Nelson, Rubin, and Fox (2005) described as a "use or lose" process in which neural connections are strengthened through an individual's experience (Huttenlocher, 1979; Huttenlocher et al.,

1983). In the adolescent prefrontal cortex, gray matter density decreases, whereas WM increases due to increased myelination, especially the myelination of those fibers connecting this brain region with others (Casey, Galvan, & Hare, 2005; Yakovlev & Lecours, 1967). Total brain volume changes little during this period (Blakenmore & Choudhury, 2006; Choudhury, Blakemore, & Charman, 2006) and these changes in gray and WM density are believed to represent a process of synaptic reorganization (Paus, 2005).

This reorganization enables greater executive control of amygdala activation by the prefrontal cortex (Yurgelun-Todd, 2007; Rubia et al., 2000; Rubia et al., 2006; Tamm, Menon, & Reiss, 2002). By adolescence, the amygdala has reached maturity whereas the prefrontal cortex has not. Increases in sex hormones occurring with puberty profoundly affect the amygdala (Nelson, Leibenluft et al., 2005). Brain imaging studies have shown that, relative to children and adults, adolescents demonstrate more pronounced amygdala activation when processing emotional information (Ernst et al., 2005; Galvan et al., 2006; Kuhnen & Knutson, 2005; Matthews, Simmons, Lane, & Paulus, 2004; Monk et al., 2003; Montague & Berns, 2002). Furthermore, amygdala activation differences can reliably differentiate adults with and without social anxiety (Birbaumer et al., 1998; Lorerbaum et al., 2004; Phan et al., 2006; Stein, Goldin, Sareen, Zorrilla, & Brown, 2002; Straube, Kolassa, Glauer, Mentzel, & Miltner, 2004; Tillfors et al., 2001; Veit et al., 2002). In the absence of top-down regulation from the prefrontal cortex, adolescents are more prone to the interference that comes from the emotional properties of social stimuli (Nelson, Leibenluft et al., 2005). Monk and colleagues (2006) noted that increases in prefrontal cortex activation were correlated with decreased subjective anxiety symptoms for those with GAD. In a related study, Monk and colleagues (2003) asked adolescents and adults to vary their attention between emotional and nonemotional aspects of a social stimulus and found that only adults demonstrated prefrontal cortex activation in response to this experimental demand. Thus, pubescent adolescents (who demonstrate more amygdala activity in response to social threat and find it difficult to disengage attention from that social threat due to the immaturity of the prefrontal cortex) appear to have a neurobiological vulnerability during this period. They can easily become preoccupied with the perception that they are being negatively evaluated by others and social anxiety concerns increase as a result (Rapee & Heimberg, 1997).

Puberty

Puberty refers to the developmental transition period marked by a cascade of biological changes resulting in sexual and physical maturation (Forbes & Dahl, 2010; Buck Louis et al., 2008). Complicating the direct effects puberty can have on biology, pubertal onset also overlaps with a crucial transitional period in which children progress through adolescence and eventually young adulthood. A healthy understanding of both the physiological changes and the shift in social demands that occurs during this development period must be considered when conceptualizing social anxiety in the adolescent population. There is some evidence suggesting that puberty may be a factor that increases the risk for many affective disorders (Angold, 2003; Angold, Costello, Erkanli, & Worthman, 1999; Angold, Erkanli, Silberg, Eaves, & Costello, 2002; Angold, Worthman, & Costello, 2003; Gunnar, Wewerka, Frenn, Long, & Griggs, 2009; Hayward, 2003). Adolescence often witnesses the onset of new, or an increase in severity of pre-existing, anxiety symptoms (Essau, Conradt, & Petermann, 1999; Reardon, Leen-Feldner, & Hayward, 2009; Schneier, Johnson, Hornig, Liebowitz, & Weissman, 1992; Wittchen, Stein, & Kessler, 1999; Zgourides & Warren, 1988). This is likely related in no small part to the fact that increases in hormone levels during puberty directly affect the response to stress in the body and brain (Chrousos, Torpy, & Gold, 1998; Spear, 2000). Also, there is growing evidence that early pubertal development may be an additional risk factor for anxiety (Hayward et al., 1997; Zehr, Culbert, Sisk, & Klump, 2007).

It warrants mentioning here that the timing of the onset of puberty is somewhat dynamic and can be influenced by such lifestyle factors as stress, diet, and exercise (Adams, 1981; Dick, Rose, Pulkkinen, & Kaprio, 2001; Gluckman & Hanson, 2006; Paikoff & Brooks-Gunn, 1991). Perhaps as a result, the onset of puberty is currently occurring earlier than was documented forty to fifty years ago (American Psychiatric Association, 2002; Anderson, Dallal, & Must, 2003; Bellis, Downing, & Ashton, 2006; Bodzsar & Susanne, 1998). Although there is some variability due to cultural factors, generally speaking, pubertal onset is now typically observed between the ages of 10–12 in males and 12–13 in females (Anderson & Must, 2005; Herman-Giddens, 2006; Whincup, Gilg, Odoki, Taylor, & Cook, 2001). One unfortunate result of the decline in average age of pubertal onset is a widening of the gap between physical and social development during adolescence. There are growing concerns that the physical maturity ushered in by puberty may now occur prior to requisite emotional development and a call has been raised to address the paucity of social support covering this gap (Dahl & Spear, 2004; Ge, Brody, Conger, & Simons, 2006; Ge, Conger, & Elder, 1996; Gluckman & Hanson, 2006). Research has demonstrated a correlation between earlier pubertal onset and a host of social and emotional risk factors in general. For example, Downing and Bellis (2009) conducted a survey in the United Kingdom and found self-reported earlier onset of puberty was a predictor of drug and alcohol abuse prior to 14 years and sexual experience including unprotected sex prior to 16 years for both sexes (see also Costello, Sung, Worthman, & Angold, 2007; Felson & Haynie, 2002). However, the timing of the onset of puberty may also have direct implications for social anxiety.

Research has demonstrated that the age of pubertal onset can affect adolescents' subjective social anxiety and self-esteem. Early-maturing girls and late-maturing boys tend to report lower self-esteem than those whose pubertal development more closely approximates the mean (Berk & Shanker, 2006).

This is often presumed to be a result of the negative attention received as a result of outward appearance (e.g., questioned machismo of less physically developed boys vs. unwanted romantic overtures towards more physically developed girls) and warrants further attention given that peer rejection and taunting have been associated with the development of social anxiety (La Greca & Harrison, 2005). Currently few studies exist examining the relationship between pubertal development and social anxiety specifically. Deardorff and colleagues (2007) studied social anxiety symptoms in adolescents and found a relationship between symptoms and pubertal status, but within the context of an interaction with gender. Advanced pubertal development was associated with increased social anxiety, but only for females. However, this study was limited by the inclusion of only a restricted range of pubertal development (9.5 through 11 years of age), its use of self-report measures, and the examination of predominantly subclinical social anxiety symptoms as measured by a questionnaire. Blumenthal, Leen-Feldner, Trainor, Babson, and Bunaciu (2009) also studied the relationship between pubertal status and social anxiety symptoms, but additionally sought to explore moderating factors. They found that early pubertal development plus interpersonal problems with peers combined to predict higher social anxiety symptoms. This study employed a larger range of the pubertal cohort (adolescents aged 10 through 17), but was similarly restricted by the reliance upon self-report measures and examination of subclinical symptoms via a single questionnaire. Further research in this area is still needed. The biological process of puberty results from hormonal changes triggered by the brain that effect the gonads, which in turn produce hormones that bring about maturational changes in other parts of the body (Buck Louis et al., 2008). As summarized in Forbes and Dahl (2010), gonadotropin-releasing hormone from the hypothalamus triggers pituitary changes in the production of luteinizing hormone and follicle-stimulating hormone. This in turn triggers maturation of the gonads and the production of the sex hormones (estradiol and testosterone). Germaine to our discussion of social anxiety, it is worth noting that the neural areas that comprise the amygdala–prefrontal cortex emotion-regulation circuit mentioned above are highly influenced by these gonadal steroids and their presence contributes to the structural and functional changes observed in that brain area during puberty (Giedd, Castellanos, Rajapakse, Vaituzis, & Rapoport, 1997; McEwen, 2001; Nelson, Leibenluft et al., 2005; Osterlund & Hurd, 2001; Romeo, Richardson, & Sisk, 2002; Stevens, 2002). Hormone levels have also been shown to exert influence over various aspects of social behavior, such as those related to approach-avoidance (Hull et al., 1999; Insel, 1997; Pfaff, Frohlich, & Morgan, 2002; Winslow & Insel, 2004) and thus suggest puberty may be a critical period for the development of patterns of adaptive adult social functioning (Flemming & Corter, 1995; Nelson, Leibenluft et al., 2005). This could in part help to explain why the prevalence of anxiety disorders rises significantly during adolescence (Pine et al., 1998; Pine, Cohen, Johnson, & Brook, 2002) and why those with pubertal onset of

SP often experience persistence of clinically significant symptoms well into adulthood (Öst, 1987; Turner & Beidel, 1989).

Gonadal sex hormones coupled with an increase in secretion of adrenal androgens result in the development of secondary sex characteristics, which are typically the most conspicuous changes adolescents face during puberty (Forbes & Dahl, 2010). Leary (1995) identified personal appearance as "perhaps the most apparent nonverbal channel of self-expression" (p. 25). Those who view their body image less favorably tend also to report elevated levels of social anxiety (Hart, Leary, & Rejeski, 1989), as is the case for those whose specific fear is related to others having a negative perception of their physical appearance (Leary & Kowalski, 1993). This concern is not entirely unfounded as attractive individuals are perceived as being more socially skilled than less attractive individuals (Feingold, 1992). Unfortunately, puberty brings with it a host of rapid physical changes for teens to view as undesirable, from growth spurts and a redistribution of body fat to cracking voices and new body hair.

As normal as the physical changes that accompany puberty may be, adolescents adjust to them with varying degrees of acceptance and occasionally normal physiological changes become the impetus for social evaluative concerns. One common example is acne vulgaris, the onset of which most commonly corresponds with the adrenarche phase of puberty, when the production of adrenal androgens fosters the development of secondary sex characteristics (Kilkenny, Merlin, Plunkett, & Marks, 1998; Stewart, 1992; Yamamoto & Ito, 1992). School-aged children with acne are often teased (Mallon et al., 1999). Loney, Arnold, and Grafman (2008) studied social anxiety resulting from acne and found it correlated negatively with self-esteem and positively with avoidance of social activities such as sports. Thomas (2004) summarized this predicament perfectly: "when teens and young adults have a need to look their best, they frequently have acne, which makes them feel and look their worst." (p. 3). Puberty is a time of heightened preoccupation with body image (Harter, 1999; Lunde, Frisén, & Hwang, 2007). Generally speaking, adolescent males try to bulk up, while on the other hand adolescent girls generally try to slim down (Muris, Meesters, van de Bloom, & Mayer, 2005). Whereas eating disorders are rarely seen in prepubertal children (Zehr, Culbert, Sisk, & Klump, 2007), evidence suggests a strong relationship between pubertal body transformation and increased body image dissatisfaction and the onset of eating disordered behavior, particularly among females (Cotrufo, Cella, Cremato, & Labella, 2007; Hayward et al., 1997; Tremblay & Lariviere, 2009).

Given that adolescence is a time of heightened self-consciousness (Elkind & Bowen, 1979; Simmons, Rosenberg, & Rosenberg, 1973), it is not surprising that we also see a jump in the prevalence of social anxiety concerns at this developmental period (Costello et al., 2002; Essau et al., 1999; Graziano, DeGiovanni, & Garcia, 1979; King, 1993; Ollendick, King, & Frary, 1989; Pine et al., 1998; Steinberg, 2005; Sumter, Bokhorst, & Westenberg, 2009). According to the self-presentation model of SP (Schlenker & Leary, 1982), social anxiety is conceptualized as the experience that results when individuals are motivated to make a desired impression on others but begin to conclude that they are not or cannot (see also Goffmann, 1959; Leary, 1995; Schlenker, 1980). As teens progress through puberty, they can experience all the key theoretical ingredients of this model of social anxiety. An increased motivation to make a desired impression (in the form of heightened teen self-consciousness and changing social demands) combines with a perceived failure to manage a favorable impression (in the form of distorted perceptions of body image and/or undesirable pubertal changes to physical appearance) and social anxiety results.

DEVELOPMENTAL FACTORS

Attachment

Immediately upon birth, infants become members of a profoundly salient social relationship – the one experienced with a caregiver, most typically a parent. It has been hypothesized that a special bond called "attachment" results between the infant and caregiver based upon the daily interaction that occurs over the first year of life (Bowlby, 1978). Attachment theory posits that the quality of this bond in childhood may serve as a contributing factor to the development of future social anxiety problems (Brumariu & Kerns, 2008; Vertue, 2003). For infants, there is inherent evolutionary survival value in the attempt to maintain close proximity to caregivers during times of threat or stress (Prior & Glaser, 2006). According to attachment theory, early caregiver availability and emotional responsiveness during attempts to maintain close proximity lead the infant to develop standards and expectations about social relationships in general, which in turn affect emotional and behavioral responses the child then displays in social situations with novel individuals (Bretherton & Munholland, 1999; Mercer, 2006; Schneider, Atkinson, & Tardif, 2001).

Four distinct infant attachment styles have been identified: secure, avoidant, ambivalent/resistant, and disorganized (Ainsworth, 1989; Ainsworth et al., 1978; Bailey, Moran, Pederson, & Bento, 2007; Madigan, Moran, & Pederson, 2006; Main & Hesse, 1990; Main & Solomon, 1986). A secure attachment style is said to develop in response to a caregiver who is reliably available to effectively soothe the child during times of stress. The remaining three represent insecure attachment styles, said to develop in response to a pattern of inconsistent, unavailable, or maladaptive caregiver response. Securely attached infants are presumed to develop into individuals who have learned how to rely upon others as calming influences and feel secure enough to explore socially, whereas insecurely attached infants learn others are unreliable, which can amplify the fear response during times of stress and foster the development of avoidance behaviors or maladaptive coping (Ainsworth et al., 1978; Bowlby, 1973; Cassidy & Berlin, 1994).

Lending support to this presumption, children with insecure attachments are viewed as less socially competent and are less well liked than those who are securely attached (Cohn, 1990; DeMulder, Denham, Schmidt, & Mitchell, 2000). Clark and Symons (2009) found a secure attachment style to be correlated not only with a child's positive self-esteem but also to more positive attributions of the social behavior of others. Raikes and Thompson (2008) found a relationship between secure attachment style and increased social problem-solving skills and decreased loneliness. Conversely, La Greca and Lopez (1998) found that adolescents who were high in social anxiety also reported a lower degree of social functioning that would appear to be reminiscent of an insecure attachment style, only with peers instead of caregivers (e.g., lower levels of peer acceptance, social support, intimacy, and companionship). Warren, Huston, Egeland, and Sroufe (1997) studied adolescents whose attachment styles had been assessed as one-year-olds. Although some children with secure attachment styles went on to develop anxiety disorders as teens, those with insecure attachment styles (especially ambivalent/resistant) doubled the risk of doing so. Finally, Irons and Gilbert (2005) found a secure attachment style to be predictive of low social anxiety and social submissiveness, whereas insecure attachment predicted the exact opposite relationship, leading the authors to speculate that an insecure attachment style fosters a preoccupation with social competition, the potential for negative social outcomes, and the need to avoid those outcomes – all key ingredients of social anxiety (Barlow, 2002; Beck, Emery, & Greenberg, 1985; Clark & Wells, 1995; Schlenker & Leary, 1982).

Temperament

Hippocrates, the father of modern medicine, proposed a theory in the fourth century BC that emotions had a predominantly physiological basis and differences were due specifically to fluctuations in body fluids called "humors." In the second century AD, the Roman physician Galen built upon Hippocratic humor theory and proposed four classic "temperamental" character styles – melancholic, phlegmatic, sanguine, and choleric. Today, the idea of an innate, constitutionally based character style persists, although considerable controversy exists (Buss & Plomin, 1984; Rothbart & Derryberry, 1981; Rothbart & Posner, 1985; Seifer & Sameroff, 1986; Strelau, 1983; Thomas & Chess, 1977). Although they are presumed to have a physiological basis, specific biological processes associated with temperament have been difficult to identify and study (Kagan, 2001). Furthermore, there is disagreement regarding the classification and number of distinct temperamental styles (cf., Goldsmith & Campos, 1982; Kagan, Reznick, & Snidman, 1988; Rothbart, 2004; Thomas, Chess, &

Birch, 1968). Temperament is generally defined as unlearned, constitutionally based individual differences in both presentation style and ability to regulate emotion, attention, and behavior (Rothbart & Bates, 2006; Rothbart, Ellis, & Posner, 2004). Simply put, developmental clinicians view temperament as a predisposing dispositional factor that can either help or hinder a child's adaptation to their environmental setting (Clark & Watson, 1999; Rothbart & Bates, 2006). A considerable research base has been devoted to the degree to which temperament serves as a risk factor for future psychopathology, either directly or indirectly through elicited changes to parental caregiving (Barron & Earls, 1984; Betts, Gullone, & Allen, 2009; Cutrona & Troutman, 1986; Essex, Klein, Slattery, Goldsmith, & Kalin, 2010; Kagan, Reznick, & Snidman, 1988; Lerner, Castellino, Patterson, Villaruel, & McKinney, 1995; Putnam, Sanson, & Rothbart, 2002). For example, Thompson, Connell, and Bridges (1988) found a fearful temperamental style had both a direct and indirect influence on children's social interaction. Eisenberg and colleagues (2001, 2005) examined a temperamental style termed "negative emotionality" (Rothbart & Bates, 2006) and found that its components contribute differently to internalizing versus externalizing problems, with internalizers more prone to fear and shyness (see also Bates, Pettit, Dodge, & Ridge, 1998; Leve, Kim, & Pears, 2005). A temperamental style marked by high negative emotionality plus physiological overarousal has been linked to anxiety problems later in life (Brown, Chorpita, & Barlow, 1998; Chorpita & Daleiden, 2002; Lonigan, Carey, & Finch, 1994; Watson, Clark, & Carey, 1988).

A considerable amount of attention has been applied to the study of BI, an anxious temperamental style marked by exaggerated physiological responding (Schmidt & Fox, 1998; Schmidt, Fox, Schulkin, & Gold, 1999; Schmidt, Fox, Sternberg et al., 1999), attentional hypervigilance (Pérez-Edgar & Fox, 2005), and an avoidant behavioral style in unfamiliar situations (Kagan et al., 1988). Several studies have identified an association between BI and an increased risk for SP later in life (Biederman et al., 2001; Caspi, Moffitt, Newman, & Silva, 1996; Chronis-Tuscano et al., 2009; Hayward, Killen, Kraemer, & Taylor, 1998; Hirshfeld et al., 1992; Muris, Merckelbach, Wessele, & Van de Ven, 1999; Muris, Merckelbach, Schmidt, Gadet, & Bogie, 2001; Reznick, Hegeman, Kaufman, Woods, & Jacobs, 1992; Schwartz, Snidman, & Kagan, 1999). In one study, 61% of children identified as being behaviorally inhibited at age 2 had social anxiety when evaluated at age 13 (compared with only 27% of those identified as being uninhibited), and this relationship was specific for generalized social anxiety but not other forms of anxiety (Kagan, 1989; Schwartz et al., 1999). Similarly, Hirshfeld-Becker and colleagues (2007) conducted a five-year follow-up of children assessed for temperament and also found that BI significantly predicted new onset of SP in middle childhood, without observing an association with this temperamental style and any other anxiety disorders. For more discussion of temperament and social anxiety, please refer to the chapter by Kagan (Chapter 12) for a more detailed review.

SOCIAL FACTORS

Parenting Style

Social learning theory (Bandura, 1977) posits learning through the observation of others. Not surprisingly, research has established a link between parenting style and internalizing problems in youth (McLeod, Weisz, & Wood, 2007; Rapee, 1997; Wood, McLeod, Sigman, Hwang, & Chu, 2003). Parents not only can serve as powerful models of social behavior for children, but also have a unique opportunity to shape their children's behavior over the course of years through parent–child interactions. Nonanxious toddlers have been shown to display anxious and avoidant behavior to a stranger after observing their mothers react fearfully (Gerull & Rapee, 2002; de Rosnay, Cooper, Tsigaras, & Murray, 2006). Murray et al. (2008) further demonstrated how mothers' anxious interactions with a stranger displayed in front of their 10-month-old children continued to predict the toddlers' avoidant responding at 14 months.

In addition to maladaptive behavioral responses, cognitive biases and catastrophic interpretations of threat are also believed to be subject to parental influence and an important factor in the development of childhood anxiety (Barrett, Rapee, Dadds, & Ryan, 1996; Dix, Ruble, Grusec, & Nixon, 1986; Joiner & Wagner, 1996). The parents of anxious youth often maintain pessimistic expectations about their children's functioning in various domains (Cobham, Dadds, & Spence, 1998; Kortlander, Kendall, & Panichelli-Mindel, 1997). Within this context, anxious children begin to demonstrate threat biases consistent with those observed with anxious adults (Hadwin, Garner, & Perez-Olivas, 2006; Muris et al., 2009), in that ambiguous situations are generally perceived as being more threatening (Barrett, Rapee, Dadds, & Ryan, 1996; Bögels & Zigterman, 2000; Dineen & Hadwin, 2004). A series of studies (Barrett et al., 1996; Chorpita, Albano, & Barlow, 1996; Dadds & Barrett, 1996) further demonstrated how a discussion with parents led anxious youth to endorse more anxious responding and choose more avoidant solutions to hypothetical threatening scenarios than they had prior to the parental influence. As previously mentioned, children with anxiety disorders often have parents who themselves have anxiety disorder diagnoses and there is a growing research base to show that adults with mental health issues demonstrate qualitatively different parenting styles compared to adults without mental health concerns (Reder, McClure, & Jolley, 2000). For example, Turner, Beidel, Roberson-Nay, and Teno (2003) discovered anxious parents to be more physically withdrawn from their children and to experience more subjective anxiety while their children engaged in nonthreatening play. Others have observed anxious parents to demonstrate less emotional warmth, more catastrophic interpretation, and more open criticism of their children (Hirshfeld, Biederman, Brody, Faraone, & Rosenbaum, 1997; Moore, Whaley, & Sigman, 2004; Whaley, Pinto, & Sigman, 1999), which likely does little to foster a sense of social competence or dispel a fear of negative evaluation in children. One final word of caution regarding the examination of the effect of parenting style upon child and adolescent social anxiety is warranted. The research base is almost completely predominated by studies examining the influence of mothers, with the influence of fathers receiving only scant attention to date.

Peer Influence

Even for nonanxious youth, one's peer standing in childhood can predict social functioning and emotional adjustment in adulthood (Gettinger, 2003; Kupersmidt, Coie, & Dodge, 1990; Kupersmidt & Dodge, 2004; Parker & Asher, 1987). For youth with SP, however, avoidance behavior is a key component of both the development and maintenance of this condition (see Vasey & Dadds, 2001). Beidel and Morris (1995) reported that the majority of children with SP described unstructured peer encounters in the school setting as their most feared of social situations, which Albano (1995) notes overlaps considerably with the social situations they most try to avoid. A pattern of social avoidance early in childhood reduces the likelihood of encountering positive social contingencies, gaining adequate social skills, or developing interpersonal relationships (Boivin, Hymel, & Burkowski, 1995; Hymel, Bowker, & Woody, 1993; Messer & Beidel, 1994), which negatively impacts social functioning over the long term (Rubin, LeMare, & Lollis, 1990; Strauss, Lahey, Frick, Frame, & Hynd, 1988). Children diagnosed with SP are less communicative and more behaviorally withdrawn and otherwise socially passive in their interactions with peers (Alfano, Beidel, & Turner, 2006; Spence, Donovan, & Brechman-Toussaint, 1999). They lack basic social skills (Beidel & Turner, 1998) and their social standing and peer relationships often suffer as a result. Socially anxious children are disliked by peers and are both passively neglected and actively rejected in social spheres (Boivin et al., 1995; Chen, DeSouza, Chen, & Wang, 2006; Deater-Deckard, 2001; Gazelle & Ladd, 2003; Ladd, 2006; Nelson et al., 2005; Newcomb, Bukowski, & Pattee, 1993; Oh et al., 2008; Ollendick, Greene, Weist, & Oswald, 1990; Rubin & Krasnor, 1986; Stewart & Rubin, 1995).

Aversive conditioning experiences have been conceptualized as avenues to the development of social anxiety (Beidel & Turner, 1998; Hofmann & Barlow, 2002). As opposed to random acts of violence, bullying can have unique social consequences that make it a potent impetus for social evaluation concerns. Bullying behavior is common in school settings (Batsche & Knoff, 1994), where it often occurs in the presence of peers and maintains humiliation of the victim as the primary goal (Smith et al., 1999; Smith & Brain, 2000). It should come as no surprise that bullying victims are at increased risk for developing anxiety problems (see Hawker & Boulton, 2000). Victims of bullying have been shown to demonstrate increased anxiety and shyness and are more withdrawn, have lower self-esteem, display poorer social skills, and experience more interpersonal difficulties than other youth (Graham, Bellmore, & Mize, 2006; Haynie et al., 2001; Hazler, 1996). Unfortunately, this relationship may be bidirectional as there is also evidence that introversion, social skills deficits, and lower self-esteem can serve as risk factors for victimization through bullying (Egan & Perry, 1998; Schwartz, Dodge, & Cole, 1993). La Greca and Harrison (2005) studied victimization among adolescents and found that even nonviolent, indirect harassment could result in high social anxiety if accompanied by a poor-quality friendship with a best friend, certainly a possibility for youth with SP who are prone to both neglect and rejection by peers. Conversely, they found the positive aspects of a close friendship to be a protective factor against social anxiety but not depression.

Unfortunately, there is often a correlation between youth who are victims of bullying by peers and their status as victims of physical, sexual, and/or emotional abuse in the home (Baldry, 2003), suggesting that these youth represent victims on a wider social scale (Gladstone, Parker, & Malhi, 2006). Chronic traumatic childhood experiences that come at the hands of influential friends or family can teach children that the social environment is a potentially dangerous place and best avoided. Gladstone and colleagues (2006) examined a sample of adults presenting to a depression clinic and found that significantly more of those who were bullied also met criteria for a diagnosis of lifetime SP as well as agoraphobia. The humiliating aspect of bullying can lead youth to conceptualize their history of abuse as the result of personal shortcomings rather than the result of the unsolicited harassment of others, fueling social anxiety concerns. For example, Singh and Bussey (2009) examined children's self-efficacy for coping with peer aggression and found increased coping self-efficacy to be associated with less social anxiety.

Adolescents begin the process of forging their independence, which involves gradually separating from the social sphere of the immediate family, assuming more autonomy over decision-making, and developing close peer and romantic relationships to increasingly rely upon for support (Choudhury, Blakemore, & Charman, 2006; Eccles et al., 1993; Steinberg & Morris, 2001). By adolescence, teens spend nearly double the time with peers that they do with parents or other adults (Csikszentmihalyi & Larson, 1984) and the presence of close friendships facilitates children's transition to adolescence (Hartup, 1996). This developmental transition is a challenging one and adolescents face more stressors on average then younger children (Colton & Gore, 1991; Compas, Hinden & Gerhardt, 1995). As the opinions and approval of peers become more relevant to the adolescent's development of a sense of self and consolidation of their social standing outside of the family unit, self-consciousness and a fear of negative evaluation become more salient stressors (Fordham & Stevenson-Hinde, 1999; Hymel, Rubin, Rowden, & LeMare, 1990; Parker & Asher, 1987; Steinberg, 2005). This period is replete with the types of social demands and developmental tasks that one would normally expect to provoke a certain degree of social anxiety (Albano & Detweiler, 2001). Some studies have noted an increase in social fears experienced during adolescence (Weems & Costa, 2005; Westenberg, Drewes, Goedhart, Siebelink, & Treffers, 2004), leading others to posit that it is an increase in avoidance observed during adolescence that results in the sudden jump in the onset of social anxiety in adolescents (Rapee & Spence, 2004; Sumter et al., 2009; see also Chartier, Hazen, & Stein, 1998; Muris, 2006; Rao et al., 2007).

THE MAINTENANCE OF CHILDHOOD SOCIAL ANXIETY: A COGNITIVE BEHAVIORAL MODEL

When left untreated, childhood social anxiety can be unremitting and persist as a chronic condition associated with psychological and physical comorbidities, as well as reduced quality of life – including decrements in social functioning, role functioning, educational attainment, and financial independence (Comer et al., in press; Mendlowicz & Stein, 2000). In fact, only 20–40% of SAD cases remit within 20 years of onset, and only 40–60% remit within 40 years (Comer & Olfson, in press). Having reviewed a number of etiological factors associated with the development of social anxiety in youth, we now turn our attention to factors that serve to maintain social anxiety. Specifically, we draw heavily on the cognitive behavioral model of social anxiety offered by Rapee and Heimberg (1997) and highlight key developmental factors to be considered when applying this maintenance model of social anxiety to youth.

What occurs when a socially anxious child confronts a situation that he or she perceives to hold the potential for negative evaluation? Evidence suggests a transactional relationship between cognitive processes and social behaviors, in which negative beliefs about social situations and others' perceptions lead to behavioral avoidance and social withdrawal, which in turn serve to further reinforce negative beliefs and perpetuate avoidance and withdrawal. Chronic avoidance of social situations denies the child important opportunities for corrective experiences that might contradict his or her negative assumptions, opportunities to master his or her anxiety in uncomfortable situations, and opportunities to learn to successfully navigate developmentally appropriate social interactions.

Rapee and Heimberg's (1997) model begins with the notion that individuals with SP attach a fundamental importance to being positively appraised by others and that such individuals assume other people are inherently critical (i.e., likely to evaluate them negatively). The model further proposes that when encountering a social situation – whether real, anticipated, or considered in retrospect – the individual forms a mental representation of his or her appearance and behavior as perceived by those around (i.e., the perceived "audience") that is informed by long-term memory (e.g., prior experiences, recollections of physical appearance), internal cues (e.g., physical symptoms), and external cues (e.g., "audience" feedback). Attentional resources are allocated simultaneously to this internal mental representation and to any perceived threat in the social environment (e.g., someone laughing). The individual also forms a mental representation of the standard against which he or she believes the audience will evaluate his or her performance. According to Rapee and Heimberg (1997), the potential for negative evaluation is assessed by evaluating the discrepancy between the mental representation of one's performance and the mental representation of the standard against which the performance is believed to be evaluated. In a SAI, a high perceived likelihood for negative evaluation, in which there is a discrepancy between the two mental representations, results in physiological (e.g., increased heart rate), cognitive (e.g., thinking "I'm making a fool of myself"), and behavioral (e.g., blushing) consequences, which in turn further color one's mental representations of oneself and the situation, and renewing the cycle.

Given the specific cognitive processes associated with the maintenance of social anxiety, it is not surprising that SAD typically onsets during adolescence. Adolescence is a developmental stage characterized by substantial advancement in perspective-taking, metacognition, self-awareness, and self-reflection (Kuhn, 2009), during which time peer-group approval increases in importance and independent social functioning is expected. Let us consider the example of a socially anxious teenager giving an oral report at the front of his classroom. As a socially anxious teen, he places a tremendous importance on being positively regarded, while at the same time he perceives his classmates to be fundamentally critical. During his oral report, he forms a mental image of how his performance is being perceived, and this image is informed by prior experiences giving oral reports (e.g., he remembers that he lost his place the last time he read out loud), internal cues (e.g., his stomach is turning and his heart is racing, which means he is not in full control of himself), and external cues (e.g., a girl in the first row just yawned). The teen also holds an image of what he believes the standard for an oral report should be (e.g., classmates hanging onto every word he speaks), and the discrepancy between this perceived standard and his image of how he is currently being perceived suggests to him that there is a high perceived likelihood for negative evaluation. This discrepancy causes the teen to have further physiological symptoms (e.g., sweating, blushing) and negative beliefs about his performance. The teen's attempt to simultaneously monitor the environment for evidence of negative evaluation *and* engage in the task of giving the oral report divides the teen's attention and actually disrupts his performance, which in turn elicits *actual* negative feedback from classmates (e.g., his classmates look puzzled or shift in their seats as he slows down, starts to mumble, and begins to sweat). This, in turn, prompts further negative mental images of his performance and increased anxiety symptoms, which further affects his performance, and the cycle is renewed.

EVIDENCE-BASED TREATMENT OF SOCIAL ANXIETY

The cognitive behavioral model of social anxiety suggests several points of intervention in the psychosocial treatment of SAD. These include (1) negative beliefs about oneself, (2) negative beliefs about social situations and other people, (3) negative predictions about the outcomes of situations in which one could be evaluated, (4) patterns of avoidance associated with these negative predictions, (5) attentional focus on social threat cues while in social situations, and (6) negative performance evaluation after engagement in social situations. A comprehensive cognitive behavioral treatment plan incorporates "skill-building" and "exposure tasks," and can be implemented in either group or individual formats (Albano & DiBartolo, 2007; Kendall & Hedtke, 2006; Beidel, Turner, & Young, 2006). We now discuss these two treatment phases in turn.

The "skill-building" phase of cognitive behavioral treatment for youth SP focuses on the acquisition of various skills that reduce anxiety and facilitate social interactions. Early skill-building sessions emphasize the cognitive components of social anxiety by first introducing the concepts of automatic thoughts and rational responses. Self-monitoring is emphasized as children are taught to identify their own anxious thoughts and thinking errors. Some treatments (e.g., Kendall & Hedtke, 2006) also introduce relaxation training during these early sessions. After children get these concepts down, therapists engage children in cognitive restructuring exercises, teaching them how to challenge their dysfunctional beliefs (e.g., a child afraid of tripping in public would be taught to ask herself "Have I ever tripped in front of others before?" "What are the realistic chances that I would trip in front of others today?" "Even if I did actually trip in front of others, would that be *so* bad?"). After cognitive restructuring is successfully addressed, treatment moves to problem-solving strategies targeted to expand the repertoire of coping behaviors available in handling problematic social situations. Typically, avoidance and social withdrawal are the only problem-solving strategies that socially anxious children have found effective in reducing their anxiety. Of course, this strategy only works in the short term, and over the long term chronic avoidance leaves the child under-equipped to master anxious experiences. The final stage of the skill-building treatment phase typically focuses on identifying and strengthening appropriate social and assertiveness skills.

The "exposure" phase of treatment builds on the socially anxious child's newly expanded repertoire of coping skills, giving them opportunities to practice these skills in increasingly fear-inducing contexts. These tasks give children practice experiencing, tolerating, enduring, and mastering distress. During CBT for SAD, the therapist and child develop a fear hierarchy of avoided social situations based on the child's idiosyncratic fears (e.g., calling a friend to get together, reading aloud, being assertive), and this hierarchy serves as an exposures roadmap. A graduated series of exposures is recommended, from lowest to highest fear-inducing situations. The goal is to always push the child further than they would naturally push themselves, while never pushing the child further than they are able to physically tolerate. Typically, exposures begin as in-session tasks, carried out in the context of a warm and therapeutic relationship, and the child is expected to increasingly engage in out-of-session exposure tasks. These out-of-session exposures are critical for generalization of gains.

Importantly, some supported treatments for SAD in youth place heavy emphasis on cognitive components (e.g., Albano & DiBartolo, 2007), whereas other successful programs place less emphasis on cognition (Beidel & Roberson-Nay, 2005). Future work is needed to better understand subpopulations of socially anxious youth for whom cognitive treatments offer improved outcomes and those youth for whom a more focused behavioral strategy may be appropriate.

A public conception may exist that exposure tasks are not appropriate (or are even cruel) within anxiety treatment, as evidenced by an editorial in The New York Times *entitled "The Cruelest Cure" that described exposure tasks within a manualized CBT for adult anxiety (Barlow, 2002) as "surprisingly simple . . . but while many clinicians praise its well-documented results, others take a dimmer view of what one clinician calls 'torture, plain and simple'" (Slater, 2003, p. 34). Such perceptions could be expected to deter practitioners from adopting exposure-based treatment for socially anxious youth, as exposure tasks might be thought to rupture the therapeutic alliance. Importantly, Kendall et al. (2009) used growth-curve modeling to examine the impact of exposure-based tasks on therapeutic alliance in the treatment of childhood anxiety disorders. Their analysis found no indication that therapeutic alliance suffers with the introduction of exposures. In fact, therapeutic alliance continued to grow across treatment after the introduction of exposure-based tasks. Given the paramount importance attributed to therapeutic alliance by a sizable proportion of mental health practitioners (e.g., Boisvert & Faust, 2006), these findings should inform dissemination efforts that promote the use of exposure-based treatments for childhood SAD. Indeed, practitioners who are hesitant to consider in-session exposure-based strategies to treat childhood social anxiety out of concern for the therapeutic relationship may more readily consider exposure tasks in the context of Kendall et al.'s findings. Moreover, public rhetoric characterizing exposure-based treatments as "torture" (e.g., Slater, 2003) appears to be quite misguided, given that alliance does not diminish following the onset of in-session exposure tasks. Regrettably, such rhetoric may deter parents of socially anxious children from enrolling their children in treatments that research evidence support.*

CBT for childhood SP can be implemented in a group or individual format. Many argue that a group treatment format for SAD is preferable (Albano & DiBartolo, 2007; Beidel et al., 2006). Many children with SAD feel isolated and have never discussed their social anxiety with a peer. A group format, in which peers share their anxious thoughts and feelings with one another, facilitates opportunities to normalize the experience of social anxiety. In addition, a group format affords in-session and natural exposures because group members can serve as role-play partners or audience members. Moreover, peer-group members can provide feedback to one another, and this feedback may be more credible than feedback provided by the adult therapist. That said, individual treatment for SAD in children and adolescents has received considerable empirical support, as well (e.g., Kendall, Hudson, Gosch, Flannery-Schroeder, & Suveg, 2008).

The role of family in the treatment of socially anxious youth merits comment and further consideration. Although family treatment modalities (i.e., treatments in which parents are present for most sessions) have shown efficacy in the treatment of children below the age of 12 (Kendall et al., 2008), when working with adolescent SAD, peer-group treatment formats or individual treatment formats with minimal parental involvement (i.e., parents are present for only a handful of sessions) are typical (Albano, Marten, Holt, Heimberg, & Barlow, 1995). However, in considering the role of parental overprotection and overcontrol in the maintenance of anxiety (Chorpita & Barlow, 1998), we offer for consideration a model of intervention focused on increasing independence on the part of the adolescent while addressing the parents' role in the maintenance of the disorder. This is especially important as adolescents will eventually need to transition to greater independent functioning by the end of high school, to meet various developmental tasks associated with emerging adulthood and role transitions (Table 9.1; see also Arnett, 2004).

The functional impairments associated with SAD may also impair an adolescent's ability to meet developmental milestones and effectively transition to more independent functioning. Amongst these anxiety-associated impairments are parents' concerns that certain opportunities will be missed; therefore, greater control and involvement in the adolescent's functioning is reinforced for fear of their failing. Consider the situation where a junior in high school – an adolescent with SAD – has difficulty with assertiveness and situations involving unfamiliar people. A college fair is being held at the school and all juniors are invited to attend to meet and ask questions of various college representatives. This particular student does not want to go and offers that "I won't know what to say." "I'm not even sure I want to go to their schools." "What if they ask me what major I want? I don't know!" While some anxiety is typical

TABLE 9.1 Developmental Tasks of Adolescents Transitioning to Adulthood

- Complete basic educational requirements
- Formulate longer-term career goals
- Enter college/workforce
- Develop independence in managing emotional and interpersonal issues
- Manage own finances
- Manage own healthcare and develop appropriate healthcare-seeking behavior and doctor–patient relations
- Develop and maintain lasting social relationships
- Develop and maintain lasting romantic relationship
- Separate successfully from parents/parental figures

for this situation for any adolescent, SAD makes the anxiety reaction much more intense and increases the pull towards avoidance. Then, instead of having the teen attend while stressed or not attend at all, a parent goes with the teen and asks all the questions, responds for the teen when a question is asked of him or her, and, essentially, the parent does all the work of signing up for catalogues and information. While this may be fine in one or two circumstances, if the parent continues to overprotect and overinvolve him- or herself on behalf of the teenager, the natural process of learning how to manage these situations while anxious (as many other people are naturally anxious in these settings) will not occur. In our practice, we see many families where the parents continue to negotiate the adolescent's world well into the college years – going so far as to contact professors for course material and to make up missed exams. In response to this overinvolvement, we propose an adaptation to traditional CBT approaches for SAD whereby, in addition to the fear and avoidance hierarchy of social situations, a developmental task hierarchy is also produced for the adolescent. This hierarchy involves tasks such as making and keeping one's own routine medical appointments, searching for a summer job on one's own, negotiating with teachers on one's own, managing a bank account, setting up college visits and interviews on one's own, and similar tasks. Teens and their parents receive several conjoint sessions to establish this hierarchy and then learn how to transfer responsibility for these tasks to the adolescent while giving the parents some support for letting consequences fall where they may as the teen learns to manage on his or her own. Figure 9.1 presents a schematic of this model of therapy.

Finally, advancements in the development of efficacious psychosocial treatments for childhood SAD have been paralleled by advances in the evaluation of psychopharmacological interventions for childhood SAD. Specifically, a number of selective serotonin reuptake-inhibitors (SSRIs) have shown efficacy in the treatment of several childhood anxiety disorders, including SAD (Birmaher et al., 2003; RUPP Anxiety Study Group, 2001). The recently completed Child-Adolescent Anxiety Multimodal Study (CAMS; Walkup et al., 2008) evaluated the comparative efficacy of CBT, sertraline, and their combination in the treatment of childhood anxiety disorders, relative to pill placebo, in a randomized sample of 488 youth treated across six treatment sites. Acute outcomes of the CAMS trial found that the combination of CBT and sertraline offered a greater treatment response (~81% of treated youth deemed to be treatment responders by blind evaluators) than either of the two monotherapies alone. Roughly 60% of anxious youth treated with CBT alone and roughly 55% of anxious youth treated with sertraline alone were deemed to be treatment responders by blind evaluators. The findings of this landmark trial document the availability of three effective short-term treatments for childhood anxiety disorders, with combination treatment offering a superior response rate to that offered by CBT or SSRI alone.

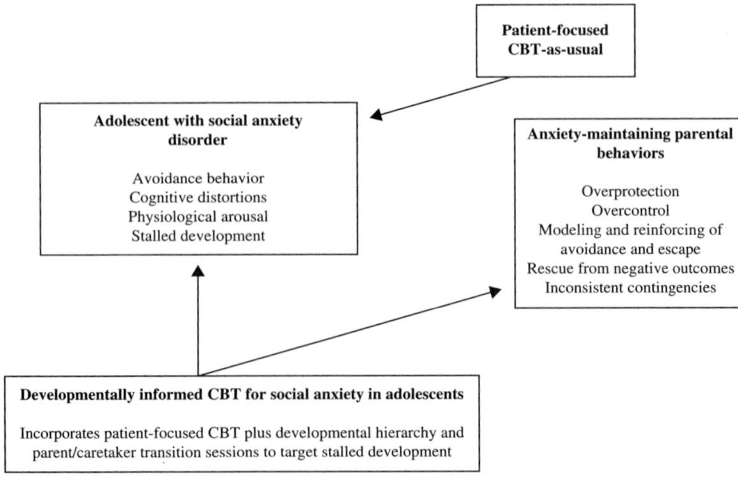

FIGURE 9.1 Adolescent social anxiety treatment model. CBT-cognitive behavioral therapy.

CONCLUSION/FUTURE DIRECTIONS

In summary, childhood social anxiety is highly prevalent and often persists as a chronic condition associated with psychological and physical comorbidities, as well as reduced quality of life, educational attainment, financial independence, and potential stalled development. Research has identified a host of biological, parenting, social, and cognitive factors associated with the development and maintenance of social anxiety in youth. Importantly, the majority of research on the development of SAD has focused exclusively on risk factor main effects (i.e., focusing on only one domain of influence, such as structural abnormalities in the brain, susceptibility genes, or distorted cognitions). Despite theoretical accounts of how these factors may interact, a new generation of research is now needed to empirically evaluate the complex interplay among risk factors and to examine how these individual domains of influence transact with one another to eventuate in childhood SAD.

Over the past decade, rapid advances in noninvasive neuroimaging technology now provide windows into the living brain in ways previously unimagined (Gerber & Peterson, 2008). These developments have greatly advanced our understanding of biological factors associated with the development of childhood SAD, but it is nonetheless important to comment on the current quality of brain images. Despite the improved resolution of images of the live brain provided by current imaging technologies over prior technologies, the pictures offered are still crude when compared to the seemingly infinite complexity and detail of the human brain (see Peterson, 2003). In addition, with current technology individuals, must lay relatively still in a laboratory when undergoing magnetic resonance imaging (MRI), and thus our window into the functioning brain does not yet reveal brain functioning in naturalistic settings while performing complex "real world" tasks. Moreover, research in molecular and population genetics has made it increasingly clear that childhood mental disorders do not exhibit simple, single-gene inheritance patterns. Research in childhood SAD needs to now shift to the search for multiple susceptibility genes that may, under specific circumstances, increase vulnerability for the development of SAD.

Despite the high prevalence and very heavy toll of childhood SAD, systematic problems with the availability, accessibility, and acceptability of effective care prevent affected youth from receiving the services they need. Epidemiological surveys document long delays in treatment-seeking and low rates of treatment among affected youth. Less than 5% of individuals with SAD make contact with a service provider within the first year of disorder onset, and the median delay of treatment initiation after initial onset of SAD is 16 years (Wang et al., 2005). Given the existence of highly effective treatments for childhood SAD (e.g., Albano & DiBartolo, 2007; Kendall & Hedtke, 2006; Beidel et al., 2006), low rates and long delays in service use underscore the need for greater efforts to increase disorder awareness, enhance treatment access, and improve clinical recognition.

Finally, investigations of social anxiety in youth have been largely confined to industrialized regions of the world. Understanding the development and phenomenology of childhood social anxiety in regions beset by economic, educational, wartime, and health-related hardships is critical to understanding cultural variations and the global burden of childhood SAD and to planning mental health service delivery in these areas. Future efforts are needed to advance research methods in developing countries and refugee populations, and to advance effective care and mental health literacy in resource-poor regions of the world.

REFERENCES

Adams, J. F. (1981). Earlier menarche, greater height and weight: A stimulation-stress factor hypothesis. *Genetic Psychological Monographs*, *104*, 3–22.

Adler, R. H. (2009). Engel's biopsychosocial model is still relevant today. *Journal of Psychosomatic Research*, *67*, 607–611.

Adolphs, R. (2001). The neurobiology of social cognition. *Current Opinion in Neurobiology*, *11*, 231–239.

Adolphs, R. (2003). Is the human amygdala specialized for processing social information? *Annals of the New York Academy of Sciences*, *985*, 326–340.

Ainsworth, M. (1989). Attachment in infancy. *American Psychologist*, *44*, 709–716.

Ainsworth, M. D., Blehar, M., Waters, E., & Wall, S. (1978). *Patterns of attachment: A psychological study of the strange situation*. Hillsdale, NJ: Lawrence Erlbaum Associates.

Albano, A. M. (1995). Treatment of social anxiety in adolescents. *Cognitive and Behavioral Practice*, *2*, 271–298.

Albano, A. M., & Detweiler, M. F. (2001). The developmental and clinical impact of social anxiety and social phobia in children and adolescents. In S. G. Hofmann & P. M. DiBartolo (Eds.), *From social anxiety to social phobia: Multiple perspectives* (pp. 162–178). Boston, MA: Allyn & Bacon.

Albano, A. M., & DiBartolo, P. M. (2007). *Cognitive-behavioral therapy for social phobia in adolescents: Stand up, speak out*. New York: Oxford University Press.

Albano, A. M., Marten, P. A., Holt, C. S., Heimberg, R. G., & Barlow, D. H. (1995). Cognitive-behavioral group treatment for social phobia in adolescents: A preliminary study. *Journal of Nervous and Mental Disease*, *183*, 685–692.

Alden, L. E., & Wallace, S. T. (1995). Social phobia and social appraisal in successful and unsuccessful social interactions. *Behaviour Research and Therapy*, *33*, 497–505.

Alfano, C. A., Beidel, D. C., & Turner, S. M. (2006). Cognitive correlates of social phobia among children and adolescents. *Journal of Abnormal Child Psychology*, *34*, 189–201.

American Psychiatric Association. (1980). *Diagnostic and statistical manual of mental disorders* (3rd ed.) (DSM-III). Washington, DC: Author.

American Psychiatric Association. (1987). *Diagnostic and statistical manual of mental disorders* (3rd ed., rev) (DSM-III-R). Washington, DC: Author.

American Psychiatric Association. (1994). *Diagnostic and statistical manual of mental disorders* (4th ed.) (DSM-IV). Washington, DC: Author.

American Psychiatric Association. (2000). *Diagnostic and statistical manual of mental disorders* (4th ed., text rev.) (DSM-IV-TR). Washington, DC: Author.

American Psychiatric Association. (2002). *Developing adolescents: A reference for professionals*. Washington, DC: Author.

Ammerlaan, E. J., Hendriks, M. P., Colon, A. J., & Kessels, R. P. (2008). Emotion perception and interpersonal behavior in epilepsy patients after unilateral amydalohippocampectomy. *Acta Neurobiologiae Experimentalis*, *68*, 214–218.

Amunts, K., Weiss, P. H., Mholberg, H., Pieperhoff, P., Eickhoff, S., Gurd, J. M., et al. (2004). Analysis or neural mechanism underlying verbal fluency in cytoarchitectonically defined stereotaxic space: The roles of Brodmann areas 44 and 45. *Neuroimage*, *22*, 42–56.

Anderson, S. E., Dallal, G. E., & Must, A. (2003). Relative weight and race influence average age at menarche: Results from two nationally representative surveys of US girls studied 25 years apart. *Pediatrics*, *111*, 844–850.

Anderson, S. E., & Must, A. (2005). Interpreting the continued decline in the average age at menarche, results from two nationally representative surveys of US girls studied 10 years apart. *Journal of Pediatrics*, *147*, 753–760.

Angold, A. (2003). Adolescent depression, cortisol and DHEA. *Psychological Medicine*, *33*, 573–581.

Angold, A., Costello, E. J., Erkanli, A., & Worthman, C. M. (1999). Pubertal changes in hormone levels and depression in girls. *Psychological Medicine*, *29*, 1043–1053.

Angold, A., Erkanli, A., Silberg, J., Eaves, L., & Costello, E. J. (2002). Depression scale scores in 8–17-year-olds: Effects of age and gender. *Journal of Child Psychology and Psychiatry*, *43*, 1052–1063.

Angold, A., Worthman, C. M., & Costello, E. J. (2003). *Puberty and depression*. New York: Cambridge University Press.

Arnett, J. J. (2004). *Emerging adulthood: The winding road from late teens through the twenties*. New York: Guilford Press.

Aron, A. R., Robbins, T. W., & Poldrack, R. A. (2004). Inhibition and the right inferior cortex. *Trends in Cognitive Science*, *8*, 170–177.

Bailey, H. N., Moran, G., Pederson, D. R., & Bento, S. (2007). Understanding the transmission of attachment using variable- and relationship-centered approaches. *Development and Psychopathology*, *19*, 313–343.

Baldry, A. C. (2003). Bullying in schools and exposure to domestic violence. *Child Abuse and Neglect*, *27*, 713–732.

Bandura, A. (1977). *Social learning theory*. New York: General Learning Press.

Barlow, D. H. (2002). *Anxiety and its disorders: The nature and treatment of anxiety and panic* (2nd ed.). New York: Guilford Press.

Barnea-Goraly, N., Menon, V., Eckert, M., Tamm, L., Bammer, R., Karchemskiy, A., et al. (2005). White matter development during childhood and adolescence: A cross-sectional diffusion tensor imaging study. *Cerebral Cortex*, *15*, 1848–1854.

Barrett, P. M., Rapee, R. M., Dadds, M. M., & Ryan, S. M. (1996). Family enhancement of cognitive style in anxious and aggressive children. *Journal of Abnormal Child Psychology*, *24*, 187–203.

Barron, A. P., & Earls, F. (1984). The relation of temperament and social factors to behavior problems in three-year-old children. *Journal of Child Psychology and Psychiatry*, *25*, 23–33.

Bates, J. E, Pettit, G. S., Dodge, K. A., & Ridge, B. (1998). Interaction of temperamental resistance to control and restrictive parenting in the development of externalizing behavior. *Developmental Psychology*, *34*, 982–995.

Batsche, G., & Knoff, H. (1994). Bullies and their victims: Understanding a pervasive problem in the schools. *School Psychology Review*, *23*, 165–174.

Baxter, M. G., Parker, A., Lindner, C. C., Izquierdo, A. D., & Murray, E. A. (2000). Control of response selection by reinforcer value requires interaction of amygdala and orbital pre-frontal context. *Journal of Neuroscience*, *20*, 4311–4319.

Beck, A. T., Emery, G., & Greenberg, R. L. (1985). *Anxiety disorders and phobias: A cognitive perspective*. New York: Basic Books.

Beesdo, K., Bittner, A., Pine, D. S., Stein, M. B., Höfler, M., Lieb, R., et al. (2007). Incidence of social anxiety disorder and the consistent risk for secondary depression in the first three decades of life. *Archives of General Psychiatry*, *64*, 903–912.

Beesdo, K., Knappe, S., & Pine, D. S. (2009). Anxiety and anxiety disorders in children and adolescents: Developmental issues and implications for DSM-V. *Psychiatric Clinics of North America*, *32*, 483–524.

Beidel, D. C. (1991). Social phobia and overanxious disorder in school-age children. *Journal of the American Academy of Child and Adolescent Psychiatry*, *30*, 545–552.

Beidel, D. C., & Morris, T. L. (1995). Social phobia. In J. S. March (Ed.), *Anxiety disorders in children and adolescents* (pp. 181–211). New York: Guilford Press.

Beidel, D. C., & Roberson-Nay, R. (2005). Treating childhood social phobia: Social effectiveness therapy for children. In E. D. Hibbs & P. S. Jensen (Eds.), *Psychosocial treatments for child and adolescent disorders* (2nd ed.) (pp. 75–96). Washington, DC: American Psychological Association.

Beidel, D. C., & Turner, S. M. (1998). *Shy children, phobic adults*. Washington, DC: American Psychological Association.

Beidel, D. C., Turner, S. M., & Young, B. J. (2006). Social effectiveness therapy for children: Five years later. *Behavior Therapy*, *37*, 416–425.

Bellis, M. A., Downing, J., & Ashton, J. A. (2006). Adults at 12? Trends in puberty and their public health consequences. *Journal of Epidemiological Community Health*, *60*, 910–911.

Bergen, S. E., Gardner, C. O., & Kendler, K. S. (2007). Age-related changes in heritability of behavioral phenotypes over adolescence and young adulthood: A meta-analysis. *Twin Research and Human Genetics*, *10*, 423–433.

Berk, L., & Shanker, S. (2006). *Child development*. Toronto, ON: Allyn & Bacon.

Bernstein, G. A., & Borchardt, C. M. (1991). Anxiety disorders of childhood and adolescence: A critical review. *Journal of the American Academy of Child and Adolescent Psychiatry*, *30*, 519–532.

Betts, J., Gullone, E., & Allen, J. S. (2009). An examination of emotion regulation, temperament, and parenting style as potential predictors of adolescent depression risk status: A correlational study. *British Journal of Developmental Psychology*, *27*, 473–485.

Biederman, J., Hirshfeld-Becker, D. R., Rosenbaum, J. F., Herot, C., Friedman, D., Snidman, N., et al. (2001). Further evidence of association between behavioural inhibition and social anxiety in children. *American Journal of Psychiatry*, *158*, 1673–1679.

Biederman, J., Rosenbaum, J. F., Bolduc, E. A., Faraone, S. V., & Hirshfeld, D. R. (1991). A high risk study of young children of parents with panic disorder and agoraphobia with and without comorbid major depression. *Psychiatry Research*, *37*, 333–348.

Birbaumer, N., Grodd, W., Diedrich, O., Klose, U., Erb, M., Lotze, M., et al. (1998). fMRI reveals amygdala activation to human faces in social phobics. *Neuroreport*, *9*, 1223–1226.

Bird, A. (2007). Perceptions of epigenetics. *Nature*, *447*, 396–398.

Birmaher, B., Axelson, D. A., Monk, K., Kalas, C., Clark, D. B., & Ehmann, M. (2003). Fluoxetine for the treatment of childhood anxiety disorders. *Journal of the American Academy of Child and Adolescent Psychiatry*, *42*, 415–423.

Blair, R. J. (2004). The roles of orbital frontal cortex in the modulation of antisocial behavior. *Brain and Cognition*, *55*, 198–208.

Blair, R. J., & Cipolotti, L. (2000). Impaired social response reversal. A case of "acquired sociopathy". *Brain*, *123*, 1122–1141.

Blair, R. J. R., Morris, J. S., Frith, C. D., Perrett, D. I., & Dolan, R. J. (1999). Dissociable neural responses to facial expressions of sadness and anger. *Brain*, *122*, 883–893.

Blakenmore, S. J., & Choudhury, S. (2006). Development of the adolescent brain: Implications for executive function and social cognition. *Journal of Child Psychology and Psychiatry*, *47*, 296–312.

Blumenthal, H., Leen-Feldner, E. W., Trainor, C. D., Babson, K. A., & Bunaciu, L. (2009). Interactive roles of pubertal timing and peer relations in predicting social anxiety symptoms among youth. *Journal of Adolescent Health*, *44*, 401–403.

Bodzsar, E. B., & Susanne, C. (Eds.) (1998). *Secular growth changes in Europe*. Budapest: Eotvos University Press.

Bögels, S. M., & Zigterman, D. (2000). Dysfunctional cognitions in children with social phobia, separation anxiety disorder, and generalized anxiety disorder. *Journal of Abnormal Child Psychology*, *28*, 205–211.

Boisvert, C. M., & Faust, D. (2006). Practicing psychologists' knowledge of general psychotherapy research findings: Implications for science-practice relations. *Professional Psychology: Research and Practice*, *37*, 708–716.

Boivin, M., Hymel, S., & Burkowski, W. M. (1995). The roles of social withdrawal, peer rejection, and victimization by peers in predicting loneliness and depressed mood in childhood. *Developmental Psychopathology*, *7*, 765–785.

Bowlby, J. (1973). *Attachment and loss: Vol 2. Separation, anxiety and danger*. New York: Basic Books.

Bowlby, J. (1978). Attachment theory and its therapeutic implications. *Adolescent Psychiatry*, *6*, 5–33.

Bretherton, I., & Munholland, K. A. (1999). Internal working models in attachment relationships: A construct revisited. In J. Cassidy & P. R. Shaver (Eds.), *Handbook of attachment: Theory, research and clinical applications* (pp. 89–114). New York: Guilford Press.

Bronson, G. (1974). The postnatal growth of visual capacity. *Child Development*, *45*, 873–890.

Brothers, L. (1990). The social brain: A project for integrating primate behavior and neurophysiology in a new domain. *Concepts in Neuroscience*, *1*, 27–51.

Brown, T. A., Chorpita, B. F., & Barlow, D. H. (1998). Structural relationships among dimensions of the DSM-IV anxiety and mood disorders and dimensions of negative affect, positive affect and autonomic arousal. *Journal of Abnormal Psychology*, *107*, 179–192.

Brumariu, L. E., & Kerns, K. A. (2008). Mother–child attachment and social anxiety symptoms in middle childhood. *Journal of Applied Developmental Psychology*, *29*, 393–402.

Buchsbaum, B. R., Greer, S., Chang, W. L., & Berman, K. F. (2005). Metal-analysis of neuroimaging studies of the Wisconsin Card-Sorting task and component processes. *Human Brain Mapping*, *25*, 35–45.

Buck Louis, G. M., Gray, L. E., Jr., Marcus, M., Ojeda, S. R., Pescovitz, O. H., Witchel, S. F., et al. (2008). Environmental factors and puberty timing: Expert panel research needs. *Pediatrics*, *121*(Suppl 3), 192–207.

Bukowski, W., Rubin, K. H., & Parker, J. (2001). Social competence. In N. J. Smelser & P. B. Baltes (Eds.), *International encyclopedia of social and behavioral sciences* (pp. 14258–14264). Oxford, UK: Elsevier.

Buss, A. H., & Plomin, R. (1984). *Temperament – Early developing personality traits*. Hillsdale, NJ: Erlbaum.

Caron, R. F., Caron, A. J., & Myers, R. S. (1985). Do infants see emotional expressions in static faces? *Child Development*, *56*, 1552–1560.

Casey, B. J., Galvan, A., & Hare, T. A. (2005). Changes in cerebral functional organization during cognitive development. *Current Opinion in Neurobiology*, *15*, 239–244.

Casey, B. J., Giedd, J. N., & Thomas, K. M. (2000). Structural and functional brain development and its relation to cognitive development. *Biological Psychology*, *54*, 241–257.

Casey, B. J., Getz, S., & Galvan, A. (2009). The adolescent brain. *Developmental Review*, *28*, 62–77.

Caspi, A., Moffitt, T. E., Newman, D. L., & Silva, P. A. (1996). Behavioral observations at age 3 years predict adult psychiatric disorders. *Archives of General Psychiatry*, *53*, 1033–1039.

Cassidy, J., & Berlin, L. J. (1994). The insecure/ambivalent pattern of attachment: Theory and research. *Child Development*, *65*, 971–991.

Cavell, T. A. (1990). Social adjustment, social performance, and social skills: A tri-component model of social competence. *Journal of Clinical Child Psychology*, *19*, 111–122.

Chartier, M. J., Hazen, A. L., & Stein, M. B. (1998). Lifetime patterns of social phobia: A retrospective study of the course of social phobia in a nonclinical population. *Depression and Anxiety*, *7*, 113–121.

Chen, X., DeSouza, A., Chen, H., & Wang, L. (2006). Reticent behavior and experiences in peer interactions in Canadian and Chinese children. *Developmental Psychology*, *42*, 656–665.

Chorpita, B. F., Albano, A. M., & Barlow, D. H. (1996). Cognitive processing in children: Relationship to anxiety and family influences. *Journal of Clinical Child Psychology*, *25*, 170–176.

Chorpita, B. F., & Barlow, D. H. (1998). The development of anxiety: The role of control in the early environment. *Psychological Bulletin*, *124*, 3–21.

Chorpita, B. F., & Daleiden, E. L. (2002). Tripartite dimensions of emotion in a child clinical sample: Measurement strategies and implications for clinical utility. *Journal of Consulting and Clinical Psychology*, *70*, 1150–1160.

Choudhury, S., Blakemore, S. J., & Charman, T. (2006). Social cognitive development during adolescence. *Social Cognitive and Affective Neuroscience*, *1*, 165–174.

Chronis-Tuscano, A., Degnan, K. A., Pine, D. S., Perez-Edgar, K., Henderson, H. A., & Diaz, Y. (2009). Stable early maternal report of behavioral inhibition predicts lifetime social anxiety disorder in adolescence. *Journal of the American Academy of Child and Adolescent Psychiatry*, *48*, 928–935.

Chrousos, G. P., Torpy, D. J., & Gold, P. W. (1998). Interactions between the hypothalamic-pituitary-adrenal axis and the female reproductive system: Clinical implications. *Annals of Internal Medicine*, *129*, 229–240.

Cicchetti, D., & Cohen, D. J. (1995). Perspectives on developmental psychopathology. In D. Cicchetti & D. J. Cohen (Eds.), *Developmental psychopathology: Vol 1 – Theory and methods* (pp. 57–80). New York: Wiley.

Cicchetti, D., & Toth, S. L. (2009). The past achievements and future promises of developmental psychopathology: The coming of age of a discipline. *Journal of Child Psychology and Psychiatry, and Allied Disciplines*, *50*, 16–25.

Clark, S. E., & Symons, D. K. (2009). Representations of attachment relationships, the self, and significant others in middle childhood. *Journal of the Canadian Academy of Child and Adolescent Psychiatry*, *18*, 316–321.

Clark, L. A., & Watson, D. (1999). Personality, disorder, and personality disorder: Towards a more rational conceptualization. *Journal of Personality Disorders*, *13*, 142–151.

Clark, D. M., & Wells, A. (1995). A cognitive model of social phobia. In R. G. Heimberg, M. R. Liebowitz, D. A. Hope, & F. R. Schneier (Eds.), *Social phobia: Diagnosis, assessment and treatment* (pp. 69–93). New York: Guilford Press.

Cobham, V. E., Dadds, M. R., & Spence, S. H. (1998). The role of parental anxiety in the treatment of childhood anxiety. *Journal of Consulting and Clinical Psychology*, *66*, 893–905.

Cohn, D. (1990). Child–mother attachment of six-year-olds and social competence at school. *Child Development*, *61*, 152–162.

Colton, M. E., & Gore, S. (1991). *Adolescent stress: Causes and consequences.* New York: Aldine De Gruyter.

Comer, J. S., Blanco, C., Grant, B., Hasin, D., Liu, S. M., Turner, J. B. et al. (in press). Health-related quality of life across the anxiety disorders. *Journal of Clinical Psychiatry.*

Comer, J. S., & Olfson, M. (in press). The epidemiology of anxiety disorders. In H. B. Simpson, F. Schneier, Y. Neria, & R. Lewis-Fernandez (Eds.), *Anxiety disorders: theory, research, and clinical perspectives.* NY: Cambridge University Press.

Compas, B. E., Hinden, B. R., & Gerhardt, C. A. (1995). Adolescent development: Pathways and processes of risk and resilience. *Annual Review of Psychology*, *46*, 265–293.

Conklin, H. K., Luciana, M., Hooper, C. J., & Yarger, R. S. (2007). Working memory performance in typically developing children and adolescents: Behavioral evidence of protracted frontal lobe development. *Developmental Neuropsychology*, *31*, 103–128.

Cooper, P. J., Fearn, V., Willetts, L., Seabrook, H., & Parkinson, M. (2006). Affective disorder in the parents of a clinic sample of children with anxiety disorders. *Journal of Affective Disorders*, *93*, 205–212.

Corden, B., Critchley, H. D., Skuse, D., & Dolan, R. J. (2006). Fear recognition ability predicts differences in social cognitive and neural functioning in men. *Journal of Cognitive Neuroscience*, *18*, 889–897.

Costello, E. J., Angold, A., Burns, B. J., Stangl, D. K., Tweed, D. L., Erkanli, A., et al. (1996). The great smoky mountains study of youth. Goals, design, methods, and the prevalence of DSM-III-R disorders. *Archives of General Psychiatry*, *53*, 1129–1136.

Costello, J., Egger, H. L., & Angold, A. (2004). Developmental epidemiology of anxiety disorders. In T. H. Ollendick & J. S. March (Eds.), *Phobic and anxiety disorders in children and adolescents* (pp. 61–91). New York: Oxford University Press.

Costello, E. J., Pine, D. S., Hammen, C., March, J. S., Plotsky, P. M., & Weissman, M. M. (2002). Development and natural history of mood disorders. *Biological Psychiatry*, *52*, 529–542.

Costello, E. J., Sung, M., Worthman, C., & Angold, A. (2007). Pubertal maturation and the development of alcohol use and abuse. *Drug and Alcohol Dependence*, *88*(Suppl), 50–59.

Cotrufo, P., Cella, S., Cremato, F., & Labella, A. G. (2007). Eating disorder attitude and abnormal eating behaviours in a sample of 11–13-year-old school children: The role of pubertal body transformation. *Eating and Weight Disorders*, *12*, 154–160.

Cox, B. J., Pagura, J., Stein, M. B., & Sareen, J. (2009). The relationship between generalized social phobia and avoidant personality disorder in a national mental health survey. *Depression and Anxiety*, *26*, 354–362.

Craske, M. G. (2003). *Origins of phobias and anxiety disorders: Why more women than men?* Amsterdam, The Netherlands: Elsevier.

Cristinzio, C., N'Diaye, K., Seeck, M., Vuilleumier, P., & Sander, D. (2010). Integration of gaze direction and facial expression in patients with unilateral amygdala damage. *Brain*, *133*(Pt 1), 248–261.

Csikszentmihalyi, M., & Larson, R. (1984). *Being adolescent*. New York: Basic Books.

Curtis, C. E., & D'Esposito, M. (2003). Persistent activity in the prefrontal cortex during working memory. *Trends in Cognitive Science*, *7*, 415–423.

Cutrona, C. E., & Troutman, B. R. (1986). Social support, infant temperament, and parenting self-efficacy: A mediational model of postpartum depression. *Child Development*, *57*, 1507–1518.

Dadds, M. R., & Barrett, P. M. (1996). Family processes in child and adolescent anxiety and depression. *Behavior Change*, *13*, 231–239.

Dahl, R. E., & Spear, L. P. (2004). Adolescent brain development. *Annals of the New York Academy of Sciences*, *1021*, 1–22.

Deardorff, J., Hayward, C., Wilson, K. A., Bryson, S., Hammer, L. D., & Agras, S. (2007). Puberty and gender interact to predict social anxiety symptoms in early adolescence. *Journal of Adolescent Health*, *41*, 102–104.

Deater-Deckard, K. (2001). Annotation: Recent research examining the role of peer relationships in the development of psychopathology. *Journal of Child Psychology and Psychiatry*, *425*, 565–579.

DeMulder, E., Denham, S., Schmidt, M., & Mitchell, J. (2000). Q-sort assessment of attachment security during the preschool years: Links from home to school. *Developmental Psychology*, *36*, 274–282.

de Rosnay, M., Cooper, P. J., Tsigaras, N., & Murray, L. (2006). Transmission of social anxiety from mother to infant: An experimental study using a social referencing paradigm. *Behaviour Research and Therapy*, *44*, 1165–1175.

Dick, D. M., Rose, R. J., Pulkkinen, L., & Kaprio, J. (2001). Measuring puberty and understanding its impact: A longitudinal study of adolescent twins. *Journal of Youth and Adolescence*, *30*, 385–399.

Dineen, K. A., & Hadwin, J. A. (2004). Anxious and depressive symptoms and children's judgements of their own and others' interpretation of ambiguous social scenarios. *Journal of Anxiety Disorders*, *18*, 499–513.

Dix, T., Ruble, D. N., Grusec, J. E., & Nixon, S. (1986). Social cognition in parents: Inferential and affective reactions to children of three age levels. *Child Development*, *57*, 879–894.

Downing, J., & Bellis, M. A. (2009). Early pubertal onset and its relationship with sexual risk taking, substance use and anti-social behaviour: A preliminary cross-sectional study. *BMC Public Health*, *9*, 446. Retrieved February 19, 2010, from www.biomedcentral.com/content/pdf/1471-2458-9-446.pdf

Drevets, W. C. (2003). Neuroimaging abnormalities in the amygdala in mood disorders. *Annals of the New York Academy of Sciences*, *985*, 420–444.

Duncan, J. (2001). An adaptive coding model of neural function in prefrontal cortex. *Nature Reviews Neuroscience*, *2*, 820–829.

Durston, S., Hilleke, E., Hulshoff, P., Casey, B. J., Giedd, J. N., Buttlelaar, J. K., et al. (2001). Anatomical MRI of the developing human brain: What have we learned? *Journal of the American Academy of Child and Adolescent Psychiatry*, *40*, 1012–1020.

Eaves, L. J., Long, J., & Heath, A. C. (1986). A theory of developmental change in quantitative phenotypes applied to cognitive development. *Behavior Genetics*, *16*, 143–162.

Eccles, J. S., Midgley, C., Wigfield, A., Buchanan, C. M., Reuman, D., Flanagan, C., et al. (1993). Development during adolescence. The impact of stage-environment fit on young adolescents' experiences in schools and in families. *American Psychologist*, *48*, 90–101.

Egan, S. K., & Perry, D. G. (1998). Does low self-regard invite victimization? *Developmental Psychology*, *34*, 299–309.

Eisenberg, N., Cumberland, A., Spinrad, T. L., Fabes, R. A., Shepard, S. A., & Reiser, M. (2001). The relations of regulation and emotionality to children's externalizing and internalizing problem behavior. *Child Development*, *72*, 1112–1134.

Eisenberg, N., Sadovsky, A., Spinrad, T. L., Fabes, R. A., Losoya, S. H., & Valiente, C. (2005). The relations of problem behavior status to children's negative emotionality, effortful control, and impulsivity: Concurrent relations and prediction of change. *Developmental Psychology*, *41*, 193–211.

Elkind, D., & Bowen, R. (1979). Imaginary audience behavior in children and adolescents. *Developmental Psychology*, *15*, 38–44.

Eley, T. C., Bolton, D., O'Connor, T. G., Perrin, S., Smith, P., & Plomin, R. (2003). A twin study of anxiety-related behaviours in pre-school children. *Journal of Child Psychology, Psychiatry, and Allied Disciplines*, *44*, 945–960.

Eley, T. C., Rijsdijk, F. V., Perrin, S., O'Connor, T. G., & Bolton, D. (2008). A multivariate genetic analysis of specific phobia, separation anxiety and social phobia in early childhood. *Journal of Abnormal Child Psychology*, *36*, 839–848.

Engel, G. L. (1977). The need for a new medical model. *Science*, *196*, 129–136.

Ernst, M., Nelson, E. E., Jazbec, S., McClure, E. B., Monk, C. S., & Leibenluft, E. (2005). Amygdala and nucleus accumbens in responses to receipt and omission of gains in adults and adolescents. *Neuroimage*, *25*, 1279–1291.

Essau, C. A., Conradt, J., & Petermann, F. (1999). Frequency and comorbidity of social phobia and social fears in adolescents. *Behaviour Research and Therapy*, *37*, 831–843.

Essex, M. J., Klein, M. H., Slattery, M. J., Goldsmith, H. H., & Kalin, N. H. (2010). Early risk factors and developmental pathways to chronic high inhibition and social anxiety disorder in adolescence. *American Journal of Psychiatry*, *167*, 40–46.

Etkin, A., & Wager, T. D. (2007). Functional neuroimaging of anxiety: A meta-analysis of emotional processing in PTSD, social anxiety disorder, and specific phobia. *American Journal of Psychiatry*, *164*, 1476–1488.

Feingold, A. (1992). Good-looking people are not what we think. *Psychological Bulletin*, *111*, 304–341.

Felson, R. B., & Haynie, D. L. (2002). Pubertal development, social factors, and delinquency among adolescent boys. *Criminology*, *40*, 967–988.

Fichter, M. M., Kohlboeck, G., Quadflieg, N., Wyschkon, A., & Esser, G. (2009). From childhood to adult age: 18-year longitudinal results and prediction of the course of mental disorders in the community. *Social Psychiatry and Psychiatric Epidemiology*, *44*, 792–803.

Flemming, A. S., & Corter, M. (1995). Psychobiology of maternal behavior in nonhuman mammals. In M. Bornstein (Ed.), *Handbook of parenting* (pp. 59–86). Hillside, NJ: Erlbaum.

Forbes, E. E., & Dahl, R. E. (2010). Pubertal development and behavior: Hormonal activation of social and motivational tendencies. *Brain and Cognition*, *72*, 66–72.

Fordham, K., & Stevenson-Hinde, J. (1999). Shyness, friendship quality, and adjustment during middle childhood. *Journal of Child Psychology, Psychiatry, and Allied Disciplines*, *40*, 757–768.

Francis, G., Last, C. G., & Strauss, C. C. (1992). Avoidant disorder and social phobia in children and adolescents. *Journal of the American Academy of Child and Adolescent Psychiatry*, *31*, 1086–1089.

Fyer, A. J., Mannuzza, S., Chapman, T. F., Liebowitz, M. R., & Klein, D. F. (1993). A direct-interview family study of social phobia. *Archives of General Psychiatry*, *50*, 286–293.

Fyer, A. J., Mannuzza, S., Chapman, T. F., Martin, L. Y., & Klein, D. F. (1995). Specificity in familial aggregation of phobic disorders. *Archives of General Psychiatry*, *52*, 564–573.

Gallagher, H. L., & Frith, C. D. (2003). Functional imaging of "theory of mind". *Trends in Cognitive Science*, *7*, 77–83.

Galvan, A., Hare, T. A., Parra, C. E., Penn, J., Voss, H., Glover, G., et al. (2006). Earlier development of the accumbens relative to orbitofrontal cortex might underlie risk-taking behavior in adolescents. *Journal of Neuroscience*, *26*, 6885–6892.

Gazelle, H., & Ladd, G. W. (2003). Anxious solitude and peer exclusion: A diathesis-stress model of internalizing trajectories in childhood. *Child Development*, *74*, 257–278.

Ge, X., Brody, G. H., Conger, R. D., & Simons, R. L. (2006). Pubertal maturation and African American children's internalizing and externalizing symptoms. *Journal of Youth and Adolescence*, *35*, 531–540.

Ge, X., Conger, R. D., & Elder, G. H. (1996). Coming of age too early: Pubertal influences on girls' vulnerability to psychological distress. *Child Development*, *67*, 3386–3400.

Gerber, A. J., & Peterson, B. S. (2008). What is an image? *Journal of the American Academy of Child and Adolescent Psychiatry*, *47*, 245–248.

Gerull, F. C., & Rapee, R. M. (2002). Mother knows best: Effects of maternal modelling on the acquisition of fear and avoidance behavior in toddlers. *Behaviour Research and Therapy*, *40*, 279–287.

Gettinger, M. (2003). Promoting social competence in an era of school reform: A commentary on Gifford-Smith and Brownell. *Journal of School Psychology*, *41*, 299–304.

Giedd, J. N. (2004). Structural magnetic resonance imaging of the adolescent brain. *Annals of the New York Academy of Sciences*, *1021*, 77–85.

Giedd, J. N., Blumenthal, J., Jeffries, N. O., Castellanos, F. X., Liu, H., Zijdenbos, A., et al. (1999). Brain development during childhood and adolescence: A longitudinal MRI study. *Nature Neuroscience*, *2*, 861–863.

Giedd, J. N., Castellanos, F. X., Rajapakse, J. C., Vaituzis, A. C., & Rapoport, J. L. (1997). Sexual dimorphism of the developing human brain. *Progress in Neuropsychopharmacology and Biological Psychiatry*, *21*, 1185–1201.

Giedd, J. N., Snell, J. W., Lange, N., Rajapakse, J. C., Casey, B. J., Kozuch, P. L., et al. (1996). Quantitative magnetic resonance imaging of human brain development: Ages 4–18. *Cerebral Cortex*, *6*, 551–560.

Gladstone, G. L., Parker, G. B., & Malhi, G. S. (2006). Do bullied children become anxious and depressed adults? A cross-sectional investigation of the correlates of bullying and anxious depression. *Journal of Nervous and Mental Disease*, *194*, 201–208.

Gluckman, P. D., & Hanson, M. A. (2006). Changing times: The evolution of puberty. *Molecular Cell Endocrinology*, *254–255*, 26–31.

Goffman, E. (1959). *The presentation of self in everyday life*. New York: Doubleday.

Goldsmith, H. H., & Campos, J. J. (1982). Toward a theory of infant temperament. In R. N. Emde & R. J. Harmon (Eds.), *The development of attachment and affiliative systems* (pp. 161–193). New York: Plenum.

Gould, R. A., Buckminster, S., Pollack, M. H., Otto, M. W., & Yap, L. (1997). Cognitive behavioral and pharmacological treatment for social phobia: A meta-analysis. *Clinical Psychology: Science and Practice*, *4*, 291–306.

Graham, S., Bellmore, A. D., & Mize, J. (2006). Peer victimization, aggression, and their co-occurrence in middle school: Pathways to adjustment problems. *Journal of Abnormal Child Psychology*, *34*, 349–364.

Graziano, A. M., DeGiovanni, I. S., & Garcia, K. A. (1979). Behavioral treatment of children's fears: A review. *Psychological Bulletin*, *86*, 804–830.

Greenberg, P. E., Sisitsky, T., Kessler, R. C., Finkelstein, S. N., Berndt, E. R., Davidson, J. R., et al. (1999). The economic burden of anxiety disorders in the 1990s. *Journal of Clinical Psychiatry*, *60*, 427–435.

Gregory, A. M., & Eley, T. C. (2007). Genetic influences on anxiety in children: What we've learned and where we're heading. *Clinical Child and Family Psychology Review*, *10*, 199–212.

Gross, C., & Hen, R. (2004). The developmental origins of anxiety. *National Review of Neuroscience*, *5*, 545–552.

Gunnar, M. R., Wewerka, S., Frenn, K., Long, J. D., & Griggs, C. (2009). Developmental changes in hypothalamus-pituitary-adrenal activity over the transition to adolescence: Normative changes and associations with puberty. *Developmental Psychopathology*, *21*, 69–85.

Hadwin, J. A., Garner, M., & Perez-Olivas, G. (2006). The development of information processing biases in childhood anxiety: A review and exploration of its origins in parenting. *Clinical Psychology Review*, *26*, 876–894.

Hare, T. A., Tottenham, N., Galvan, A., Voss, H. U., Glover, G. H., & Casey, B. J. (2008). Biological substrates of emotional reactivity and regulation in adolescence during an emotional go-nogo task. *Biological Psychiatry*, *63*, 927–934.

Hariri, A. R., Mattay, V. S., Tessitore, A., Fera, F., & Weinberger, D. R. (2003). Neurocortical modulation of the amygdale response to fearful stimuli. *Biological Psychiatry*, *53*, 494–501.

Hart, E. A., Leary, M. R., & Rejeski, W. J. (1989). The measurement of social physique anxiety. *Journal of Sport and Exercise Psychology*, *11*, 94–104.

Harter, S. (1999). *The construction of the self: A developmental perspective*. New York: Guilford Press.

Hartup, W. W. (1996). "The company they keep." Friendships and their development significance. *Child Development*, *67*, 1–13.

Hasselmo, M. E., Rolls, E. T., & Baylis, G. C. (1989). The role of expression and identity in the face-selective responses of neurons in the temporal visual cortex of the monkey. *Behavioural Brain Research*, *32*, 203–218.

Hawker, D. S. J., & Boulton, M. J. (2000). Twenty years' research on peer victimization and psychosocial maladjustment: A meta-analytic review of cross-sectional studies. *Journal of Child Psychology and Psychiatry*, *41*, 441–455.

Haxby, J. V., Hoffman, E. A., & Gobbini, M. I. (2002). Human neural systems for face recognition and social communication. *Biological Psychiatry*, *51*, 59–67.

Haynie, D. L., Nansel, T., Eitel, P., Crump, A. D., Saylor, K., Yu, K., et al. (2001). Bullies, victims, and bully/victims: Distinct groups of youth at risk. *Journal of Early Adolescence*, *21*, 29–49.

Hayward, C. (2003). *Gender differences at puberty*. Cambridge, UK: Cambridge University Press.

Hayward, C., Killen, J. D., Kraemer, H. C., & Taylor, C. B. (1998). Linking self-reported childhood behavioral inhibition to adolescent social phobia. *Journal of the American Academy of Child and Adolescent Psychiatry*, *37*, 1308–1316.

Hayward, C., Killen, J. D., Wilson, D. M., Hammer, L. D., Litt, I. F., Kraemer, H. C., et al. (1997). Psychiatric risk associated with early puberty in adolescent girls. *Journal of the American Academy of Child and Adolescent Psychiatry*, *36*, 255–262.

Hazler, R. J. (1996). *Breaking the cycle of violence: Interventions for bullying and victimization*. Athens, OH: Ohio University Press.

Heimberg, R. G., Stein, M. B., Hiripi, E., & Kessler, R. C. (2000). Trends in the prevalence of social phobia in the United States: A synthetic cohort analysis of changes over four decades. *European Psychiatry*, *2000*(15), 29–37.

Herman-Giddens, M. E. (2006). Recent data on pubertal milestones in United States children: The secular trend toward earlier development. *International Journal of Andrology*, *29*, 241–246.

Hirshfeld, D. R., Biederman, J., Brody, L., Faraone, S. V., & Rosenbaum, J. F. (1997). Expressed emotion toward children with behavioural inhibition: Associations with maternal anxiety disorder. *Journal of the American Academy of Child and Adolescent Psychiatry*, *36*, 910–917.

Hirshfeld, D. R., Rosenbaum, J. F., Biederman, J., Bolduc, E. A., Faraone, S. V., Snidman, N., et al. (1992). Stable behavioral inhibition and its association with anxiety disorders. *Journal of the American Academy of Child and Adolescent Psychiatry*, *31*, 103–111.

Hirshfeld-Becker, D. R., Biederman, J., Henin, A., Faraone, S. V., Davis, S., Harrington, K., et al. (2007). Behavioral inhibition in preschool children at risk is a specific predictor of middle childhood social anxiety: A five-year follow-up. *Journal of Developmental and Behavioral Pediatrics*, *28*, 225–233.

Hofmann, S. G., & Barlow, D. H. (2002). Social phobia (social anxiety disorder). In D. H. Barlow (Ed.), *Anxiety and its disorders: The nature and treatment of anxiety and panic* (2nd ed.) (pp. 454–476). New York: Guilford Press.

Holmbeck, G. N., & Updegrove, A. L. (1995). Clinical-development interface: Implications of developmental research for adolescent psychotherapy. *Psychotherapy*, *32*, 16–33.

Hope, D. A., Heimberg, R. G., & Bruch, M. A. (1995). Dismantling cognitive-behavioral group therapy for social phobia. *Behaviour Research and Therapy*, *33*, 637–650.

Hugdahl, K., & Nordby, H. (1994). Electrophysiological correlates to cued attentional shifts in the visual and auditory modalities. *Behavioral and Neural Biology*, *62*, 21–32.

Hull, E. M., Lorraine, D. S., Du, J., Matuszewich, L., Lumley, L. A., Putnam, S. K., et al. (1999). Hormone-neurotransmitter interactions in the control of sexual behavior. *Behavioural Brain Research*, *105*, 105–116.

Huttenlocher, P. R. (1979). Synaptic density in human frontal cortex – developmental changes and effects of aging. *Brain Research*, *163*, 195–205.

Huttenlocher, P. R., De Courten, C., Garey, L. J., & van Der Loos, H. (1983). Synaptic development in human cerebral cortex. *International Journal of Neurology*, *16–17*, 144–154.

Hymel, S., Bowker, A., & Woody, E. (1993). Aggressive versus withdrawn unpopular children: Variations in peer and self-perceptions in multiple domains. *Child Development*, *64*, 879–896.

Hymel, S., Rubin, K. H., Rowden, L., & LeMare, L. (1990). Children's peer relationships: Longitudinal prediction of internalising and externalising problems from middle to late childhood. *Child Development*, *61*, 2004–2021.

Insel, T. R. (1997). A neurobiological basis for attachment. *American Journal of Psychiatry*, *154*, 726–735.

Irons, C., & Gilbert, P. (2005). Evolved mechanisms in adolescent anxiety and depression symptoms: The role of the attachment and social rank systems. *Journal of Adolescence*, *28*, 325–341.

Jacobson, R. (1986). Disorders of facial recognition, social behaviour and affect after combined bilateral amygdalotomy and subcaudate tractotomy – A clinical and experimental study. *Psychological Medicine*, *16*, 439–450.

Joiner, T. E., & Wagner, K. D. (1996). Parental, child-centered attributions and outcome: A meta-analytic review with conceptual and methodological implications. *Journal of Abnormal Child Psychology*, *24*, 37–52.

Joseph, R. (1999). Environmental influences on neural plasticity, the limbic system, emotional development and attachment: A review. *Child Psychiatry and Human Development*, *29*, 189–208.

Kagan, J. (1989). Temperamental contributions to social behavior. *American Psychologist*, *22*, 668–674.

Kagan, J. (2001). Temperamental contributions to affective and behavioral profiles in childhood. In S. G. Hofmann & P. M. DiBartolo (Eds.), *From social anxiety to social phobia: Multiple perspectives* (pp. 216–234). Boston, MA: Allyn & Bacon.

Kagan, J., Reznick, J. S., & Snidman, N. (1988). Biological bases of childhood shyness. *Science*, *240*, 167–171.

Kandel, E. R., Schwartz, J. H., & Jessell, T. M. (2000). *Principles of neural science* (4th ed.). New York: McGraw–Hill.

Kendall, P. C., Comer, J. S., Marker, C. D., Creed, T. A., Puliafico, A. C., Hughes, A. A., et al. (2009). In-session exposure tasks and therapeutic alliance across the treatment of childhood anxiety disorders. *Journal of Consulting and Clinical Psychology*, *77*, 517–525.

Kendall, P. C., & Hedtke, K. (2006). *Coping Cat Workbook* (2nd ed.). Ardmore, PA: Workbook Publishing.

Kendall, P. C., Hudson, J. L., Gosch, E., Flannery-Schroeder, E., & Suveg, C. (2008). Cognitive-behavioral therapy for anxiety disordered youth: A randomized clinical trial evaluating child and family modalities. *Journal of Consulting and Clinical Psychology*, *76*, 282–297.

Kendall, P. C., & Warman, M. J. (1997). Anxiety disorders in youth: Diagnostic consistency across DSM-III-R and DSM-IV. *Journal of Anxiety Disorders*, *10*, 453–463.

Kendler, K. S., Gardner, C. O., & Lichtenstein, P. (2008). A developmental twin study of symptoms of anxiety and depression: Evidence for genetic innovation and attenuation. *Psychological Medicine*, *38*, 1567–1575.

Kendler, K. S., Neale, M. C., Kessler, R. C., Heath, A. C., & Eaves, L. J. (1992). The genetic epidemiology of phobias in women: The interrelations of agoraphobia, social phobia, situational phobia, and simple phobia. *Archives of General Psychiatry*, *49*, 273–281.

Kessler, R. C., Berglund, P. A., Demler, O., Jin, R., Merikangas, K. R., & Walters, E. E. (2005). Lifetime prevalence and age-of-onset distributions of DSM-IV disorders in the National Comorbidity Survey Replication (NCS-R). *Archives of General Psychiatry*, *62*, 593–602.

Kessler, R. C., Chiu, W. T., Demler, O., & Walters, E. E. (2005). Prevalence, severity, and comorbidity of twelve-month DSM-IV disorders in the National Comorbidity Survey Replication (NCS-R). *Archives of General Psychiatry*, *62*, 617–627.

Kilkenny, M., Merlin, K., Plunkett, A., & Marks, R. (1998). The prevalence of common skin conditions in Australian school students. 3. Acne vulgaris. *British Journal of Dermatology*, *139*, 840–845.

King, N. J. (1993). Simple and social phobias. In T. H. Ollednick & R. J. Prinz (Eds.), *Advances in child clinical psychology: Vol. 15* (pp. 305–341). New York: Plenum Press.

Kortlander, E., Kendall, P. C., & Panichelli-Mindel, S. M. (1997). Maternal expectations and attributions about coping in anxious children. *Journal of Anxiety Disorders*, *11*, 297–315.

Kringelbach, M. L., & Rolls, E. T. (2003). Neural correlates of rapid reversal learning in a simple model of social interaction. *Neuroimage*, *20*, 1371–1383.

Kuhn, D. (2009). Adolescent thinking. In R. M. Lerner & L. Steinberg (Eds.), *Handbook of adolescent psychology: Vol. 1 – Individual bases of adolescent development*. New York: Wiley.

Kuhnen, C. M., & Knutson, B. (2005). The neural basis of financial risk taking. *Neuron, 47*, 763–770.

Kupersmidt, J. B., Coie, J. D., & Dodge, K. A. (1990). The role of poor peer relationships in the development of disorder. In S. R. Asher & J. D. Coie (Eds.), *Peer rejection in childhood* (pp. 274–305). New York: Cambridge University Press.

Kupersmidt, J. B., & Dodge, K. A. (Eds.), (2004). *Children's peer relations: From development to intervention*. Washington, DC: American Psychological Association.

Ladd, G. W. (2006). Peer rejection, aggressive or withdrawn behavior, and psychological maladjustment from ages 5 to 12: An examination of four predictive models. *Child Development, 77*, 822–846.

La Greca, A. M., & Harrison, H. (2005). Adolescent peer relations, friendships and romantic relationships: Do they predict social anxiety and depression? *Journal of Clinical Child and Adolescent Psychology, 34*, 49–61.

La Greca, A. M., & Lopez, N. (1998). Social anxiety among adolescents: Linkages with peer relations and friendships. *Journal of Abnormal Child Psychology, 26*, 83–94.

Langenecker, S. A., Nielson, K. A., & Rao, S. M. (2004). fMRI in healthy older adults during Stroop interference. *Neuroimage, 21*, 192–200.

Last, C. G., Hersen, M., Kazdin, A. E., Francis, G., & Grubb, H. J. (1987). Psychiatric illness in the mothers of anxious children. *American Journal of Psychiatry, 144*, 1580–1583.

Last, C. G., Hersen, M., Kazdin, A. E., Orvaschel, H., & Perrin, S. (1991). Anxiety disorders in children and their families. *Archives of General Psychiatry, 48*, 928–939.

Leary, M. R. (1995). *Self-presentation: Impression management and interpersonal behavior.* Boulder, CO: Westview Press.

Leary, M. R., & Kowalski, R. M. (1993). The Interaction Anxiousness Scale: Current and criterion-related validity. *Journal of Personality Assessment, 61*, 136–146.

Lerner, R. M., Castellino, D. R., Patterson, T. A., Villaruel, F. A., & McKinney, M. H. (1995). Developmental contextual perspective on parenting. In M. H. Bornstein (Ed.), *Handbook of parenting* (pp. 285–309). Hillsdale, NJ: Lawrence Erlbaum Associates, Publishers.

Leve, L. D., Kim, H. K., & Pears, K. C. (2005). Childhood temperament and family environment as predictors of internalizing and externalizing trajectories from ages 5 to 17. *Journal of Abnormal Child Psychology, 33*, 505–520.

Loney, T., Arnold, M. C., & Grafman, J. (2008). Not just "skin deep": Psychosocial effects of dermatological-related social anxiety in a sample of acne patients. *Journal of Health Psychology, 13*, 47–54.

Lonigan, C. J., Carey, M. P., & Finch, A. J. (1994). Anxiety and depression in children and adolescents: Negative affectivity and the utility of self-reports. *Journal of Consulting and Clinical Psychology, 62*, 1000–1008.

Lorerbaum, J. P., Kose, S., Johnson, M. R., Arana, G. W., Sullivan, L. K., Hamner, M. B., et al. (2004). Neural correlates of speech anticipatory anxiety in generalized social phobia. *Neuroreport, 15*, 2701–2705.

Lunde, C., Frisén, A., & Hwang, C. P. (2007). Ten-year-old girls' and boys' body composition and peer victimization experiences: Prospective associations with body satisfaction. *Body Image, 4*, 11–28.

Madigan, S., Moran, G., & Pederson, D. R. (2006). Unresolved states of mind, disorganized attachment relationships, and disrupted interactions of adolescent mothers and their infants. *Developmental Psychology, 42*, 293–304.

Mah, L., Arnold, M. C., & Grafman, J. (2004). Impairments of social perception associated with lesions of the prefrontal cortex. *American Journal of Psychiatry*, *161*, 1247–1255.

Main, M., & Hesse, E. (1990). Parents' unresolved traumatic experiences are related to infant disorganized attachment status: Is frightened and/or frightening parental behavior the linking mechanism? In M. T. Greenberg, D. Cicchetti, & E. M. Cummings (Eds.), *Attachment in the preschool years: Theory, research, and intervention* (pp. 161–182). Chicago, IL: University of Chicago Press.

Main, M., & Solomon, J. (1986). Discovery of an insecure disoriented attachment pattern: Procedures, findings and implications for the classification of behavior. In T. Brazelton & M. Youngman (Eds.), *Affective development in infancy* (pp. 121–160). Norwood, NJ: Ablex.

Mallon, E., Newton, J. N., Klassen, A., Stewart-Brown, S. L., Ryan, T. J., & Finlay, A. Y. (1999). The quality of life in acne: A comparison with general medical conditions using generic questionnaires. *British Journal of Dermatology*, *140*, 672–676.

Mancini, C., van Ameringen, M., Szatmari, P., Fugere, C., & Boyle, M. (1996). A high risk pilot study of the children of adults with social phobia. *Journal of the Academy of Child and Adolescent Psychiatry*, *35*, 1511–1517.

Mannuzza, S., Schneier, F. R., Chapman, T. F., Liebowitz, M. R., Klein, D. F., & Fyer, A. J. (1995). Generalized social phobia. Reliability and validity. *Archives of General Psychiatry*, *52*, 230–237.

Matthews, S. C., Simmons, A. N., Lane, S. D., & Paulus, M. P. (2004). Selective activation of the nucleus accumbens during risk-taking decision making. *Neuroreport*, *15*, 2123–2127.

Mayberg, H. S. (1997). Limbic-cortical dysregulation: A proposed model of depression. *Journal of Neuropsychiatry and Clinical Neuroscience*, *9*, 471–481.

Mayberg, H. S. (2007). Defining the neural circuitry of depression: Toward a new nosology with therapeutic implications. *Biological Psychiatry*, *61*, 729–730.

McClure, E. B., Monk, C. S., Nelson, E. E., Parrish, J. M., Adler, A., Blair, R. J., et al. (2007). Abnormal attention modulation of fear circuit function in pediatric generalized anxiety disorder. *Archives of General Psychiatry*, *64*, 97–106.

McEwen, B. S. (2001). Estrogen effects on the brain: Multiple sites and molecular mechanisms. *Journal of Applied Physiology*, *91*, 2785–2801.

McLeod, B. D., Weisz, J. R., & Wood, J. J. (2007). Examining the association between parenting and childhood depression: A meta-analysis. *Clinical Psychology Review*, *27*, 986–1003.

Mendlowicz, M. V., & Stein, M. B. (2000). Quality of life in individuals with anxiety disorders. *American Journal of Psychiatry*, *157*, 669–682.

Mercer, J. (2006). *Understanding attachment: Parenting, child care, and emotional development*. Westport, CT: Praeger Publishers.

Messer, S. C., & Beidel, D. C. (1994). Psychosocial correlates of childhood anxiety disorders. *Journal of the American Academy of Child and Adolescent Psychiatry*, *33*, 975–983.

Monk, C. S., McClure, E. B., Nelson, E. E., Zarhn, E., Bilder, R. M., Leibenluft, E., et al. (2003). Adolescent immaturity in attention-related brain engagement to emotional facial expressions. *Neuroimage*, *20*, 420–428.

Monk, C. S., Nelson, E. E., McClure, E. B., Mogg, K., Bradley, B. P., Leibenluft, E., et al. (2006). Ventrolateral prefrontal cortex activation and attentional bias in response to angry faces in adolescents with generalized anxiety disorder. *American Journal of Psychiatry*, *163*, 1091–1097.

Montague, P. R., & Berns, G. S. (2002). Neural economics and the biological substrates of valuation. *Neuron*, *36*, 265–284.

Moore, P. S., Whaley, S. E., & Sigman, M. (2004). Interactions between mothers and children: Impacts of maternal and child anxiety. *Journal of Abnormal Psychology*, *113*, 471–476.

Mori, E., & Yamadori, A. (1989). Rejection behaviour: A human homologue of the abnormal behaviour of Denny-Brown and Chambers' monkey with bilateral parietal ablation. *Journal of Neurology, Neurosurgery, and Psychiatry*, *52*, 1260–1266.

Morris, J. S., Frith, C. D., Perrett, D. I., Rowland, D., Young, A. W., Calder, A. J., et al. (1996). A differential neural response in the human amygdala to fearful and happy facial expressions. *Nature*, *383*, 812–815.

Moss, H., & Damasio, A. (2001). Emotion and the human brain. *Annals of the New York Academy of Sciences*, *935*, 101–106.

Muris, P. (2006). The pathogenesis of childhood anxiety disorders: Considerations from a developmental psychopathology perspective. *International Journal of Behavioral Development*, *30*, 5–11.

Muris, P., Meesters, C., van de Bloom, W., & Mayer, B. (2005). Biological, psychological, and sociocultural correlates of body change strategies and eating problems in adolescent boys and girls. *Eating Behaviors*, *6*, 11–22.

Muris, P., Merckelbach, H., Schmidt, H., Gadet, B., & Bogie, N. (2001). Anxiety and depression as correlates of self-reported behavioural inhibition in normal adolescents. *Behaviour Research and Therapy*, *39*, 1051–1061.

Muris, P., Merckelbach, H., Wessele, I., & Van de Ven, M. (1999). Psychopathological correlates of self-reported behavioural inhibition in normal children. *Behaviour Research and Therapy*, *37*, 575–584.

Muris, P., Rassin, E., Mayer, B., Smeets, G., Huijding, J., Remmerswaal, D., et al. (2009). Effects of verbal information on fear-related reasoning biases in children. *Behaviour Research and Therapy*, *47*, 206–214.

Murray, L., DeRosnay, M., Pearson, J., Bergeron, C., Schofield, L., Royal-Lawson, M., et al. (2008). Intergenerational transmission of maternal social anxiety: The role of the social referencing process. *Child Development*, *79*, 1049–1064.

Murray, L., Creswell, C., & Cooper, P. J. (2009). The development of anxiety disorders in childhood: An integrative review. *Psychological Medicine*, *39*, 1413–1423.

Nelson, E. E., Leibenluft, E., McClure, E. B., & Pine, D. S. (2005). The social re-orientation of adolescence: A neuroscience perspective on the process and its relation to psychopathology. *Psychological Medicine*, *35*, 163–174.

Nelson, L. J., Rubin, K. H., & Fox, N. A. (2005). Social and nonsocial behaviors and peer acceptance: A longitudinal model of the development of self-perceptions in children ages 4 to 7 years. *Early Education and Development*, *20*, 185–200.

Newcomb, A. F., Bukowski, W. M., & Pattee, L. (1993). Children's peer relations: A meta-analyic review of popular, rejected, neglected, controversial, and average sociometric status. *Psychological Bulletin*, *113*, 99–128.

Ogliari, A., Citterio, A., Zanoni, A., Fagnani, C., Patriarca, V., & Cirrincione, R. (2006). Genetic and environmental influences on anxiety dimensions in Italian twins evaluated with the SCARED questionnaire. *Journal of Anxiety Disorders*, *20*, 760–777.

Oh, W., Rubin, K. H., Bowker, J. C., Booth-LaForce, C. L., Rose-Krasnor, L., & Laursen, B. (2008). Trajectories of social withdrawal from middle childhood to early adolescence. *Journal of Abnormal Child Psychology*, *36*, 553–566.

Ojeda, S. R., Lomniczi, A., Sandau, U., & Matagne, V. (2010). New concepts on the control of the onset of puberty. *Endocrine Development*, *17*, 44–51.

Ollendick, T. H., Greene, R. W., Weist, M. D., & Oswald, D. P. (1990). The predictive validity of teacher nominations: A five-year follow up of at-risk youth. *Journal of Abnormal Child Psychology*, *18*, 699–713.

Ollendick, T. H., & Hirshfeld-Becker, D. R. (2002). The developmental psychopathology of social anxiety disorder. *Biological Psychiatry*, *51*, 44–58.

Ollendick, T. H., King, N. J., & Frary, R. B. (1989). Fears in children and adolescents: Reliability and generalizability across gender, age, and nationality. *Behaviour Research and Therapy*, *27*, 19–26.

Öst, L. G. (1987). Age of onset in different phobias. *Journal of Abnormal Psychology*, *96*, 223–229.

Osterlund, M. K., & Hurd, Y. L. (2001). Estrogen receptors in the human forebrain and the relation to neuropsychiatric disorders. *Progress in Neurobiology*, *64*, 251–267.

Ozmen, M., Erdogan, A., Duvenci, S., Ozyurt, E., & Ozkara, C. (2004). Excessive masturbation after epilepsy surgery. *Epilepsy Behavior*, *5*, 133–136.

Paikoff, R. L., & Brooks-Gunn, J. (1991). Do parent–child relationships change during puberty? *Psychological Bulletin*, *110*, 47–66.

Parker, J., & Asher, S. R. (1987). Peer acceptance and later personal adjustment: Are low-accepted children "at risk"? *Psychological Bulletin*, *102*, 357–389.

Paus, T. (2005). Mapping brain maturation and cognitive development during adolescence. *Trends in Cognitive Sciences*, *9*, 60–68.

Pérez-Edgar, K., & Fox, N. A. (2005). Temperament and anxiety disorders. *Child and Adolescent Psychiatric Clinics of North America*, *14*, 681–706.

Pérez-Edgar, K., Roberson-Nay, R., Hardin, M. G., Poeth, K., Guyer, A. E., & Nelson, E. E. (2007). Attention alters neural responses to evocative faces in behaviorally inhibited adolescents. *Neuroimage*, *35*, 1538–1546.

Peterson, B. S. (2003). Conceptual, methodological, and statistical challenges in brain imaging studies of developmentally based psychopathologies. *Development and Psychopathology*, *15*, 811–832.

Pezawas, L., Meyer-Lindenberg, A., Drabant, E. M., Verchinski, B. A., Munoz, K. E., Kolachana, B. S., et al. (2005). 5-HTTLPR polymorphism impacts human cingulate-amygdala interactions: A genetic susceptibility mechanism for depression. *Nature Neuroscience*, *8*, 828–834.

Pfaff, D., Frohlich, J., & Morgan, M. (2002). Hormonal and genetic influences on arousal – sexual and otherwise. *Trends in Neuroscience*, *25*, 45–50.

Phan, K. L., Fitzgerald, D. A., Nathan, P. J., & Tancer, M. E. (2006). Association between amygdala hyperactivity to harsh faces and severity of social anxiety in generalized social phobia. *Biological Psychiatry*, *59*, 424–429.

Pine, D. S., Cohen, P., Gurley, D., Brook, J., & Ma, Y. (1998). The risk for early-adulthood anxiety and depressive disorders in adolescents with anxiety and depressive disorders. *Archives of General Psychiatry*, *55*, 56–64.

Pine, D. S., Cohen, P., Johnson, J. G., & Brook, J. S. (2002). Adolescent life events as predictors of adult depression. *Journal of Affective Disorders*, *68*, 49–57.

Prior, V., & Glaser, D. (2006). *Understanding attachment and attachment disorders: Theory, evidence and practice*. Philadelphia, PA: Jessica Kingsley.

Putnam, S., Sanson, A. V., & Rothbart, M. K. (2002). Child temperament and parenting. In M. H. Bornstein (Ed.), *Handbook of parenting: Vol. 1* (2nd ed.) (pp. 255–277). Hillsdale, NJ: Lawrence Erlbaum Associates.

Raikes, H. A., & Thompson, R. A. (2008). Attachment security and parenting quality predict children's problem-solving, attributions, and loneliness with peers. *Attachment and Human Development*, *10*, 319–344.

Rao, P. R., Beidel, D. C., Turner, S. M., Ammerman, R. T., Crosby, L. E., & Sallee, F. R. (2007). Social anxiety disorder in childhood and adolescence: Descriptive psychopathology. *Behaviour Research and Therapy*, *45*, 1181–1191.

Rapee, R. M. (1997). Potential role of childrearing practices in the development of anxiety and depression. *Clinical Psychology Review*, *17*, 47–67.

Rapee, R. M., & Heimberg, R. G. (1997). A cognitive-behavioral model of anxiety in social phobia. *Behaviour Research and Therapy*, *35*, 741–756.

Rapee, R. M., & Spence, S. H. (2004). The etiology of social phobia: Empirical evidence and the initial model. *Clinical Psychology Review*, *24*, 737–767.

Rauch, S. L., Shin, L. M., & Phelps, E. A. (2006). Neurocircuitry models of posttraumatic stress disorder and extinction: Human neuroimaging research – past, present, and future. *Biological Psychiatry*, *60*, 376–382.

Reardon, L. E., Leen-Feldner, E. W., & Hayward, C. (2009). A critical review of the empirical literature on the relation between anxiety and puberty. *Clinical Psychology Review*, *29*, 1–23.

Reder, P., McClure, M., & Jolley, A. (2000). Interfaces between child and adult mental health. In P. Reder, M. McClure, & A. Jolley (Eds.), *Family matters: Interfaces between child and adult mental health* (pp. 3–20). London: Routledge.

Reich, J. H., & Yates, W. (1988). Family history of psychiatric disorders in social phobia. *Comprehensive Psychiatry*, *29*, 72–75.

Reiss, A. L., Abrams, M. T., Singer, H. S., Ross, J. L., & Denckla, M. B. (1996). Brain development, gender, and IQ in children: A volumetric imaging study. *Brain*, *119*, 1763–1774.

Reznick, J. S., Hegeman, I. M., Kaufman, E., Woods, S. W., & Jacobs, M. (1992). Retrospective and concurrent self-report of behavioural inhibition and their relation to adult mental health. *Developmental Psychology*, *4*, 301–321.

Romeo, R. D., Richardson, H. N., & Sisk, C. L. (2002). Puberty and the maturation of the male brain and sexual behavior: Recasting a behavioral potential. *Neuroscience and Biobehavioral Reviews*, *26*, 381–391.

Rosen, J. B., & Schulkin, J. (1998). From normal fear to pathological anxiety. *Psychological Review*, *105*, 325–350.

Rothbart, M. K. (2004). Commentary: Differentiated measures of temperament and multiple pathways to childhood disorders. *Journal of Clinical Child and Adolescent Psychology*, *33*, 82–87.

Rothbart, M. K., & Bates, J. E. (2006). Temperament. In W. Damon & N. Eisenberg (Eds.), *Handbook of child psychology: Vol. 3 – Social, emotional and personality development* (6th ed.) (pp. 99–166). New York: Wiley.

Rothbart, M. K., & Derryberry, D. (1981). Development of individual differences in temperament. In M. E. Lamb & A. L. Brown (Eds.), *Advances in developmental psychology: Vol. 1* (pp. 37–86). Hillsdale, NJ: Lawrence Erlbaum Associates.

Rothbart, M. K., Ellis, L. K., & Posner, M. I. (2004). Temperament and self-regulation. In R. F. Baumeister & K. D. Vohs (Eds.), *Handbook of self-regulation: Research theory and applications* (pp. 283–300). New York: Guilford Press.

Rothbart, M. K, & Posner, M. I. (1985). Temperament and the development of self-regulation. In L. C. Hartlage & C. F. Telzrow (Eds.), *The neuropsychology of individual differences: A developmental perspective* (pp. 93–123). New York: Plenum.

Rubia, K., Overmeyer, S., Taylor, E., Brammer, M., Williams, S. C., Simmons, A., et al. (2000). Functional frontalisation with age: Mapping neurodevelopmental trajectories with fMRI. *Neuroscience and Biobehavioral Reviews*, *24*, 13–19.

Rubia, K., Smith, A. B., Woolley, J., Nosarti, C., Heyman, I., Taylor, E., et al. (2006). Progressive increase of frontostriatal brain activation from childhood to adulthood during event-related tasks of cognitive control. *Human Brain Mapping*, *27*, 973–993.

Rubin, K. H., Bukowski, W., & Parker, J. (2006). Peer interactions, relationships, and groups. In N. Eisenberg (Ed.), *Handbook of child psychology: Social, emotional, and personality development* (6th ed.) (pp. 571–645). New York: Wiley.

Rubin, K. H., & Krasnor, L. R. (1986). Social-cognitive and social behavioral perspectives on problem solving. In M. Perlmutter (Ed.), *Cognitive perspectives on children's social and behavioral development. The Minnesota symposia on child psychology: Vol. 18* (pp. 1–68). Hillsdale, NJ: Erlbaum.

Rubin, K. H., LeMare, L. J., & Lollis, S. (1990). Social withdrawal in childhood: Developmental pathways to peer rejection. In S. R. Asher & J. D. Coie (Eds.), *Peer rejection in childhood* (pp. 217–249). Cambridge, UK: Cambridge University Press.

RUPP Anxiety Study Group. (2001). Fluoxamine for the treatment of anxiety disorders in children and adolescents. *New England Journal of Medicine, 344*, 1279–1285.

Santrock, J. W. (2007). *A topical approach to human life-span development* (3rd ed.). St Louis, MO: McGraw–Hill.

Schaffer, H. R. (1966). The onset of fear of strangers and the incongruity hypothesis. *Journal of Child Psychology. Psychiatry and Allied Disciplines, 7*, 95–106.

Schlenker, B. R. (1980). *Impression management: The self-concept, social identity and interpersonal relations*. Monterey, CA: Brooks/Cole.

Schlenker, B. R., & Leary, M. R. (1982). Social anxiety and self-presentation: A conceptualization model. *Psychological Bulletin, 92*, 641–669.

Schmidt, L. A., & Fox, N. A. (1998). Fear-potentiated startle responses in temperamentally different human infants. *Developmental Psychobiology, 32*, 113–120.

Schmidt, L. A., Fox, N. A., Schulkin, J., & Gold, P. W. (1999). Behavioral and psychophysiological correlates of selfpresentation in temperamentally shy children. *Developmental Psychobiology, 35*, 119–135.

Schmidt, L. A., Fox, N. A., Sternberg, E. M., Gold, P. W., Smith, C. C., & Schulkin, J. (1999). Adrenocortical reactivity and social competence in seven-year-olds. *Personality and Individual Differences, 26*, 977–985.

Schneider, B. H., Atkinson, L., & Tardif, C. (2001). Child–parent attachment and children's peer relations: A quantitative review. *Developmental Psychology, 37*, 86–100.

Schneier, F. R. (2006). Clinical practice. Social anxiety disorder. *New England Journal of Medicine, 355*, 1029–1036.

Schneier, F. R., Johnson, J., Hornig, C. D., Liebowitz, M. R., & Weissman, M. M. (1992). Social phobia: Comorbidity and morbidity in an epidemiologic sample. *Archives of General Psychiatry, 49*, 282–288.

Schwartz, C. E., Snidman, N., & Kagan, J. (1999). Adolescent social anxiety as an outcome of inhibited temperament in childhood. *Journal of the American Academy of Child and Adolescent Psychiatry, 38*, 1008–1015.

Schwartz, D., Dodge, K., & Cole, J. (1993). The emergence of chronic peer victimization in boys' play groups. *Child Development, 64*, 1755–1772.

Scott, S. K., Young, A. W., Calder, A. J., Hellawell, D. J., Aggleton, J. P., & Johnson, M. (1997). Impaired auditory recognition of fear and anger following bilateral amygdala lesions. *Nature, 385*, 254–257.

Seifer, R., & Sameroff, A. J. (1986). The concept, measurement, and interpretation of temperament in young children: A survey of research issues. In M. L. Wolraich & D. Routh (Eds.), *Advances in developmental and behavioral pediatrics: Vol. 7* (pp. 1–43). Greenwich, CT: JAI.

Shaw, P., Lawrence, E. J., Radbourne, C., Bramham, J., Polkey, C. E., & David, A. S. (2004). The impact of early and late damage to the human amygdale on "theory of mind" reasoning. *Brain, 127*, 1535–1548.

Shin, L. M., & Liberzon, I. (2010). The neurocircuitry of fear, stress, and anxiety disorders. *Neuropsychopharmacology, 35*, 169–191.

Simmons, R., Rosenberg, R., & Rosenberg, M. (1973). Disturbance in the self-image at adolescence. *American Sociological Review*, *38*, 553–568.

Singh, P., & Bussey, K. (2009). The development of a Peer Aggression Coping Self-Efficacy Scale for adolescents. *The British Journal of Developmental Psychology*, *27*(Pt 4), 971–992.

Slater, L. (2003, November 2). The cruelest cure. *The New York Times*, p. 34.

Smith, P., & Brain, P. (2000). Bullying in schools: Lessons from two decades of research. *Aggressive Behavior*, *26*, 1–9.

Smith, P., Morita, Y., Junger-Tas, J., Olweus, D., Catalano, R., & Slee, P. (Eds.), (1999). *The nature of school bullying: A crossnational perspective*. New York: Routledge.

Sowell, E. R., Peterson, B. S., Thompson, P. M., Welcome, S. E., Henkenius, A. L., & Toga, A. W. (2003). Mapping cortical changes across the life span. *Nature and Neuroscience*, *6*, 309–315.

Sowell, E. R., Thompson, P. M., Holmes, C. J., Jernigan, T. L., & Toga, A. W. (1999). In vivo evidence for post-adolescent brain maturation in frontal and striatal regions. *Nature and Neuroscience*, *2*, 859–861.

Sowell, E. R., Thompson, P. M., Tessner, K. D., & Toga, A. W. (2001). Mapping continued brain growth and gray matter density reduction in dorsal frontal cortex: Inverse relationships during postadolescent brain maturation. *Journal of Neuroscience*, *21*, 8819–8829.

Spear, L. P. (2000). The adolescent brain and age-related behavioral manifestations. *Neuroscience and Biobehavioral Reviews*, *24*, 417–463.

Spence, S. H., Donovan, C., & Brechman-Toussaint, M. (1999). Social skills, social outcomes, and cognitive features of childhood social phobia. *Journal of Abnormal Psychology*, *108*, 211–221.

Spezio, M. L., Huang, P. Y., Castelli, F., & Adolphs, R. (2007). Amygdala damage impairs eye contact during conversations with real people. *Journal of Neuroscience*, *27*, 3994–3997.

Sripada, C. S., Angstadt, M., Banks, S., Nathan, P. J., Liberzon, I., & Phan, K. L. (2009). Functional neuroimaging of mentalizing during the trust game in social anxiety disorder. *Neuroreport*, *20*, 984–989.

Stein, M. B., Chartier, M. J., Hazen, A. L., Kozak, M. V., Tancer, M. E., Lander, S., et al. (1998). A direct-interview family study of generalized social phobia. *American Journal of Psychiatry*, *155*, 90–97.

Stein, M. B., Chavira, D. A., & Jang, K. L. (2001). Bringing up bashful baby: Developmental pathways to social phobia. *Psychiatric Clinics of North America*, *24*, 661–675.

Stein, M. B., Goldin, P. R., Sareen, J., Zorrilla, L. T., & Brown, G. G. (2002). Increased amygdala activation to angry and contemptuous faces in generalized social phobia. *Archives of General Psychiatry*, *59*, 1027–1034.

Steinberg, L. (2005). Cognitive and affective development in adolescence. *Trends in Cognitive Sciences*, *9*, 69–74.

Steinberg, L., & Morris, A. S. (2001). Adolescent development. *Annual Review of Psychology*, *52*, 83–110.

Stevens, J. R. (2002). Schizophrenia: Reproductive hormones and the brain. *American Journal of Psychiatry*, *159*, 713–719.

Stewart, M. E. (1992). Sebaceous gland lipids. *Seminars in Dermatology*, *11*, 100–105.

Stewart, S. L., & Rubin, K. H. (1995). The social problem solving skills of anxious-withdrawn children. *Developmental Psychopathology*, *7*, 323–336.

Straube, T., Kolassa, I. T., Glauer, M., Mentzel, H. J., & Miltner, W. H. (2004). Effect of task conditions on brain responses to threatening faces in social phobics: An event-related functional magnetic resonance imaging study. *Biological Psychiatry*, *56*, 921–930.

Strauss, C. C., Lahey, B. B., Frick, P., Frame, C. L., & Hynd, G. W. (1988). Peer social status of children with anxiety disorders. *Journal of Consulting and Clinical Psychology*, *56*, 137–141.

Strelau, J. (1983). *Temperament personality activity*. New York: Academic Press.

Sumter, S. R., Bokhorst, C. L., & Westenberg, P. M. (2009). Social fears during adolescence: Is there an increase in distress and avoidance? *Journal of Anxiety Disorders*, *23*, 897–903.

Tamm, L., Menon, V., & Reiss, A. L. (2002). Maturation of brain function associated with response inhibition. *Journal of the American Academy of Child and Adolescent Psychiatry*, *41*, 1231–1238.

Thomas, A., & Chess, S. (1977). *Temperament and development.* New York: Brunner/Mazel.

Thomas, A., Chess, S., & Birch, H. G. (1968). *Temperament and behavior disorders in children.* New York: New York University Press.

Thomas, D. R. (2004). Psychosocial effects of acne. *Journal of Cutaneous Medicine and Surgery*, *8*(Suppl 4), 3–5.

Thompson, R. A., Connell, J. P., & Bridges, L. J. (1988). Temperament, emotion, and social interactive behavior in the strange situation: A component process analysis of attachment system functioning. *Child Development*, *59*, 1102–1110.

Tillfors, M., Furmark, T., Marteinsdottir, I., Fischer, H., Pissiota, A., Långström, B., et al. (2001). Cerebral blood flow in subjects with social phobia during stressful speaking tasks: A PET study. *American Journal of Psychiatry*, *158*, 1220–1226.

Tillfors, M., Furmark, T., Marteinsdottir, I., & Fredrikson, M. (2002). Cerebral blood flow during anticipation of public speaking in social phobia: A PET study. *Biological Psychiatry*, *52*, 1113–1119.

Toga, A. W., Thompson, P. M., & Sowell, E. R. (2006). Mapping brain maturation. *Trends in Neurosciences*, *29*, 148–159.

Tottenham, N., Tanaka, J. W., Leon, A. C., McCarry, T., Nurse, M., Hare, T. A., et al. (2009). The NimStim set of facial expressions: Judgments from untrained research participants. *Psychiatry Research*, *168*, 242–249.

Tranel, D., & Hyman, B. T. (1990). Neuropsychological correlates of bilateral amygdala damage. *Archives of Neurology*, *47*, 349–355.

Tremblay, L., & Lariviere, M. (2009). The influence of puberty onset, body mass index, and pressure to be thin on disordered eating behaviors in children and adolescents. *Eating Behaviors*, *10*, 75–83.

Turner, S. M., & Beidel, D. C. (1989). Social phobia: Clinical syndrome, diagnosis, and comorbidity. *Clinical Psychology Review*, *9*, 3–18.

Turner, S. M., Biedel, D. C., & Costello, A. (1987). Psychopathology in the offspring of anxiety disordered patients. *Journal of Consulting and Clinical Psychology*, *55*, 229–235.

Turner, S. M., Beidel, D. C., Roberson-Nay, R., & Tervo, K. (2003). Parenting behaviours in parents with anxiety disorders. *Behaviour Research and Therapy*, *41*, 541–554.

Vasey, M. W., & Dadds, M. R. (2001). *The developmental psychopathology of anxiety*. New York: Oxford University Press.

Veit, R., Flor, H., Erb, M., Hermann, C., Lotze, M., & Grodd, W. (2002). Brain circuits involved in emotional learning in antisocial behavior and social phobia in humans. *Neuroscience Letters*, *328*, 233–236.

Vertue, F. M. (2003). From adaptive emotion to dysfunction: An attachment perspective on social anxiety disorder. *Personality and Social Psychology Review*, *7*, 170–191.

Walkup, J., Albano, A. M., Piacentini, J. P., Birmaher, B., Compton, S., Sherrill, J., et al. (2008). *New England Journal of Medicine*, *359*, 2753–2766.

Wang, P. S., Berglund, P., Olfson, M., Pincus, H. A., Wells, K. B., & Kessler, R. C. (2005). Failure and delay in initial treatment contact after first onset of mental disorders in the National Comorbidity Survey Replication. *Archives of General Psychiatry*, *62*, 603–613.

Warner, V., Mufson, L., & Weissman, M. M. (1995). Offspring at low and high risk for depression and anxiety: Mechanisms of psychiatric disorder. *Journal of the Academy of Child and Adolescent Psychiatry, 34*, 786–797.

Warren, S. L., Huston, L., Egeland, B., & Sroufe, A. (1997). Child and adolescent anxiety disorders and early attachment. *Journal of the American Academy of Child and Adolescent Psychiatry, 36*, 637–644.

Waters, E., Matas, L., & Sroufe, L. A. (1975). Infants' reactions to an approaching stranger: Description, validation, and functional significance of wariness. *Child Development, 46*, 348–356.

Watson, D., Clark, L. A., & Carey, G. (1988). Positive and negative affectivity and their relation to anxiety and depressive disorders. *Journal of Abnormal Psychology, 97*, 346–353.

Weems, C. F., & Costa, N. M. (2005). Developmental differences in the expression of childhood anxiety symptoms and fears. *Journal of the American Academy of Child and Adolescent Psychiatry, 44*, 656–663.

Weissman, M. M., Leckman, J. F., Merikangas, K. R., Gammon, G. D., & Prusoff, B. A. (1984). Depression and anxiety disorders in parents and children. *Archives of General Psychiatry, 41*, 845–852.

Westenberg, P. M., Drewes, M. J., Goedhart, A. W., Siebelink, B. M., & Treffers, P. D. (2004). A developmental analysis of self-reported fears in late childhood through mid-adolescence: Social-evaluative fears on the rise? *Journal of Child Psychology, Psychiatry, and Allied Disciplines, 45*, 481–495.

Whaley, S. E., Pinto, A., & Sigman, M. (1999). Characterising interactions between anxious mothers and their children. *Journal of Consulting and Clinical Psychology, 67*, 826–836.

Whincup, P. H., Gilg, J. A., Odoki, K., Taylor, S. J. C., & Cook, D. G. (2001). Age of menarche in contemporary British teenagers: Survey of girls born between 1982 and 1986. *British Medical Journal, 322*, 1095–1096.

White, L. K., Helfinstein, S. M., Reeb-Sutherland, B. C., Degnan, K. A., & Fox, N. A. (2009). Role of attention in the regulation of fear and anxiety. *Developmental Neuroscience, 31*, 309–317.

Whitelaw, N. C., & Whitelaw, E. (2006). How lifetimes shape epigenotype within and across generations. *Human Molecular Genetics, 1*(Spec No. 2), R131–137.

Winslow, J. T., & Insel, T. R. (2004). Neuroendocrine basis or social recognition. *Current Opinion in Neurobiology, 14*, 248–253.

Wittchen, H-U., & Fehm, L. (2003). Epidemiology and natural course of social fears and social phobia. *Acta Psychiatrica Scandinavica, 108*(Suppl 417), 4–18.

Wittchen, H-U., Nelson, C. B., & Lachner, G. (1998). Prevalence of mental disorders and psychosocial impairments in adolescents and young adults. *Psychological Medicine, 28*, 109–126.

Wittchen, H-U., Stein, M. B., & Kessler, R. C. (1999). Social fears and social phobia in a community sample of adolescents and young adults: Prevalence, risk factors, and co-morbidity. *Psychological Medicine, 29*, 309–323.

Wood, J. G., McLeod, B. D., Sigman, M., Hwang, W.-C., & Chu, B. C. (2003). Parenting and childhood anxiety: Theory, empirical findings and future directions. *Journal of Child Psychology and Psychiatry, 44*, 134–151.

Wright, C. I., Fischer, H., Whalen, P. J., McInerney, S. C., Shin, L. M., & Rauch, S. L. (2001). Differential prefrontal cortex and amygdala habituation to repeatedly presented emotional stimuli. *Brain Imaging, 12*, 379–383.

Yakovlev, P. I., & Lecours, A. R. (1967). The myelogenetic cycles of regional maturation of the brain. In A. Minkowski (Ed.), *Regional development of the brain early in life* (pp. 3–170). Oxford: Blackwell.

Yamamoto, A., & Ito, M. (1992). Sebaceous gland activity and urinary androgen levels in children. *Journal of Dermatological Science, 4*, 98–104.

Yeates, K. O., Bigler, E. D., Dennis, M., Gerhardt, C. A., Rubin, K. H., & Stancin, T. (2007). Social outcomes in childhood brain disorder: A heuristic integration of social neuroscience and developmental psychology. *Psychological Bulletin*, *133*, 535–556.

Yurgelun-Todd, D. (2007). Emotional and cognitive changes during adolescence. *Current Opinions in Neurobiology*, *17*, 251–257.

Zehr, J. L., Culbert, K. M., Sisk, C. L., & Klump, K. L. (2007). An association of early puberty with disordered eating and anxiety in a population of undergraduate women and men. *Hormones and Behavior*, *52*, 427–435.

Zgourides, G. D., & Warren, R. (1988). Prevalence of panic in adolescents: A brief report. *Psychological Reports*, *62*, 935–937.

Part II

Theoretical Perspectives

Chapter 10

Neuroendocrinology and Neuroimaging Studies of Social Anxiety Disorder

K. Luan Phan[1] and Heide Klumpp[2]

[1]Department of Psychiatry, University of Michigan, Ann Arbor, MI 48109; Mental Health Service, VA Ann Arbor Healthcare System, MI 48105, [2]Department of Psychiatry, University of Michigan, Ann Arbor, MI 48109-2700

INTRODUCTION

Social anxiety disorder (SAD), otherwise known as SP, is a common anxiety disorder characterized by an intense, irrational, and persistent fear of being scrutinized or negatively evaluated by others (American Psychiatric Association, 1994). Patients with SAD fear social or performance situations that typically provoke an immediate anxious reaction ranging from diffuse apprehension to situational panic. When faced with social scrutiny, patients with SAD respond with signs of hyperarousal (e.g., blushing, increased heart rate, shaking, sweating). Situations that evoke anxiety and fear are often avoided, for fear of embarrassment in the context of perceived threat and/or criticism. Over time, a stimulus–response association develops akin to fear conditioning and aversive learning. As such, it has also been proposed that individuals with social anxiety have difficulty in the way in which social and emotion-laden information is processed (Clark & McManus, 2002) and/or have enhanced memory for negative events (Amir, Foa, & Coles, 2000).

Given the response to social threat in SAD, several complementary theories exist about the neuropathophysiology of SP. First, the brain and body's neuroendocrine system, which is activated when a person comes under threat, may be dysregulated. Second, the amygdala and associated paralimbic brain regions, which govern fear perception, memory, responding, and learning, may be hyper-sensitive to information that conveys the *potential* for threat or may be hyper-reactive during situations that involve public scrutiny. Third, the frontal and associative cortices, which control cognition and executive function, may exhibit deficient functioning when incoming social signals require complex interpretation and/or when negative feedback requires reappraisal.

Social Anxiety: Clinical, Developmental, and Social Perspectives. DOI: 10.1016/B978-0-12-375096-9.00010-9

Collectively, these theories are based on the proposition that SAD involves aberrant social cognitive affective functioning. For example, patients with SAD are hypervigilant for social signals that covey threat or criticism, such as "harsh" (e.g., angry, afraid, contemptuous, disgusted) faces (Mogg & Bradley, 2002; Mogg, Philippot, & Bradley, 2004); pay more attention to those threatening stimuli (Amir, Elias, Klumpp, & Przeworski, 2003; Bogels & Mansell, 2004); and tend to *mis*interpret ambiguous interpersonal situations as threatening (Amir, Beard, & Przeworski, 2005; Hirsch & Clark, 2004; Stopa & Clark, 2000; Yoon & Zinbarg, 2008). If these social cognitive affective processes are abnormal in SAD, then examining the stress-related neuroendocrine system on the structure and/or function of relevant brain areas may further our knowledge about the underlying biological mechanisms that cause and/or maintain the symptoms and behaviors of patients with the disorder.

In the past two decades, substantial advances have been made in the neurobiology of stress and of fear from animal, lesion, and human studies. By extension, these advances have been translated into clinical investigations of patients with SAD. In this chapter, we provide a qualitative review and synthesis of the extant literature on the neuroendocrinology and neuroanatomy of SAD.

NEUROENDOCRINOLOGY OF SOCIAL ANXIETY DISORDER

The neuroendocrine response to stress involves the activation of the hypothalamic-pituitary-adrenal (HPA) axis, represented by a cascade of interactive neuroactive hormones, starting with the peptide corticotropin-releasing hormone (CRH) from the hypothalamus, which stimulates release of adrenocorticotropin hormone (ACTH) from the pituitary gland, which in turn evokes adrenal release of glucocorticoids such as cortisol. Cortisol is an extensively used stress marker as it modulates mental and physical states associated with stress.

Methods of evaluating HPA axis function include the measurement of stress hormones in the context of diurnal variation (i.e., basal levels) (Brown, Koob, & Rivier, 1991; Erickson, Drevets, & Schulkin, 2003; Khan, King, Abelson, & Liberzon, 2009). Normal HPA activity is associated with circadian rhythm and therefore fluctuates, with relatively elevated levels in the early morning and low levels in the evening. Another measure of HPA function is the dexamethasone suppression test (DST), which involves the administration of a synthetic glucocorticoid that suppresses plasma ACTH and cortisol concentrations. Behavioral challenges (a "psychological stressor" such as public speaking) permit investigation of endogenous cortisol levels in response to stress. Additionally, the administration of exogenous glucocorticoids (e.g., cortisone), which is metabolized into endogenous cortisol or pharmacological panicogens (e.g., pentagastrin) allows for the manipulation of stress hormones.

With regard to basal state, a number of studies have failed to find evidence of abnormal HPA activity in terms of circadian or morning cortisol levels (Furlan, DeMartinis, Schweizer, Rickels, & Lucki, 2001; Potts, Davidson,

Krishnan, Doraiswamy, & Ritchie, 1991; Uhde, Tancer, Gelernter, & Vittone, 1994; van Veen et al., 2008). Moreover, Uhde and colleagues (1994) reported an absence of HPA-axis over under-activity from DST challenge in SP patients. One subsequent DST study (van Veen et al., 2008) reported that SAD patients had normal levels of cortisol but higher diurnal and post-dexamethasone alpha-amylase (sAA) levels, a putative index of ANS stimulation, suggesting a relatively increased activity of the ANS as compared to the HPA axis, in line with the observed hyperarousal in SAD.

Unlike basal-state studies, cortisol reactivity in response to psychological stressors that often provoke anxiety may capture HPA axis dysregulation in SAD and reflect the real-life social situations feared and avoided by patients. Furlan and colleagues (2001) investigated salivary cortisol reactivity in SAD subjects while performing a speech task and showed mixed results. Although some patients exhibited enhanced cortisol release, more than half exhibited a similar or lower cortisol response relative to controls. Interestingly, those subjects who "responded" to the stressor showed a robust (90%) increase in cortisol from public speaking, in the context of similar state anxiety levels to controls. Interestingly, social phobics did not differ from controls in terms of their cortisol response to a physical exercise (nonsocial) challenge. Subsequently, Condren, O'Neill, Ryan, Barrett, & Thakore (2002) had subjects perform cognitive tasks (i.e., subtraction and digit span), instead of public speaking, in front of an audience; the authors showed that the SAD group exhibited increased cortisol levels (in terms of greater delta max cortisol response). More recently, Roelofs and colleagues (2009) investigated whether increased cortisol stress-responsiveness is linked to increased social avoidance behavior in SAD patients. The study involved two tasks: a social approach-avoidance task (AA-task) in a baseline condition and in a social stress condition (Trier Social Stress Test; TSST). The authors showed that patients with SAD had exaggerated cortisol responses to the TSST and that the extent of cortisol reactivity was positively associated with extent of social avoidance behavior in patients with SAD.

Although the above studies suggest some consistency, other studies have reported *under*-reactivity of the HPA stress response during public speaking. For example, Beaton et al. (2006) showed that SAD patients had lower salivary cortisol levels than controls, before and after a speech task. Similarly, in a study of male college students (Shirotsuki et al., 2009), those with high trait social anxiety exhibited lower cortisol reactivity to a psychosocial stressor compared to those with low trait social anxiety.

Given that SAD often appears before adulthood, two studies have investigated HPA axis reactivity to public speaking in children and adolescents. First, Martel and colleagues (1999) measured salivary cortisol levels during normal daily activities and immediately before and after a modified Trier Social Stress Test TSST, which involves performance tasks (i.e., an unprepared speech mental arithmetic task) in front of a panel/audience conveying no feedback. Both

SP subjects and controls showed significant elevations in cortisol levels prior to the TSST and prior to attending school, but no between-group differences were detected. More recently, elevated cortisol reactivity to public speaking was also observed in prepubertal subjects with SAD compared to controls; in that study, trait, but not state, anxiety was associated with HPA reactivity, indicating that subjects may have been predisposed to develop SAD (van West, Sulon, & Deboutte, 2008).

To complement "psychosocial" stressors, some investigators have pursued paradigms that involve pharmacological induction or mimic of the stress response. In one study (Katzman, Koszycki, & Bradwejn, 2004), the panicogenic sensitivity to CCK-tetrapeptide (CCK-4) was not observed in SAD; moreover, CCK-4 did not induce enhanced cortisol release. Soravia et al. (2006) demonstrated that a low dose of exogenous glucocorticoids (i.e., cortisone administration) versus placebo on stress response in individuals with SAD while undergoing the TSST reduced subjective fear.

The Roelofs et al. (2009) study reported that patients with SAD showed greater cortisol reactivity to social stress than patients with PTSD, another anxiety disorder in which a preponderance of evidence exists for an HPA axis dysregulation. Elzinga, Spinhoven, Berretty, de Jong, and Roelofs, 2009 examined HPA sensitization due to early aversive events by measuring cortisol response to an TSST challenge in individuals with SAD with a history of childhood abuse (SAD + CA), SA individuals without such a history (SAD – CA), individuals with PTSD, and healthy controls. Results showed that the SAD + CA group had significantly elevated cortisol to the threat-relevant stressor compared to the SAD – CA PTSD control group and healthy control group, despite similar self-reported anxiety among the patient groups relative to the control group.

In summary, studies of HPA reactivity have examined basal cortisol levels, reactivity in response to stress, and administration of glucocorticoid. Findings indicate basal cortisol levels are normal in SAD (Furlan et al., 2001; Potts et al., 1991; Uhde et al., 1994; van Veen et al., 2008) even in the context of exaggerated autonomic activity (van Veen et al., 2008). In contrast, studies on cortisol responses to stress challenges (e.g., public speaking/TSST) have shown an inconsistent set of findings, suggesting that the role of HPA reactivity to social threat paradigms may be more complex.

The absence of clear and convincing evidence of an enhanced sensitivity to public speaking and other performance-related tasks is puzzling given that fear of public scrutiny is a core clinical feature of SAD. In a recent meta-analysis, Dickerson and Kemeny (2004) showed that tasks containing both uncontrollable and social-evaluative elements, such as the TSST, were associated with the most robust cortisol and ACTH changes and the longest times to recovery, compared to those that simply evoke subjective distress (without threat to self-esteem/fear of negative evaluation) and fatigue. Therefore, one possible explanation for the absence of findings of exaggerated cortisol reactivity to public performance in SAD is the "ceiling" effect; that is, since both control and SAD participants exhibit such a pronounced cortisol response to tasks such as the TSST, the detection of a group difference becomes more difficult. That said, Young, Abelson, and Cameron (2004) showed that SAD subjects with comorbid depression *did* show enhanced HPA axis reactivity to public speaking but "pure" social phobics did not, which a "ceiling" effect would account for. The Soravia et al. (2006) study hints at a complex interaction between social stress, subjective fear, and cortisol. In that report, stress-induced cortisol release was *negatively* correlated with self-rated fear, and exogenous administration one hour prior to public performance reduced fear during anticipation, exposure, and recovery. These data suggest that cortisol may not be a biomarker of fear/anxiety from social stress but rather may serve a protective role in situations involving social stress.

The finding that SAD with aversive childhood experiences had increased cortisol reactivity relative to SA individuals without a past of abuse may also contribute to mixed findings (Elzinga et al., 2009). Furthermore, individual differences such as repressive coping style, characterized by elevated autonomic physiological responses to stress but reduced self-reported anxiety (Weinberger, Schwartz, & Davidson, 1979), may be related to cortisol effects, as evidenced in healthy controls (Brown et al., 1996). In general, inconsistent results suggest that discrete branches of the stress system are involved in adaptation to stress contributing to either increased or decrease cortisol reactivity. Individual differences in response to symptom provocation (e.g., avoidance behavior, attentional vigilance, or self-focus; Bogels & Mansell, 2004; Rapee & Heimberg, 1997) and chronicity of perceived stress may also relate to the variability in the extent of dysregulation of HPA axis function.

Moreover, the presence of comorbidity such as depression as shown in the Young et al. (2004) study, may impact HPA reactivity. Therefore, the findings noted above may or may not be specific to SAD, given that it often co-occurs with other anxiety disorders (e.g., generalized anxiety, PD) and mood disorders such as depression. That said, the HPA profile in SAD may differ to that in other stress-related disorders such as PTSD. For example, unlike SAD, PTSD is associated with lower basal cortisol levels than controls and appears to have a cortisol profile (e.g., HPA sensitization) that differs from that of depression (for review see Handwerger, 2009). Although Elzinga et al. (2009) did not find cortisol reactivity in response to stress in PTSD, they propose this may have been due to differences in the types and severity of abuse and trauma between PTSD patients and SAD patients. In general, PTSD is associated with HPA axis hyperactivity (Khan et al., 2009). Regarding PD, there is evidence of HPA axis hyperactivity (Abelson, Khan, Liberzon, & Young, 2007), yet panic attacks in panic patients and normal individuals do not appear to activate the HPA axis (Graeff, Garcia-Leal, Del-Ben, & Guimaraes, 2005); therefore, general phobic fear of panic attacks may relate to HPA axis hyperactivity. Although further study is needed to draw conclusions regarding the specificity of neuroendocrine dysregulation in SAD, limited findings indicate that cortisol reactivity to stress from social evaluative threat stress may be a promising biomarker in a subset of individuals with SAD. In particular, the cortisol reactivity has been shown to predict stress-induced increase in social avoidance tendencies over and above the effects of blood pressure and subjective anxiety (Roelofs et al., 2009). Indeed, future studies are needed to pursue the role of HPA function in the context of aberrant social behavior (e.g., avoidance) and/or cognitive processing (e.g., misinterpretation of social events) in SAD. Such studies may be more fruitful than those that attempt to differentiate groups with and without the disorder.

NEUROANATOMY OF SOCIAL ANXIETY DISORDER

Brain Imaging and Neurophysiological Approaches

Human brain imaging provides a unique opportunity to examine the integrity of these neural substrates in psychiatric disorders *in vivo* by providing data on structural and/or morphometric changes, functional neuroanatomy, neurochemistry, and brain receptor systems (Frackowiack, Zeki, Ashburner, Friston, & Frith, 2003; Friston, 1998; Gordon, 1999). As one of the first brain imaging techniques used in psychiatric research, computerized axial tomography can be used to measure total brain volumes and the size of brain structures and ventricles. However, its utility in assessing brain morphology is somewhat limited by its resolution, including separation of white and gray matter, and by its exposure to radiation. Some of these limitations were overcome by MRI, which provides a higher resolution anatomical image and does not require the use of radiation, and via diffusion tensor imaging (DTI), which avails the opportunity to examine the structural integrity and pathways of WM tracts that represent connections between regions. Functional brain imaging depicts the brain as it carries out a particular activity in terms of changes in regional metabolism, blood flow, or oxygenation. Current technologies include positron emission tomography (PET) and single photon emission computed tomography (SPECT), which use radionuclide-labeled tracer molecules to measure regional cerebral blood flow (rCBF) and functional MRI (fMRI), which uses the paramagnetic properties of deoxyhemoglobin to mark blood oxygenation changes (referred to as blood oxygen level-dependent (BOLD) signal). All of these serve as, arguably distal, indices of neuronal activity. Coupled with a neurobehavioral task, these techniques can probe anatomic structures that may serve a particular cognitive, affective, or sensory functions. PET also allows for regional measures of brain metabolism (typically by measuring cerebral glucose metabolic rate (GMR)) and neuroreceptor occupancy (receptor PET); PET imaging coupled with a neuropharmacological probe and/or challenge also can be used to activate a specific neurotransmitter system or elicit a set of psychiatric and/or mood symptoms. In addition, techniques such as PET radioligand binding and MRS can be used to quantify neurochemical receptor systems and neurochemistry, respectively. Lastly, complementary measures of cortical brain activity also can be elucidated by electroencephalography (EEG) and similar techniques that measure event-related potentials (ERP).

It should be noted that the preponderance of our knowledge of the "neuroanatomy" of SP is derived from functional neuroimaging studies that probe brain "activation" in response to a stimulus and/or psychological task. Because SAD is an illness marked with abnormal fear response to social-evaluative threat, sensitivity to facial expressions, particularly those that convey negative feedback (i.e., threat, criticism, disapproval) may play a critical role. As such, a number of fMRI studies have employed tasks that have participants view and process emotional expressions from photographs of faces. Also, given that patients with SAD find public performance anxiety-provoking, another often-used functional imaging (PET, fMRI) paradigm is to have participants listen to anxiety-relevant scripts and perform imagery, anticipate the act of public speaking, and give a speech in front of an audience. Moreover, given the idea that anxiety patients have exaggerated aversive learning, some studies have used fear-conditioning paradigms. Other 'tasks' that do not involve fear perception and learning, emotion processing, or anxiety-symptom provocation have probed cognitive and/or social-cognitive function (e.g., sequence learning, mentalizing, appraising negative remarks) or general brain function while at "rest" (while not engaged in a task).

As noted above, dysregulated fear perception and/or affective responding and/or aberrant cognitive functioning (e.g., misinterpretation) may underlie the phenomenological features of SAD. Therefore, using brain imaging and studying the structural and functional integrity of relevant brain areas may further our knowledge about the underlying neuropathophysiology of SP. These domains of brain function (emotion, cognition, social cognition) have been functionally linked to specific neural circuits in humans (Lieberman, 2007; Miller & Cohen, 2001; Ochsner & Gross, 2005; Phan, Wager, Taylor, & Liberzon, 2002), which may differ between patients and healthy controls at the level of structure, function, or neurochemistry. For example, limbic (amygdala) and paralimbic (insula, orbitofrontal cortex (OFC), medial prefrontal cortex (MPFC), rostral anterior cingulate cortex (rACC), retrosplenial cortex including the posterior cingulate cortex (PCC) and adjacent precuneus) brain regions may subserve emotional or affective processing, including the generation and control of emotional (i.e., anxiety) states and emotional memory (Barrett, Mesquita, Ochsner, & Gross, 2007; Davidson, 2002; Maddock, 1999; Paulus & Stein, 2006; Phan et al., 2002). Similarly, the frontal cortex, including the dorsolateral prefrontal cortex (DLPFC), ventrolateral prefrontal cortex (VLPFC), and dorsal portions of the ACC (dACC), have been implicated in studies of working memory, executive function, attention, impulse control, and cognitive control of behavior (Miller & Cohen, 2001). Social neuroscience (Lieberman, 2007) attempts to integrate emotional and cognitive functioning in the context of the individual and her surrounding social environment (e.g., perception of social cues, social interactions), and has highlighted the role of the MPFC, amygdala, and superior temporal sulcus (STS) in governing these functions (Ochsner, 2004). Characterization of the interplay among social, cognitive, and emotional processes poses a major challenge going forward for disciplines engaged in brain imaging of normal human behavior and of patients with psychiatric disorders.

Below, we structure our review of the literature in terms of various types of neuroimaging methodologies: (1) structural brain imaging studies (CT, MRI); (2) functional "activation" studies, which probe areas engaged in relation to a particular affective, cognitive, and/or social task (rCBF PET, fMRI); (2) functional imaging studies of rest disassociated from task demands (GMR PET, fMRI); (3) neurochemical (MRS) and neuroreceptor (receptor PET) imaging studies; and (4) electrophysiological imaging studies (EEG, ERP). Given the scope of this chapter, we will focus on regions commonly highlighted across studies that have been implicated in affective, cognitive, and/or social function.

Structural Brain Imaging

Relative to other anxiety disorders (particularly PTSD) (Ferrari, Busatto, McGuire, & Crippa, 2008), CT and MRI have scarcely been employed to examine volumetric abnormalities in SAD. In the first and only MRI study specific to SAD, Potts and colleagues observed no differences in cerebral, caudate, putamen, or thalamic volumes between SAD subjects and controls (Potts, Davidson, Krishnan, & Doraiswamy, 1994). Although age-related reductions in putamen volumes were greater in SAD (than controls), the extent of this reduction was not associated with symptomatology. Subsequently, using MRI voxel-based morphometry (VBM), Milham and colleagues reported reduced amygdala (only left-sided) in a cohort of pediatric anxiety patients (9 of 17 who carried a SAD diagnosis); a full-brain exploration revealed only subthreshold decreases in gray matter volume in the bilateral VLPFC and precuneus (Milham et al., 2005). However, given the heterogeneity of the sample, specificity to SAD cannot be determined.

Hence, data on structural deficits in SAD are very limited and no studies have specifically implicated abnormal volumes in brain regions associated with affective, cognitive, and/or social function. Our group, using DTI to evaluate microstructural WM connectivity, observed a local reduction in fractional anisotropy (FA), an index of axonal organization, within the uncinate fasciculus, the main WM tract linking the amygdala and OFC (Ghashghaei, Hilgetag, & Barbas, 2007), in SAD patients (relative to controls) (Phan et al., 2009). This finding is consistent with the hypothesis that impaired frontal–amygdala interactions contribute to the hyperactive amygdala reactivity to threat in SAD observed in functional neuroimaging studies (discussed below). Interestingly, Kim and Whalen (2009) recently showed that individual differences in the structural integrity (FA) of this putative amygdala–prefrontal pathway (the uncinate fasciculus) were inversely correlated with trait anxiety levels (i.e., higher FA predicted lower anxiety). Although requiring replication, these findings suggest that structural abnormalities are more likely to be found in the WM tracts that connect limbic and frontal regions than in the absolute volumes of discrete structures.

Functional Brain Imaging: Task-related "Activation" Studies

The amygdala has been under intense focus in a number of functional brain-imaging studies of SAD. In support of this "amygdala-centric" search, findings from animal, human lesion, and nonclinical populations have consistently implicated the amygdala in fear perception, memory/learning, and responding, including aversive conditioning (Davis & Whalen, 2001; LeDoux, 2000; Whalen, 1998; Zald, 2003). Moreover, the amygdala is central to the processing of social signals (e.g., facial expressions, gestures) that convey threat and danger in the immediate environment (Adolphs, 2002). Specifically, humans with bilateral damage of the amygdala are impaired in making accurate judgments on trustworthiness and approachability (from photographs of faces) (Adolphs, Tranel, & Damasio, 1998; Adolphs, Tranel, Damasio, & Damasio, 1994, 1995), and macaque monkeys with neonatal amygdala lesions have enhanced social fear (Emery et al., 2001; Prather et al., 2001). Brain imaging with PET and fMRI has consistently identified amygdala activation to facial expressions of threat/danger (e.g., fear) (Morris et al., 1996; Phillips et al., 2001; Whalen et al., 1998) and to socially threatening/negative faces (e.g., anger, disgust) (Adams, Gordon, Baird, Ambady, & Kleck, 2003; Anderson, Christoff, Panitz, de Rosa, & Gabrieli, 2003; Hariri, Bookheimer, & Mazziotta, 2000; Sato, Yoshikawa, Kochiyama, & Matsumura, 2004; Schienle et al., 2002). Furthermore, the amygdala is activated during evaluative judgments of trust, and the intensity of amygdala activation is related to the level of trustworthiness (Winston, Strange, O'Doherty, & Dolan, 2002). The extent of amygdala reactivity to social stimuli has been shown to predict trait/state anxiety (Somerville, Kim, Johnstone, Alexander, & Whalen, 2004; Stein, Simmons, Feinstein, & Paulus, 2007) and extraversion (Canli, Sivers, Whitfield, Gotlib, & Gabrieli, 2002). There is also evidence that the amygdala plays a critical role in processing social information (Adolphs, 2003), in heightening general vigilance (Davis & Whalen, 2001), and in the perception of emotionally salient, arousing stimuli (Sander, Grafman, & Zalla, 2003; Zald, 2003). A number of clinical studies would therefore support the notion that amygdala dysfunction may underlie the symptoms and behavior of patients with SP. Individuals with SAD exhibit an attentional and recall bias towards threat-related material (Amir et al., 2000, 2003; Mogg & Bradley, 2002; Mogg et al., 2004; Pishyar, Harris, & Menzies, 2004); recall all faces in general better than nonanxious controls (Foa, Gilboa-Schechtman, Amir, & Freshman, 2000); recall negative faces in particular better than accepting (e.g., happy) emotional faces (Foa et al., 2000); and have a recognition bias for critical faces relative to nonanxious controls (Coles & Heimberg, 2005; Lundh & Ost, 1996). Moreover, patients exhibit avoidance of social situations that are anxiety-provoking (Amir, Foa, & Coles, 1998; Ly & Roelofs, 2009); and often mistrust and/or misinterpret social information as threatening (Hirsch & Clark, 2004). As such, there is good reason to expect that aberrant amygdala function in threat and social processing may underlie the sensitivity, biases, hypervigilance, and phobic avoidance observed in patients with SP.

Besides the amygdala, there is increasing interest in improving our understanding of the role of the insula in SAD and other anxiety disorders (Paulus & Stein, 2006). The insula is a part of the paralimbic cortex with substantial reciprocal connections with the amygdala (Augustine, 1996). It is integral to mind-body interactions (Craig, 2002), as evidenced by its involvement in the interplay of threat perception and bodily states of arousal, which contribute to aversive emotional experiences (Critchley, Mathias, & Dolan, 2002). Additionally, it is proposed to link emotion processing with cognitive and behavioral responses (Nitschke, Sarinopoulos, Mackiewicz, Schaefer, & Davidson, 2006); specifically, anticipation of an aversive body state triggers an increase in anxiety and worry and promotes avoidance behaviors (Paulus & Stein, 2006). According to the cognitive model of Clark and Wells, attention to internal physiological cues plays a central role in maintaining social anxiety, as self-focused attention interferes with the processing of nonthreatening information (Clark & McManus, 2002; Clark & Wells, 1995). Therefore, this enhanced self-focus on one's own bodily sensations (flushing, heart racing, sweating) may be represented by insular hypersensitivity in SAD.

Dysfunction of the frontal cortex (including the ACC, OFC, MPFC, VLPFC, and DLPFC) is also predicted in the pathophysiology of SAD. Taken together, this constellation of regions is well known for its role in attention and vigilance, cognitive control of behavior, and integration of cognitive-emotion function (Bush, Luu, & Posner, 2000), as well as in the regulation of emotional responding and of fear learning (Ochsner & Gross, 2005; Quirk & Beer, 2006), processes relevant to anxiety disorders in general (Shin & Liberzon, 2009). In particular, MPFC has been implicated in social cognition, particularly in mentalizing (the ability to understand the mental states of others), which may be related to the accurate interpretation of social signals, a process that may be dysfunctional in SAD (Clark & McManus, 2002).

In addition, reward circuitry and regions that regulate motor control/learning such as the basal ganglia (dorsal and ventral striatum, caudate, putamen) may be relevant in SAD. This notion is supported by studies showing a high incidence of SP in persons with Parkinson's disease, a hypodopaminergic disorder localized to the striatum (Richard, Schiffer, & Kurlan, 1996; Stein, Heuser, Juncos, & Uhde, 1990). Also, treatment of Tourette's disorder with dopamine (DA) antagonists can induce social anxiety (Mikkelsen, Detlor, & Cohen, 1981).

Animal models such as subordination implicated low levels of striatal DA (Grant et al., 1998).

Emotional Face Processing

Facial expressions are potent nonverbal cues that facilitate social communication and motivate approach or avoidance behaviors (Ekman, 2003), and serve as ecologically valid probes of social anxiety symptoms. In particular, reliable circuitry is engaged in processing the social information decoded from faces, including the amygdala, fusiform gyrus (fusiform face area (FFA)), inferior frontal gyrus (IFG)/OFC, and STS (Adolphs, 1999, 2002).

In an fMRI study of patients with GSP engaged in the processing of emotional faces, Stein and colleagues were among the first to demonstrate that the amygdala exhibits greater activation to "harsh" (angry, fearful, and contemptuous) faces that convey negative feedback than those that connote acceptance/approval (happy); in addition, the authors observed greater BOLD response in the dorsal MPFC, IFG, uncus, and parahippocampal gyrus (pHG) (Stein, Goldin, Sareen, Zorrilla, & Brown, 2002). Interestingly, it was noted that significant group differences in amygdala reactivity were specific to angry and contemptuous faces, although the pattern for fearful faces was similar in direction (GSP > controls).

Using a similar set of "harsh" faces, our laboratory has also shown that the amygdala reactivity to "harsh" faces is enhanced in patients with GSP (relative to controls) (Phan, Fitzgerald, Nathan, & Tancer, 2006). Importantly, no group differences in the amygdala were noted in the happy (vs. control radio stimuli) or in the neutral (vs. control radio stimuli) faces, suggesting that the observed differences in activation to the harsh faces between GSP and HC subjects were not contributed to by differences between these groups during the reference/control conditions. Each of the three "harsh" expressions (fearful, angry, disgusted) separately evoked greater amygdala activation in the GSP group (relative to controls). Outside the amygdala, we also observed hyper-reactivity in the postcentral sulcus, pHG, and dorsal ACC.

Other studies have examined brain reactivity more specifically to certain negative expressions (disgusted faces, fearful faces, and angry faces separately). Amir and colleagues showed that patients with SAD exhibited greater activation to disgusted (vs. neutral) faces in rACC, dACC, caudate, insula, lingual gyrus, pHG, STG, and middle frontal gyrus most consistently across "runs" within the fMRI session (Amir, Klumpp, et al., 2005). Using a novel schematic face paradigm, Evans and colleagues (2008) demonstrated greater response to angry (vs. neutral) faces in the amygdala, superior frontal cortex, and ACC, and to angry (vs. happy) faces in the lingual gyrus, fusiform gyrus, precentral gyrus, insula, PCC, middle frontal gyrus, and middle temporal gyrus. Similarly, Straube and coauthors also observed greater amygdala activation to angry and fearful faces (but not neutral ones) in social phobics (relative to controls)

(Straube, Mentzel, & Miltner, 2005). Increased insula activation to angry faces (vs. neutral faces) was also observed in SAD patients while they explicitly assessed either emotional expression or nonemotional aspects of faces (Straube, Kolassa, Glauer, Mentzel, & Miltner, 2004). In an implicit task in which subjects were asked to identify whether the stimulus was a photograph or a schematic, subjects with SAD also showed more insular activation to photographic angry faces (Straube et al., 2004). Similarly, under a passive viewing condition, individuals with SAD demonstrated increased bilateral insula activation in response to angry faces but not to neutral or happy faces (Straube et al., 2005). These patterns found by Straube and colleagues were not observed in the control groups. Blair and colleagues recently reported that GSP subjects show greater amygdala and frontal polar/MPFC reactivity to fearful, but not angry, faces (vs. neutral faces) than controls (Blair, Shaywitz, et al., 2008). Collectively, these studies demonstrate that, relative to happy and/or neutral faces, those that express negative affect (anger, fear, and/or disgust) evoke a greater response from the amygdala in adults with SAD (Blair, Shaywitz, et al., 2008; Evans et al., 2008; Phan et al., 2006; Straube et al., 2005). Moreover, three of these studies showed that the extent of amygdala response to these threatening social signals predicts the level of social anxiety (Evans et al., 2008; Phan et al., 2006) or of general anxiety (Blair, Shaywitz, et al., 2008).

Interestingly, in the Blair, Shaywitz et al. study, the authors also observed that SAD had greater reactivity to fear (vs. neutral) faces in the middle frontal gyrus/frontal polar cortex, lateral frontal cortex, anterior cingulate cortex, and temporal cortex compared to generally anxious (GAD) patient controls and psychiatrically healthy controls. Although exaggerated amygdala activation to fear faces was observed in SAD subjects, the GAD group demonstrated reduced amygdala activation to fear faces compared to SAD and healthy controls, suggesting that limbic, namely amygdala, function in response to social threat appears to differ between SAD and GAD.

There have been relatively fewer studies of children and adolescents with SP, though there is some evidence that this pattern of amygdala hyperreactivity to negative faces exists in younger participants. First, adolescents with anxiety (SAD and/or GAD) exhibit greater amygdala reactivity to fearful (than happy) faces (Beesdo et al., 2009). Second, amygdala activity to fearful faces in adolescents has also positively correlated with social/interpersonal scales (e.g., peer rejection, humiliation, performing in public) but not with nonsocial dimensions of anxiety (Killgore & Yurgelun-Todd, 2005). Taken together, there is substantial evidence that both youth and adult patients with SAD have a hypersensitive amygdala response to negative feedback, as conveyed from fearful, angry, and/or contemptuous faces.

Although most studies have shown hyperactive amygdala reactivity to these harsh/negative faces, there is evidence that amygdala reactivity in SAD to other facial expressions may also be exaggerated, as shown by a number of studies that have focused on amygdala function. Initially, Birbaumer and colleagues

(1998) observed that patients with SP, but not controls, showed an amygdala response to "neutral" faces paired with an aversive odor. Interestingly, this group reported that the SP group exhibited this hyperactive amygdala response to neutral faces even *prior* to aversive condition and continued to exhibit amygdala hyper-reactivity during the "habituation" phase (Veit et al., 2002). More recently, Cooney, Atlas, Joormann, Eugene, and Gotlib (2006) showed that SAD participants had greater amygdala reactivity to neutral faces during an appraisal task and were more likely to assign a negative valence to these faces (although not significantly more so than controls). Complementary facial cues such as the direction of eye gaze also may also convey a sense of "threat" from an otherwise neutral face. In support of this notion, Schneier, Kent, Star, and Hirsch (2009) found that patients with SAD had greater amygdala activation to neutral faces when the eye gaze was directed at them as opposed to away from them; this study also reported greater responses in the insula, associated frontal regions (rACC, MPFC), and FFA in SAD in response to direct gaze. There is an increasing appreciation that "neutral" expressions confer ambiguity and evoke amygdala response in the service of decoding the information from a "neutral" face (Somerville et al., 2004; Wright & Liu, 2006). Given that SAD is associated with negative bias from "neutral" and/or ambiguous social signals (Amir, Beard, et al., 2005), it would be sensible to expect an enhanced amygdala response to neutral expressions.

It can be posited that patients with SAD have acquired an aversive response to "neutral" faces. Beyond processing social information from faces, the amygdala is also critical to fear learning (e.g., conditioning). Consistent with animal studies (LeDoux, 2000), a number of human neuroimaging studies have observed amygdala reactivity during the acquisition of fear, for example when an association is formed between a previously unconditioned neutral stimulus (CS; e.g., a tone) with an aversive unconditioned stimulus (US; e.g., a shock) (see reviews by Phelps, 2004; Sehlmeyer et al., 2009). Consistently with the view that SAD involves exaggerated aversive learning (and subsequent avoidance), amygdala reactivity appears to be enhanced during fear conditioning in SAD patients, particularly when presented with a "neutral" face previously paired with an aversive event (e.g., aversive odor) (Birbaumer et al., 1998; Schneider et al., 1999; Veit et al., 2002). However, all of these fear-conditioning paradigms involved "neutral" faces as the CS and no study has employed nonface CS stimuli, and thus these findings cannot be fully generalizable to fear conditioning in general.

Furthermore, there are at least two studies that have demonstrated enhanced amygdala responsivity to happy faces in SAD (Evans et al., 2008; Straube et al., 2005). It has previously been suggested that the amygdala in SAD participants does not activate to happy faces because such faces convey a tone of acceptance and approval (Phan et al., 2006; Stein, Goldin, et al., 2002); these subsequent findings would therefore contradict that idea. Initially, Straube et al. (2005) demonstrated that social phobics, relative to controls, had greater amygdala reactivity to happy (but not neutral) faces. Evans and colleagues (2008) also showed that SAD patients had greater amygdala responses to happy (relative to neutral) schematic faces than control subjects. One explanation for these findings is that the amygdala, which does appear to activate to happy faces in healthy volunteers (Fitzgerald, Angstadt, Jelsone, Nathan, & Phan, 2006; Yang, Menon, Reid, Gotlib, & Reiss, 2003), may show greater reactivity in phobic participants because it is responding to the arousal dimension of affective stimuli rather than their valence (i.e., negative vs. positive) (Liberzon, Phan, Decker, & Taylor, 2003; Phan et al., 2003) and/or to the attention or task demands (Williams, McGlone, Abbott, & Mattingley, 2005). Supportive of this notion, we have previously shown that individuals with SAD, compared with healthy controls, exhibited greater amygdala response to faces expressing emotions at high (vs. moderate) intensity (Yoon, Fitzgerald, Angstadt, McCarron, & Phan, 2007). An alternative interpretation recently emerged from Campbell and colleagues (2009), who showed that individuals with GSP rated happy faces as less approachable than controls and that higher social anxiety severity was associated with lower approachability ratings; they proposed that patients with GSP have explicit, subjective social interpretation biases to overtly presented positive feedback. Complementary research has suggested that happy faces may be interpreted as reflecting mockery or misrepresented as another form of threat signal (e.g., social dominance, higher social expectations, disingenuous expression) (Alden & Taylor, 2004; Coles & Heimberg, 2005; Yoon & Zinbarg, 2007).

As noted, numerous studies have observed impaired amygdala and/or frontal cortical function when processing faces that convey negative feedback in SAD. There is increasing evidence that amygdala–frontal interactions are critical during emotion processing, particular when the regulation of negative emotional states is required (Banks, Eddy, Angstadt, Nathan, & Phan, 2007; Ochsner & Gross, 2005; Wager, Davidson, Hughes, Lindquist, & Ochsner, 2008). Among the first to extend these emotion regulation "activation" paradigms into SAD, Goldin, Manber, Hakimi, Canli, and Gross (2009) deployed a well-validated emotion regulation technique (e.g., reappraisal; Gross, 1999) and examined amygdala and frontal function while subjects with SAD attempted to reduce negative affect evoked by "harsh" face stimuli and negative nonsocial images. Correlational analysis showed a positive relationship between SAD symptom severity and activity in the amygdala and middle occipital gyrus when viewing harsh faces, consistent with prior studies (Evans et al., 2008; Phan et al., 2006), but not when viewing negative scenes or during emotion regulation. Additionally, for viewing harsh faces (vs. neutral scenes), SAD patients compared to controls exhibited exaggerated activation in OFC, ACC, and pHG, again consistent with prior studies (Phan et al., 2006; Stein, Goldin, et al., 2002). Unlike controls, SAD patients failed to engage the DLPFC, dACC, and PCC (and the dorsal parietal, fusiform, and superior temporal gyrus) when instructed to reappraise harsh faces. For violent scenes, the reappraisal task engaged greater activation of the DLPFC and lentiform/caudate in SAD subjects (vs. controls). These findings represent the first evidence of dysfunctional frontal cortical function during the cognitive regulation of negative social cues in SAD.

Symptom Provocation – Public Speaking

As previously stated, the key feature of SAD is excessive anxiety about embarrassment in situations in which there is potential scrutiny. Therefore, it is no surprise that neuroimaging studies in SAD have utilized several provocation paradigms to induce social and performance anxiety, with the assumption that the symptom induction would evoke neural substrates responsible for the generation of social anxiety symptoms. Specifically, these studies involve anticipation of and/or participation in public speaking, which reliably evokes anxiety and psychological distress in patients with SAD.

In a PET study, Tillfors and colleagues (2001) found that, during public versus private speaking, subjective anxiety increased more in the social phobics (than controls) and that there was enhanced blood flow to the amygdaloid complex in the social phobics relative to the comparison subjects. In the orbitofrontal, temporal, and insular cortices, rCBF decreased in the SAD group, whereas there was an increase in rCBF in these areas in the control group during public compared to private speaking. Additionally, the SAD group had less increase in rCBF in the parietal and secondary visual cortices compared to the controls. Likewise, rCBF in the perirhinal and retrosplenial cortices increased in the control group, but not in the SAD group.

In a follow-up PET study, these authors also scanned SAD subjects while speaking alone either before or after speaking in public and showed that anticipatory anxiety was associated with increased heart rate, subjective anxiety, and enhanced rCBF in the left amygdaloid-hippocampal region, which was accompanied by enhanced cerebral blood flow in the right DLPFC and left inferior temporal cortex (Tillfors, Furmark, Marteinsdottir, & Fredrikson, 2002). These observations have been replicated by Lorberbaum and colleagues (2004) who measured BOLD-fMRI brain activity and showed that GSP patients (more so than controls) activated the amygdala while anticipating making public speeches. Moreover, these authors reported greater subcortical, limbic, and paralimbic activity (pons, striatum, uncus/anterior parahippocampus, insula, temporal pole), and less frontal cortical activity (dorsal ACC, MPFC, DLPFC), suggesting that, in the context of anticipation-related anxiety, less frontal activity is engaged for cognitive processing in social phobics, or, alternatively, less frontal engagement leads to greater limbic reactivity.

Interestingly, Furmark and colleagues (2002) have also shown that "responders" to treatment with the SSRI citalopram medication and cognitive behavioral group therapy (CBGT) exhibited a decreased rCBF response to public speaking bilaterally in the amygdale. Between-group comparisons confirmed that rCBF in these regions decreased significantly more in treated groups than in wait-list control subjects and in responders than nonresponders; moreover, the degree of amygdala attenuation was associated with clinical improvement when these subjects were reassessed a year later (Furmark, 2002). In the CBGT group, rCBF also decreased in the periaqueductal gray area, while increases were noted in the right cerebellum and the secondary visual cortex. In the citalopram group, rCBF decreased in the left thalamus and left IFG. Responders exhibited rCBF decreases in the right IFG, DLPFC, and ACC. In the between-group comparison, rCBF decreased more in responders than nonresponders in the right DLPFC and ACC. These treatment-mediated effects were replicated in a subsequent randomized double-blind placebo-controlled study involving the NK1 antagonist GR205171 and citalopram in which the authors demonstrated that symptom improvement was accompanied by reduced rCBF response to public speaking in the amygdala and nearby parahippocampal–hippocampal regions (Furmark et al., 2005).

Based on the notion that individuals with SAD tend to focus on themselves (e.g., attend to interoceptive cues and negative thoughts (Clark & McManus, 2002; Clark & Wells, 1995)), van Ameringen et al. (2004) diverted from traditional speech paradigms and instructed participants to watch a videotape of either (1) a socially competent stranger giving a talk (baseline condition) or (2) themselves giving a talk in the presence of three confederates (exposure condition). Compared to the baseline condition, there was a significant decrease in rCBF in the right lingual gyrus and the right medial frontal gyrus during the exposure condition, which the authors suggest reflects the possibility that individuals with GSP were diverting their attention away from the anxiety-provoking stimuli (i.e., video clips of themselves giving an impromptu speech). Due to the absence of a normal control group, however, it is not clear whether the deactivation found in the GSP is an abnormal response specific to social anxiety psychopathology.

Symptoms in response to threatening stimuli frequently include hyperarousal (e.g., increased heart rate) and anxiety disorders are associated with cardiac disease. In a study by Ahs, Sollers, Furmark, Fredrikson, and Thayer (2009), PET was used to examine high-frequency heart rate variability (HF-HRV) and brain function during public speaking in SAD. The results revealed positive correlations between HF-HRV and cerebral blood flow in the ACC, caudate head, and MPFC extending into the DLPFC in SAD; no significant negative correlations were revealed.

It should be noted that not all studies of public performance have observed amygdala hyper-reactivity in SAD patients. Using PET, Kilts and colleagues (2006) examined rCBF during script-guided mental imagery of an anxiogenic social situation and a confrontational mental arithmetic task before and after treatment with nefazodone. SAD subjects exhibited increased activity in the left postcentral gyrus and lenticulate and the right inferior frontal and middle temporal gyri to the social imagery task, and activation of the MPFC, DLPFC, cerebellum, thalamus, insula, and ventral striatum to the arithmetic task. Interestingly, both tasks were associated with relative *decreases* in activity in the right amygdala and the hippocampus. The authors also observed greater activity in the precentral gyrus, insula, midbrain/hypothalamus, and middle frontal and anterior cingulate gyrus prior to treatment, and greater activity in the left middle occipital and bilateral lingual gyri, postcentral gyrus, gyrus rectus, and hippocampus after treatment. The authors suggest that the distributed neural activity is consistent with cognitive models of SAD during these tasks and adaptive decreases in amygdala activity in response to the provocation of social anxiety.

In summary, there is some evidence of increased limbic reactivity and reduced cortical activation in response to the anxiety-provoking stress of public speaking and its anticipation. Additionally, some evidence of reduced frontal cortical activation during anticipation and anticipation of a speech task has been proposed to reflect dysregulated control of attention or impaired cognitive function when regulation of stress is needed. This pattern deactivation of cortical areas relevant to emotional appraisal and regulation could indicate possible deficits in cognitive evaluative or self-regulatory processes in SAD under stress.

Social Interactions

Little information about the psychological processes of appraisal and interpretation can be ascertained by examining brain response to static face photographs. The underlying cause of the exaggerated social fear response is unknown but could partly be due to deficits in social cognition that manifest as a tendency towards inaccurate and distorted interpretations of the beliefs and intentions of others during interpersonal interactions (Hirsch & Clark, 2004). However, the use of static face stimuli in elucidating social cognitive deficits in GSAD is likely to be limited, since they primarily engage *perception* of emotional signals and do not reflect real-world social interactions that are inherently dynamic and interactive. To address this critical gap in knowledge, Guyer and colleagues (2008) developed an fMRI paradigm to examine fear-circuitry dysfunction in the context of anticipated social evaluation, which may result in the misperception of threat from peers, to determine whether photographs of negatively evaluated smiling peers viewed during anticipated social evaluation engage the amygdala in adolescents with and without social anxiety. Here, the participants classified photos of same-age peers on whether they would or would not like to engage in a social interaction. The authors demonstrated that socially anxious adolescents had a greater (than nonanxious controls) amygdala, ACC, and middle frontal gyrus response when anticipating interactions and evaluations previously classified as undesirable to interact with. Given the nature of the paradigm, the authors were able to examine functional amygdala–frontal connectivity and observed a positive correlation between the right amygdala seed and left VLPFC while appraising low-versus-high-desirability peers (observed only in patients during appraisal of low-desirability peers) and observed that lower self-esteem and higher anxiety severity were associated with the pattern of positive connectivity.

Along the lines of heightened sensitivity to perceived threat, individuals may have difficulty making context-dependent assumptions about others' behaviors, as evidenced by nonimaging studies that show negative interpretive bias in SAD (Amir et al., 1998; Hirsch & Mathews, 1997; Hirsch & Clark, 2004; Stopa & Clark, 2000). With this background, we recently employed an "interactive" social task (e.g., the trust game) (Sripada et al., 2009) in which participants engage in an economic exchange with fictive partners who vary in the likelihood of reciprocity (e.g., sharing invested money) and probe the ability of participants to predict another player's actions based on reputation built over time ("mentalizing"). Human (vs. computer) results included the finding that the SAD group had greater activation in the middle frontal gyrus and supplementary motor area than controls. Moreover, patients exhibited hyporeactive (less activity than controls) responses in the MPFC, IFG, cuneus, postcentral gyrus, and middle occipital gyrus to human (vs. computer) partners, whereas controls had less activity than patients in the supplementary motor area, middle frontal gyrus, and supramarginal gyrus. We interpret that the deficient activation of the MPFC, a region increasingly implicated by social neuroscience as part of the brain's social-cognitive network and particularly critical to mentalizing and forming impressions about others (Frith & Frith, 2006; Gallagher & Frith, 2003; Mitchell, Neil Macrae, & Banaji, 2005), may partly explain tendencies of patients with GSAD to form distorted impressions about how others judge them and about social events more generally (Stopa & Clark, 2000). Preliminary analyses (unpublished data) of this task also show that the amygdala response when interacting with "unfair" partners (those who exhibit low probability of reciprocity) is greater in SAD than control subjects (Phan et al., 2007). Future studies such as these that model real-life and/or socially interactive formats are much needed to model the complexity of social exchange between individuals (Ochsner, 2004).

Negative Emotional Processing

A few studies have implicated limbic and paralimbic frontal dysfunction using nonface, or nonsocial stimuli. In a novel design, Blair, Shaynitz, and colleagues (2008) exposed SAD subjects to negative (e.g., "you are ugly") comments and showed enhanced amygdala and MPFC response in patients to such comments (but not to neutral or positive comments), particularly when those comments were referring to themselves (rather than other people). Given that MPFC regions are involved in representations of the self (Schmitz & Johnson, 2006; van Overwalle, 2008), it might be suggested that this enhanced response, along with amygdala activation, reflects a negative self-image, particularly when faced with self-critical comments. Interestingly, examination of amygdala–frontal connectivity showed that the strength of amygdala–MPFC connectivity was significantly greater for the GSP group relative to the HC group for negative comments about the self, but not for other comment categories.

Another important aspect of interpretation of social situations is appropriate comprehension of emotional prosody. To determine whether neural impairment underlies emotional prosody in SAD, participants performed an emotion-identification task and a gender-identification task during fMRI (Quadflieg, Mohr, Mentzel, Miltner, & Straube, 2008). For the former task, participants identified the emotion conveyed by the utterance and for the latter task the gender of the speaker was determined. All participants showed activation in the amygdala, insula, striatum, and frontotemporal regions in response to angry relative to neutral prosody. However, SAD patients, compared to controls, exhibited greater activation in the OFC across task condition, indicating altered comprehension of emotional prosody in SAD. In prior studies of healthy subjects, the OFC has been previously implicated in processing and regulating responses to angry faces and anger (Blair, Morris, Frith, Perrett, & Dolan, 1999; Coccaro, McCloskey, Fitzgerald, & Phan, 2007; Dougherty et al., 1999).

Our laboratory has also shown that SAD patients show an enhanced amygdala and insula response to nonsocial, negative emotional (aversive, disgust, and fear-inducing) images and that the extent of amygdala activation was associated with social anxiety severity (Shah, Klumpp, Angstadt, Nathan, & Phan, 2009), suggesting a broader implication of amygdala and insular hyper-reactivity in the pathophysiology of SAD. However, given that this was not observed in the study by Goldin and colleagues (2009), who employed "violent" images from the same stimulus set, the findings require replication.

Nonemotional, Nonsocial Cognitive Studies

In an fMRI study that focused on the striatal function, SAD and control participants performed similarly a serial reaction time task (i.e., implicit learning) (Sareen et al., 2007); however, patients had significantly reduced neural activation related to implicit learning in the caudate head, insula, and inferior parietal lobe compared to the control group. This observation of striatal dysfunction fits well with growing evidence from DA receptor PET studies but also with complementary reward-related paradigms. For example, a recent study showed that adolescents who were characterized as behavioral inhibited (a vulnerability trait for subsequent development of SAD), relative to noninhibited adolescents, showed enhanced activation in the ventral striatum when they believed their selection of an action would influence the likelihood of reward but not when actions were predetermined to result in reward or randomly resulted in reward (Guyer et al., 2006). These findings suggest a link between inhibited temperament and altered striatal responses to reward–contingency cues, which have not been explored in patients with SAD.

Summary of "Activation" Studies

In summary, individuals with SAD exhibit exaggerated amygdala reactivity to harsh faces, which is consistent with the notion that these faces convey criticism and negative feedback. Some studies have observed similar reactivity in the amygdala to neutral and happy expressions. Few studies have specifically examined the temporal profile of amygdala reactivity to faces, though there is evidence to suggest that amygdala responses in participants with GSP occurred later (than those observed in controls) (Campbell et al., 2007). In addition, amygdala and insula reactivity to public speaking (performing and anticipation) tasks appear to be enhanced in SAD. Whereas MPFC and other frontal cortical regions (ACC, DLPFC, OFC) are engaged by SAD patients differently nonanxious controls, when presented with self-relevant negative criticism and in the context of peer and human partner interactions, the directionality (increased vs. decreased) of frontal activation patterns has been inconsistent, likely due to methodological (e.g., task-related) differences, and requires further clarification. In relation, future studies are needed to ascertain the underlying social cognitive processes (appraisal/interpretation, and reappraisal) that may occur after stimulus presentation. PEP may account for why "neutral" and happy faces acquire a negative bias (or fail to evoke a positive bias) after or in the context of a dynamic social interaction in patients with SAD; the Goldin et al. (2009) study suggests dysfunction in the cognitive network that subseries the regulation and adaptive processing of negative social cues. Indeed, how patients "internalize" social signals and relate the signals to themselves may influence amygdala and prefrontal reactivity; the Blair, Geraci, et al. (2008) study supports this notion. Moreover, interactive designs (e.g., having patients engage in a social exchange) coupled with fMRI may be better suited to probing the neural mechanisms of these social cognitive process that unfold after the initial perception/processing of cues from a facial expression. We also know very little about the underlying structural anatomy and neurochemistry of the amygdala itself, partly due to lack of investigation, lack of evidence, and/or methodological constraints of brain imaging. Some emerging data exist on aberrant amygdala–cortical/frontal structural and functional relationships, but a more comprehensive understanding of these interactions awaits further studies and advances in signal processing analytic approaches (Wager et al., 2008). Also, it would be relevant to ascertain whether heightened amygdala and insula reactivity and aberrant frontal cortical function is specific to SAD, given that other anxiety disorders such PTSD are also associated with these observations (for review see Etkin & Wager, 2007; Shin & Liberzon, 2009). Interestingly, in the context of emotional face processing, some evidence suggests that amygdala hyper-reactivity to social threat is *not* observed in PD (Pillay, Gruber, Rogowska, Simpson, & Yurgelun-Todd, 2006), specific phobia (Wright, Martis, McMullin, Shin, & Rauch, 2003), and OCD (Cannistraro et al., 2004). Therefore, amygdala hyper-responsivity to social signals may be relatively specific to social anxiety, or anxiety related to social/interpersonal interactions, such as that often observed in PTSD (Hofmann, Litz, & Weathers, 2003). However, few studies to date have directly compared amygdala reactivity to faces or during several emotional, cognitive, and social tasks, across anxiety disorders.

Functional Brain Imaging: 'Resting State' Studies

Though relatively few studies have investigated neural processes in SAD when participants are at rest – that is, not engaged in emotional or cognitive tasks – such investigations are of increasing scientific interest because they permit the examination of potential anomalies that may be masked during activation paradigms. It has been proposed that the brain has an organized, baseline default mode of function that represents its intrinsic state (Raichle et al., 2001). This explanation arose from the consistent observation that activity decreases in functional neuroimaging data when the control state was passive visual fixation or eyes-closed resting or when the brain is actively engaged by a cognitive task (Raichle & Snyder, 2007). Areas that constitute this default mode network (MPFC, PCC, precuneus) can be modulated by different factors such as emotional states, cognitive load of the task, and psychopathology, including anxiety, and, as noted above, these areas play a pivotal role in social cognition.

In one of the first "resting state" studies, Stein and Leslie showed that SAD patients did not differ from controls on basal metabolic cerebral perfusion using SPECT and technetium-99m-hexamethyl-propylenamineoxime (^{99m}Tc-HMPAO) (Stein & Leslie, 1996); however, it should be noted that the authors used an *a priori* region of interest (ROI) analysis based on brain regions previously observed to be abnormal in OCD. In a subsequent SPECT resting perfusion scan in adult subjects with generalized SAD, Warwick, Carey, Jordaan, Dupont, and Stein (2008) showed that SAD subjects had increased resting perfusion in the frontal cortex and right cerebellum and decreased perfusion in the pons, left cerebellum, and right precuneus. Moreover, the authors reported that social anxiety severity correlated positively with left frontal cortex resting perfusion and negatively with right fusiform and right lingual perfusion.

In a previous (^{99m}Tc-HMPAO) SPECT study, Warwick and colleagues measured resting perfusion before and after eight weeks of treatment with either citalopram or the reversible inhibitor of monoamine oxidase (MAOI) moclobemide, and showed in SAD patients in both treatment groups a decrease in rCBF in the insula post-therapy corresponding with symptom improvement; there was a significant relationship between the magnitude of deactivation and the change in symptom severity. Subjects receiving citalopram had decreased superior cingulate rCBF after therapy compared to those receiving moclobemide.

To examine the effects of pharmacotherapy on resting perfusion in SAD, patients with a number of anxiety disorders including SAD were SPECT scanned before and after eight weeks of pharmacotherapy with the SSRI citalopram (Carey et al., 2004). Citalopram treatment resulted in significant deactivation in the superior and anterior cingulate, right thalamus, and left hippocampus. The authors observed that deactivation within the left precentral, right mid-frontal, right inferior frontal, left prefrontal and right precuneus was more marked in treatment responders; however, no pattern of baseline activation distinguished responders from nonresponders in subsequent pharmacotherapy.

Using a similar approach but with [^{18}F] fluorodeoxyglucose (FDG) PET, Evans et al. (2009) examined resting state and treatment effects on regional cerebral metabolic rate of glucose uptake (rCMRglu) before and after treatment with tiagabine, a gamma-aminobutyric acid (GABA) reuptake inhibitor, in SAD patients. Compared to the controls, individuals with gSAD demonstrated less pretreatment rCMRglu within the ACC and ventral MPFC at baseline. Following tiagabine treatment, ventral MPFC rCMRglu increased significantly in the patient group, and treatment response was inversely correlated with pretreatment resting metabolism in this region.

Recently, using fMRI, Gentili and colleagues (2009) examined task-induced deactivations within the default network by examining "activity" in these areas during a conventional face-processing task in patients with SAD. The authors reported that, although both groups exhibited the typical pattern of deactivation observed in MPFC, ACC, and PCC, the SAD group, relative to controls, showed a lower deactivation in the precuneus and posterior cingulate regions (PCC, precuneus) during task conditions. Given the role of the PCun/PCC in self-state perception and attribution and more generally in social cognition, the authors speculated that its impairment in SAD might be relevant in the development worries others' regarding evaluation/judgment and self-focused attention.

An increasing number of fMRI BOLD "resting state" (eyes closed, no task) studies are being conducted in healthy volunteers (Greicius, Krasnow, Reiss, & Menon, 2003) and in individuals with neuropsychiatric disorders such as autism and Alzheimer's disease (Broyd et al., 2009; Buckner, Andrews-Hanna, & Schacter, 2008; Greicius, Srivastava, Reiss, & Menon, 2004; Monk et al., 2009). However, to date, no study has specifically measured fMRI BOLD during rest in patients with SAD.

Neurochemical and Neuroreceptor Brain Imaging

Dopamine System

Striatal and basal ganglia (caudate and putamen) regions are rich in DA receptors, and the DA system has been hypothesized to be abnormal in SAD (Stein, et al. 2002), given that DA levels are reduced in timid mice, striatal DA receptor binding is reduced in subordinate monkeys, SP is associated with Parkinson's disease, and dopaminergic agents are particularly efficacious in SAD (reviewed in D. J. Stein et al., 2002). In a symptom provocation study of dopaminergic effects (Hood et al., 2008), untreated patients with SAD and those treated with an SSRI, with remitted symptoms, engaged in a behavioral challenge that comprised an impromptu speech and listening to an anxiety-provoking autobiographical script. Results showed DA activation with pramipexole and DA depletion with sulpiride were associated with increased anxiety during symptom-provocation in the untreated SAD group. Regarding the remitted patient group, anxiety during the behavioral challenges was reduced compared with the untreated group and particularly for pramipexole. Thus, there is reason to suspect that SAD patients would exhibit a deficient DA system. In support of this hypothesis, a SPECT study using [^{123}I]β-CIT, a specific ligand for the DA transporter, found a decrease in striatal DA reuptake sites among individuals with SAD compared to healthy volunteers (Tiihonen et al., 1997). However, a recent [^{123}I]β-CIT SPECT study showed that SAD patients exhibited higher (compared to controls) striatal binding ratios, suggesting an *increased* number of DA reuptake sites. In a different study, Schneier et al. (2000) reported that reduced D_2-receptor binding in the striatum was found in individuals with SAD compared to controls, suggesting dopaminergic hypofunction in the striatum. In addition, the level of social anxiety in the SAD group was negatively correlated, although nonsignificantly, with D_2-binding potential. In support of this, a subsequent study showed that striatal postsynaptic D_2-receptor binding has been associated with severity of SAD (unpublished data; for review see Li, Chokka, & Tibbo, 2001).

Collectively, these findings are supported by complementary studies that show that D_2-receptor density is positively correlated with the detachment scale of the Karolinska Scales of Personality (KSP), which taps into social avoidance (Farde, Gustavsson, & Jonsson, 1997). Similarly, DA transporter binding in the putamen correlated negatively with detachment scores on the KSP in a different PET study (Laakso et al., 2000). As noted above, an MRI study measuring brain volumes found greater age-related reductions in putamen volumes in individuals with SAD compared with controls, though there were no significant differences between the two groups in total cerebral, caudate, putamen, and thalamic volumes (Potts et al., 1994).

A recent study by Schneier, Abi-Dargham, et al. (2009) measured baseline D2-receptor availability with [^{11}C]raclopride and a repeat scan after intravenous administration of d-amphetamine to study DA release. SAD subjects were also scanned with [^{123}I]β-CIT to assess DAT availability. The results contrasted with demonstrations of abnormal D_2-receptor binding in previous studies. The authors found no significant between-group differences (SAD vs. control) in D_2-receptor binding potential or amphetamine-induced decrease in D_2-receptor binding in the striatum; additionally, receptor availability and change after d-amphetamine were not significantly associated with severity of social anxiety or trait detachment.

In summary, these studies suggest equivocal evidence of dopaminergic dysfunction in SAD. Interpretation of results includes the proposition by van der Wee et al. (2008) that SAD is associated with reduced extracellular DA, increased density of the DA transporter, or a combination of both mechanisms. Furthermore, Bell, Malizia, and Nutt (1999) suggest that decreased binding potentials reflect *increased* levels of free DA in the vicinity of D_2-receptors, altered affinity of D_2-receptors for DA, or some combination of these factors.

Lastly, differences in imaging methods or characteristics of samples or sample size may contribute to the lack of replication across studies (Schneier, Abi-Dargham, et al., 2009). Further studies are needed to clarify the role of the DA system.

Serotonin System

Besides dopamine, serotonin (5-HT) is also implicated in SAD (see review by D. J. Stein et al., 2002), particularly because it plays a role in social dominance and affiliation (Knutson et al., 1998) and SSRI treatments are efficacious for SAD (Schneier, 2006; Stein & Stein, 2008). Moreover, SSRIs have been shown to attenuate amygdala reactivity to fearful, and other negative, faces (Arce, Simmons, Lovero, Stein, & Paulus, 2008; Harmer, Mackay, Reid, Cowen, & Goodwin, 2006). Although SSRIs have also been shown to attenuate amygdala hyper-reactivity in SAD, this PET study was isolated to a public speaking task (Furmark et al., 2002); in other words, no SSRI pre-post treatment fMRI study has been conducted using emotional face-processing tasks. Interestingly, allelic variation in the gene that codes the 5-HT transporter (SERT) functionality influences the extent of amygdala reactivity during a public speaking task in SAD individuals (Furmark et al., 2004). Further supporting the role of 5-HT in SAD during stress, it has been observed that SSRI-remitted, SAD patients reported increased anxiety during a behavioral challenge (e.g., fearful autobiographic script) after tryptophan depletion (TD) relative to a control, non-TD day (Argyropoulos et al., 2004), suggesting that TD reverses the therapeutic effect of SSRIs in SAD. Thus, there is reason to expect 5-HT abnormalities in SAD.

In an early study, Miner and colleagues (1995) measured brain concentrations of fluoxetine using fluorine ^{19}F-MRS following an open trial of the SSRI fluoxetine; treatment responders ($n = 5$) had higher, albeit nonsignificant, fluoxetine/norfluoxetine concentrations than nonresponders ($n = 3$). Although this study implicates the involvement of the serotonergic system in SAD, variable dosage levels and treatment duration (8–20 weeks) and the small number of patients make it difficult to interpret the results.

To investigate the effects of the SSRI paroxetine on the occupancy of the 5-HT reuptake transporter, Kent et al. (2002) studied patients with SAD with [^{11}C](+)-McN 5652 PET after three to six months of treatment. All five patients were considered to have significantly improved, and occupancy of the 5-HT reuptake transporter was high and in regions of the highest known 5-HT transporter density (i.e., midbrain, thalamus, striatum, hippocampus, amygdala, and cingulate), suggesting that paroxetine at therapeutic doses achieves very high occupancy levels of the SERT.

In a study of the 5-HT receptor system, Lanzenberger et al. (2007) evaluated 5-HT_{1A} binding potential in the ACC, OFC, insula, amygdala, and hippocampus. Results showed that the greatest decrease in 5-HT_{1A} binding in SAD compared to controls was in the amygdale, though significantly lower 5-HT_{1A} binding potential was also evident in the ACC, insula, and dorsal raphe nuclei. On the other hand, a SPECT study by van der Wee et al. (2008) demonstrated that SAD patients, relative to controls, had significantly higher [^{123}I]β-CIT binding ratios, specific for 5-HT transporter (5-HTT), in the thalamus without correlation to severity of SAD symptoms. Further serotonergic findings include a PET study using the [^{11}C]-5-hydroxy-L-tryptophan tracer, which showed a lower uptake of the tracer mainly in the temporal lobe in SAD patients compared to controls (Marteinsdottir et al., 2001).

In conclusion, based on a limited number of studies, there is support for attenuated 5-HT neurotransmission in cortical and subcortical regions in SAD, though results have been inconsistent. Van der Wee et al. (2008) hypothesized that their finding of higher 5-HTT binding potential were the result of increased densities of 5-HTT in SAD patients due to a "higher homeostatic tone of the serotonergic system (with concomitant lower densities of 5-HT receptors)" (p. 761). Additionally, the attenuated accumulation of the immediate precursor of 5-HT (i.e., 5-HTP) in the temporal lobe might indicate regionally specific 5-HT synthesis suppressions in SAD (Marteinsdottir et al., 2001). However, other studies are needed to further delineate 5-HT receptor subtypes involved in SAD and elucidate neurotransmission mechanisms.

Other Neurotransmitter–Neurochemical Systems

In addition to possible differences in dopaminergic and serotonergic functions, differences in levels of other neuroactive metabolites have been found in patients with SAD. In an early ^{1}H-MRS study, Davidson et al. (1993) reported that SAD patients (vs. controls) had a decrease in choline and creatine signal-to-noise ratios in the subcortical, thalamic, and caudate areas. Similarly, using ^{1}H-MRS at high-field (4 Telsa), we had previously reported that subjects with SAD had a significantly decreased choline/creatine ratios in the ACC (Phan et al., 2005). However, Tupler et al. (1997) had previously observed that patients with SAD had higher choline/creatine levels in cortical gray matter. Of particular note, in that study, severity of social anxiety symptoms were correlated with decreased choline/creatine ratios in subcortical gray matter.

The results are somewhat inconsistent regarding N-acetylaspartate (NAA), a putative marker of neuronal viability/density. Some spectroscopic studies have reported increased absolute NAA and/or NAA/creatine concentrations in the frontal cortex of anxious subjects without psychopathology (Grachev & Apkarian, 2000a, 2000b) and in the ACC of subjects with SAD (Phan et al., 2005). There was consistently a significant positive correlation between severity of social anxiety symptoms and NAA/creatine ratios in cortical gray matter (Tupler et al., 1997). Another study using a similar approach, however, found lowered NAA signal-to-noise ratios in cortical and subcortical regions among individuals with SAD (Davidson et al., 1993). In addition, *myo*-inositol/

creatine ratios have been found to be significantly increased in subcortical gray matter and in WM in the SAD group (Tupler et al., 1997).

In our high-field ^{1}H-MRS, we had previously reported that subjects with SAD had a significantly higher glutamate/creatine ratio in the perigenual ACC than the normal controls, but no differences were found in glutamate/creatine ratio in the occipital cortex, which served as a control region (Phan et al., 2005). Furthermore, we observed that SAD symptom severity was positively correlated with glutamate/creatine ratio in the anterior cingulate cortex but not in the occipital cortex. In support of this, increased glutamatergic transmission and/or excessive glutamate release within the limbic system might be involved in anxiety (Cortese & Phan, 2005; Walker & Davis, 2002). Sustained levels of anxiety might increase excitatory neurotransmitter release (localized to limbic/paralimbic regions) and lead to a subsequent neuronal reorganization and an increase in the number of axons and synaptic connections, reflected by increased levels of NAA (Grachev & Apkarian, 2000a, 2000b). Studies thus far indicate that metabolite differences, if any, in SAD concentrate more in gray matter than in WM. Even with some inconsistencies, it is difficult to derive definitive conclusions from the existing MRS studies because most results are based on the patterns of ratios rather than absolute values. That is, for example, it is difficult to conclude that SAD is associated with increased glutamate levels *per se*, because lower level of creatine in SAD subjects could lead to similar findings. Given the inconsistent results, however, more studies are needed to confirm the putative link between NAA and glutamate and pathological anxiety including SAD. Thus, more studies and advances in MRS methodology are needed, not only to resolve inconsistencies between previous findings but also to obtain absolute quantification of these relevant metabolites.

INTEGRATING NEUOROENDOCRINE AND NEUROANATOMICAL STUDIES

Systematic integration of findings and approaches across disciplines is critical to a comprehensive understanding of the neurobiology of SAD. Evidence of neuroendocrine dysregulation in SAD, particularly in response to stress, indicates potential neural abnormality in regions associated with the HPA axis. However, few studies have attempted to link HPA axis measures of stress responsivity and brain "activation" measures related to stress (fear perception, symptom provocation, etc.). In one such study, Ahs et al. (2006) investigated the association between rCBF and cortisol reactivity during a speech task in SAD and reported no evidence of an increase in cortisol level from baseline to speech despite an increase in subjective anxiety. Nevertheless, a positive covariation between rCBF in the hypothalamus and salivary cortisol was found during the stress task. In addition, cortisol and rCBF were shown to covary negatively in an area encompassing the MPFC and premotor/motor cortices.

A recent study by van Peer, Spinhoven, van Dijk, and Roelofs (2009) investigated the effects of cortisol administration on approach and avoidance tendencies in SAD while measuring ERPs during a reaction-time task in which patients evaluated the emotional expression of photographs of happy and angry faces by making an approaching (flexion) or avoiding (extension) arm movement. The authors showed a significant interaction of condition by severity of social anxiety on early positive (P150) amplitudes during avoidance compared to approach, indicating that cortisol enhances early processing of social stimuli (in particular angry faces) during avoidance. This finding suggests cortisol-induced increase in processing of angry faces in SAD. Interestingly, the P1 ERP component is proposed to reflect enhanced sensory processing of emotional stimuli due to projections from the amygdala (Pizzagalli, Regard, & Lehmann, 1999). Consistent with attentional hypervigilance models (Bogels & Mansell, 2004), individuals with SAD exhibit enhanced P1 amplitudes, in a modified probe detection task, for angry – neutral face pairs versus happy – neutral face pairs (Mueller et al., 2009). Within the SAD group, enhanced activation for angry–neutral versus happy–neutral face pairs was localized to the right middle temporal gyrus area, which included the fusiform gyrus. Furthermore, the SAD group showed greater activation than controls at the right fusiform gyrus.

These two studies suggest the potential utility of combining methodological approaches and integrating neuroendocrine stress systems and neural circuits that mediate stress response and social threat. Interestingly, there is emerging evidence that HPA axis reactivity may be related to the limbic–paralimbic reactivity to emotional and stress-related processing (King et al., 2009; King & Liberzon, 2009; Liberzon et al., 2007).

GENERAL CONCLUSIONS

Neurobiological investigations of SAD, a disorder of abnormal fear of social and performance situations, show that evidence of neuroendocrine dysregulation in response to stress though the pattern of cortisol reactivity has been inconsistent. Moreover, anomalous reactivity may be limited to a subset of individuals with SAD and may reflect individual variability in the stress response. The finding that early aversive experiences (e.g., childhood abuse) contribute to cortisol reactivity in SAD and the possibility that individual differences in coping style (e.g., repressors) may affect cortisol levels suggest that more study in the area of individual differences in HPA axis reactivity and their relation to social anxiety is warranted.

Although gross structural deficits are not evident in SAD, a growing number of functional neuroimaging techniques (PET, fMRI) show abnormalities in discrete brain regions involve affective, cognitive, and social functioning. Most consistent is hyperactive amygdala reactivity to signals of social threat such as harsh faces and during the anticipation and act of public speaking.

There is also evidence of enhanced insula and ACC activation in SAD to social threat stimuli and during symptom provocation, though few studies have focused on these areas. Taken together, hyperactivation in "bottom-up" limbic/paralimbic regions (involved in threat perception, fear responding, anxious states, etc.) and hyporeactivity of "top-down" frontal cortical regions involved in appraisal and affect regulation may contribute to excessive fear and avoidance behaviors in SAD and manifest in information-processing biases and misinterpretation of social information. Frontal function requires further clarification in future studies, as current methodological differences across tasks/paradigms may contribute to the disparity in observations. Most relevant appears to be the relationship between cortical and subcortical regions as it pertains to PEP, emotion regulation, and "real-life" social interactions. Although there is a suggestion that structural connectivity between amygdala and frontal cortex is altered in SAD, little known is about "effective" connectivity (the direct and dynamic influence of one region over another) in the context of maintaining social phobic cognitions and behaviors.

FUTURE DIRECTIONS

Given the rapid emergence of novel techniques and discoveries from basic animal and human neuroscience, our field is poised to study domains previously unexplored. Although some evidence exists for the amelioration of neuroendocrine, neuroanatomic, and neurochemical abnormalities, the majority of studies have focused on pharmacotherapy. Given that cognitive therapy has been shown to reduce cortisol levels in generally anxious patients (Tafet, Feder, Abulafia, & Roffman, 2005) and that cognitive strategies can reduce both cortisol and ACTH responses to anxiogenic pharmacological challenges (Abelson, Khan, Liberzon, Erickson, & Young, 2008; Abelson, Liberzon, Young, & Khan, 2005), more studies coupling cognitive therapy and/or attentional training with neuroendocrine and neuroimaging studies would facilitate a biological mechanism to explain the symptoms and behavior of SAD patients.

The emerging field of functional genomics, together with neuroimaging (Hariri, 2009; Hariri, Drabant, & Weinberger, 2006) ("imaging genetics"), offers the opportunity to explore the relationships between genes, brain, and behavior, and it will be important to discover molecular underpinnings of vulnerability to disease. For example, we know that BI observed at infancy is a risk factor for the development of SP later in life and is associated with amygdala hyper-reactivity to social cues (Schwartz, Wright, Shin, Kagan, & Rauch, 2003); longitudinal neuroimaging designs coupled with genetic analyses could elucidate predictive biological markers to identify those at high risk of developing SAD for early, preventive interventions.

As we refine our brain models of SAD, it is critical to exploit these mechanisms to improve our understanding of how and why treatment works, and for whom it works. As such, coupling clinical trials (from treatment development to efficacy studies) will allow us to identify brain markers that predict therapeutic success and failure. First, this may stimulate the development of new treatments aimed at neuromodulation of discrete brain areas or circuits. Second, valid and reliable brain markers can guide patients towards the most optimal treatment strategies on a personalized basis.

Much more progress is urgently needed in integrating imaging modalities so that we can link functional neuroanatomical findings with underlying neurochemical (and molecular) mechanisms. Moreover, there is increasing awareness of the importance of interactions among brain regions (as circuits and networks), and advances in signal processing and improvements in temporal and spatial resolution will expedite a more complete understanding of normal brain function. From there, we will be able to explore more specific and direct questions about alterations in brain function in patients with SAD.

REFERENCES

Abelson, J. L., Khan, S., Liberzon, I., Erickson, T. M., & Young, E. A. (2008). Effects of perceived control and cognitive coping on endocrine stress responses to pharmacological activation. *Biological Psychiatry*, *64*(8), 701–707.

Abelson, J. L., Khan, S., Liberzon, I., & Young, E. A. (2007). HPA axis activity in patients with panic disorder: Review and synthesis of four studies. *Depression and Anxiety*, *24*(1), 66–76.

Abelson, J. L., Liberzon, I., Young, E. A., & Khan, S. (2005). Cognitive modulation of the endocrine stress response to a pharmacological challenge in normal and panic disorder subjects. *Archives of General Psychiatry*, *62*(6), 668–675.

Adams, R. B., Jr., Gordon, H. L., Baird, A. A., Ambady, N., & Kleck, R. E. (2003). Effects of gaze on amygdala sensitivity to anger and fear faces. *Science*, *300*(5625), 1536.

Adolphs, R. (1999). Social cognition and the human brain. *Trends in Cognitive Science*, *3*(12), 469–479.

Adolphs, R. (2002). Neural systems for recognizing emotion. *Current Opinions in Neurobiology*, *12*(2), 169–177.

Adolphs, R. (2003). Is the human amygdala specialized for processing social information? *Annals of the New York Academy of Sciences*, *985*, 326–340.

Adolphs, R., Tranel, D., & Damasio, A. R. (1998). The human amygdala in social judgment. *Nature*, *393*(6684), 470–474.

Adolphs, R., Tranel, D., Damasio, H., & Damasio, A. (1994). Impaired recognition of emotion in facial expressions following bilateral damage to the human amygdala. *Nature*, *372*(6507), 669–672.

Adolphs, R., Tranel, D., Damasio, H., & Damasio, A. R. (1995). Fear and the human amygdala. *Journal of Neuroscience*, *15*(9), 5879–5891.

Ahs, F., Furmark, T., Michelgard, A., Langstrom, B., Appel, L., Wolf, O. T., et al. (2006). Hypothalamic blood flow correlates positively with stress-induced cortisol levels in subjects with social anxiety disorder. *Psychosomatic Medicine*, *68*(6), 859–862.

Ahs, F., Sollers, J. J., 3rd, Furmark, T., Fredrikson, M., & Thayer, J. F. (2009). High-frequency heart rate variability and cortico-striatal activity in men and women with social phobia. *Neuroimage*, *47*(3), 815–820.

Alden, L. E., & Taylor, C. T. (2004). Interpersonal processes in social phobia. *Clinical Psychology Review*, *24*(7), 857–882.

American Psychiatric Association. (1994). *Diagnostic and statistical manual of mental disorders* (4th ed.) (DSM-IV). Washington, DC: Author.

Amir, N., Beard, C., & Przeworski, A. (2005). Resolving ambiguity: The effect of experience on interpretation of ambiguous events in generalized social phobia. *Journal of Abnormal Psychology*, *114*(3), 402–408.

Amir, N., Elias, J., Klumpp, H., & Przeworski, A. (2003). Attentional bias to threat in social phobia: Facilitated processing of threat or difficulty disengaging attention from threat? *Behaviour Research and Therapy*, *41*(11), 1325–1335.

Amir, N., Foa, E. B., & Coles, M. E. (1998). Automatic activation and strategic avoidance of threat-relevant information in social phobia. *Journal of Abnormal Psychology*, *107*(2), 285–290.

Amir, N., Foa, E. B., & Coles, M. E. (2000). Implicit memory bias for threat-relevant information in individuals with generalized social phobia. *Journal of Abnormal Psychology*, *109*(4), 713–720.

Amir, N., Klumpp, H., Elias, J., Bedwell, J. S., Yanasak, N., & Miller, L. S. (2005). Increased activation of the anterior cingulate cortex during processing of disgust faces in individuals with social phobia. *Biological Psychiatry*, *57*(9), 975–981.

Anderson, A. K., Christoff, K., Panitz, D., de Rosa, E., & Gabrieli, J. D. (2003). Neural correlates of the automatic processing of threat facial signals. *Journal of Neuroscience*, *23*(13), 5627–5633.

Arce, E., Simmons, A. N., Lovero, K. L., Stein, M. B., & Paulus, M. P. (2008). Escitalopram effects on insula and amygdala BOLD activation during emotional processing. *Psychopharmacology (Berlin)*, *196*(4), 661–672.

Argyropoulos, S. V., Hood, S. D., Adrover, M., Bell, C. J., Rich, A. S., Nash, J. R., et al. (2004). Tryptophan depletion reverses the therapeutic effect of selective serotonin reuptake inhibitors in social anxiety disorder. *Biological Psychiatry*, *56*(7), 503–509.

Augustine, J. R. (1996). Circuitry and functional aspects of the insular lobe in primates including humans. *Brain Research, Brain Research Reviews*, *22*(3), 229–244.

Banks, S. J., Eddy, K. T., Angstadt, M., Nathan, P. J., & Phan, K. L. (2007). Amygdala–frontal connectivity during emotion regulation. *Social Cognitive Affective Neuroscience*, *2*, 303–312.

Barrett, L. F., Mesquita, B., Ochsner, K. N., & Gross, J. J. (2007). The experience of emotion. *Annual Review of Psychology*, *58*, 373–403.

Beaton, E. A., Schmidt, L. A., Ashbaugh, A. R., Santesso, D. L., Antony, M. M., McCabe, R. E., et al. (2006). Low salivary cortisol levels among socially anxious young adults: Preliminary evidence from a selected and a non-selected sample. *Personality and Individual Differences*, *41*, 1217–1228.

Beesdo, K., Lau, J. Y., Guyer, A. E., McClure-Tone, E. B., Monk, C. S., et al. (2009). Common and specific amygdala-function perturbations in depressed vs anxious adolescents. *Archives of General Psychiatry*, *66*(3), 275–285.

Bell, C. J., Malizia, A. L., & Nutt, D. J. (1999). The neurobiology of social phobia. *European Archives of Psychiatry and Clinical Neurosciences*, *249*(Suppl 1), S11–S18.

Birbaumer, N., Grodd, W., Diedrich, O., Klose, U., Erb, M., Lotze, M., et al. (1998). fMRI reveals amygdala activation to human faces in social phobics. *Neuroreport*, *9*(6), 1223–1226.

Blair, K., Geraci, M., Devido, J., McCaffrey, D., Chen, G., Vythilingam, M., et al. (2008). Neural response to self- and other referential praise and criticism in generalized social phobia. *Archives of General Psychiatry*, *65*(10), 1176–1184.

Blair, K., Shaywitz, J., Smith, B. W., Rhodes, R., Geraci, M., Jones, M., et al. (2008). Response to emotional expressions in generalized social phobia and generalized anxiety disorder: Evidence for separate disorders. *American Journal of Psychiatry*, *165*, 1193–1202.

Blair, R. J., Morris, J. S., Frith, C. D., Perrett, D. I., & Dolan, R. J. (1999). Dissociable neural responses to facial expressions of sadness and anger. *Brain*, *122*(Pt 5), 883–893.

Bogels, S. M., & Mansell, W. (2004). Attention processes in the maintenance and treatment of social phobia: Hypervigilance, avoidance and self-focused attention. *Clinical Psychology Review*, *24*(7), 827–856.

Brown, L. L., Tomarken, A. J., Orth, D. N., Loosen, P. T., Kalin, N. H., & Davidson, R. J. (1996). Individual differences in repressive-defensiveness predict basal salivary cortisol levels. *Journal of Personality and Social Psychology*, *70*(2), 362–371.

Brown, M. R., Koob, G. F., & Rivier, C. (1991). *Stress: Neurobiology and neuroendocrinology*. New York: Dekker.

Broyd, S. J., Demanuele, C., Debener, S., Helps, S. K., James, C. J., & Sonuga-Barke, E. J. (2009). Default-mode brain dysfunction in mental disorders: A systematic review. *Neuroscience and Biobehavioral Reviews*, *33*(3), 279–296.

Buckner, R. L., Andrews-Hanna, J. R., & Schacter, D. L. (2008). The brain's default network: Anatomy, function, and relevance to disease. *Annals of the New York Academy of Sciences*, *1124*, 1–38.

Bush, G., Luu, P., & Posner, M. I. (2000). Cognitive and emotional influences in anterior cingulate cortex. *Trends in Cognitive Science*, *4*(6), 215–222.

Campbell, D. W., Sareen, J., Paulus, M. P., Goldin, P. R., Stein, M. B., & Reiss, J. P. (2007). Time-varying amygdala response to emotional faces in generalized social phobia. *Biological Psychiatry*, *62*(5), 455–463.

Campbell, D. W., Sareen, J., Stein, M. B., Kraretsky, L. B., Paulus, M. P., Hassard, S. T., et al. (2009). Happy but not so approachable: The social judgments of individuals with generalized social phobia. *Depression and Anxiety*, *26*(5), 419–424.

Canli, T., Sivers, H., Whitfield, S. L., Gotlib, I. H., & Gabrieli, J. D. (2002). Amygdala response to happy faces as a function of extraversion. *Science*, *296*(5576), 2191.

Cannistraro, P. A., Wright, C. I., Wedig, M. M., Martis, B., Shin, L. M., Wilhelm, S., et al. (2004). Amygdala responses to human faces in obsessive-compulsive disorder. *Biological Psychiatry*, *56*(12), 916–920.

Carey, P. D., Warwick, J., Niehaus, D. J., van der Linden, G., van Heerden, B. B., Harvey, B. H., et al. (2004). Single photon emission computed tomography (SPECT) of anxiety disorders before and after treatment with citalopram. *BMC Psychiatry*, *4*, 30.

Clark, D. M., & McManus, F. (2002). Information processing in social phobia. *Biological Psychiatry*, *51*(1), 92–100.

Clark, D. M., & Wells, A. (Eds.), (1995). *A cognitive model of social phobia*. New York: Guilford Press.

Coccaro, E. F., McCloskey, M. S., Fitzgerald, D. A., & Phan, K. L. (2007). Amygdala and orbitofrontal reactivity to social threat in individuals with impulsive aggression. *Biological Psychiatry*, *62*(2), 168–178.

Coles, M. E., & Heimberg, R. G. (2005). Recognition bias for critical faces in social phobia: A replication and extension. *Behaviour Research and Therapy*, *43*(1), 109–120.

Condren, R. M., O'Neill, A., Ryan, M. C. M., Barrett, P., & Thakore, J. H. (2002). HPA axis response to a psychological stressor in generalised social phobia. *Psychoneuroendocrinology*, *27*, 693–703.

Cooney, R. E., Atlas, L. Y., Joormann, J., Eugene, F., & Gotlib, I. H. (2006). Amygdala activation in the processing of neutral faces in social anxiety disorder: Is neutral really neutral? *Psychiatry Research*, *148*(1), 55–59.

Cortese, B. M., & Phan, K. L. (2005). The role of glutamate in anxiety and related disorders. *CNS Spectrums*, *10*(10), 820–830.

Craig, A. D. (2002). How do you feel? Interoception: The sense of the physiological condition of the body. *National Reviews in Neuroscience*, *3*(8), 655–666.

Critchley, H. D., Mathias, C. J., & Dolan, R. J. (2002). Fear conditioning in humans: The influence of awareness and autonomic arousal on functional neuroanatomy. *Neuron*, *33*(4), 653–663.

Davidson, J. R., Krishnan, K. R., Charles, H. C., Boyko, O., Potts, N. L., Ford, S. M., et al. (1993). Magnetic resonance spectroscopy in social phobia: Preliminary findings. *Journal of Clinical Psychiatry*, *54*(Suppl), 19–25.

Davidson, R. J. (2002). Anxiety and affective style: Role of prefrontal cortex and amygdala. *Biological Psychiatry*, *51*(1), 68–80.

Davis, M., & Whalen, P. J. (2001). The amygdala: Vigilance and emotion. *Molecular Psychiatry*, *6*(1), 13–34.

Dickerson, S. S., & Kemeny, M. E. (2004). Acute stressors and cortisol responses: A theoretical integration and synthesis of laboratory research. *Psychological Bulletin*, *130*(3), 355–391.

Dougherty, D. D., Shin, L. M., Alpert, N. M., Pitman, R. K., Orr, S. P., Lasko, M., et al. (1999). Anger in healthy men: A PET study using script-driven imagery. *Biological Psychiatry*, *46*(4), 466–472.

Ekman, P. (2003). *Emotions revealed: Recognizing faces and feelings to improve communication and emotional life*. New York: Henry Holt.

Elzinga, B. M., Spinhoven, P., Berretty, E., de Jong, P., & Roelofs, K. (2009). The role of childhood abuse in HPA-axis reactivity in social anxiety disorder: A pilot study. *Biological Psychology*, *83*(1), 1–.

Emery, N. J., Capitanio, J. P., Mason, W. A., Machado, C. J., Mendoza, S. P., & Amaral, D. G. (2001). The effects of bilateral lesions of the amygdala on dyadic social interactions in rhesus monkeys *(Macaca mulatta)*. *Behavioral Neuroscience*, *115*(3), 515–544.

Erickson, K., Drevets, W., & Schulkin, J. (2003). Glucocorticoid regulation of diverse cognitive functions in normal and pathological emotional states. *Neuroscience and Biobehavioral Reviews*, *27*(3), 233–246.

Etkin, A., & Wager, T. D. (2007). Functional neuroimaging of anxiety: A meta-analysis of emotional processing in PTSD, social anxiety disorder, and specific phobia. *American Journal of Psychiatry*, *164*(10), 1476–1488.

Evans, K. C., Simon, N. M., Dougherty, D. D., Hoge, E. A., Worthington, J. J., Chow, C., et al. (2009). A PET study of tiagabine treatment implicates ventral medial prefrontal cortex in generalized social anxiety disorder. *Neuropsychopharmacology*, *34*(2), 390–398.

Evans, K. C., Wright, C. I., Wedig, M. M., Gold, A. L., Pollack, M. H., & Rauch, S. L. (2008). A functional MRI study of amygdala responses to angry schematic faces in social anxiety disorder. *Depression and Anxiety*, *25*(6), 496–505.

Farde, L., Gustavsson, J. P., & Jonsson, E. (1997). D2 dopamine receptors and personality traits. *Nature*, *385*(6617), 590.

Ferrari, M. C., Busatto, G. F., McGuire, P. K., & Crippa, J. A. (2008). Structural magnetic resonance imaging in anxiety disorders: An update of research findings. *Revista brasileira de psiquiatria (Saõ Paulo)*, *30*(3), 251–264.

Fitzgerald, D. A., Angstadt, M., Jelsone, L. M., Nathan, P. J., & Phan, K. L. (2006). Beyond threat: Amygdala reactivity across multiple expressions of facial affect. *Neuroimage*, *30*(4), 1441–1448.

Foa, E. B., Gilboa-Schechtman, E., Amir, N., & Freshman, M. (2000). Memory bias in generalized social phobia: Remembering negative emotional expressions. *Journal of Anxiety Disorders*, *14*(5), 501–519.

Frackowiack, R., Zeki, S., Ashburner, J., Friston, K. J., & Frith, C. D. (2003). *Human brain function* (2nd ed.). San Diego, CA: Academic Press.

Friston, K. J. (1998). Imaging neuroscience: Principles or maps? *Proceedings of the National Academy of Sciences of the USA*, *95*(3), 796–802.

Frith, C. D., & Frith, U. (2006). The neural basis of mentalizing. *Neuron*, *50*(4), 531–534.

Furlan, P. M., DeMartinis, N., Schweizer, E., Rickels, K., & Lucki, I. (2001). Abnormal salivary cortisol levels in social phobic patients in response to acute psychological but not physical stress. *Biological Psychiatry*, *50*(4), 254–259.

Furmark, T., Appel, L., Michelgard, A., Wahlstedt, K., Ahs, F., Zancan, S., et al. (2005). Cerebral blood flow changes after treatment of social phobia with the neurokinin-1 antagonist GR205171, citalopram, or placebo. *Biological Psychiatry*, *58*(2), 132–142.

Furmark, T., Tillfors, M., Garpenstrand, H., Marteinsdottir, I., Langstrom, B., Oreland, L., et al. (2004). Serotonin transporter polymorphism related to amygdala excitability and symptom severity in patients with social phobia. *Neuroscience Letters*, *362*(3), 189–192.

Furmark, T., Tillfors, M., Marteinsdottir, I., Fischer, H., Pissiota, A., Langstrom, B., et al. (2002). Common changes in cerebral blood flow in patients with social phobia treated with citalopram or cognitive-behavioral therapy. *Archives of General Psychiatry*, *59*(5), 425–433.

Gallagher, H. L., & Frith, C. D. (2003). Functional imaging of "theory of mind". *Trends in Cognitive Science*, *7*(2), 77–83.

Gentili, C., Ricciardi, E., Gobbini, M. I., Santarelli, M. F., Haxby, J. V., Pietrini, P., et al. (2009). Beyond amygdala: Default mode network activity differs between patients with social phobia and healthy controls. *Brain Research Bulletin*, *79*(6), 409–413.

Ghashghaei, H. T., Hilgetag, C. C., & Barbas, H. (2007). Sequence of information processing for emotions based on the anatomic dialogue between prefrontal cortex and amygdala. *Neuroimage*, *34*(3), 905–923.

Goldin, P. R., Manber, T., Hakimi, S., Canli, T., & Gross, J. J. (2009). Neural bases of social anxiety disorder: Emotional reactivity and cognitive regulation during social and physical threat. *Archives of General Psychiatry*, *66*(2), 170–180.

Gordon, E. (1999). Brain imaging technologies: How, what, when and why? *Australia and New Zealand Journal of Psychiatry*, *33*(2), 187–196.

Grachev, I. D., & Apkarian, A. V. (2000a). Anxiety in healthy humans is associated with orbital frontal chemistry. *Molecular Psychiatry*, *5*(5), 482–488.

Grachev, I. D., & Apkarian, A. V. (2000b). Chemical mapping of anxiety in the brain of healthy humans: An in vivo 1H-MRS study on the effects of sex, age, and brain region. *Human Brain Mapping*, *11*(4), 261–272.

Graeff, F. G., Garcia-Leal, C., Del-Ben, C. M., & Guimaraes, F. S. (2005). Does the panic attack activate the hypothalamic-pituitary-adrenal axis? *Anais da Academia Brasileira de Ciencias*, *77*(3), 477–491.

Grant, K. A., Shively, C. A., Nader, M. A., Ehrenkaufer, R. L., Line, S. W., Morton, T. E., et al. (1998). Effect of social status on striatal dopamine D2 receptor binding characteristics in cynomolgus monkeys assessed with positron emission tomography. *Synapse*, *29*(1), 80–83.

Greicius, M. D., Krasnow, B., Reiss, A. L., & Menon, V. (2003). Functional connectivity in the resting brain: A network analysis of the default mode hypothesis. *Proceedings of the National Academy of Sciences of the USA*, *100*(1), 253–258.

Greicius, M. D., Srivastava, G., Reiss, A. L., & Menon, V. (2004). Default-mode network activity distinguishes Alzheimer's disease from healthy aging: Evidence from functional MRI. *Proceedings of the National Academy of Sciences of the USA*, *101*(13), 4637–4642.

Gross, J. J. (1999). Emotion regulation: Past, present, future. *Cognition and Emotion*, *13*(5), 551–573.

Guyer, A. E., Lau, J. Y., McClure-Tone, E. B., Parrish, J., Shiffrin, N. D., Reynolds, R. C., et al. (2008). Amygdala and ventrolateral prefrontal cortex function during anticipated peer evaluation in pediatric social anxiety. *Archives of General Psychiatry*, *65*(11), 1303–1312.

Guyer, A. E., Nelson, E. E., Perez-Edgar, K., Hardin, M. G., Roberson-Nay, R., Monk, C. S., et al. (2006). Striatal functional alteration in adolescents characterized by early childhood behavioral inhibition. *Journal of Neuroscience*, *26*(24), 6399–6405.

Handwerger, K. (2009). Differential patterns of HPA activity and reactivity in adult posttraumatic stress disorder and major depressive disorder. *Harvard Review of Psychiatry*, *17*(3), 184–205.

Hariri, A. R. (2009). The neurobiology of individual differences in complex behavioral traits. *Annual Review of Neuroscience*, *32*, 225–247.

Hariri, A. R., Bookheimer, S. Y., & Mazziotta, J. C. (2000). Modulating emotional responses: Effects of a neocortical network on the limbic system. *Neuroreport*, *11*(1), 43–48.

Hariri, A. R., Drabant, E. M., & Weinberger, D. R. (2006). Imaging genetics: Perspectives from studies of genetically driven variation in serotonin function and corticolimbic affective processing. *Biological Psychiatry*, *59*(10), 888–897.

Harmer, C. J., Mackay, C. E., Reid, C. B., Cowen, P. J., & Goodwin, G. M. (2006). Antidepressant drug treatment modifies the neural processing of nonconscious threat cues. *Biological Psychiatry*, *59*(9), 816–820.

Hirsch, C. R., & Clark, D. M. (2004). Information-processing bias in social phobia. *Clinical Psychology Review*, *24*(7), 799–825.

Hirsch, C., & Mathews, A. (1997). Interpretive inferences when reading about emotional events. *Behaviour Research and Therapy*, *35*, 1123–1132.

Hofmann, S. G., Litz, B. T., & Weathers, F. W. (2003). Social anxiety, depression, and PTSD in Vietnam veterans. *Journal of Anxiety Disorders*, *17*(5), 573–582.

Hood, S., Potokar, J., Davies, S., Hince, D., Morris, K., Seddon, K. M., et al. (2008). Dopaminergic challenges in social anxiety disorder: Evidence for dopamine D3 desensitisation following successful treatment with serotonergic antidepressants. *Journal of Psychopharmacology*, *24*, 709–716.

Katzman, M. A., Koszycki, D., & Bradwejn, J. (2004). Effects of CCK-tetrapeptide in patients with social phobia and obsessive-compulsive disorder. *Depression and Anxiety*, *20*(2), 51–58.

Kent, J. M., Coplan, J. D., Lombardo, I., Hwang, D. R., Huang, Y., Mawlawi, O., et al. (2002). Occupancy of brain serotonin transporters during treatment with paroxetine in patients with social phobia: A positron emission tomography study with 11C McN 5652. *Psychopharmacology (Berlin)*, *164*(4), 341–348.

Khan, S., King, A. P., Abelson, J. L., & Liberzon, I. (2009). Neuroendocrinology of anxiety disorders. In M. Anthony & M. B. Stein (Eds.), *Oxford handbook of anxiety and related disorders* (pp. 111–122). New York: Oxford University Press.

Killgore, W. D., & Yurgelun-Todd, D. A. (2005). Social anxiety predicts amygdala activation in adolescents viewing fearful faces. *Neuroreport*, *16*(15), 1671–1675.

Kilts, C. D., Kelsey, J. E., Knight, B., Ely, T. D., Bowman, F. D., Gross, R. E., et al. (2006). The neural correlates of social anxiety disorder and response to pharmacotherapy. *Neuropsychopharmacology*, *31*(10), 2243–2253.

Kim, M. J., & Whalen, P. J. (2009). The structural integrity of an amygdala-prefrontal pathway predicts trait anxiety. *Journal of Neuroscience*, *29*(37), 11614–11618.

King, A. P., Abelson, J. L., Britton, J. C., Phan, K. L., Taylor, S. F., & Liberzon, I. (2009). Medial prefrontal cortex and right insula activity predict plasma ACTH response to trauma recall. *Neuroimage*, *47*(3), 872–880.

King, A. P., & Liberzon, I. (2009). Assessing the neuroendocrine stress response in the functional neuroimaging context. *Neuroimage*, *47*(3), 1116–1124.

Knutson, B., Wolkowitz, O. M., Cole, S. W., Chan, T., Moore, E. A., Johnson, R. C., et al. (1998). Selective alteration of personality and social behavior by serotonergic intervention. *American Journal of Psychiatry*, *155*(3), 373–379.

Laakso, A., Vilkman, H., Kajander, J., Bergman, J., Paranta, M., Solin, O., et al. (2000). Prediction of detached personality in healthy subjects by low dopamine transporter binding. *American Journal of Psychiatry*, *157*(2), 290–292.

Lanzenberger, R. R., Mitterhauser, M., Spindelegger, C., Wadsak, W., Klein, N., Mien, L. K., et al. (2007). Reduced serotonin-1A receptor binding in social anxiety disorder. *Biological Psychiatry*, *61*(9), 1081–1089.

LeDoux, J. E. (2000). Emotion circuits in the brain. *Annual Review of Neuroscience*, *23*, 155–184.

Li, D., Chokka, P., & Tibbo, P. (2001). Toward an integrative understanding of social phobia. *Journal of Psychiatry and Neuroscience*, *26*(3), 190–202.

Liberzon, I., King, A. P., Britton, J. C., Phan, K. L., Abelson, J. L., & Taylor, S. F. (2007). Paralimbic and medial prefrontal cortical involvement in neuroendocrine responses to traumatic stimuli. *American Journal of Psychiatry*, *164*(8), 1250–1258.

Liberzon, I., Phan, K. L., Decker, L. R., & Taylor, S. F. (2003). Extended amygdala and emotional salience: A PET activation study of positive and negative affect. *Neuropsychopharmacology*, *28*(4), 726–733.

Lieberman, M. D. (2007). Social cognitive neuroscience: A review of core processes. *Annual Review of Psychology*, *58*, 259–289.

Lorberbaum, J. P., Kose, S., Johnson, M. R., Arana, G. W., Sullivan, L. K., Hamner, M. B., et al. (2004). Neural correlates of speech anticipatory anxiety in generalized social phobia. *Neuroreport*, *15*(18), 2701–2705.

Lundh, L. G., & Ost, L. G. (1996). Recognition bias for critical faces in social phobics. *Behaviour Research and Therapy*, *34*(10), 787–794.

Ly, V., & Roelofs, K. (2009). Social anxiety and cognitive expectancy of aversive outcome in avoidance conditioning. *Behaviour Research and Therapy*, *47*(10), 840–847.

Maddock, R. J. (1999). The retrosplenial cortex and emotion: New insights from functional neuroimaging of the human brain. *Trends in Neuroscience*, *22*(7), 310–316.

Marteinsdottir, I., Furmark, T., Tillfors, M., Agren, H., Hartvig, P., Fredrikson, M., et al. (2001). Presynaptic serotonin imaging in social phobia using [3-llC]-5-hydroxy-L-tryptophan and PET. *Neuroimage*, *13*(6), S1070.

Martel, F. L., Hayward, C., Lyons, D. M., Sanborn, K., Varady, S., & Schatzberg, A. F. (1999). Salivary cortisol levels in socially phobic adolescent girls. *Depression and Anxiety*, *10*(1), 25–27.

Mikkelsen, E. J., Detlor, J., & Cohen, D. J. (1981). School avoidance and social phobia triggered by haloperidol in patients with Tourette's disorder. *American Journal of Psychiatry*, *138*(12), 1572–1576.

Milham, M. P., Nugent, A. C., Drevets, W. C., Dickstein, D. P., Leibenluft, E., Ernst, M., et al. (2005). Selective reduction in amygdala volume in pediatric anxiety disorders: A voxel-based morphometry investigation. *Biological Psychiatry*, *57*(9), 961–966.

Miller, E. K., & Cohen, J. D. (2001). An integrative theory of prefrontal cortex function. *Annual Review of Neuroscience*, *24*, 167–202.

Miner, C. M., Davidson, J. R., Potts, N. L., Tupler, L. A., Charles, H. C., & Krishnan, K. R. (1995). Brain fluoxetine measurements using fluorine magnetic resonance spectroscopy in patients with social phobia. *Biological Psychiatry*, *38*(10), 696–698.

Mitchell, J. P., Neil Macrae, C., & Banaji, M. R. (2005). Forming impressions of people versus inanimate objects: Social-cognitive processing in the medial prefrontal cortex. *Neuroimage*, *26*(1), 251–257.

Mogg, K., & Bradley, B. P. (2002). Selective orienting of attention to masked threat faces in social anxiety. *Behaviour Research and Therapy*, *40*(12), 1403–1414.

Mogg, K., Philippot, P., & Bradley, B. P. (2004). Selective attention to angry faces in clinical social phobia. *Journal of Abnormal Psychology*, *113*(1), 160–165.

Monk, C. S., Peltier, S. J., Wiggins, J. L., Weng, S. J., Carrasco, M., Risi, S., et al. (2009). Abnormalities of intrinsic functional connectivity in autism spectrum disorders. *Neuroimage*, *47*(2), 764–772.

Morris, J. S., Frith, C. D., Perrett, D. I., Rowland, D., Young, A. W., Calder, A. J., et al. (1996). A differential neural response in the human amygdala to fearful and happy facial expressions. *Nature*, *383*(6603), 812–815.

Mueller, E. M., Hofmann, S. G., Santesso, D. L., Meuret, A. E., Bitran, S., & Pizzagalli, D. A. (2009). Electrophysiological evidence of attentional biases in social anxiety disorder. *Psychological Medicine*, *39*(7), 1141–1152.

Nitschke, J. B., Sarinopoulos, I., Mackiewicz, K. L., Schaefer, H. S., & Davidson, R. J. (2006). Functional neuroanatomy of aversion and its anticipation. *Neuroimage*, *29*(1), 106–116.

Ochsner, K. N. (2004). Current directions in social cognitive neuroscience. *Current Opinions in Neurobiology*, *14*(2), 254–258.

Ochsner, K. N., & Gross, J. J. (2005). The cognitive control of emotion. *Trends in Cognitive Science*, *9*(5), 242–249.

Paulus, M. P., & Stein, M. B. (2006). An insular view of anxiety. *Biological Psychiatry*, *60*(4), 383–387.

Phan, K. L., Angstadt, M., Fitzgerald, D. A., McCarron, R., Nathan, P. J., Cacioppo, J. T., et al. (2007). Limbic reactivity to partner reputation and rejection in social phobia: fMRl of the trust game. *Biological Psychiatry*, *61*(8), 183S.

Phan, K. L., Fitzgerald, D. A., Cortese, B. M., Seraji-Bozorgzad, N., Tancer, M. E., & Moore, G. J. (2005). Anterior cingulate neurochemistry in social anxiety disorder. *1H-MRS at 4 Tesla. Neuroreport*, *16*(2), 183–186.

Phan, K. L., Fitzgerald, D. A., Nathan, P. J., & Tancer, M. E. (2006). Association between amygdala hyperactivity to harsh faces and severity of social anxiety in generalized social phobia. *Biological Psychiatry*, *59*(5), 424–429.

Phan, K. L., Orlichenko, A., Boyd, E., Angstadt, M., Coccaro, E. F., Liberzon, I., et al. (2009). Preliminary evidence of white matter abnormality in the uncinate fasciculus in generalized social anxiety disorder. *Biological Psychiatry*, *66*(7), 691–694.

Phan, K. L., Taylor, S. F., Welsh, R. C., Decker, L. R., Noll, D. C., Nichols, T. E., et al. (2003). Activation of the medial prefrontal cortex and extended amygdala by individual ratings of emotional arousal: A functional magnetic resonance imaging study. *Biological Psychiatry*, *53*, 211–215.

Phan, K. L., Wager, T., Taylor, S. F., & Liberzon, I. (2002). Functional neuroanatomy of emotion: A meta-analysis of emotion activation studies in PET and fMRI. *Neuroimage*, *16*(2), 331–348.

Phelps, E. A. (2004). Human emotion and memory: Interactions of the amygdala and hippocampal complex. *Current Opinion Neurobiology*, *14*(2), 198–202.

Phillips, M. L., Medford, N., Young, A. W., Williams, L., Williams, S. C., Bullmore, E. T., et al. (2001). Time courses of left and right amygdalar responses to fearful facial expressions. *Human Brain Mapping*, *12*(4), 193–202.

Pillay, S. S., Gruber, S. A., Rogowska, J., Simpson, N., & Yurgelun-Todd, D. A. (2006). fMRI of fearful facial affect recognition in panic disorder: The cingulate gyrus-amygdala connection. *Journal of Affective Disorders*, *94*(1–3), 173–181.

Pishyar, R., Harris, L. M., & Menzies, R. G. (2004). Attentional bias for words and faces in social anxiety. *Anxiety, Stress & Coping: An International Journal*, *17*(1), 23–36.

Pizzagalli, D., Regard, M., & Lehmann, D. (1999). Rapid emotional face processing in the human right and left brain hemispheres: An ERP study. *Neuroreport*, *10*(13), 2691–2698.

Potts, N. L., Davidson, J. R., Krishnan, K. R., & Doraiswamy, P. M. (1994). Magnetic resonance imaging in social phobia. *Psychiatry Research*, *52*(1), 35–42.

Potts, N. L., Davidson, J. R., Krishnan, K. R., Doraiswamy, P. M., & Ritchie, J. C. (1991). Levels of urinary free cortisol in social phobia. *Journal of Clinical Psychiatry*, *52*(Suppl), 41–42.

Prather, M. D., Lavenex, P., Mauldin-Jourdain, M. L., Mason, W. A., Capitanio, J. P., Mendoza, S. P., et al. (2001). Increased social fear and decreased fear of objects in monkeys with neonatal amygdala lesions. *Neuroscience*, *106*(4), 653–658.

Quadflieg, S., Mohr, A., Mentzel, H. J., Miltner, W. H., & Straube, T. (2008). Modulation of the neural network involved in the processing of anger prosody: The role of task-relevance and social phobia. *Biological Psychology*, *78*(2), 129–137.

Quirk, G. J., & Beer, J. S. (2006). Prefrontal involvement in the regulation of emotion: Convergence of rat and human studies. *Current Opinion in Neurobiology*, *16*(6), 723–727.

Raichle, M. E., MacLeod, A. M., Snyder, A. Z., Powers, W. J., Gusnard, D. A., & Shulman, G. L. (2001). A default mode of brain function. *Proceedings of the National Academy of Sciences of the USA*, *98*(2), 676–682.

Raichle, M. E., & Snyder, A. Z. (2007). A default mode of brain function: A brief history of an evolving idea. *Neuroimage*, *37*(4), 1083–1090.

Rapee, R. M., & Heimberg, R. G. (1997). A cognitive-behavioral model of anxiety in social phobia. *Behaviour Research and Therapy*, *35*(8), 741–756.

Richard, I. H., Schiffer, R. B., & Kurlan, R. (1996). Anxiety and Parkinson's disease. *Journal of Neuropsychiatry and Clinical Neuroscience*, *8*(4), 383–392.

Roelofs, K., van Peer, J., Berretty, E., Jong, P., Spinhoven, P., & Elzinga, B. M. (2009). Hypothalamus-pituitary-adrenal axis hyperresponsiveness is associated with increased social avoidance behavior in social phobia. *Biological Psychiatry*, *65*(4), 336–343.

Sander, D., Grafman, J., & Zalla, T. (2003). The human amygdala: An evolved system for relevance detection. *Reviews in the Neurosciences*, *14*(4), 303–316.

Sareen, J., Campbell, D. W., Leslie, W. D., Malisza, K. L., Stein, M. B., Paulus, M. P., et al. (2007). Striatal function in generalized social phobia: A functional magnetic resonance imaging study. *Biological Psychiatry*, *61*(3), 396–404.

Sato, W., Yoshikawa, S., Kochiyama, T., & Matsumura, M. (2004). The amygdala processes the emotional significance of facial expressions: An fMRI investigation using the interaction between expression and face direction. *Neuroimage*, *22*(2), 1006–1013.

Schienle, A., Stark, R., Walter, B., Blecker, C., Ott, U., Sammer, G., et al. (2002). The insula is not specifically involved in disgust processing: An fMRI study. *Neuroreport*, *13*(16), 2023–2026.

Schmitz, T. W., & Johnson, S. C. (2006). Self-appraisal decisions evoke dissociated dorsal-ventral aMPFC networks. *Neuroimage*, *30*(3), 1050–1058.

Schneider, F., Weiss, U., Kessler, C., Muller-Gartner, H. W., Posse, S., Salloum, J. B., et al. (1999). Subcortical correlates of differential classical conditioning of aversive emotional reactions in social phobia. *Biological Psychiatry*, *45*(7), 863–871.

Schneier, F. R. (2006). Clinical practice. Social anxiety disorder. *New England Journal of Medicine*, *355*(10), 1029–1036.

Schneier, F. R., Abi-Dargham, A., Martinez, D., Slifstein, M., Hwang, D. R., Liebowitz, M. R., et al. (2009). Dopamine transporters, D2 receptors, and dopamine release in generalized social anxiety disorder. *Depression and Anxiety*, *26*(5), 411–418.

Schneier, F. R., Kent, J. M., Star, A., & Hirsch, J. (2009). Neural circuitry of submissive behavior in social anxiety disorder: A preliminary study of response to direct eye gaze. *Psychiatry Research*, *173*(3), 248–250.

Schneier, F. R., Liebowitz, M. R., Abi-Dargham, A., Zea-Ponce, Y., Lin, S. H., & Laruelle, M. (2000). Low dopamine D(2) receptor binding potential in social phobia. *American Journal of Psychiatry*, *157*(3), 457–459.

Schwartz, C. E., Wright, C. I., Shin, L. M., Kagan, J., & Rauch, S. L. (2003). Inhibited and uninhibited infants "grown up": Adult amygdalar response to novelty. *Science*, *300*(5627), 1952–1953.

Sehlmeyer, C., Schoning, S., Zwitserlood, P., Pfleiderer, B., Kircher, T., Arolt, V., et al. (2009). Human fear conditioning and extinction in neuroimaging: A systematic review. *PLoS One*, *4*(6), e5865.

Shah, S. G., Klumpp, H., Angstadt, M., Nathan, P. J., & Phan, K. L. (2009). Amygdala and insula response to emotional images in patients with generalized social anxiety disorder. *Journal of Psychiatry and Neuroscience*, *34*(4), 296–302.

Shin, L. M., & Liberzon, I. (2009). The neurocircuitry of fear, stress, and anxiety disorders. *Neuropsychopharmacology*, *35*(2), 169–191.

Shirotsuki, K., Izawa, S., Sugaya, N., Yamada, K. C., Ogawa, N., Ouchi, Y., et al. (2009). Salivary cortisol and DHEA reactivity to psychosocial stress in socially anxious males. *International Journal of Psychophysiology*, *72*(2), 198–203.

Somerville, L. H., Kim, H., Johnstone, T., Alexander, A. L., & Whalen, P. J. (2004). Human amygdala responses during presentation of happy and neutral faces: Correlations with state anxiety. *Biological Psychiatry*, *55*(9), 897–903.

Soravia, L. M., Heinrichs, M., Aerni, A., Maroni, C., Schelling, G., Schelling, G., et al. (2006). Glucocorticoids reduce phobic fear in humans. *Proceedings of the National Academy of Sciences of the USA*, *103*(14), 5585–5590.

Sripada, C. S., Angstadt, M., Banks, S., Nathan, P. J., Liberzon, I., & Phan, K. L. (2009). Functional neuroimaging of mentalizing during the trust game in social anxiety disorder. *Neuroreport*, *20*(11), 984–989.

Stein, D. J., Westenberg, H. G., & Liebowitz, M. R. (2002). Social anxiety disorder and generalized anxiety disorder: Serotonergic and dopaminergic neurocircuitry. *Journal of Clinical Psychiatry*, *63*(Suppl 6), 12–19.

Stein, M. B., Goldin, P. R., Sareen, J., Zorrilla, L. T., & Brown, G. G. (2002). Increased amygdala activation to angry and contemptuous faces in generalized social phobia. *Archives of General Psychiatry*, *59*(11), 1027–1034.

Stein, M. B., Heuser, I. J., Juncos, J. L., & Uhde, T. W. (1990). Anxiety disorders in patients with Parkinson's disease. *American Journal of Psychiatry*, *147*(2), 217–220.

Stein, M. B., & Leslie, W. D. (1996). A brain single photon-emission computed tomography (SPECT) study of generalized social phobia. *Biological Psychiatry*, *39*(9), 825–828.

Stein, M. B., Simmons, A. N., Feinstein, J. S., & Paulus, M. P. (2007). Increased amygdala and insula activation during emotion processing in anxiety-prone subjects. *American Journal of Psychiatry*, *164*(2), 318–327.

Stein, M. B., & Stein, D. J. (2008). Social anxiety disorder. *Lancet*, *371*(9618), 1115–1125.

Stopa, L., & Clark, D. M. (2000). Social phobia and interpretation of social events. *Behaviour Research and Therapy*, *38*(3), 273–283.

Straube, T., Kolassa, I. T., Glauer, M., Mentzel, H. J., & Miltner, W. H. (2004). Effect of task conditions on brain responses to threatening faces in social phobics: An event-related functional magnetic resonance imaging study. *Biological Psychiatry*, *56*(12), 921–930.

Straube, T., Mentzel, H. J., & Miltner, W. H. (2005). Common and distinct brain activation to threat and safety signals in social phobia. *Neuropsychobiology*, *52*(3), 163–168.

Tafet, G. E., Feder, D. J., Abulafia, D. P., & Roffman, S. S. (2005). Regulation of hypothalamic-pituitary-adrenal activity in response to cognitive therapy in patients with generalized anxiety disorder. *Cognitive, Affective and Behavioral Neuroscience*, *5*(1), 37–40.

Tiihonen, J., Kuikka, J., Bergstrom, K., Lepola, U., Koponen, H., & Leinonen, E. (1997). Dopamine reuptake site densities in patients with social phobia. *American Journal of Psychiatry*, *154*(2), 239–242.

Tillfors, M., Furmark, T., Marteinsdottir, I., Fischer, H., Pissiota, A., Langstrom, B., et al. (2001). Cerebral blood flow in subjects with social phobia during stressful speaking tasks: A PET study. *American Journal of Psychiatry*, *158*(8), 1220–1226.

Tillfors, M., Furmark, T., Marteinsdottir, I., & Fredrikson, M. (2002). Cerebral blood flow during anticipation of public speaking in social phobia: A PET study. *Biological Psychiatry*, *52*(11), 1113–1119.

Tupler, L. A., Davidson, J. R., Smith, R. D., Lazeyras, F., Charles, H. C., & Krishnan, K. R. (1997). A repeat proton magnetic resonance spectroscopy study in social phobia. *Biological Psychiatry*, *42*(6), 419–424.

Uhde, T. W., Tancer, M. E., Gelernter, C. S., & Vittone, B. J. (1994). Normal urinary free cortisol and postdexamethasone cortisol in social phobia: Comparison to normal volunteers. *Journal of Affective Disorders*, *30*(3), 155–161.

van Ameringen, M., Mancini, C., Szechtman, H., Nahmias, C., Oakman, J. M., Hall, G. B., et al. (2004). A PET provocation study of generalized social phobia. *Psychiatry Research*, *132*(1), 13–18.

van der Wee, N. J., van Veen, J. F., Stevens, H., van Vliet, I. M., van Rijk, P. P., & Westenberg, H. G. (2008). Increased serotonin and dopamine transporter binding in psychotropic medication-naive patients with generalized social anxiety disorder shown by 123I-beta-(4-iodophenyl)-tropane SPECT. *Journal of Nuclear Medicine*, *49*(5), 757–763.

van Overwalle, F. (2008). Social cognition and the brain: A meta-analysis. *Human Brain Mapping*, *30*, 829–858.

van Peer, J. M., Spinhoven, P., van Dijk, J. G., & Roelofs, K. (2009). Cortisol-induced enhancement of emotional face processing in social phobia depends on symptom severity and motivational context. *Biological Psychology*, *81*(2), 123–130.

van Veen, J. F., van Vliet, I. M., DeRijk, R. H., van Pelt, J., Mertens, B., & Zitman, F. G. (2008). Elevated alpha-amylase but not cortisol in generalized social anxiety disorder. *Psychoneuroendocrinology*, *33*, 1313–1321.

van West, D., S. C., Sulon, J., & Deboutte, D. (2008). Hypothalamic-pituitary-adrenal reactivity in prepubertal children with social phobia. *Journal of Affective Disorders*, *111*, 281–290.

Veit, R., Flor, H., Erb, M., Hermann, C., Lotze, M., Grodd, W., et al. (2002). Brain circuits involved in emotional learning in antisocial behavior and social phobia in humans. *Neuroscience Letters*, *328*(3), 233–236.

Wager, T. D., Davidson, M. L., Hughes, B. L., Lindquist, M. A., & Ochsner, K. N. (2008). Prefrontal–subcortical pathways mediating successful emotion regulation. *Neuron*, *59*(6), 1037–1050.

Walker, D. L., & Davis, M. (2002). The role of amygdala glutamate receptors in fear learning, fear-potentiated startle, and extinction. *Pharmacology, Biochemistry and Behavior*, *71*(3), 379–392.

Warwick, J. M., Carey, P., Jordaan, G. P., Dupont, P., & Stein, D. J. (2008). Resting brain perfusion in social anxiety disorder: A voxel-wise whole brain comparison with healthy control subjects. *Progress in Neuropsychopharmacology and Biological Psychiatry*, *32*(5), 1251–1256.

Weinberger, D. A., Schwartz, G. E., & Davidson, R. J. (1979). Low-anxious, high-anxious, and repressive coping styles: Psychometric patterns and behavioral and physiological responses to stress. *Journal of Abnormal Psychology*, *88*(4), 369–380.

Whalen, P. J. (1998). Fear, vigilance, and ambiguity: Intial neuroimaging studies of the human amygdala. *Current Directions in Psychological Science*, *7*(6), 177–188.

Whalen, P. J., Rauch, S. L., Etcoff, N. L., McInerney, S. C., Lee, M. B., & Jenike, M. A. (1998). Masked presentations of emotional facial expressions modulate amygdala activity without explicit knowledge. *Journal of Neuroscience*, *18*(1), 411–418.

Williams, M. A., McGlone, F., Abbott, D. F., & Mattingley, J. B. (2005). Differential amygdala responses to happy and fearful facial expressions depend on selective attention. *Neuroimage*, *24*(2), 417–425.

Winston, J. S., Strange, B. A., O'Doherty, J., & Dolan, R. J. (2002). Automatic and intentional brain responses during evaluation of trustworthiness of faces. *Nature Neuroscience*, *5*(3), 277–283.

Wright, C. I., Martis, B., McMullin, K., Shin, L. M., & Rauch, S. L. (2003). Amygdala and insular responses to emotionally valenced human faces in small animal specific phobia. *Biological Psychiatry*, *54*(10), 1067–1076.

Wright, P., & Liu, Y. (2006). Neutral faces activate the amygdala during identity matching. *Neuroimage*, *29*(2), 628–636.

Yang, T. T., Menon, V., Reid, A. J., Gotlib, I. H., & Reiss, A. L. (2003). Amygdalar activation associated with happy facial expressions in adolescents: A 3-T functional MRI study. *Journal of American Academy of Child and Adolescent Psychiatry*, *42*(8), 979–985.

Yoon, K. L., Fitzgerald, D. A., Angstadt, M., McCarron, R. A., & Phan, K. L. (2007). Amygdala reactivity to emotional faces at high and low intensity in generalized social phobia: A 4-Tesla functional MRI study. *Psychiatry Research*, *154*(1), 93–98.

Yoon, K. L., & Zinbarg, R. E. (2007). Threat is in the eye of the beholder: Social anxiety and the interpretation of ambiguous facial expressions. *Behaviour Research and Therapy*, *45*(4), 839–847.

Yoon, K. L., & Zinbarg, R. E. (2008). Interpreting neutral faces as threatening is a default mode for socially anxious individuals. *Journal of Abnormal Psychology*, *117*(3), 680–685.

Young, E. A., Abelson, J. L., & Cameron, O. G. (2004). Effect of comorbid anxiety disorders on the hypothalamic-pituitary-adrenal axis response to a social stressor in major depression. *Biological Psychiatry*, *56*(2), 113–120.

Zald, D. H. (2003). The human amygdala and the emotional evaluation of sensory stimuli. *Brain Research, Brain Research Reviews*, *41*(1), 88–123.

Chapter 11

Genetic Basis of Social Anxiety Disorder

Murray B. Stein[1] and Joel Gelernter[2]
[1]University of California, San Diego La Jolla, CA 92093, [2]Yale University School of Medicine, VA CT Healthcare Center, West Haven, CT 06516

INTRODUCTION

There are several reasons to focus on a genetic basis for SAD. First and foremost is the fact that SAD runs in families (Stein, Chartier, Hazen et al., 1998) and is strongly believed to have a heritable basis (e.g., Hettema, Neale, & Kendler, 2001). That is, genes account for at least some of the tendency for SAD to run in families. Second, the relationship between certain heritable quantitative traits (e.g., social interactional anxiety) and SAD provides an opportunity to find linkage and/or association to a phenotype that may be closer to biological reality than that provided by DSM-IV (Stein, Chartier, Lizak, & Jang, 2001; Stein, Chavira, & Jang, 2001; Stein, Gelernter, & Smoller, 2004). Such traits are often called "endophenotypes" or "intermediate phenotypes." There have recently been published several reviews on the molecular genetics of anxiety disorders (Norrholm & Ressler, 2009; Hamilton, 2009; Smoller, Block, & Young, 2009) including one of our own (Gelernter & Stein, 2009). Accordingly, in this chapter, we focus our review on the small but growing literature suggesting a relationship between particular genes and SAD or related phenotypes such as introversion and BI.

LINKAGE STUDIES IN SOCIAL ANXIETY DISORDER

In earlier work, we were able to provide evidence excluding linkage of the generalized type of SAD to the 5-HT transporter promoter, 5-HT_{2A} receptor, and to a series of DA receptor genes in a particular set of families (Stein, Chartier, Kozak et al., 1998; Kennedy et al., 2001). These studies, which were designed in the early 1990s, had power only to detect major susceptibility loci, now believed to be inadequate for what is almost certainly a complex disease or trait (Colhoun, McKeigue, & Smith, 2003; Risch, 2000). We subsequently

Social Anxiety: Clinical, Developmental, and Social Perspectives. DOI: 10.1016/B978-0-12-375096-9.00011-0

conducted a genome-wide linkage analysis at 10 cM (centiMorgan) resolution for SAD in a set of extended pedigrees (approximately 160 individuals) (Gelernter, Page, Stein, & Woods, 2004). The most promising results were observed on chromosome 16 where a nonparametric lod score of 3.41 was observed at position 62.3 cM ($p = 0.0003$) within a 53.3 cM region that spans from position 40.6 to 93.9. These results may be considered suggestive of linkage to this region (Lander & Kruglyak, 1995). The most obvious candidate gene mapped in this region is SLC6A2 ("solute carrier family 6 member 2"), the NE transporter protein locus (protein product, NET1), which maps close to D16S3136 (within the ROI, but not at the linkage peak). These preliminary observations indicate the need for larger, better-powered studies to replicate and extend this work, and for fine-mapping and association studies to confirm the identity of susceptibility gene(s).

To the best of our knowledge, no linkage studies have been published reporting on the SAD phenotype in approximately the past decade. Investigators looking at many of the neuropsychiatric disorders have largely switched to the techniques that were for a period of time considered better suited for the study of complex traits: genetic association studies, which are increasingly being conducted at the genome-wide level (McCarthy et al., 2008).

ASSOCIATION STUDIES IN SAD

Although there are dozens of published association studies in other anxiety disorders such as PD (Hamilton, 2009), there are very few association studies of SAD *per se*. Following is a summary of association studies that have focused on various aspects of the SAD phenotype or have included SAD among the phenotypes of interest as part of a broader approach to anxiety phenotypes.

Furmark et al. (2004) studied amygdala activation using [H2(15)O] PET during social anxiety provocation in relation to affective ratings and 5HTTLPR genetic variation in 17 patients with SAD. 5HTTLPR is a frequently studied genetic polymorphism at the 5-HT transporter protein (*SLC6A4*) genetic locus. Individuals with one or two copies of the short ("s") allele had significantly increased levels of anxiety-related traits, state anxiety, and enhanced right amygdala responding to anxiety provocation compared with subjects homozygous for the long ("l") allele. In this study, then, 5HTTLPR variation was associated with symptom severity and amygdala hyperactivity in SAD.

Domschke et al. (2009) studied 62 patients with SAD and 62 age- and sex-matched healthy controls for the influence of serotonin transporter (5HTT) gene variation (5-HTTLPR, rs25531) on tendency to blush. This is considered a very small sample size for a complex trait association study. The authors concluded that this study warranted replication and encouraged genetic analyses of further intermediate phenotypes of SAD.

Finnish researchers took a cross-species approach to identifying genes that regulate anxiety-like behavior, using inbred mouse strains that differ in their innate anxiety levels as a model system. They had previously identified 17 genes with expression levels that correlate with anxiety behavior across the studied strains (Hovatta et al., 2005). In this study they tested for association a total of 208 single-nucleotide polymorphisms (SNPs) in their 13 known human homologues as candidate genes for human anxiety disorders in a sample derived from a Finnish population-based cohort (Donner et al., 2008). Specific alleles and haplotypes of 6 of the 13 genes revealed some evidence for association ($p \leqslant 0.01$) with the strongest evidence for association with SAD found for $p = 0.0009$ with *ALAD* (delta-aminolevulinate dehydratase) ($p = 0.0009$).

In a recent follow-up to that study the investigators tested for association between anxiety disorders and circadian genes, reasoning that circadian disturbances (manifested as sleep problems) were common in persons with anxiety disorders (Sipila et al., 2010). They analyzed 131 SNPs from 13 circadian clock-related genes in the same Finnish sample of 321 persons with anxiety disorders and 653 healthy controls used in the aforementioned study. They found SNPs in two genes that showed evidence of association to SAD: in *ARNTL2* rs2306073 ($p = 0.0099$) and in *DRD2* rs7131056 ($p = 0.0084$). These findings have yet to be replicated.

ASSOCIATION STUDIES IN TRAITS OF POTENTIAL RELEVANCE TO SAD

Shyness

A polymorphism of the 5-HT transporter promoter region polymorphism (a 44-base-pair insertion deletion discussed above, usually referred to as 5HTTLPR) was reported to be related to shyness in a sample of 98 Israeli children attending second grade (Arbelle et al., 2003). This polymorphism has been the focus of considerable prior scrutiny, much of it focused on neuroticism, where numerous associations (and nonreplications) have been reported over the past decade (Schinka, Busch, & Robichaux-Keene, 2004; Sen, Burmeister, & Ghosh, 2004). To the best of our knowledge, the shyness study has not been replicated.

Neuroticism

Neuroticism is a nonspecific, underlying characteristic of many of the mood and anxiety disorders including SAD (Andrews, 1996; Andrews, Slade; Bienvenu, Brown et al., 2001; Hirschfeld et al., 1989; Issakidis, 2002 & Ormel, Oldehinkel, & Brilman, 2001;). Clarifying the genetic architecture of neuroticism and better understanding its molecular basis is likely to yield new insights into the etiology of these disorders (Bienvenu & Stein, 2003). In one study (Hettema, Neale, Myers, Prescott, & Kendler, 2006), the investigators examined how genetic and environmental factors shared by neuroticism and various internalizing disorders (which included major depression, GAD, PD, and phobias including SAD) might explain their comorbidity. Neuroticism and lifetime history of each of these disorders were assessed in over 9000 twins. Using multivariate structural equation modeling, the investigators determined that the genetic correlations between neuroticism and each disorder were high, but not complete, helping to explain the high rates of comorbidity between neuroticism and each of these disorders. The authors stated that these findings suggest that the search for genes for these disorders would benefit from an approach that acknowledges the likelihood that risk genes for each disorder are largely shared among the internalizing disorders.

There have been several genome-wide studies of trait neuroticism (Terracciano et al., 2008; van den Oord et al., 2008; Wray et al., 2008). A genome-wide association scan (GWAS) of 3792 individuals from the genetically isolated population of Sardinia, Italy, found a nonsignificant association of neuroticism with SNAP25 (rs362584, point $P = 5 \times 10(-5)$) (Terracciano et al., 2008). Another study used a sample of 1227 healthy individuals ascertained from a US national sampling frame and available from the National Institute of Mental Health genetics repository; the most promising markers were subsequently tested in a German replication sample of 1880 healthy individuals (van den Oord et al., 2008). The most promising results to emerge were SNPs in the gene *MAMDC1*. The authors noted that small effect sizes may limit the usefulness of SNP markers such as those in *MAMDC1* but that the study did demonstrate the potential of the GWAS approach in detecting potentially important pathogenic pathways.

Yet another study used a genome-wide approach to the topic of neuroticism, but in this instance a linkage approach was used (Wray et al., 2008). The investigators genotyped microsatellite markers in 5069 sibling pairs from Australia and the Netherlands. They found one chromosomal region that exceeded empirically derived thresholds for suggestive linkage using mean neuroticism scores that retained significance after correction for multiple testing: 14q 103 cM (in the Dutch study sample). Linkage intervals for this region overlap with regions identified in other studies of neuroticism or related traits and/or in studies of anxiety in mice. The investigators concluded that these regions may contain causal variants for neuroticism and its related psychiatric disorders and might be useful in prioritizing results from GWAS studies.

Extraversion

Another personality trait that is of equal or greater relevance to SP is extraversion (Bienvenu & Stein, 2003). Bienvenu, Nestadt et al. (2001) found in a general population sample that individuals with SAD or agoraphobia were low in extraversion (almost 1 standard deviation below the mean). Studies in clinical and nonclinical (e.g., college-age student) samples similarly found that persons with anxiety disorders are low in extraversion and high on a conceptually and psychometrically related construct that combines aspects of neuroticism and introversion: harm avoidance (Samuels et al., 2000; Trull & Sher, 1994;). Relatives of probands with SAD show increased levels of harm avoidance compared to relatives of comparison subjects (Stein, Chartier et al., 2001). These observations suggest that the study of extraversion, as a complement to the study of neuroticism, is likely to be of considerable importance in our understanding of the genetics of SAD. In a recent population-based study using a twin registry, Bienvenu, Hettema, Neale, Prescott, and Kendler, (2007) examined the extent to which these two personality dimensions (neuroticism and extraversion) indexed genetic and environmental risk for SAD (and two other phobic disorders, agoraphobia and animal phobia) among 7800 twins. The investigators found that genetic correlations were moderate and negative between extraversion and SAD, and high and positive between neuroticism and SAD. Genetic factors that influenced individual variation in extraversion and neuroticism appeared to account entirely for the genetic liability to SAD, thereby highlighting the importance of maintaining a perspective on the molecular genetics of both introversion (i.e., low extraversion) and neuroticism in SAD.

Compared to neuroticism, relatively little work has been done looking at genetic aspects of extraversion. Most work in this area has been limited to investigation of the relationship between the dopamine D4 receptor gene (*DRD4*) and harm avoidance (which combines aspects of neuroticism and extraversion) (Zohar et al., 2003) or novelty-seeking (which itself shares variance with extraversion) (Costa & McCrae, 1992; Livesley & Jang, 1998). We evaluated the association between allelic variation leading to functional alteration in beta-1-adrenergic function and extraversion (Stein, Schork, & Gelernter, 2004). In a sample of 504 undergraduate college students, we found that a functional serine/glycine substitution at amino acid 49 (Ser49Gly) was associated with an increase in the odds of having low or very low extraversion (odds ratio = 1.68, 95% confidence interval 1.05–2.71). Formal testing showed that population structure did not explain the findings. We suggested that these findings should be replicated and extended to the study of psychiatric disorders marked by low extraversion, namely SAD and other phobic disorders. As of this date, we are not aware of such replications having been attempted. We have also noted an association between the gene encoding regulator of G protein signaling 2 (*RGS2*) and extraversion (Smoller et al., 2008), making it a compelling candidate gene for human anxiety phenotypes (see further discussion of this gene, below).

Several studies have taken a genome-wide approach to the study of extraversion (which, it should be noted, is also the study of introversion; i.e., low levels of extraversion). In one of the aforementioned studies, which also measured neuroticism (Terracciano et al., 2008), a widely studied Val66Met (rs6265) SNP in the gene that codes for brain-derived neurotrophic factor (*BDNF*, a regulator of synaptic plasticity) was associated with extraversion (i.e., Met carriers were more introverted), as were two cadherin genes (*CDH13* and *CDH23*). In a follow-up to that study, the investigators examined the association between *BDNF* and personality traits using a sample from Sardinia ($n = 1560$) and a sample from the Baltimore Longitudinal Study of Aging ($n = 1131$) (Terracciano et al., 2010). Consistent with their aforementioned GWAS results, they found that *BDNF* Met carriers were more introverted. They subsequently explored an interaction between Val66Met and 5HTTLPR in a larger Sardinian sample ($n = 2333$) and found that 5-HTTLPR LL carriers scored lower on neuroticism in the presence of the *BDNF* Val variant but scored higher on neuroticism in the presence of the *BDNF* Met variant. The authors proposed that their findings not only support an association between the *BDNF* Met variant and introversion but also further suggest an interaction between *BDNF* and 5HTTLPR to influence neuroticism. Given these rather complex putative interactions between *BDNF* and 5HTTLPR, replication is in order, but the possibility that these genes may influence traits that underlie SAD is worth further study.

Further genetic investigation of extraversion is, in our opinion, likely to be of considerable value for the understanding of susceptibility for SAD and other anxiety disorders.

Behavioral Inhibition

May represent an "intermediate phenotype" for panic and phobic anxiety disorders that may be more amenable to genetic dissection than the DSM diagnoses (Smoller et al., 2009). In an initial study, researchers conducted family-based association analyses of BI using four genes derived from genetic studies of mouse models of BI (Smoller et al., 2001). The sample included families of 72 children classified as inhibited by structured behavioral assessments. The investigators observed modest evidence of association ($p = 0.05$) between BI and the glutamic acid decarboxylase gene (65 kDA isoform) that encodes an enzyme involved in GABA synthesis.

Subsequently, this research team genotyped a marker tightly linked to the CRH locus in 85 families of children who underwent laboratory-based behavioral assessments of BI (Smoller et al., 2003). Using family-based association analyses, they observed an inverse association between an allele of the CRH-linked locus and BI ($p = 0.015$).

More recently, investigators evaluated the association between RGS2 (discussed above in the section on extraversion) and BI in a family-based sample ($n = 119$ families) of children who underwent laboratory-based assessments of BI (Smoller et al., 2008). Markers spanning *RGS2* were found to be associated with childhood BI (haplotype $P = 3 \times 10^{-5}$; odds ratio, 2.99 in complete trios).

Given the strong, longitudinal association between BI and SAD (Essex, Klein, Slattery, Goldsmith, & Kalin, 2010), this work suggests that the CRH and RGS2 loci should be further scrutinized as potential risk factors for SAD. Moreover, these data further illustrate the potential utility of studying anxiety-related traits as an approach to identifying loci involved in SAD and related anxiety disorders.

CONCLUSIONS

Studies aimed at improving understanding of the genetic basis of SAD have, surprisingly, been scarce. Most of the molecular studies published to date have been seriously underpowered by current standards. As for many of the mental disorders (Craddock et al., 2009), there is uncertainty about the precise delineation of the phenotype, and this may have hindered molecular genetic studies in SAD (and other anxiety disorders) (Smoller et al., 2009). Recent twin studies show, however, that there is much shared genetic liability across the anxiety disorders (Tambs et al., 2009), suggesting that it may be most fruitful in future molecular genetic studies to focus on these common risk genes.

REFERENCES

Andrews, G. (1996). Comorbidity and the general neurotic syndrome. *British Journal of Psychiatry*, *30*, 76–84.

Andrews, G., Slade, T., & Issakidis, C. (2002). Deconstructing current comorbidity: Data from the Australian National Survey of Mental Health and Well-Being. *British Journal of Psychiatry*, *181*, 306–314.

Arbelle, S., Benjamin, J., Golin, M., Kremer, I., Belmaker, R. H., & Ebstein, R. P. (2003). Relation of shyness in grade school children to the genotype for the long form of the serotonin transporter promoter region polymorphism. *American Journal of Psychiatry*, *160*, 671–676.

Bienvenu, O. J., Brown, C., Samuels, J. F., Liang, K. Y., Costa, P. T., Eaton, W. W., et al. (2001). Normal personality traits and comorbidity among phobic, panic, and major depressive disorders. *Psychiatry Research*, *102*, 73–85.

Bienvenu, O. J., Hettema, J. M., Neale, M. C., Prescott, C. A., & Kendler, K. S. (2007). Low extraversion and high neuroticism as indices of genetic and environmental risk for social phobia, agoraphobia, and animal phobia. *American Journal of Psychiatry*, *164*, 1714–1721.

Bienvenu, O. J., Nestadt, G., Samuels, J. F., Howard, W. T., Costa, P. T., Jr., & Eaton, W. W. (2001). Phobic, panic, and major depressive disorders and the five-factor model of personality. *Journal of Nervous and Mental Disease*, *189*, 154–161.

Bienvenu, O. J., & Stein, M. B. (2003). Personality and anxiety disorders: A review. *Journal of Personal Disorder*, *17*, 139–151.

Colhoun, H. M., McKeigue, P. M., & Smith, G. D. (2003). Problems of reporting genetic associations with complex outcomes. *Lancet*, *361*, 865–872.

Costa, P. T., Jr., & McCrae, R. R. (1992). *NEO PI-R Professional Manual*. Odessa, FL: Psychological Assessment Resources, Inc.

Craddock, N., Kendler, K., Neale, M., Nurnberger, J., Purcell, S., Rietschel, M., et al. (2009). Dissecting the phenotype in genome-wide association studies of psychiatric illness. *British Journal of Psychiatry*, *195*, 97–99.

Domschke, K., Stevens, S., Beck, B., Baffa, A., Hohoff, C., Deckert, J., et al. (2009). Blushing propensity in social anxiety disorder: Influence of serotonin transporter gene variation. *Journal of Neural Transmission, 116*, 663–666.

Donner, J., Pirkola, S., Silander, K., Kananen, L., Terwilliger, J. D., Lonnqvist, J., et al. (2008). An association analysis of murine anxiety genes in humans implicates novel candidate genes for anxiety disorders. *Biological Psychiatry, 64*, 672–680.

Essex, M. J., Klein, M. H., Slattery, M. J., Goldsmith, H. H., & Kalin, N. H. (2010). Early risk factors and developmental pathways to chronic high inhibition and social anxiety disorder in adolescence. *American Journal of Psychiatry, 167*, 40–46.

Furmark, T., Tillfors, M., Garpenstrand, H., Marteinsdottir, I., Langstrom, B., Oreland, L., et al. (2004). Serotonin transporter polymorphism related to amygdala excitability and symptom severity in patients with social phobia. *Neuroscience Letters, 362*, 189–192.

Gelernter, J., Page, G. P., Stein, M. B., & Woods, S. W. (2004). Genome-wide linkage scan for loci predisposing to social phobia: Evidence for a chromosome 16 risk locus. *American Journal of Psychiatry, 161*, 59–66.

Gelernter, J., & Stein, M. B. (2009). Heritability and genetics of anxiety disorders. In M. M. Antony & M. B. Stein (Eds.), *Handbook of Anxiety Disorders*. New York: Oxford University Press.

Hamilton, S. P. (2009). Linkage and association studies of anxiety disorders. *Depression and Anxiety, 26*, 976–983.

Hettema, J. M., Neale, M. C., & Kendler, K. S. (2001). A review and meta-analysis of the genetic epidemiology of anxiety disorders. *American Journal of Psychiatry, 158*, 1568–1578.

Hettema, J. M., Neale, M. C., Myers, J. M., Prescott, C. A., & Kendler, K. S. (2006). A population-based twin study of the relationship between neuroticism and internalizing disorders. *American Journal of Psychiatry, 163*, 857–864.

Hirschfeld, R. M., Klerman, G. L., Lavori, P., Keller, M. B., Griffith, P., & Coryell, W. (1989). Premorbid personality assessments of first onset of major depression. *Archives of General Psychiatry, 46*, 345–350.

Hovatta, I., Tennant, R. S., Helton, R., Marr, R. A., Singer, O., Redwine, J. M., et al. (2005). Glyoxalase 1 and glutathione reductase 1 regulate anxiety in mice. *Nature, 438*, 662–666.

Kennedy, J. L., Neves-Pereira, M., King, N., Lizak, M. V., Basile, V. S., Chartier, M. J., et al. (2001). Dopamine system genes not linked to social phobia. *Psychiatric Genetics, 11*, 213–217.

Lander, E., & Kruglyak, L. (1995). Genetic dissection of complex traits: Guidelines for interpreting and reporting linkage results. *Nature Genetics, 11*, 241–247.

Livesley, W. J., & Jang, K. L. (1998). Toward an empirically based classification of personality disorder. *Journal of Personality Disorders, 14*, 137–151.

McCarthy, M. I., Abecasis, G. R., Cardon, L. R., Goldstein, D. B., Little, J., Ioannidis, J. P., et al. (2008). Genome-wide association studies for complex traits: Consensus, uncertainty and challenges. *Nature Reviews Genetics, 9*, 356–369.

Norrholm, S. D., & Ressler, K. J. (2009). Genetics of anxiety and trauma-related disorders. *Neuroscience, 164*, 272–287.

Ormel, J., Oldehinkel, A. J., & Brilman, E. (2001). The interplay and etiological continuity of neuroticism, difficulties, and life events in the etiology of major and subsyndromal, first and recurrent depressive episodes in later life. *American Journal of Psychiatry, 158*, 885–891.

Risch, N. J. (2000). Searching for genetic determinants in the new millenium. *Nature, 405*, 847–856.

Samuels, J., Nestadt, G., Bienvenu, O. J., Costa, P. T., Jr., Riddle, M. A., Liang, K.-Y., et al. (2000). Personality disorders and normal personality dimensions in obsessive-compulsive disorder. *British Journal of Psychiatry, 177*, 457–462.

Schinka, J. A., Busch, R. M., & Robichaux-Keene, N. (2004). A meta-analysis of the association between the serotonin transporter gene polymorphism (5-HTTLPR) and trait anxiety. *Molecular Psychiatry*, *9*, 197–202.

Sen, S., Burmeister, M., & Ghosh, D. (2004). Meta-analysis of the association between a serotonin transporter promoter polymorphism (5-HTTLPR) and anxiety-related personality traits. *American Journal of Medical Genetics*, *127B*, 85–89.

Sipila, T., Kananen, L., Greco, D., Donner, J., Silander, K., Terwilliger, J. D., et al. (2010). An association analysis of circadian genes in anxiety disorders. *Biological Psychiatry*, *67*, 1163–1170.

Smoller, J. W., Block, S. R., & Young, M. M. (2009). Genetics of anxiety disorders: The complex road from DSM to DNA. *Depression and Anxiety*, *26*, 965–975.

Smoller, J. W., Paulus, M. P., Fagerness, J. A., Purcell, S., Yamaki, L. H., Hirshfeld-Becker, D., et al. (2008). Influence of RGS2 on anxiety-related temperament, personality, and brain function. *Archives of General Psychiatry*, *65*, 298–308.

Smoller, J. W., Rosenbaum, J. F., Biederman, J., Kennedy, J., Dai, D., Racette, S. R., et al. (2003). Association of a genetic marker at the corticotropin-releasing hormone locus with behavioral inhibition. *Biological Psychiatry*, *54*, 1376–1381.

Smoller, J. W., Rosenbaum, J. F., Biederman, J., Susswein, L. S., Kennedy, J., Kagan, J., et al. (2001). Genetic association analysis of behavioral inhibition using candidate loci from mouse models. *American Journal of Medical Genetics (Neuropsychiatric Genetics)*, *105*, 226–235.

Stein, M. B., Chartier, M. J., Hazen, A. L., Kozak, M. V., Tancer, M. E., Lander, S., et al. (1998). A direct-interview family study of generalized social phobia. *American Journal of Psychiatry*, *155*, 90–97.

Stein, M. B., Chartier, M. J., Kozak, M. V., Hazen, A. L., King, N., & Kennedy, J. L. (1998). Genetic linkage to the serotonin transporter and 5HT2A receptor excluded in generalized social phobia. *Psychiatry Research*, *81*, 283–291.

Stein, M. B., Chartier, M. J., Lizak, M. V., & Jang, K. L. (2001). Familial aggregation of anxiety-related quantitative traits in generalized social phobia: Clues to understanding "disorder" heritability? *American Journal of Medical Genetics (Neuropsychiatric Genetics)*, *105*, 79–83.

Stein, M. B., Chavira, D. A., & Jang, K. L. (2001). Bringing up bashful baby: Developmental pathways to social phobia. *Psychiatric Clinics of North America*, *24*, 661–675.

Stein, M. B., Gelernter, J., & Smoller, J. W. (2004). Genetic aspects of social anxiety and related traits. In B. Bandelow & D. J. Stein (Eds.), *Social anxiety disorder: More than shyness* (pp. 197–214). New York, NY: Marcel Dekker, Inc.

Stein, M. B., Schork, N. J., & Gelernter, J. (2004). A polymorphism of the beta(1)-adrenergic receptor is associated with low extraversion. *Biological Psychiatry*, *56*, 217–224.

Tambs, K., Czajkowsky, N., Roysamb, E., Neale, M. C., Reichborn-Kjennerud, T., Aggen, S. H., et al. (2009). Structure of genetic and environmental risk factors for dimensional representations of DSM-IV anxiety disorders. *British Journal of Psychiatry*, *195*, 301–307.

Terracciano, A., Sanna, S., Uda, M., Deiana, B., Usala, G., Busonero, F., et al. (2008). Genome-wide association scan for five major dimensions of personality. *Molecular Psychiatry, 15*(6), 647–650.

Terracciano, A., Tanaka, T., Sutin, A. R., Deiana, B., Balaci, L., Sanna, S., et al. (2010). BDNF Val66Met is associated with introversion and interacts with 5-HTTLPR to influence neuroticism. *Neuropsychopharmacology*, *35*, 1083–1089.

Trull, T. J., & Sher, K. J. (1994). Relationship between the five-factor model of personality and axis I disorders in a non-clinical sample. *Journal of Abnormal Psychology*, *103*, 350–360.

van den Oord, E. J., Kuo, P. H., Hartmann, A. M., Webb, B. T., Moller, H. J., Hettema, J. M., et al. (2008). Genomewide association analysis followed by a replication study implicates a novel candidate gene for neuroticism. *Archives of General Psychiatry*, *65*, 1062–1071.

Wray, N. R., Middeldorp, C. M., Birley, A. J., Gordon, S. D., Sullivan, P. F., Visscher, P. M., et al. (2008). Genome-wide linkage analysis of multiple measures of neuroticism of 2 large cohorts from Australia and the Netherlands. *Archives of General Psychiatry*, *65*, 649–658.

Zohar, A. H., Dina, C., Rosolio, N., Osher, Y., Gritsenko, I., Bachner-Melman, R., et al. (2003). Tridimensional personality questionnaire trait of harm avoidance (anxiety proneness) is linked to a locus on chromosome 8p21. *American Journal of Medical Genetics*, *117B*, 66–69.

Chapter 12

Temperamental Contributions to the Development of Psychological Profiles

Jerome Kagan
Department? Harvard University, Cambridge, MA 02138

Most scientists define a temperamental bias as a biologically based susceptibility for particular feelings and actions, usually appearing during early childhood, that experiences sculpt into a large, but limited, number of possible personality traits. The affective components of each bias include the ease and intensity with which particular feelings are experienced and the individual's ability to regulate them. I have suggested that, although most temperamental biases are the result of heritable variation in brain neurochemistry, some temperaments can be produced by prenatal events that are not strictly genetic, including season of conception and maternal infections or stressors that alter the chemical environment during gestation (Kagan & Snidman, 2004).

Because the number of possible biological foundations for a temperament is very large, the majority of biases remain undiscovered. Some of these biases will be rare and others relatively common. There are over 290000 combinations of the 12 blood types and their variants and the probability that any two people will have the same combination is 3 out of 10000 (Lewontin, 1995). Because there are many more distinct neurochemical profiles than there are blood types, the chance of any two individuals having the same pattern of temperaments should be far less than 3 out of 10000. Newton's inverse square law explained why there are seasons; Darwinian theory provided an account of the similarities and differences among animals; the concept of "temperament" helps to explain why fraternal twins develop different personalities and why only some individuals exposed to a stressor acquire a form of psychopathology.

HOW MANY TEMPERAMENTS?

Infants vary in a relatively small number of behaviors that appear to be temperamental in origin. The most obvious refer to reactions to the uncomfortable

Social Anxiety: Clinical, Developmental, and Social Perspectives. DOI: 10.1016/B978-0-12-375096-9.00012-2

states of pain, cold, and hunger. Infants vary in both the intensity and duration of distress to aversive events, as well as in the ease of being soothed; hence, there should be at least four different temperamental biases: (1) infants who cry intensely and do not soothe easily; (2) infants who cry intensely but are soothed with minimal effort; (3) infants who are not seriously distressed but, nonetheless, do not soothe easily; and, finally (4), those who are minimally distressed and easily soothed.

Another quartet of temperaments is defined by reactions to unfamiliar or unexpected events that are neither painful nor frustrating. These include new foods, smells, sounds, and sights. Some infants become motorically active to these incentives; others remain still; some cry; others are quiet. The combinations of these reactions generate four additional temperaments. Infants also vary in their reaction to frustrations, such as losing the nipple they were sucking or being restrained by a blanket or hands. The combination of vigorous motor activity and crying to these frustrations yields an additional four temperaments. Four additional biases are defined by the degree of lability or predictability of the infant's behavior, as well as the frequency of spontaneous babbling, smiling, or limb movements that occur without any external incentive.

These 16 temperaments are defined by the infants' behavior rather than by private psychological states that are not easily observed. It is likely, however, that infants also vary in the intensity of hedonic pleasure or pain they experience to sweet tastes and gentle caresses, or bitter tastes and rough handling. Some infants have a larger-than-expected number of taste buds for sweet or bitter substances and should experience more intense sensations to ice cream or turnips (Zhang et al., 2009).

Thus, future investigators may add these 2 biases to the 16 that are detected more easily. However, 18 is a small number considering the large number of possible temperaments with a biological foundation. Hence, it is relevant to ask why psychologists have observed such a small number of temperamental biases when, potentially, there could be several thousand. First, many potential brain profiles probably have no implications for temperament. Second, there may be subtypes within each bias. Perhaps some infants scream to the pain of a diaper pin but do not cry when hungry; some may smile when they see their mothers but not while playing peek-a-boo. Future research will discover many more temperaments than those nominated.

Although scientists will eventually discover the genes that predispose a child to a particular pattern of temperaments, it will be impossible to predict their later personality because each pattern leads to different combinations of emotions and habits depending on life experiences. No scientist has discovered any gene, or set of genes, that is consistently associated with a particular personality independent of the child's gender, ethnicity, and life history.

GENES AND NEUROCHEMISTRY

There are at least 150 different brain molecules, along with the density and location of their receptors, that could be the foundation of a human temperament. These molecules include norepinephrine, DA, 5-HT, CRH, GABA, opioids, vasopressin, oxytocin, prolactin, monoamine oxidase, and the sex hormones.

First, some brain molecules and the neuronal clusters they influence are excitatory and some inhibitory, and a balance between excitation and inhibition determines the brain state that might lead to a behavior. For example, the balance between opioids and CRH in the locus ceruleus influences the organism's reactions to a stressor (van Bockstaele, Bajic, Proudfit, & Valentino, 2001). Endogenous opioids are more effective in muting unpleasant states in males than in females because estrogen dilutes but androgen potentiates the effectiveness of the opioids.

Second, variation in the density of receptors can be independent of the concentration of the molecule that binds to it. If we assume that the concentration of a particular neurotransmitter or neuromodulator, as well as the density of their receptors, can be low, moderate, or high, there can be nine possible profiles for each molecule. Hence, 150 different molecules would yield at least 1400 neurochemical profiles that could reciprocally influence each other. This claim implies a very large number of temperaments.

Examples of modest relations between neurochemistry and behaviors related to temperament have been discovered. Norepinephrine is secreted by the locus ceruleus, which sends axons to sites that affect alertness and the ability to detect a subtle stimulus in a noisy background.

5-HT, secreted by the raphe nucleus, suppresses neuronal excitability and infants or children with lower levels of brain 5-HT tend to be more distressed. The duration of 5-HT activity in the synapse is affected by the presence of the 5-HT transporter molecule, which absorbs 5-HT from the synapse. Children inherit varied alleles of the gene for this molecule that influence the amount of transporter produced. Two of these alleles, called short and long, are located in the promoter region of the gene. The short allele is associated with less effective transcription of the gene and therefore there is less transporter and 5-HT remains active for a longer time. It is believed, however, that this state leads to suppression of the raphe and, as a result, a lower tonic level of 5-HT and greater excitability in the circuit that connects the amygdala and the prefrontal cortex (Green et al., 2008; Pezawas et al., 2005). Adults with the short allele have greater amygdalar activity to fear-provoking events than those with the long allele (Hariri et al., 2002). Asians are much more likely than Europeans and Africans to possess the short allele and Asian infants and children react differently from Caucasians to unfamiliar events (Gelernter et al., 1999; Kagan & Snidman, 2004).

The different classes of neuropeptides, secreted in the hypothalamus but stored in the pituitary, are relevant for temperaments. One function of the opioids is to modulate the medulla, which receives information from the body and transmits it to the amygdala and cortex. Variation in the density of opioid receptors in the medulla will affect the intrusiveness of bodily states into consciousness. Infants born with a high density should experience less-frequent and less-intense changes in feeling tone than those with fewer receptors, who will be vulnerable to conscious feelings of arousal that they may interpret as anxiety or dysphoria (McNally & Westbrook, 2003). Those with greater opioid activity might experience more moments of serenity (Miyawaki, Goodchild, & Pilowsky, 2002).

The neuropeptide oxytocin mutes tension and contributes to close emotional relationships with others. The females of most species have greater oxytocin activity than males and women in most cultures establish closer relationships with family, peers, and romantic partners than men. Infants born with a lower level of oxytocin or a smaller density of receptors might form less intense bonds to their parents despite affectionate care.

The peptide vasopressin has an excitatory effect on neurons and its activity is greater in males than females.

GABA, one of the most prevalent molecules, inhibits neuronal excitability. The amygdala, which mediates signs of fear and anxiety, has a dense set of GABA receptors and infants born with a lower density should be more vulnerable to states of fear or anxiety. The speculation that infants born with a compromise in the effectiveness of either GABA-ergic or serotonergic circuits should be less able to modulate distress finds support in the fact that very irritable two-year-olds, compared with relaxed toddlers, possessed the shorter form of an allele in the promoter region for the 5-HT transporter gene (Auerbach et al., 1999).

Variation in DA release and the density of its varied receptors contribute to cortical excitability, intensity of sensory pleasure, and reaction to novelty. However, the surge in DA to an unexpected event that is desired is inversely related to the tonic level of DA activity, especially in the striatum. The lower the tonic level, the larger the surge in DA and the greater the probability that the individual will report a feeling of pleasure. These facts suggest that children with smaller surges of dopaminergic activity might derive less pleasure from experiences most enjoy. Some infants rarely smile or laugh to a surprise or a sweet food and occasionally display a frown on their face. But those with a lower tonic level who experience a large surge should have a stronger preference for novel experiences. It is relevant that females, both animals and humans, have more DA receptors in the striatum that are occupied and, therefore, fewer receptors are available for activation. This state is due, in part, to the fact that estrogen inhibits the DA transporter molecule (Becker, 1999). It may not be a coincidence that fewer females than males prefer high-risk novel experiences such as sport parachuting, drag racing, or high-stakes gambling.

These relations represent only a small number of the possible neurochemical profiles that might contribute to a temperament. Unfortunately, the current immaturity of our knowledge frustrates any synthetic attempt to posit any specific relation between a neurochemical profile and a temperament. Because genes appear to account for less than 10% of the variation in most complex behaviors that have been studied, it is unlikely that a single allele, molecule, or receptor distribution can create a temperamental type independent of the person's social class, gender, and life history (Manuck, Flory, Ferrell, & Muldoon, 2004). It is impossible, at the present time, to define a temperament in terms of a neurobiological profile. Furthermore, the number of possible neurochemical profiles that could affect behavior is larger than the number of behavioral profiles. There is, after all, a limited number of ways in which a child can display timidity with other children on a playground. A large number of neurochemical patterns could accompany standing apart from the group, remaining quiet, playing alone, or staring vigilantly at other children.

Furthermore, it is likely that combinations of alleles, rather than single alleles, will be more predictive of a temperamental type. One-year-olds with extreme levels of avoidant behavior to a stranger possessed both the two short alleles of the 5-HT transporter gene, as well as the seven-repeat polymorphism of the dopamine D4 receptor. Minimally avoidant children combined the two long forms of the 5-HT transporter gene with the seven-repeat polymorphism (Lakatos et al., 2003). The combined effects of 19 different brain molecules were required to account for 60% of the variation in avoidant behavior in a sample of rats (Ray, Hansen, & Waters, 2006). It is likely that the many inconsistencies reported across different laboratories reflect the investigator's decision to measure only one allele, rather than several simultaneously (Arbelle et al., 2003).

OTHER ORIGINS OF TEMPERAMENT

Although inherited variation in brain chemistry is probably the most frequent basis for a temperament, it is not the only source. Identical twins do not have identical fingerprints or moods, and the first kitten cloned from one of its mother's cells had a coat color and personality that differed from these characteristics in the mother.

Season of conception might contribute to a select number of temperaments because the pregnant mother's physiology is influenced by the rate of change in the hours of daylight that occur during the spring and fall. When daylight is decreasing faster than usual, from early September to late October in the northern hemisphere, mothers secrete larger amounts of melatonin and women differ in the amount of melatonin they secrete as dusk approaches. Embryos conceived from late February to late April, when the hours of daylight are increasing, are exposed to smaller amounts of melatonin. Melatonin has profound influences on the embryo's brain and body, including the activation or silencing of genes and the synthesis of molecules, such as cortisol, that influence the developing brain (Chotai & Asberg, 1999; Torres-Farfan et al., 2004). Thus, embryos with genes that rendered them especially vulnerable to high or low concentrations of melatonin should be affected by the season of conception. The evidence supports that conviction. Children conceived during the fall in the northern hemisphere are at a slightly higher risk for becoming extremely shy and for having suicidal thoughts as adults (Gortmaker, Kagan, Caspi, & Silva, 1997).

In addition, maternal infections, extreme stress, or the mother's abuse of alcohol or drugs during pregnancy could create conditions that lead to neurochemical, anatomical, or immune disturbances that can create psychological biases in the infant. Unborn infants whose mothers were exposed to the flu are at a slightly higher risk for developing schizophrenia because the mother's immune system responds to the infection by producing cytokines, which affect the developing fetus (Patterson, 2006).

SOURCES OF EVIDENCE

The source of evidence used to define a temperamental bias remains controversial. The validity of every inference in every domain of science is influenced by the method that generated the observation. Therefore, the validity of a conclusion can change when the source of evidence is altered, even though investigators might continue to use the same construct. Verbal reports continue to be the most frequent source of evidence for human temperaments, either verbal descriptions of young children provided by a parent or reports provided by older children and their teachers or peers. A less frequent source comes from behavioral observations in the laboratory, or, less often, at home or in the school setting. The least frequent source refers to biological measures, such as vagal tone, heart rate, or cortisol level. Behavioral observations are not a good proxy for parental descriptions; biological measures are not a valid proxy for behavior or parent reports; and parent reports are not a good proxy for behavioral observations.

Investigators who rely only on parent reports assume that the parent's descriptions correspond closely to what they would find if they observed the infant directly. Unfortunately, this assumption is overly optimistic. The degree of correspondence is modest at best; hence, conclusions based only on parental descriptions have a special meaning and limited validity.

At least six conditions compromise the accuracy of parental report. First, the parents' descriptions are influenced by their conceptions of the ideal child. Those who want sociable children will be threatened by a very quiet infant and may deny their child's timidity while exaggerating their sociability. Second, parents are sensitive to the logical consistency of their multiple answers to a questionnaire. If a mother says that her daughter smiles a lot on an early question, she might resist acknowledging on later questions that her child shows signs of sadness or anxiety.

Third, the nouns and verbs on questionnaires refer to abstract behavioral categories; hence, it is difficult for a parent to describe blends of behaviors or emotions. There is no English word that describes the emotion generated in a child who hopes for parental forgiveness for a misdemeanor but is afraid of being punished. Human languages are simply not rich enough to capture the important emotions and behaviors that are essential parts of the human competence.

Fourth, every question requires informants to make a comparison. When parents read, "Does your child like to go to parties?" they unconsciously compare that preference with that for other activities their child might enjoy. If one parent compares "going to parties" with an activity that the child dislikes whereas a second parent compares "going to parties" with another activity the child prefers, the former is more likely than the latter to endorse that item strongly, even though both children might like going to parties to an equivalent degree. Fifth, young parents who have not had extensive experience with infants or children have a less accurate basis for judging their first child than those who have had two or three children.

Finally, parents differ in their understanding of the meanings of the words on questionnaires. One of my students once asked adolescents who had watched two actors compete in a laboratory film, "Which actor was more anxious?" Some adolescents interpreted the word "anxious" as meaning "eager to perform well;" others interpreted the same word as meaning "they were fearful." Some mothers interpret the word "shy" as implying that their child is very sensitive to peers; others interpret the same word as meaning that their child is cautious when interacting with others; still others interpret the word "shy" as if it meant "fear of all unfamiliar adults."

These are only some reasons why parental answers to questionnaires have only a poor to modest correspondence with comparable information based on direct behavioral observations (Kagan, 1998; Klein, 1991; Seifer, Sameroff, Barrett, & Krafchuk, 1994). A nice example of the imperfect relation between what people say, and presumably what they believe is true, and their brain state is seen in the difference between a subjective feeling and the brain's reaction to a painful source of heat applied to the arm. Although all adults were told they would be receiving acupuncture to reduce the pain produced by the heat, only some received the acupuncture. Although the adults in both groups who thought they were receiving acupuncture reported an equivalent reduction in pain, only those who actually received the acupuncture showed reduced activation of the brain areas that mediate pain (Kong et al., 2009).

The ambiguous meaning of a person's verbal statement is revealed by a comment Ludwig Wittgenstein made to a relative as the philosopher lay dying. As some readers may know, Wittgenstein was profoundly depressed and anxious most of his life and had written in a notebook years earlier that he could not imagine a future that contained any joy or friendships. Nonetheless, one of his last comments before dying was: "Tell them I've had a wonderful life" (Waugh, 2008). So much for the meaning and validity of verbal reports.

Psychologists must exploit multiple sources of evidence in order to understand most phenomena. If they do not they resemble blind adults, some with scissors and others with a jackknife, trying to separate an intact rose from the other parts of the plant. All will come away with a different part of the flower but all will be convinced they have extracted a perfect example of a rose.

The candidates for human temperaments that are based on adult answers to questionnaires are, in reality, personality traits. Adult descriptions of their feelings, moods, and behaviors represent different combinations of childhood temperaments, life histories, and private interpretations of their actions in the settings in which they live. A person can report chronic unhappiness because of persistent poverty and marginalization or a neurochemistry characterized by low levels of 5-HT and DA. No astrophysicist would restrict the evidence to observations made with optical telescopes in order to understand the universe; no biologist would rely only on basal metabolic rate to understand human physiology; and no social scientist should rely only on verbal answers to questionnaires in order to understand temperaments or personality types.

VARIATION IN REACTIONS TO THE UNFAMILIAR

Two important temperamental biases refer to the reactions of children to unexpected changes in the sensory surround and to events that deviate from the agent's acquired representations. Both events automatically alert the individual and provoke attempts to relate the unexpected experience to the local context and their knowledge. The brain/mind of an animal or human is always prepared for a particular envelope of events that is most likely to occur in a particular context. An adult wearing a clown costume entering a room in which a child is playing lies outside the envelope of expected events and elicits automatic vigilance, immobility, and, in a small proportion of children, crying. This profile defines what psychologists call "event uncertainty" or "fear to novelty." The fact that some children cry intensely and remain frozen whereas others stare for a few moments and then smile or approach the clown requires an explanation.

The reaction to events that are deviant from acquired knowledge creates a state of uncertainty that differs from the surprise and startle provoked by an unexpected change in the sensory surround originating in the unexpected occurrence of a familiar stimulus (i.e., a sudden clap of thunder). In addition, by six or seven years of age, children can recognize that they have to select one response from a set of alternatives and often are not certain which one is most appropriate. This state, called "response uncertainty," can activate the amygdala (Hsu, Bhatt, Adolphs, Tranel, & Caamerer, 2005).

I have suggested that a temperamental bias favoring high or low reactivity, which can be detected during infancy, is the basis for the variation in infant behavior to events that deviate from acquired knowledge, and could be the foundation of a salient state of response uncertainty during adolescence (Kagan & Fox, 2006; Kagan & Snidman, 2004). Infants who are easily aroused by unfamiliar events could become one of a large, but nonetheless limited, number of personality types depending on their past experiences. Every psychological quality can be likened to a fabric woven from very thin black threads representing biology and very thin white ones representing experience. However, the cloth appears pale gray because the separate black and white threads are impossible to detect once the weaving is complete. Similar variation in the behavioral reactions to unfamiliar events have been observed in mice, rats, voles, dogs, cows, monkeys, birds, and fish (LeDoux, 1996).

Behavioral observations of a large sample of identical and fraternal twins at 14, 20, 24, and 36 months revealed that a timid–shy or a bold–sociable profile had a heritable component (Kagan & Saudino, 2001; Robinson, Kagan, Reznick, & Corley, 1992). Timid children, called "inhibited," remain close to their mother and avoid playing with unfamiliar toys or children. Bold, sociable children, called "uninhibited," display the opposite profile. The heritability values for inhibited and uninhibited behavior were higher when the sample was restricted to children who were extreme on either trait in a play session with two unfamiliar children (DiLalla, Kagan, & Reznick, 1994).

Many children who developed PTSD following a trauma had been vulnerable to anxiety before the trauma occurred. A group of fourth- and fifth-grade children living in south Florida had been assessed for anxiety 15 months before Hurricane Andrew struck the area in which they lived. The 11% who remained anxious seven months after the storm had been categorized as highly anxious prior to the hurricane (LaGreca, Silverman, & Wassastein, 1998). During the bombings of London during World War II, those children under age five who became extremely fearful when taken from their homes had displayed signs of anxiety long before the bombing raids began (John, 1941).

Freud dismissed unfamiliarity as a source of anxiety because he was concerned with chronic, rather than acute, anxiety. Most adults are not afraid of meeting strangers or visiting new places. Therefore, it was easy for Freud to conclude that a child's fear of the unfamiliar was a transient property. In addition, Freud's wish to be loyal to the principle of parsimony motivated him to posit only one type of anxiety. The aesthetic appeal of his ideas would have been diluted if he had nominated several different types of anxiety, each with a distinct origin. A similar aesthetic standard motivated the Greeks to assume there were only four temperamental types to match the number of combinations of the qualities warm–cold and dry–moist. Freud and the Greeks failed to heed Francis Bacon's warning, "Let every student of nature take this as his rule, that whatever the mind seizes upon with particular satisfaction is to be held in suspicion."

HIGH- AND LOW-REACTIVE INFANTS

Extensive research with animals reveals that the amygdala responds to unfamiliar or unexpected events, even if the event is not aversive. This structure also mediates the acquisition of conditioned responses, such as freezing and changes in autonomic activity, to an aversive unconditioned stimulus (LeDoux, 1996). The amygdala contains several distinct neuronal clusters and receptors for a variety of neurotransmitters and neuromodulators relevant to the emotions and behaviors that define a temperament (Amaral, Price, Pitkanen, & Carmichael, 1992). These facts imply that infants who become distressed to unfamiliar events possess a neurochemistry that renders the amygdala and its projections excitable. Infants who inherit this neurochemistry should display behaviors consistent with that assumption.

One important clue as to the infant behaviors that might predict future inhibited or uninhibited profiles is the discovery that the basolateral area of the amygdala sends projections to the striatum which, in turn, mediates limb movements in animals (Rolls, 1992). The amygdala is also the origin of a pathway to the central gray that mediates arching of the back and body immobility, and a pathway to the nucleus ambiguus that mediates distress cries. Therefore, an infant with a neurochemistry that produces a lower threshold of excitability in the amygdala should display vigorous limb movements, arching of the back, and crying to unfamiliar events. Infants who display this profile, called "high-reactive," should be especially vulnerable to becoming avoidant to, and distressed by, unfamiliar events later in life; that is, they should become inhibited children. By contrast, infants born with a different neurochemistry that raises the threshold of the amygdala should display minimal motor activity and little crying and, after the first birthday, should be uninhibited.

My colleagues and I administered a battery of unfamiliar visual, auditory, and olfactory stimuli to 462 healthy, Caucasian, middle-class, four-month-old infants (Kagan, 1994). The unexpected events included the mother looking down at the infant but not talking, brief sentences played through a speaker baffle without the support of a human face, colorful mobiles moving in front of the infant's face, a cotton swab dipped in dilute butyl alcohol applied to the nostrils, and tape-recorded nonsense syllables played at three different levels of loudness. The 20% of the sample who combined vigorous motor activity, including arching of the back, and crying were classified as high-reactive. The 40% who showed little motor activity and minimal distress were classified as low-reactive. The remaining 40% of the sample belonged to two other temperamental categories. Fox and colleagues at the University of Maryland reported similar proportions based on their longitudinal study of a large number of Maryland infants (Calkins & Fox, 1992).

ASSESSMENT IN THE SECOND YEAR

About 80% of this sample returned to the laboratory at 14 and 21 months and they were exposed to a variety of unfamiliar social and nonsocial events (Kagan, 1994). The episodes included (1) rotation of small plastic objects in a metal wheel, (2) an examiner who frowned and spoke to the child in a serious voice, (3) the placement of electrodes for heart rate and a blood pressure cuff, (4) an unfamiliar woman who invited the child to imitate some novel actions and accept liquid on the tongue, and (5) a stranger and clown who invited the child to approach and a moving robot the examiner asked the child to touch. Each episode was scored for the presence of fear, where fear was defined as fretting or crying to an unfamiliar incentive or failing to approach the stranger, clown, or robot despite a friendly invitation to do so.

The 30% of the children who showed four or more fears at both 14 and 21 months were regarded as displaying a high level of fear (the mean number of fears was 2.6 at 14 months and 2.7 at 21 months). One-half of the high-reactive infants had four or more fears at both ages, compared with only 10% of the low-reactives. By contrast, 75% of the children who had been low-reactive showed zero or only one fear at both ages. These results suggest that the high- and low-reactive categories predict a tendency to be fearful or fearless to unfamiliar experiences in the second year of life.

ASSESSMENT AT FOUR-AND-A-HALF YEARS

Most four-year-old children have gained control over the display of extreme distress to unfamiliarity; hence, it is difficult to provoke unambiguous signs of fear without violating ethical standards. However, two behaviors that might index these biases are absence of spontaneous talking and smiling when interacting with an unfamiliar child or adult. If we assume that becoming quiet in an unfamiliar social setting is analogous to an animal freezing in an unfamiliar context, children who had been high-reactive should be less talkative and smile less often with an unfamiliar adult than those who had been low-reactive. Each 4.5-year-old child interacted with an unfamiliar female examiner during a 60-minute battery that included cognitive tests and measurements of autonomic function. We coded the videotapes of these sessions for the number of spontaneous comments and smiles.

Behavior with unfamiliar children should also be a sensitive sign of the two temperaments. About three to six weeks after the laboratory session, each child returned for a play session with two other unfamiliar peers of the same sex and age while the three parents sat on a coach in a playroom containing age-appropriate toys. At the end of a half-hour of play, an adult dressed in a gorilla costume carrying toys entered the room and, after a minute, invited the children to play with the toys. The entire corpus was coded for whether the child was sociable and spontaneous (uninhibited), shy and quiet (inhibited), or belonged to neither category.

About one-half of the children were classified as uninhibited, one-quarter as inhibited, and the remaining quarter belonged to neither category. Forty-six percent of the four-year-olds who had been high-reactive were classified as inhibited, compared with only 10% of the low-reactives. By contrast, two-thirds of low-reactives, but only one-quarter of high-reactives, were uninhibited. Only 4% displayed a profile that was inconsistent with their temperamental category at four months (Kagan, Snidman, & Arcus, 1998).

The four-year-olds who had been high-reactive were also more intimidated by the examiner. In one episode, the examiner asked the child to perform some actions that most parents would prohibit. For example, she opened a photo album containing pictures of herself, took out a large color photograph and as she handed it to the child said, "This is my favorite picture; tear up my favorite picture." More low- than high-reactives either asked her why they should perform that act or, in the case of five low-reactives, refused to do so. This resistance was not accompanied by anxiety; these low-reactives were simply less afraid of disobeying the request of an authority figure when the request required them to violate a norm they had accepted. Almost all the high-reactives were reluctant to disobey and, after a short delay, tore a small corner from the photograph.

Not one high-reactive four-year-old showed a profile of low fear in the second year and uninhibited behavior at 4.5 years. A bias to be high- or low-reactive constrains a child from developing the complementary profile. Thus, it is easy to sculpt high- or low-reactive infants into children who are neither extremely inhibited nor extremely uninhibited but it is more difficult to produce a consistently uninhibited profile in high-reactives or a consistently inhibited profile in those who had been low-reactive infants.

ASSESSMENT AT SEVEN-AND-A-HALF YEARS

A sample of 164 children were evaluated again when they were 7.5 years old. Mothers first filled out a questionnaire inquiring about their children's fears. The parents who described their child as highly anxious were interviewed on the telephone to ensure that their descriptions were accurate. After the interview, we selected the children whom we believed were anxious and asked their teachers to rank each child with respect to all children of the same sex in that classroom for the traits of shyness, fearfulness, aggression, and distractibility. If mother and teacher agreed that the child was anxious, we placed the child in a group labeled "anxious." Forty-three children, about one-quarter, were classified as anxious.

The high-reactives were most likely to be classified as anxious (45% of high-reactives vs. 15% of low-reactives). A good predictor of being classified as anxious was inhibition with the unfamiliar peers at 4.5 years of age. Eighteen percent of high-reactives had been highly fearful in the second year, inhibited at 4.5 years, and classified as anxious at 7.5 years, and not one high-reactive showed the complementary profile of consistently uninhibited and nonanxious behavior. Twenty-nine percent of low-reactives were uninhibited in the second year and at 4.5 years, and were not anxious at 7 years, compared with only 2% of high-reactives. Once again, being classified as high- or low-reactive constrained the probability of developing the opposite profile.

More high-reactive children who were anxious, compared with high-reactives who were not anxious, had (1) a narrow face based on the ratio of the width of the face at its broadest part divided by the height of the face, (2) high sitting diastolic blood pressure, and (3) greater cooling of the temperature of the fingertips while they listened to a series of digits they had to remember. The difference in facial skeleton warrants a comment. The 14- and 21-month-olds with a narrow face were more inhibited than those who had broad faces. The seven-year-olds with narrow faces and high fear scores in the second year made fewer impulsive errors when they had to inhibit the natural reflex of looking in the direction of a light that suddenly came on. This result implies that the gene that controls the growth of the bones of the face (derivatives of the cells in the neural crest) might also contribute to high and low reactivity (Kagan, 2010).

ASSESSMENT AT 11 YEARS

A sample of 237 children returned to our laboratory at 11 years of age for an evaluation that included quantification of a large number of biological variables under the direct or indirect influence of the amygdala, as well as their tendency to talk and smile while interacting with an interviewer.

As anticipated, more high-reactives were quiet and nonsmiling with the examiner; more low-reactives were talkative and smiled frequently. About one-third of high- and one-third of low-reactives behaved in ways that were in accord with their infant temperament, compared with only 16% who were inconsistent. Once again, the number of spontaneous smiles was a particularly sensitive sign of their infant temperament (Kagan & Snidman, 2004).

The selection of biological measures was guided by our hypothesis of differential amygdala excitability. We measured asymmetry of activation in the EEG; desynchronization of alpha frequencies is regarded as an index of activation. The left frontal area is usually more active than the right when individuals are relaxed, but the right is more active than the left when they are in a state of uncertainty or anxiety (Davidson, 2003; Fox, 1994). This asymmetry is moderately heritable and stable over intervals of one to three years (Anokhin, Heath, & Myers, 2006; Vuga et al., 2006). Children and adults who show right frontal activation are more likely to react to unfamiliar events with greater dysphoria and/or anxiety; those with left frontal activation show the complementary pattern of a relaxed, happy mood (Schmidt & Fox, 1994).

The high-reactives showed greater activation of the right, compared with the left, hemisphere, as well as a larger increase in the higher frequency beta band when asked to reflect on and later recite the thoughts they had had as they drove with their parent to the laboratory. This result is in accord with data reported by Fox, Henderson, Rubin, Caalkins, and Schmidt (2001).

The biological measure that best separated the high- from the low-reactives was the magnitude of the brain stem-evoked potential from the inferior colliculus, which is the fifth structure in the auditory chain. The waveform generated by the colliculus, called Wave 5, occurs within 6 ms of the onset of a sound. Amygdala activity enhances the excitability of the inferior colliculus through projections to the locus ceruleus and the central gray, which synapse on the colliculus. This fact means that children with a more excitable amygdala should have a larger Wave 5 to a series of clicks. The high-reactives displayed a larger Wave 5 than the low-reactives, and the high-reactives who had been most inhibited with peers at 4.5 years of age had larger Wave 5 values than the small number of high-reactives who had been more sociable.

The third variable separating high- from low-reactives was the magnitude of the event-related potential (ERP) to unfamiliar scenes. The amygdala sends projections to the locus ceruleus, ventral tegmentum, and basal nucleus of Meynert, which project to cortical neurons that mediate the magnitude of the ERP. Children with a more excitable amygdala should show larger P300 or N400 waveforms to unfamiliar events. Once again, the data affirmed our expectation, as high-reactives showed larger N400 waveforms to ecologically invalid scenes (i.e., a child's head on an animal's body) than low-reactives.

Finally, sympathetic activity in the cardiovascular system, which reflects amygdala activity, separated the two groups. A spectral analysis of supine heart rate revealed that more high- than low-reactives had more power in the lower frequency band of the spectrum, which reflects sympathetic and parasympathetic activity, and less power in the higher-frequency band, which reflects vagal activity. The combination of greater power in the low-frequency band and a high resting heart rate characterized one of every three high-reactives, but only one of five low-reactives. By contrast, one of every two low-reactives but only one of 16 high-reactives displayed greater power in the higher frequency vagal band and, in addition, had a low heart rate (Kagan & Snidman, 2004).

It is worth noting that high-reactives did not display larger potentiation of the eye-blink startle to a loud sound when they saw a light that warned of the possible delivery of an aversive air puff to the throat or when they were looking at unpleasant scenes. This finding is inconsistent with the popular assumption that potentiated startle to aversive events is larger in those who are acutely or chronically anxious (Bradley, Cuthbert, & Lang, 1999). Moreover, the experimental induction of an unpleasant feeling state by regular administration of corticosteroids, which produces greater activation of the right frontal lobe, had no effect on the magnitude of potentiated startle (Schmidt, Fox, Schultkin, & Gold, 1999). In addition, potentiated startle is observed when individuals are engaged in thought (Lipp, Siddle, & Dall, 2000). My colleagues and I have unpublished data suggesting that startle is potentiated when adults are trying to solve difficult anagrams or arithmetic problems, and the magnitude of the startle response was equivalent to the value observed when subjects were looking at unpleasant pictures. Thus, investigators should reflect before they use the paradigm of potentiated startle as an index of acute or chronic anxiety.

A slightly shorter stature, lighter weight, and blue eyes were also a little more frequent among high- than low-reactives. The modest relation between eye color and temperament is not original. Other investigators have reported that shy, school-aged, Caucasian children are more often blue- than brown-eyed, and a collaborative study with psychiatrists at the Massachusetts General Hospital revealed that 10 girls from a large group of 148 middle-class, Caucasian children were extremely shy with the examiner and had a parent with PD – all 10 girls had very light blue eyes (Kagan & Snidman, 2004). Finally, college-age males who were shy and had blue eyes had lower thresholds for olfactory stimuli than sociable, brown-eyed men (Herbener, Kagan, & Cohen, 1989).

ASSESSMENT AT 15 YEARS

A sample of 146 15-year-olds (59 low-reactives, 49 high-reactives, and 38 who were neither) were visited at home for a lengthy interview. In addition, 72 children from this group were also seen in the laboratory. The videotapes of the home interviews revealed that the high-reactives showed more nervous hand and leg movements and greater postural tension than the low-reactives. High-reactive boys talked less often and were more inhibited than low-reactive boys. About two-thirds of high-reactives were extremely inhibited during the home interview compared with only 10% of low-reactives (Kagan, Snidman, Kahn & Towsley, 2007).

Sources of Worry

Three questions the interviewer posed at different times asked the same question in different ways; namely, to report the targets of their worries. The questions were: "What things make you nervous or anxious?," "What do you worry about?," and "Can you name two times when you were worried over the past few months?" The major targets of worry were (1) performance in school or in extra-curricular activities; (2) uncertainty over meeting unfamiliar people or going to unfamiliar places; (3) social rejection and maintaining friendships; (4) physical harm; and (5) the health of a close relative.

Competent performance was the most frequent target of worry (54% cited only this concern) and low-reactives were more likely than high-reactives to nominate this concern as their only source of anxiety (61 vs. 37%). By contrast, two-thirds of high-reactives said they worried about being in crowds, interacting with unfamiliar peers, visiting new cities, or not knowing what might happen in the future, compared with only 20% of low-reactives. Some excerpts from the interviews illustrate this concern: "In a crowd I feel isolated and left out; I don't know what to pay attention to because it is all too ambiguous;" "I worry about the future, over not knowing what will happen next;" "I like being alone and, therefore, horses are my hobby; I don't have to worry about fitting in with others when I'm with my horses;" and "I get nervous with every vacation because I don't know what will happen." One high-reactive adolescent who had been very inhibited in the second year told the interviewer that she did not like spring because of the unpredictable changes in weather. Statements with this content were rare among low-reactives.

Most middle-class adolescents from nurturant families know their level of talent, do not expect to fail seriously, and understand that a less than excellent school performance could affect their vocational future. Hence, there is minimal ambiguity surrounding these worries. By contrast, encountering strangers, visiting new places, or coping with unfamiliar challenges are more ambiguous, and serious failure is possible. The high-reactive adolescents who reported unrealistic worries are unsure of the personal qualities others might judge, do not know how they will react, and believe there is not much they can do to reduce the possibility of inappropriate behavior. Therefore, the level of uncertainty is probably higher than it is in adolescents who are concerned only with school or athletic performance. Perhaps that is why twice as many high- as low-reactive adolescents were deeply religious. A survey of the fears of college students from seven different societies revealed no significant cultural or gender differences in the incidence of realistic fears of dangerous animals, but significant cultural and sex differences for less realistic fears of cockroaches, worms, and rats (Davey et al., 1998); unrealistic fears have higher heritability values than realistic fears (Sundet, Skre, Okkenhaug, & Tamds, 2003).

Each adolescent was given a set of 20 statements descriptive of personality and asked to rank them from most to least characteristic of the self. We created an index of a sanguine, compared with a dour, mood by averaging the ranks of four highly correlated items: "I am pretty serious;" "I think too much before deciding what to do;" "I wish I were more relaxed;" and the reverse of the score for the item "I am easy-going." High scores reflected a sanguine mood whereas low scores reflected a dour mood. Low-reactives were much more likely than high-reactives to describe themselves as sanguine. The two groups also differed in the rank they assigned to a single item: "Most of the time I'm happy." High-reactives were less likely to endorse this trait. The statement, "I'm happy most of the time," had also been administered in a Q-sort given at 11 years of age and more low- than high-reactives reported being happy at both ages.

Biology

The biological assessment at age 15 was similar to the one administered at 11 years of age. The display of left or right frontal activation in the EEG was moderately stable from 11 to 15 years ($r = 0.4$) and more high-reactives showed greater activation of the right frontal lobe at both ages whereas more low-reactives were left-frontal-active at both ages. The magnitude of the brain stem auditory-evoked potential (Wave 5) was also stable ($r = 0.64$) and 40% of high-reactives but not one low-reactive had large Wave 5 magnitudes at both ages.

The high-reactives continued to maintain larger ERP waveforms to unfamiliar scenes. In the procedure at age 15, blocks of 20 ecologically valid pictures alternated with blocks of 20 invalid pictures (blocks 1, 3, and 5 displayed pictures that were familiar to the adolescent while blocks 2, 4, and 6 displayed unfamiliar pictures that were ecologically invalid). Each picture was unique and none suggested disgust, fear, anger, or sadness. The high-reactives had the shallowest slope of habituation of the N400 waveform to the invalid pictures; that is, more high- than low-reactives showed larger differences in the N400 between the valid scenes on block 5 and the invalid pictures on block 6. These high-reactives with a shallow habituation of the N400 also had a large Wave 5 and a relatively unique behavioral profile during the interview. Two of these adolescents were reluctant to look at the interviewer and four reported atypical fears. One adolescent boy was afraid of another terrorist attack; one girl became anxious when she thought someone might touch her; a third worried about a school trip to Washington, DC; and a fourth confessed, "I feel vulnerable when I'm with people I don't know because I don't know what to do or what to say" (Kagan et al., 2007).

A final pair of observations provides persuasive support for the suggestion that high- and low-reactives possess differentially excitable circuits connecting the amygdala and prefrontal cortex. Carl Schwartz, a psychiatrist at Massachusetts General Hospital, recorded brain activity and structure in our high- and low-reactives at 18 years of age. The adolescents first saw a set of faces with neutral expressions repeatedly, followed unexpectedly by a new set of faces, also with neutral expressions. The high-reactive 18-year-olds showed greater amygdalar activation to the unexpected change than the low-reactives. Recall that the high-reactive 11- and 15-year-olds showed a larger ERP waveform to unfamiliar pictures.

A second difference between the two groups involves cortical thickness values in two sites in the prefrontal cortex. One cluster of neurons in the ventromedial prefrontal cortex contributes to conscious feelings of tension that adolescents might interpret as anxiety because this site sends projections to the hypothalamus, amygdala, central gray, and sympathetic nervous system. The 47 high-reactive 18-year-olds had a significantly thicker cortex in this region than the 54 low-reactives with a thinner cortex in this location. A second site in the OFC sends fibers to the intercalated neurons of the amygdala, which inhibit the neurons in the central nucleus that are responsible for the behavioral and biological signs of fear or anxiety. The high-reactives had a thinner cortex in this site in the left hemisphere whereas the low-reactives had a thicker cortex.

About one-half of high-reactives, but not one low-reactive, had a thicker cortex in the medial site of the right hemisphere than in the orbitofrontal site in the left hemisphere. These high-reactives displayed the most frequent arching of the back at 4 months, and at age 11 years displayed very few smiles and had ectomorphic body builds. The 12 low-reactives who had a clearly thicker cortex in the orbitofrontal area in the left hemisphere than in the medial location in the right hemisphere did not show any fear responses to the unfamiliar episodes at 14 months and displayed left frontal activation in the EEG during the 11-year assessment (Schwartz et al., 2010).

These intriguing facts, together with the fact that cortical thickness in this area has a heritability value of about 0.2 (Lenroot et al., 2008), imply that the brains of high- and low-reactives may have been different at as early as four months of age and biased high-reactives to become fearful one-year-olds and anxious 15-year-olds, and biased low-reactives to become fearless one-year-olds and happy-go-lucky adolescents. It may not be a coincidence that scientists at the University of Iowa have reported that, among a group of healthy boys aged 7 to 17 years, those who were most likely to be cautious before acting had more brain tissue in the medial portion of the prefrontal cortex of the right hemisphere, close to the site where high-reactive 18-year-olds had a thick cortex (Boes et al., 2009). Additional support comes from a study of the offspring of parents or grandparents who had been diagnosed as depressed. The offspring had a thicker cortex in the area of the right ventromedial prefrontal cortex, close to the site where the high-reactives had thicker values (Peterson et al., 2009). Patients with lesions of the ventromedial prefrontal cortex report less depressed moods (Koenigs et al., 2008), and rats with lesions of the right ventromedial cortex show less fear and less avoidance of a bitter taste (Sullivan & Gratton, 2002).

Implications

Because all adolescents meet new people and visit unfamiliar places, it is important to ask why high-reactives mentioned these experiences as primary sources of worry. One possible answer is that they are more susceptible to spontaneous visceral feedback from the body, which pierces consciousness to create a state of uncertainty that shares features with the state evoked when, as children, they encountered unfamiliar people or situations. Because the amygdala contributes to both states, it is possible that the psychological state created by unexpected visceral feedback and the state that accompanies encounters with strangers or novel places became associated because the neuronal clusters of each state were oscillating at the same frequency. Buzsaki (2006) has argued that clusters of neurons that oscillate at the same frequency are likely to bind together.

High-reactives in American society are biased to interpret the feeling evoked by unexpected visceral feedback as implying that they are worried about their ability to cope with a future challenge, and the folk theory they learned implies that their feelings of uncertainty reflect a compromise in their personal characteristics. Members of other cultures might impose different interpretations on similar visceral sensations. Cambodian refugees living in Massachusetts interpret an unexpected bout of tachycardia as implying a weak heart caused by a loss of energy that is due to a lack of sleep or a diminished appetite (Hinton & Hinton, 2002).

Social anxiety is especially salient in societies like our own because encounters with strangers are frequent and social acceptance is an important goal. Thus, high-reactives are at a higher risk for developing SAD than other anxiety disorders. Serious depression, although infrequent in our sample, also occurred more often among high- than low-reactives.

We believe that encounters with the unfamiliar generate a more salient and intense psychobiological state in high- than low-reactives because of differences in brain neurochemistry. Temperaments render individuals especially vulnerable to several members of a family of emotions; the person's life history selects a specific emotion from that family. Occupational and social failure in contemporary America have replaced the seven traditional sins of pride, anger, envy, avarice, sloth, gluttony, and lust as incentives for anxiety or guilt.

Perhaps the most significant implication of the temperamental biases for high- or low-reactivity is that each prevents the development of the contrasting profile. The probability that a high-reactive will not become a consistently exuberant, sociable, fearless child with a minimally excitable amygdala is very high – this prediction was correct for about 90% of high-reactives. But the probability that these infants will become extremely shy, fearful, socially anxious adolescents with amygdala excitability held for only 20% of high-reactives. By contrast, over 90% of low-reactives were neither extremely shy nor showed signs of amygdala excitability, but only 40% were consistently sociable, exuberant, and had a minimally excitable amygdala.

Contemporary psychiatry is more concerned with extreme levels of anxiety than with equally intense levels of anger, boredom, or sexual frustration. Epidemiological surveys ask informants about their worries and fears but less often inquire about the frequency of other equally unpleasant emotions. Although ancient societies regarded extreme anger as the most dangerous emotion, contemporary Americans and Europeans have been persuaded that anxiety is the cardinal villain. This judgment implies that these scholars regard anxiety as a greater obstacle to adaptation in contemporary society than anger, boredom, or sexual frustration. It is not obvious that this assumption is correct.

The anger felt by marginalized adults living in poverty might be a more frequent source of debilitating symptoms than anxiety over meeting strangers. I do not suggest that we ignore the 20% of the population who report high levels of anxiety that interfere with their daily responsibilities; these individuals should be helped. However, a large proportion of the population also experience high levels of anger at the unjust or uncivil behavior of others, extreme boredom at work, or prolonged frustration of their sexual motives. These emotions are not necessarily less serious intrusions into a feeling of serenity than anxiety over being part of a crowd.

Finally, the evidence supports the suggestion that high- and low-reactivity should be regarded as categories rather than ends of a continuum of reactivity to unfamiliarity. Extreme values on behavioral or biological measures often separated high- and low-reactives better than average scores. For example, 10% of high-reactives, but not one low-reactive, had a standard score equal to or greater than 0.5 on the four differentiating biological variables of EEG asymmetry, Wave 5, ERP waveforms, and sympathetic activity in the cardiovascular system. Ax (1953) reported years ago that the highest value attained on autonomic responsivity better differentiated the emotional states of fear and anger than the mean values. We also found that the highest heart rate a child attained across a battery better differentiated high- from low-reactives than mean heart rate values. Persistent aggression is also characteristic of only a small group of children (only 4% of a very large sample) (Brody et al., 2003).

Psychologists prefer continua over categories because the statistics they use most often, especially regression and analysis of variance, are most sensitive when used with continuous variables rather than qualitative categories. However, nonlinear functions are common in biology and the social sciences and qualitatively distinct phenotypes often emerge at transition points. The behavior of a small number of ants appears random and without coherence, but the apparent chaos becomes orderly and rhythmic patterns emerge over the colony when the density of the ants in the colony reaches a critical value. One biologist phrased the case for qualitative categories as follows: "The study of biological form begins to take us in the direction of the science of qualities that is not an alternative to, but complements and extends, the science of quantities" (Goodwin, 1994, p. 198).

Temperamental categories, like high- and low-reactives, emerge from a cascade that began in a neuronal cluster that became part of a circuit that was recruited into a module of circuits to generate the behaviors that define a particular temperament. A word in a sentence that is part of a paragraph in an essay provides an analogy.

The data and ideas in this chapter support the usefulness of combining behavioral and biological evidence. The history of all the sciences is replete with examples of the progress that can occur when previously isolated domains of inquiry probe a common problem. A child's temperament and life history operating together determine the ease with which particular events activate brain structures and subsequent emotions. We must now search for the integrative profiles that emerge when particular temperamental predispositions encounter environmental events, and should resist the aesthetic urge to simplify the problem by assuming we can arrive at a quantitative estimate of the separate contributions of temperament and life history to a type of personality or form of psychopathology.

REFERENCES

Amaral, D. G., Price, J. L., Pitkanen, A., & Carmichael, S. T. (1992). Anatomical organization of the primate amygdaloid complex. In J. T. Aggleton (Ed.), *The amygdala* (pp. 1–166). New York: Wiley-Liss.

Anokhin, A. P., Heath, A. C., & Myers, E. (2006). Genetic and environmental influences on frontal EEG asymmetry: A twin study. *Biological Psychology*, *71*(3), 289–295.

Arbelle, S., Benjamin, J., Galin, M., Kremer, P., Belmaker, R. H., & Ebstein, R. P. (2003). Relation of shyness in grade school children to the genotype for the long form of the serotonin transporter promoter region polymorphism. *American Journal of Psychiatry*, *160*, 671–676.

Auerbach, J., Geller, V., Lezer, S., Shinwell, E., Belmaker, R. H., & Levin, J. (1999). Dopamine D4 receptor (D4DR) and serotonin transporter promoter (5-HTTLPR) polymorphisms in the determination of temperament in 2-month-old infants. *Molecular Psychiatry*, *4*, 369–373.

Ax, A. F. (1953). The physiological association between fear and anger in humans. *Psychosomatic Medicine*, *15*, 433–442.

Becker, J. B. (1999). Gender differences in dopaminergic function in striatum and nucleus accumbens. *Pharmacology Biochemistry & Behavior*, *64*, 803–812.

Boes, A. D., Bechara, A., Tranel, D., Anderson, S. W., Richman, L., & Nopoulos, P. (2009). Right ventromedial prefrontal cortex: A neuroanatomical correlate of impulse control in voles. *Social, Cognitive, and Affective Neuroscience*, *4*, 1–9.

Bradley, M. M., Cuthbert, B. N., & Lang, P. J. (1999). Affect and the startle reflex. In M. E. Dawson, A. M. Shell, & A. N. Bohmalt (Eds.), *The startle modification* (pp. 157–183). New York: Cambridge University Press.

Brody, L. M., Tremblay, R. E., Brane, B., Fergusson, D., Horwood, J. L., Dodge, K. A., et al. (2003). Developmental trajectories of childhood disruptive behaviors and adolescent delinquency. *Developmental Psychology*, *39*, 222–245.

Buzsaki, G. (2006). *Rhythms of the brain*. New York: Oxford University Press.

Calkins, S., & Fox, N. A. (1992). The relations among infant temperament, security of attachment, and behavioral inhibition at 24 months. *Child Development*, *63*, 1456–1472.

Chotai, J., & Asberg, M. (1999). Variations in CSF monoamine metabolites according to the season of birth. *Neuropsychobiology*, *39*, 57–62.

Davey, G. C., McDonald, A. S., Hirisade, U., Pravhu, G. G., Iwawaki, S., Jim, C. I., et al. (1998). A cross cultural study of animal fears. *Behavioral Research & Therapy*, *36*, 735–750.

Davidson, R. J. (2003). Affective neuroscience and psychophysiology. *Psychophysiology*, *40*, 655–665.

DiLalla, L. F., Kagan, J., & Reznick, J. S. (1994). Genetic etiology of behavioral inhibition among 2-year-old children. *Infant Behavior & Development*, *17*, 401–408.

Fox, N. A. (1994). Dynamic cerebral processes: Emotional regulation. *Monographs of the Society for Research in Child Development*, *59*(240), 52–166.

Fox, N. A., Henderson, N. A., Rubin, K. H., Caalkins, S. D., & Schmidt, L. A. (2001). Continuity and discontinuity of behavioral inhibition and exuberance. *Child Development*, *72*, 1–21.

Gelernter, J., Cubella, J. F., Kidd, J. R., Pakstis, A. J., & Kidd, K. K. (1999). Population studies of polymorphisms of the serotonin transporter protein gene. *American Journal of Medical Genetics*, *88*, 61–66.

Goodwin, B. (1994). *How the leopard changed its spots*. New York: Scribners Sons.

Gortmaker, S. L., Kagan, J., Caspi, A., & Silva, P. A. (1997). Daylight during pregnancy and shyness in children. *Developmental Psychobiology*, *31*, 107–114.

Green, A. E., Munafo, M. R., DeYoung, C. G., Fossella, J. A., Fan, J., & Gray, J. R. (2008). Using data in cognitive neuroscience. *Nature Reviews: Neuroscience*, *9*, 710–720.

Hariri, A. R., Mattoy, B. S., Tessitore, A., Fera, F., Smith, W. T., & Weinberger, D. R. (2002). Extroamphetamine modulates the response of the human amygdala. *Neurosystems Pharmacology*, *27*, 1036–1040.

Herbener, E. S., Kagan, J., & Cohen, M. (1989). Shyness and olfactory threshold. *Personality and Individual Differences*, *10*, 1159–1163.

Hinton, D., & Hinton, S. (2002). Panic disorder, somatization, and the new cross-cultural psychiatry. *Culture, Medicine, and Psychiatry*, *26*, 155–178.

Hsu, M., Bhatt, M., Adolphs, R., Tranel, D., & Caamerer, C. F. (2005). Neural systems responding to degrees of uncertainty in human decision-making. *Science*, *310*, 1680–1683.

John, E. M. (1941). A study of the effects of evacuation and air raids on children in pre-school age. *British Journal of Educational Psychology*, *11*, 173–182.

Kagan, J. (1994). *Galen's prophecy*. New York: Basic Books.

Kagan, J. (1998). Biology and the child. In W. Damon (Editor-in-Chief) & N. Eisenberg (Vol. Ed.) *Handbook of child psychology: Vol. 3* (5th ed) (pp. 177–201). New York: Wiley.

Kagan, J. (2010). *The temperamental thread*. Washington, DC: Dana Press.

Kagan, J., & Fox, N. A. (2006). Biology, culture and temperamental biases. In N. Eisenberg (Vol. Editor); W. Damon & R. M. Lerner (Editors-in-Chief), *Handbook of child psychology: Vol. 3*, (6th ed) (pp. 167–225). New York: Wiley.

Kagan, J., & Saudino, K. J. (2001). Behavioral inhibition and related temperament. In R. M. Emde & J. K. Hewitt (Eds.), *Infancy to early childhood* (pp. 111–119). New York: Oxford University Press.

Kagan, J., & Snidman, N. (2004). *The long shadow of temperament.* Cambridge, MA: Harvard University Press.

Kagan, J., Snidman, N., & Arcus, D. (1998). Childhood derivatives of high- and low-reactivity in infancy. *Child Development*, *69*, 1483–1493.

Kagan, J., Snidman, N., Kahn, V., & Towsley, S. (2007). The preservation of two infant temperaments into adolescence. *Monographs of the Society for Research in Child Development*, *72*, 2.

Klein, R. G. (1991). Parent–child agreement in clinical assessment of anxiety and other psychopathology. *Journal of Anxiety*, *5*, 182–198.

Koenigs, M., Huey, E. D., Calamia, M., Raymont, V., Tranel, D., & Grafman, J. (2008). Distinct regions of prefrontal cortex mediate resistance and vulnerability to depression. *Journal of Neuroscience*, *28*, 12341–12348.

Kong, J., Kaptchuk, T. J., Polich, G., Kirsch, I., Vangel, M., Zyloney, C., et al. (2009). Expectancy and treatment interactions: A dissociation between acupuncture and analgesia and expectancy evoked placebo analgesia. *Neuroimage*, *15*, 940–949.

LaGreca, A. M., Silverman, W. K., & Wassastein, S. B. (1998). Children's predisaster functioning as a predictor of post-traumatic stress following Hurricane Andrew. *Journal of Consulting & Clinical Psychology*, *66*, 883–892.

Lakatos, K., Memoda, Z., Dirkas, E., Ronai, Z., Kovacs, E., Ney, K., et al. (2003). Association of D4 dopamine receptor gene and serotonin transporter promoter polymorphism – infants' response to novelty. *Molecular Psychiatry*, *8*, 90–98.

LeDoux, J. E. (1996). *The emotional brain*. New York: Simon & Schuster.

Lenroot, R. K., Schmitt, J. E., Ordaz, S. J., Wallace, G. L., Neale, M. C., Lerch, J. P., et al. (2008). Differences in genetic and environmental influences on the human cerebral cortex associated with development during childhood and adolescence. *Human Brain Mapping*, *30*, 163–174.

Lewontin, R. (1995). *Human diversity*. New York: Scientific American.

Lipp, O. V., Siddle, D. A. T., & Dall, P. J. (2000). The effect of morning stimulus modality on blink startle modification in reaction time tasks. *Psychophysiology*, *37*, 55–64.

Manuck, S. B., Flory, J. D., Ferrell, R. E., & Muldoon, M. F. (2004). Socio-economic status covaries with central nervous system serotonergic responsivity as a function of allelic variation in the serotonin transporter gene-linked polymorphic region. *Psychoneuroendocrinology*, *29*, 651–668.

McNally, G. T., & Westbrook, R. F. (2003). Opioid receptors regulate the extinction of Pavlovian fear conditioning. *Behavioral Neuroscience*, *117*, 1292–1301.

Miyawaki, T., Goodchild, A. K., & Pilowsky, P. M. (2002). Activation of mu-opioid receptors in rat ventrolateral medulla selectively block baroreceptor reflexes while activation of delta opioid receptors blocks somato-sympathetic reflexes. *Neuroscience*, *109*, 132–144.

Patterson, P. H. (2006). Pregnancy, immunity, schizophrenia, and autism. *Engineering & Science, 10*, 11–21.

Peterson, B. S., Warner, V., Bansal, R., Zhu, H., Hao, X., Liu, J., et al. (2009). Cortical thinning in persons at increased familial risk for major depression. *Proceedings of the National Academy of Sciences, 106*, 6273–6278.

Pezawas, L., Meyer-Lindenberg, A., Drabant, E. M., Verchinski, B. A., Munoz, K. E., Kolachana, B. S., et al. (2005). 5-HTTLPR polymorphism impacts human cingulated-amygdala interactions. *Nature Neuroscience, 8*, 828–834.

Ray, J., Hansen, S., & Waters, N. (2006). Links between temperamental dimensions and brain monoamines in the rat. *Behavioral Neuroscience, 120*, 85–92.

Robinson, J. L., Kagan, J., Reznick, S., & Corley, R. (1992). The heritability of inhibited and uninhibited behavior. *Developmental Psychology, 28*, 1030–1037.

Rolls, E. T. (1992). Neurophysiology and functions of the primate amygdala. In J. P. Aggleton (Ed.), *The amygdala* (pp. 143–166). New York: Wiley–Liss.

Schmidt, L., & Fox, N. A. (1994). Patterns of corticoelectrophysiology and autonomic activity in adult shyness and sociability. *Biological Psychology, 38*, 183–198.

Schmidt, L. A., Fox, N. A., Schultkin, J., & Gold, P. W. (1999). Behavioral and psychophysiological correlates of self-presentation in temperamentally shy children. *Developmental Psychobiology, 35*, 119–135.

Schwartz, C. E., Kunwar, P. S., Greve, D. N., Moran, L. R., Viner, J. C., Covino, J. M., et al. (2010). Structural differences in adult orbital and ventromedial prefrontal cortex predicted by infant temperament at 4 months of age. *Archives of General Psychiatry, 67*, 78–84.

Seifer, R., Sameroff, A. J., Barrett, L. C., & Krafchuk, E. (1994). Infant temperament measured by multiple observations and mother reports. *Child Development, 65*, 1478–1490.

Sullivan, R. M., & Gratton, A. (2002). Behavioral effects of excitotoxic lesions of ventral prefrontal cortex in the rat are hemisphere dependent. *Brain Research, 927*, 69–79.

Sundet, J. M., Skre, I., Okkenhaug, J. J., & Tamds, K. (2003). Genetic and environmental causes of the inter-relationships between self-reported fears. *Scandinavian Journal of Psychology, 44*, 97–106.

Torres-Farfan, C., Richter, H. G., Germain, A. M., Valenzuela, G. J., Campino, C., Rojas-García, P., et al. (2004). Maternal melatonin selectively inhibits cortisol production in the primate fetal adrenal gland. *Journal of Physiology, 554*, 841–856.

van Bockstaele, E. J., Bajic, D., Proudfit, H., & Valentino, R. J. (2001). Topographic architecture of stress-related pathways targeting the noradrenergic locus ceruleus. *Physiology & Behavior, 73*, 273–283.

Vuga, M., Fox, N. A., Cohn, J. F., George, C. J., Levenstein, R. M., & Kovacs, M. (2006). Long-term stability of frontal electroencephalographic asymmetry in adults with a history of depression and controls. *International Journal of Psychophysiology, 59*, 107–115.

Waugh, A. (2008). *The House of Wittgenstein*. New York: Doubleday.

Zhang, G. H., Zhang, H. U., Wang, X. F., Zhan, Y. H., Deng, S. P., & Qin, Y. M. (2009). The relationship between fungiform papillae density and detection threshold for sucrose in the young males. *Chemical Senses, 34*, 93–99.

Chapter 13

Basic Behavioral Mechanisms and Processes in Social Anxieties and Social Anxiety Disorders

Daniel W. McNeil[1], C.W. Lejuez[2], and John T. Sorrell[3]

[1]Anxiety, Psychophysiology, and Pain Research Laboratory, Department of Psychology, West Virginia University, Morgantown, WV 26506, [2]Department of Psychology, University of Maryland, MD 20742, [3]Department of Anaesthesia, School of Medicine, Stanford University, CA 94305

INTRODUCTION

Various behaviorally oriented theoretical perspectives on social anxieties and SADs (SPs) have been forwarded over the past four decades, since Isaac Marks's pioneering (1969, 1970; Marks & Gelder, 1966) and subsequent work (Marks, 1985, 1987). Using early conditioning theories as a basis and expanding into new dimensions, a host of cognitive behavioral and cognitive theories of SAD have been developed (Clark & Wells, 1995; Hofmann, 2007; Hofmann & Barlow, 2002; Moscovitch, 2009; Rapee & Heimberg, 1997). Neurobiological theories also are an area of focus (e.g., Liebowitz, Gorman, Fyer, & Klein, 1985; Tancer, Lewis, & Stein, 1995; Schneier & Welkowitz, 1996). Evolutionary, genetic, and ethological data and theories (Ohman, Dimberg, & Ost, 1985; Trower & Gilbert, 1989; Weeks, Rodebaugh, Heimberg, Norton, & Jakatdar, 2009) are a fascinating foray into broad, distal determinants of social behavior. Nevertheless, exclusively (Beidel & Turner, 1998) or predominantly (Barlow, 2002), behavioral and conditioning models (Mineka & Sutton, 2006) continue to be important for the field. Although the early history of behavioral theories emphasized an extreme nurture position in the "nature versus nurture" debate, contemporary behavioral theories of anxieties and fears incorporate both learning and biogenetic influences (Eelen & Vervliet, 2006).

Early behavioral models for social and other phobias focused on stimulus–response relations (Pavlov, 1927; Watson & Rayner, 1920) and two-factor theory (Mowrer, 1947), providing a primarily respondent conditioning-based behavioral analysis of the factors that give rise to and maintain the disorder. These conditioning models were refined to include indirect conditioning

Social Anxiety: Clinical, Developmental, and Social Perspectives. DOI: 10.1016/B978-0-12-375096-9.00013-4

(Rachman, 1976, 1977). Nevertheless, the idea of direct traumatic conditioning predominated, but many limitations of purely respondent conditioning approaches were identified in trying to explain the development of anxieties, fears, and phobias (Mineka & Sutton, 2006). As an alternative, Mineka and colleagues (Mineka & Sutton, 2006; Mineka & Zinbarg, 1995, 1996) have presented models of conditioning from an ethological perspective that also emphasize experiential variables (e.g., prior experience with the conditioned stimulus, inflation of fear after exposure to a more intense unconditioned stimulus), preparedness (e.g., angry facial expressions), and genetic/temperamental variables (e.g., BI). The evolutionary focus, with the addition of cognitive elements, was earlier used with basic learning principles in attempting to explain the development and maintenance of SAD (Trower & Gilbert, 1989; Trower, Gilbert, & Sherling, 1990; Trower & Turland, 1984). In addition to the idea of direct traumatic conditioning, Mineka and colleagues have included observational or vicarious conditioning, and verbal or instructional learning, as two other associative pathways that can lead to the development of phobias (Mineka & Sutton, 2006). These other types of learning seem particularly relevant to SAD in that the influence of parents and caregivers, and other aspects of the learning environment, likely are involved in the development of this syndrome, particularly early in life (Bögels et al., 2010). A further behavioral model of anxieties and fears in general has been proposed by Öhman and Mineka (2001; Mineka & Öhman, 2002) in an "evolved fear module." This evolutionarily shaped behavioral system incorporates the three associative pathways, as well as the preparedness of eliciting stimuli, automaticity in responding, encapsulation from higher-order cognitions, and its own neural circuitry in the amygdala (Mineka & Sutton, 2006). Such a model might be specifically and fruitfully applied to social fears and anxieties.

Behavioral models have emphasized social skills deficits in the formulation of SAD (e.g., Marks, 1985). The disorder has been regarded as being the result of social skills deficits (primary deficit), or as the result of anxiety related to social behavior despite the knowledge of fluent social functioning (secondary deficit), or a combination of these factors (tertiary deficit) (Hopko, McNeil, Zvolensky, & Eifert, 2001). Both skills deficits and anxiety are useful intervening variables (cf. MacCorquodale & Meehl, 1948) as they can be used as a summary label for the actual environmental variables that produce patterns of behavior referred to as SAD (see Masia & Morris, 1998). For example, an individual whose SAD involves being "so nervous [she] can't talk at parties" may be labeled as anxious. Likewise, an individual who says he "just doesn't know what to say when around new people at a party" may be thought to have a skills deficit. Using the labels "anxiety" or "skills deficit" as hypothetical constructs (i.e., actual entities with causal status), however, provides little explanation of the variables controlling the anxious responses. For example, suggesting that an individual did not go to a party because of anxiety provides no more information about the setting events and maintaining variables than simply saying that the individual did not attend the party. Instead, a more parsimonious and useful analysis would focus on the environment–behavior relations (e.g., type of party, number of people attending who were well known or unknown) leading to the pattern of behavior (e.g., increased heart rate, phobic cognitions, and overt avoidance) referred to as SAD. In such a case, anxiety and skills deficits simply are summary terms for these relations, and not the cause. For example, if an individual reports being "anxious" when in social settings, one should assess for the particular characteristics of that situation, seek to determine other events that may provoke anxiety, and attempt to identify stimulus or functional similarities across situations that may represent the controlling variables (e.g., presence of an authority figure). Similarly, regarding skills deficits, one should consider the various situations that require social functioning, knowledge, and prior learning of social skills, and the current options to keep them "polished."

Following from a focus on environment–behavior relations, the importance of situation specificity becomes clearer. Individuals with SAD vary in the number and type of situations that evoke anxiety and fear (e.g., conversations in groups, public speaking, blushing after being embarrassed) (Bögels et al., 2010); the scope and severity of these social fears and anxieties are highly related to particular situational variables (Holt, Heimberg, Hope, & Liebowitz, 1992). SAD is influenced by biological and developmental factors, but certainly also is under environmental control and may manifest differently across settings. For example, when there is an informal party associated with one's workplace, an individual may engage in avoidance or escape because he has found that he does not know what to say or do, and so attending the party is not reinforcing. Additionally, when exposed to a social situation in which an individual previously was criticized and ridiculed, he also may engage in avoidance or escape. In both cases, the structure of the resulting (avoidance) behavior is similar, but the function clearly differs. In contrast to situations in which escape or avoidance does occur, the same individual may experience little anxiety or social difficulty in a situation in which he has had positive and comfortable prior exposure. Although the first part of this example could be labeled as consistent with SAD due to a skills deficit, the second as reflective of possible SAD due to anxiety, and the third as an absence of SAD, looking beyond labels and focusing on environment–behavior relations may allow for the particular situational variables supporting SAD to be identified and targeted more easily and accurately.

Consistent with the cognitive zeitgeist in psychology (Eifert & Plaud, 1998), SAD often is considered to be a result of cognitive processes (e.g., anxious anticipation of negative evaluation by others); these variables are endowed with causal status and are regarded as primary determinants of the disorder (e.g., Barlow, 2002; Beck & Emery, 1985; Clark & Wells, 1995; Rapee & Heimberg, 1997). In general, purely behavioral theories of psychopathology often are dismissed as they traditionally have focused upon simple instances of conditioning and ignored the role of cognitions and other private events (Anderson,

Hawkins, & Scotti, 1997). In response to such criticisms, comprehensive behavioral theories of psychopathology have been proposed (e.g., Lejuez, Schaal, & O'Donnell, 1998; Lewinsohn, 1974). We believe that such behavioral approaches also have relevance for the understanding and treatment of SAD. In fact, although the issue is far from resolved, research suggests that the behavioral components of SAD treatments are underutilized (e.g., Strahan & Conger, 1998); yet, they may account for a considerable percentage of treatment gain (Emmelkamp & Mersch, 1982; Feske & Chambless, 1995; Hope, Heimberg, & Bruch, 1995; Scholing & Emmelkamp, 1996). Furthermore, significant improvement in cognitive symptoms of SAD has been found with purely behavioral treatment protocols (Newman, Hofmann, Trabert, Roth, & Taylor, 1994).

As a result of such findings, it is important that theoreticians re-examine the potential for understanding the nature of SAD from behavioral perspectives. Current behavioral theorizing incorporates the development of more comprehensive learning principles to explain complex phenomena once thought to be accessible only through cognitive explanations. Furthermore, recent far-reaching extrapolations of these behavioral principles (e.g., functional equivalence, the matching law, and experiential avoidance) will be discussed to show how a comprehensive theory of SAD is possible within a strictly behavioral framework. Such formulations, however, can include cognitive responses as important elements. To enhance the utility of behavioral theories, an exclusive focus on simple, isolated conditioning explanations with little or no recognition of cognitions or other more complex variables has been replaced by more thorough and comprehensive formulations that remain consistent with a behavioral framework.

CURRENT STATUS OF BEHAVIORAL THEORY OF SOCIAL ANXIETIES AND SOCIAL ANXIETY DISORDER

The most comprehensive specifically behavioral formulation of SAD that has been provided to date is that of Beidel and Turner (1998). In presenting a behavioral account of SAD, they proposed a model that outlines several ways in which SAD may develop and be maintained. Similar to other contemporary theorists, they emphasize that the etiology and maintenance of SAD is multidimensional. In clinical endeavors, these interacting multiple determinants of psychological disorders (and adaptive human behavior) are best approached by an idiographic approach to assessment and treatment (Eifert, Schulte, Zvolensky, Lejuez, & Lau, 1997).

Beidel and Turner (1998) identify psychological factors as one broad class of contributors to SAD, specifically listing direct conditioning, observational learning, and information transfer as components. Direct respondent conditioning events (see Miller, 1977; Pavlov, 1927; Skinner, 1953; Wolpe, 1958) appear to determine initial development of SAD (Öst & Hugdahl, 1981) in about half the cases (Mineka & Zinbarg, 1995), although such findings are not entirely consistent (Hofmann, Ehlers, & Roth, 1995). Interestingly, the specific subtype of SAD is more associated with traumatic conditioning experiences than the generalized subtype (Stemberger, Turner, Beidel, & Calhoun, 1995). Similarly to Mineka and colleagues (Mineka & Sutton, 2006; Mineka & Zinbarg, 1995, 1996), Beidel and Turner discuss the limitations of direct conditioning explanations of SAD and propose vicarious conditioning as a supplementary explanation. Additionally, Beidel and Turner discuss information transfer in terms of accounting for instances of SAD that appear to be verbally transmitted. For example, a child who frequently hears a parent using phrases such as, "Be polite!" and "What will your teacher think?," may come to associate social situations as consistently having strict rules and being highly evaluative. Moreover, frequently overhearing one's caregivers utter phrases like "Going to this ceremony is going to be painful; I don't want to go!" and "Do I have to take [child's name] to her friend's birthday party? It's going to be miserable," suggest social events are uncomfortable and that avoidance is a coping strategy to consider. Information transfer is but one aspect of the broader area of language-based learning, which is extremely complex; this latter topic is discussed in greater detail in a subsequent section.

Beidel and Turner (1998) also emphasize genetic and biological factors, citing both twin and family studies. Despite inconclusive results, they suggest at least some evidence for a genetic component to SAD. Available data suggest that SAD, like other anxiety disorders, is somewhat familial, with a degree of genetic influence. As a separate categorization, Beidel and Turner also consider other predispositional factors and trait variables that increase the likelihood of SAD and serve to maintain it. Family environment, peer relationships and loneliness, cognitive development, temperament (specifically BI), shyness, early attachment, and social skill all are cited as factors that can contribute to SAD. In accordance with this work, Beidel, Morris, and Turner (2004) outline the developmental role of parenting factors, as well as peer relations. Along these lines, loneliness and peer relations are considered in terms of inability to receive social reinforcement from peers, leading rejected children to seek reinforcement outside the social environment, thus producing a cycle of avoidant behavior and social neglect. Similarly, Barrett, Rapee, Dadds, and Ryan (1996) found that both clinically anxious children and their parents predominantly chose avoidant solutions to ambiguous social situations, relative to aggressive and typical children.

A broad array of psychological and biological factors are appropriately considered in Beidel and Turner's (1998) formulation of SAD. Consistent with a diathesis–stress model of psychopathology (e.g., Barlow, 2992), it is recognized that an individual with a genetic predisposition for anxiety, fear, or panic, including SAD, is more susceptible to environmental influences that could lead to the development of the disorder. Conversely, certain biological substrates might lead to a resistance to certain environmental influences, or a resiliency in response to stressors. Nevertheless, in some individuals, only environmental influences are necessary to elicit psychopathology. In most cases, however, it is not the independent effects of psychological or biological factors but instead the interaction of the two that drives the development and maintenance of SAD. Contemporary formulations strongly suggest that numerous environmental, biological, and developmental factors combine in a variety of arrays to produce anxiety, fear, and associated disorders (Mineka & Sutton, 2006). Although Beidel and Turner (1998) currently provide the most comprehensive purely behavioral view, there still are contemporary learning principles that can further add to our understanding of social anxiety and phobia. Rather than attempting to provide an overall, integrated model, we instead propose a number of mechanisms and processes that may help account for the development, generalization, and maintenance of SAD (as well as other forms of psychopathology). Integration of these ideas awaits further development of theory.

CONTEMPORARY BEHAVIORAL PRINCIPLES AS A BASIS FOR THE FURTHER DEVELOPMENT OF THEORIES OF SOCIAL ANXIETIES AND SOCIAL ANXIETY DISORDER

Current theories of SAD are well constructed and are increasingly comprehensive, yet in many cases the basic behavioral principles that underlie these formulations have not been clearly delineated. It should be noted that the field of behavior analysis is a natural science approach to behavior, including social behavior (e.g., Guerin, 1994), that provides one background for the exposition of these principles. Knowledge regarding these underlying principles allows for the further evolution of a formulation, including etiology and treatment, without moving in a direction that is inconsistent with the underlying framework of the formulation itself. As such, we present a number of behavior analytic principles, including some of the research support for them, that are relevant to a behavioral formulation of social anxiety and phobia. Furthermore, we use social anxiety and phobia examples to highlight the understanding of these principles and their role in the development and maintenance of SAD.

Initiation of Social Anxiety and Phobia

Any theory of SAD must account for the early learning of socially anxious/avoidant responses in childhood and adolescence, given that the typical age of onset is in the mid-teens, although it sometimes occurs earlier in childhood (Hofmann, Heinrichs, & Moscovitch, 2004). The role of temperament is well documented, with behaviorally inhibited children being especially likely to develop SAD (Schwartz, Snidman, & Kagan, 1999). Experiential variables, resulting in individual differences in vulnerability and protective factors, also are important in the development of SAD in childhood and adolescence. Harsh, criticizing, and controlling parenting styles are associated with the development of social anxieties and fears (Greco & Morris, 2002). Also, as noted by Mineka and Sutton (2006), rapid observational learning of fears and anxieties may occur in children as a result of parental modeling. Additionally, instructional or verbal learning can occur. Again, as suggested by Mineka and Sutton (2006), "negative information may primarily set up negative expectancies that then potentiate the outcome of direct or conditioning episodes" (pp. 78–79). So, negative information from parents about social events and social interactions may create a stimulus situation in which social conditioning episodes may result in anxiety and fear, and associated avoidance.

There are numerous opportunities in childhood for naturalistically occurring events that serve as "conditioning trials" for social anxiety. For example, there may be traumatic conditioning associated with an event that is social in nature (Marks, 1987; Stemberger et al., 1995; Wolpe, 1958). It may happen that, an individual mispronounces words or "freezes" while speaking in front of peers, consequently receiving ridicule for the poor performance. As a result, future instances involving similar stimuli (e.g., speaking when peers are listening) may produce a fear response (e.g., physiological arousal) despite the absence of ridicule. Furthermore, the negative reinforcement via escape or avoidance, and positive reinforcement (e.g., compassion from concerned friends or family members) following reports or observable instances of fear, may strengthen these initial patterns of behavior, therefore producing further phobic behavior. The resulting limited contact with social stimuli may produce anxious apprehension and further decrements in social skills.

Despite the simplicity of a basic conditioning interpretation, explaining why some individuals develop SAD and others do not is far from simple. For example, some individuals develop SAD in the absence of recalled traumatic conditioning events, whereas others experience social trauma (e.g., by committing a faux pas) and do not develop SAD or even social anxieties that persist beyond a few hours. Although the absence of recall identification does not preclude the possibility that direct conditioning occurred, other plausible causes are necessary to strengthen a behavioral theory of SAD. Information transfer and vicarious conditioning are possible mechanisms (Beidel & Turner, 1998; Mineka & Zinbarg, 1995, 1996), but they have not been fully integrated with the current research involving language-based learning. As a complementary analysis, rule-governed behavior consists of responses that an individual emits that are not the result of direct exposure to a conditioning event, but instead are a result of verbally transmitted reports of other individuals' experiences (Hayes, Zettle, & Rosenfarb, 1989). For example, an individual who hears reports of others experiencing an embarrassing social situation, such as through a faux pas, may attempt to avoid such situations, despite the fact that he or she never had such experiences. Thus, despite the absence of a direct conditioning event, the individual behaves in a manner in which one might expect had she or he had such an experience. Although rules could be considered to mediate the individual's behavior in response to particular environmental contingencies, research has shown that rule-following itself is selected and maintained by the contingencies for following or complying with rules, and thereby is subject to environmental control (Catania, Matthews, & Shimoff, 1982; Galizio, 1979). An individual will only continue to follow a rule if rule-following under similar circumstances previously was reinforced.

As an example of rule-governed social behavior, suppose a heterosexual adolescent boy operates under a rule, based on embarrassing anecdotes from same-sex peers, that he will approach a girl to talk (and express interest in her) only if he "knows" for certain that she currently does not have a romantic partner and very likely will not "turn down" his advances. The rule may function to prevent the embarrassment of rejection, but unfortunately also operates to insulate the boy from contacting positive, developmentally growth-inducing socialization. That is, the potentially positive outcomes associated with approach towards and interaction with potential romantic partners are not contacted, and thus the frequency of such behavior is not subject to being increased via positive reinforcement. As a result, this individual's behavior is under the control of contingencies for following rules regarding the avoidance of aversive experiences and the consequences of negative social evaluation. Individuals may be more aware of the contingencies supporting rule-governed behavior due to learning through observation or verbal communication as opposed to direct experience, but, similar to other conditioned behavior, awareness is not necessary for the occurrence of the behavior in question (Miller, 1977). As such, rule-governance describes the way in which environmental contingencies may be learned indirectly. Rule governance does not, however, describe a determinant of behavior that overrides environmental control.

Both direct and indirect respondent and operant conditioning provide examples in which behavioral principles successfully may be used to explain more complex behavior without ascribing causal status to cognitive variables. Nevertheless, the principles discussed in this section might only explain initial development of SAD. In the following sections, we examine behavioral principles that underlie both the generalization of SAD to contexts in which it has not previously been directly or indirectly conditioned, and the maintenance of SAD within those contexts.

Generalization of Social Anxiety Disorder

As children, adolescents, and young adults move through developmental phases in life, they encounter social situations that evolve in complexity and import. Avoidance of interactions with peers during childhood may then generalize to avoidance of encounters with potential romantic partners, and to peer relationships in education, training, or employment. As demands for independent functioning increase over the early part of the lifespan, in SAD, there is likely to be generalization to social situations that are new and not previously encountered.

Phobic behavior may occur under conditions in which conditioned stimuli are absent (i.e., respondent conditioning) and such behavior has yet to be reinforced (i.e., operant conditioning). These instances appear to present difficulties for a behavioral view, and neither direct respondent nor operant conditioning principles alone can explain the occurrence of this behavior in such situations. Principles based upon stimulus control, however, provide a solid foundation for explaining such instances of behavior.

Stimulus Generalization

Stimulus generalization occurs when a response that has been reinforced in the presence of one stimulus occurs for the first time in the presence of a structurally similar stimulus (Fields, Reeve, Adams, & Verhave, 1991; see Honig & Urcuioli, 1981, for a review). For example, consider an individual having an embarrassing experience in a nightclub (e.g., being "turned down" when requesting to dance with someone). If the individual worries that "everyone in the nightclub saw this interaction and is now laughing" at him, feelings of relief likely will result after leaving the situation (i.e., negative reinforcement via escape). Because of this history of negative reinforcement, the individual may leave future situations at the first instance of distress or even come to avoid such situations altogether (e.g., avoidance of inviting someone to dance, or avoidance of the nightclub altogether). Following from these experiences, a stimulus generalization account of SAD helps to explain why *structurally* similar settings such as parties or informal social gatherings may result in escape or complete avoidance for this individual even though these situations had not previously produced anxiety, as with the embarrassing experience at the nightclub in the example above.

Thus, stimulus generalization is a useful concept that describes how a response may begin to occur in a variety of contexts without being directly reinforced in those contexts. Consequently, this concept provides the basic explanation of how SAD may generalize without any further operant or respondent conditioning events. The processes underlying generalization, however, often are considerably more complex than simple structural similarities. As a result, more complex behavior principles are needed.

Stimulus Equivalence

According to Hayes, Kohlenberg, and Hayes (1991), more sophisticated behavioral principles are necessary to provide for an adequate analysis of the role of verbal behavior and its relation to psychopathology than can be provided with the principle of stimulus generalization alone. Whereas stimulus generalization requires physical similarity between stimuli, stimulus equivalence describes the formation of a relation between unpaired stimuli based on their trained relation to the same stimuli (Barnes, 1994; Sidman, Wynne, Maguire, & Barnes, 1989). That is, if through experience stimulus A is paired with stimulus B, and stimulus B is paired with stimulus C, then a relation can occur between stimuli A and C, even though that relation has not been directly trained. An example adapted from Masia, McNeil, Cohn, and Hope (1999), based on semantic conditioning, may exemplify this principle most clearly. Suppose that the word "evaluation" (stimulus A) is paired with "social" (stimulus B). Further suppose that "evaluation" (stimulus A) and "negative" (stimulus C) are paired. Then, if new bidirectional relations occur, "social" (stimulus B) and "negative" (stimulus C) might be related, even though that equivalence was never specifically taught. Such conditioning could then lead to generalization across social situations, not just ones involving evaluation. There are other, detailed processes of conditioning that occur in stimulus equivalence that are beyond the scope of this chapter (Barnes, 1994). Although it is conceivable how relations among otherwise structurally dissimilar stimuli may be formed, the most central feature of social anxiety and phobia may be the functional qualities shared by stimuli, which may be best accounted for by the principle of functional equivalence.

Functional Equivalence

Similarly to stimulus equivalence, generalization may occur in relation to function, not as a result of structural similarity among stimuli. The end result is the transfer of function across stimulus class members, but the method by which this process occurs is unique from stimulus equivalence (Augustson & Dougher, 1997; Hayes et al., 1991; Sidman et al., 1989).

Defined briefly, a functional stimulus class is a set of structurally dissimilar stimuli that are grouped together because of similar discriminative stimulus functions (Dougher & Markham, 1994; Hayes et al., 1991; Sidman et al., 1989; Vaughan, 1988). Thus, unlike stimulus equivalence, relations are formed via functional similarities among the stimuli. For example, a graduate seminar, a formal party, and a picnic all may belong in the same functional stimulus class because outgoing and talkative behavior is reinforced in each setting (e.g., the teacher engaging in eye contact and saying "right" after the individual provides a comment or an answer to a question in a graduate seminar, or people laughing after the individual tells a joke at a party or picnic). Although these settings all may share structural stimulus properties (e.g., large groups of people), a stimulus generalization explanation may not be sufficient in all cases because the key aspect of these situations is the social/evaluative nature. Thus, the social/evaluative aspect distinguishes this functional class from other situations involving large groups of people (i.e., the structural similarity), such as those in libraries or at funerals, in which outgoing and talkative behavior is rarely reinforced, and in most cases punished.

Once a functional class is established, patterns of behavior other than that underlying the functional class membership may begin to occur across each of the situations. This "transfer of function" may explain the occurrence of SAD in new contexts for which no other obvious reason is available (see Augustson & Dougher, 1997; Sidman et al., 1989). Considering the previous example, if an individual is ridiculed while answering a question in a graduate seminar, speaking as little as possible when in class allows the individual to avoid most potential ridicule. Because that avoidance behavior is negatively reinforced, avoidance also may begin to occur in association with picnics and parties, but not in regard to libraries or funerals. Thus, behavior may occur for the first time in the presence of a particular stimulus if that behavior has been reinforced in the presence of another stimulus that is a member of the same functional class (Dougher & Markham, 1994).

Stimulus generalization, stimulus equivalence, and functional equivalence provide an explanation for the emergence of phobic behavior across several situations that appear to be unrelated to outside observers. Generalization also may occur, however, across responses within a particular context.

Response Generalization

Response generalization can be used to explain how phobic behavior changes and persists over several contexts and how it can be extinguished across these contexts. As SAD develops in an individual, there likely is generalization of avoidance responding, with learning that avoidance of social interactions and/or other social situations is (temporarily) reinforcing due to lessened anxiety. Nevertheless, it is virtually impossible in most lifestyles to completely avoid social interactions. The typical latency between onset of SAD and initial treatment for it is longer than that many other anxiety disorders. Since social avoidance is partially successful, extended time may elapse before sufficient misery and comorbid disorders (e.g., depression) are manifested, thus prompting treatment.

The neobehavioral concept of experiential avoidance (Forsyth, Eifert, & Barrios, 2006) may be explained by response generalization. Defined as a process that involves both an unwillingness to have and an effort to control or escape from unwanted thoughts, emotions, and physiological sensations, experiential avoidance has gained a great deal of attention over the past decade (e.g., Hayes, Strosahl, & Wilson, 1999). Across situations that individuals with SAD find phobic, both overt and subtle avoidance strategies are learned. Limiting one's social interactions to restrict either the number of contacts or sustained contact, or both, allows one to not encounter the negative aspects of experiencing anxiety, in an attempt to down-regulate fear conditioning (Forsyth et al., 2006). Nevertheless, it also disallows the potentially therapeutic results of exposure (McNeil & Kyle, 2009). Experiential avoidance, when generally, excessively, and rigidly applied across (potential) social encounters, results in the individual with SAD maintaining her problems, leading to constriction of life functioning, decreased contact with important life values, and eventually leading to chronic suffering (Forsyth et al., 2006).

As with all patterns of behavior, each instance of a particular behavior may be slightly different from previous instances. When a particular response that once produced reinforcement no longer does so, behavioral variability occurs such that other functionally similar patterns of behavior may emerge in the place of the no-longer-reinforced pattern. For example, consider a highly socially anxious student who initially is able to keep an instructor from calling on her by looking down throughout class. If the instructor begins calling on the student despite this subtle avoidance strategy, the student may try other similar responses to avoid this unwanted attention until one of the somewhat random strategies (e.g., taking or pretending to take notes) starts to work (i.e., is reinforced) on a regular basis.

It should be noted, however, that although such instances of subtle avoidance often are a reasonable alternative to more overt avoidance, subtle avoidance also may produce negative consequences or it may not always provide for the successful avoidance of the aversive stimuli. For example, individuals who make little eye contact may be considered to be less socially skilled and can be thought of less favorably than individuals who make appropriate eye contact. Furthermore, the student in the prior example may be called on regardless of where her attention is focused. Thus, it is likely that if instances of subtle avoidance engendered via response generalization do not provide the desired result, the new strategies may involve a type of "escalation" leading to more overt and extreme forms of avoidance (e.g., avoiding attending the class altogether).

Maintenance of Social Anxiety and Phobia

The combination of principles based on generalization and equivalence provide an explanation for the emergence of numerous forms of phobic behavior across several situations that, on the surface, may appear to be unrelated. Once particular patterns of phobic behavior have begun to occur in a new context, it is then the consequences provided for such behavior and the relative consequences provided for alternative (i.e., nonphobic) behavior that determine its persistence. As such, principles that consider contextual variables are relevant.

Matching Law

We argue that the basic assumption within a behavioral formulation is that phobic behavior occurs more frequently when it produces greater reinforcement value than all other possible forms of nonphobic behavior. Value is defined as the interaction of several parameters of reinforcement including frequency, magnitude, duration, immediacy, and certainty. Application of the matching law (Herrnstein, 1961, 1970), a behavioral model of choice behavior, more specifically suggests that the relative frequency of phobic behavior, compared to nonphobic behavior, is proportional to the relative value of reinforcement for phobic behavior compared to nonphobic behavior.

In other words, if the value of reinforcers for phobic behavior is increased, the relative value of reinforcers for nonphobic behavior must decrease. Consequently, the likelihood of future phobic behavior will increase, while the likelihood of future nonphobic behavior will decrease. Conversely, if the individual encounters less frequent reinforcement for phobic behavior than nonphobic behavior, nonphobic behavior will occur more frequently. In both cases, the shift in relative reinforcement frequency will be correlated with the shift in relative preference. For example, if reinforcement is obtained for phobic behavior at twice the frequency of reinforcement for nonphobic behavior, phobic behavior should occur twice as often.

The matching law typically is considered in terms of reinforcers, yet the role of punishers may be accounted for in a similar way, such that the presence of punishers diminishes the relative value of an alternative (Deluty, 1978). Thus, in a more complex system than that described previously, the value of an alternative is a combination of the obtained reinforcers (increasing value) and punishers (decreasing value), relative to the combination of the obtained reinforcers (increasing value) and punishers (decreasing value) for other alternatives.

Although the precision of the behavioral account provided by the matching law is necessarily reduced in the natural environment, this limitation does not preclude its usefulness in applied settings. The matching law has not yet been applied to SAD, but its clinical utility has been asserted (McDowell, 1982) and demonstrated in areas such as social behavior. For example, Conger and Killeen (1974) found that, when given a chance to speak with two experimental confederates, individuals would spend more time conversing with the confederate that provided more frequent praise. Furthermore, the ratio of conversation directed at the two confederates was proportional to the ratio of praise.

Related to social fears, consider an individual with GSAD who is offered a job promotion providing considerably more prestige and salary. Taken alone, such reinforcers would be thought to make taking such a job highly desirable. Accepting the new position, however, also would present potential punishers such as increased public speaking responsibilities. Thus, not taking the position would be negatively reinforced, as instances of public speaking and other social stressors would be avoided, reducing the relative frequency of aversive work-related social situations. Additionally, positive reinforcers such as continued opportunity to interact with coworkers with whom the individual is well acquainted may increase the value of not taking the new position. As a result, although there may be several potential benefits of taking the new position, the associated benefits of not taking the position and therefore avoiding novel social and evaluative situations may be relatively greater.

Thus, the matching law suggests that the frequency of phobic and nonphobic patterns of behavior should conform to the relative value obtained for those alternatives. Nevertheless, it remains unclear why an individual might continue with a particular pattern of behavior and not engage in others that potentially might produce greater gain. This question may be answered by considering the matching law's focus on obtained as opposed to available reinforcers. For example, going to a party potentially may provide a high level of reinforcement, making it a desirable alternative; however, if the individual avoids parties and has not experienced the available reinforcers, there is no "obtained" reinforcer for going to parties. As a result, the temporary relief via cessation of physiological and cognitive responses produced by avoidance of feared stimuli, although resulting in long-term negative effects, continues to have greater relative obtained value than party attendance.

Rule-governed Behavior

In addition to its applicability to initial instances of behavior, rule-governance also may be used to explain the persistence of ineffective patterns of behavior. Research has shown that, under certain conditions, individuals will continue to behave in accordance with an initially provided rule despite the fact that the rule may no longer provide for the most conducive pattern of behavior. For example, Galizio (1979) found that, when given a "strategy" for successful participation in a contrived game situation, participants would use these strategies and often not ever contact the actual contingencies, even when the provided strategy was not optimal. Nonetheless, the influence of rules should not be considered independently of the associated environmental contingencies. That is, an individual who follows a rule that is contrary to the environmental contingencies often does so because the potential reinforcers available in the avoided situation have not been contacted. Thus, when Galizio's participants engaged in a strategy (often by accident on its first instance of use) that was more effective than the strategy given to them, the influence of rule governance was weakened and new strategies developed.

For reasons related to rule-governance, exposure therapy has value beyond extinction of conditioned fear responses. For example, if an individual avoids a situation because of a rule and not because the situation is actually dangerous or threatening, repeatedly exposing the individual to the situation will allow for contact with the reinforcers available in that situation. For example, an individual with circumscribed public speaking phobia may operate under a rule that indicates: "I am poor at delivering speeches, so I should make every effort to avoid formal speaking opportunities, even if my career is hurt in the long-term." Either with or without the presence of significant public speaking skills deficits, systematic therapeutic exposure should help to counteract this rule. More sophisticated speaking skills may be developed, and positive comments from the therapist (and, through modeling and shaping, the individual himself) should result in greater reinforcement for public speaking, first in the therapy situation and later in the natural environment. As discussed regarding the matching law, this increase in obtained reinforcers should increase the likelihood of the socially positive behavior in question. It should be noted, however, that repeated exposure to positive consequences of new (healthy) behavior patterns often is necessary to counteract previous longstanding patterns of old (unhealthy) behavior, especially considering that these old patterns of behavior may be strengthened by coincidental instances of intermittent reinforcement (e.g., occasional subtle negative facial expressions in some audience members).

In addition to rule governance, other factors may possibly explain the occurrence of less adaptive behavior. Basic operant studies in the area of delay and certainty of reinforcement (also referred to as self-control and impulsivity) provide possible answers to this question.

Delay, Amount, and Certainty of Reinforcement

Delayed events (positive or negative) impact behavior less than immediate events (Bjorkman, 1984; Renner, 1964; Tarpy & Sawabini, 1974). Preference for small immediate rewards as opposed to delayed larger rewards has been defined as impulsivity (Ainslie, 1975; Rachlin & Green, 1972). Although not explicitly outlined in any current theory of SAD, this definition of impulsivity can be used to better understand some of the variables controlling socially mediated phobic avoidance and escape. Specifically, phobic avoidance and escape result in immediate negative reinforcement through terminated or prevented contact with a feared stimulus, whereas entering or remaining in an anxiety-provoking situation may produce a larger, but considerably more delayed, reinforcer. For example, a phobic individual may avoid going to parties because of the potential for negative evaluation, even though such avoidance prevents the attainment of a variety of social reinforcers including engaging in rewarding conversations and possibly developing friendships. To obtain such reinforcers, the individual must endure any pre-party anxiety that may increase as the time of the party approaches. Furthermore, many social reinforcers often are not immediately obtained. For example, it may take lengthy conversations and numerous encounters before a comfortable relationship is developed between the phobic individual and another person. Thus, the larger, more delayed rewards obtained by going to parties often are less preferred compared to the immediate, yet small and temporary, negative reinforcement provided by avoidance.

Although less empirical support has been provided, the same general processes also appear to be evident for punishment. Regarding punishment, self-control involves the choice of an immediate small punisher as opposed to a delayed large punisher (Deluty, 1978). For example, an individual with SAD may prematurely terminate a presentation that is proceeding poorly, and then leave the room abruptly. Although the consequences of leaving may be greater than finishing the presentation, the consequences in the former (e.g., ultimate loss of job) are delayed whereas the consequences for the latter are occurring at that moment (e.g., negative nonverbal feedback from audience members).

Organisms often behave impulsively in regard to both reinforcement and punishment, but these outcomes can be changed. First, the value of a delayed reinforcer can be increased. For example, a phobic individual is less likely to avoid a public speaking presentation if a substantial promotion, as opposed to only employer praise, eventually will result following completion of the task.

Second, the value of a delayed reinforcer can be increased if the delay to the more immediate reinforcer is increased. Grusec (1968) examined the behavior of third-grade children given actual choices between immediate and delayed reinforcers and punishers. As the delay to reinforcement for the immediate reward was increased, participants preferred the larger, more delayed reinforcers over the smaller, less delayed reinforcers. Additionally, participants preferred the smaller, more immediate punisher to the larger, more delayed punishers after the delay to the larger punisher was shortened. Not surprisingly, increasing the delay of a smaller reinforcer will limit impulsivity; however, the same result may be obtained by increasing the delay to both reinforcers by the same absolute amount (Rachlin & Green, 1972).

This work on delay and amount of reinforcement may help to explain a common occurrence in which a commitment to a social engagement may be made a week or more prior to the event, yet, as the event approaches, the avoidance option is selected, perhaps utilizing a socially acceptable excuse ("I'm not feeling well"). In such an example, a person with GSAD may promise to attend a party with a strong, stated intention to follow through with this agreement to a casual friend. On an immediate basis, there is positive (e.g., enthusiastic encouragement) and negative (e.g., cessation of cajoling) reinforcement from the friend for agreeing to attend the event. Consequently, less reinforcement is then available for a stated decision to not attend (i.e., avoid) at that point. Yet, in the hours just before the party, reinforcement is then immediate for avoidance (e.g., through termination of the worry regarding adequacy of her social interactions at the party) and considerably delayed for attendance (e.g., through satisfying relationships potentially developing in the future), beyond the lesser negative social repercussions from the casual friend. Consequently, the individual is then considerably more likely to avoid. Although beyond the scope of this chapter, a quantitative model predicting choice based on reinforcer magnitude and delay duration is provided by Rachlin and Baum (1972). Additionally, a similar model is presented substituting aversive events for reinforcers (Deluty, 1978).

A less obvious method for decreasing impulsivity involves the presence of stimuli that signal reinforcement. Basic research suggests that impulsive behavior may be reduced if the delay to reinforcement is accompanied by a constant or reoccurring signal (e.g., Schaal & Branch, 1990; Schaal, Schuh, & Branch, 1992). The value of a repeated signal can be considered in the context of an individual with SAD who is more likely to attend a party, given continued reassurance from friends as opposed to one discrete instance of reassurance. A signal may have an effect simply because it serves as a conditioned reinforcer and/or a discriminative stimulus for when reinforcement will occur. A signal acquires such stimulus functions, however, only if its presence in the past has been paired with reinforcer delivery. For example, a person with SAD may be more likely to attend a party if frequently told that several friends will be at the party; such information serves as a constant signal that reinforcers such as enjoyable conversation, although delayed, are very likely to be obtained by attending the party. Furthermore, the signal itself may come to be valued, assuming that such information has been accurate and has reliably been followed by reinforcer delivery. Similar to the discussion of rule-governed behavior, if such information in the past has not led to reinforcer delivery (e.g., although the individual is told that friends will be at a party, the friends never show up), such information in the future will most likely not serve as a discriminative stimulus or conditioned reinforcer, the delay will not be mediated, and most importantly the individual will not attend the party.

Although this discussion is focused on delay to reinforcement/punishment, it is difficult to consider delay irrespective of certainty and uncertainty. Considering the prior examples, there often are no guarantees that going to a party will produce the desired reinforcers, even after a long delay. For example, attempts to interact with others at a party may be ignored or deflected, or may even lead to the delivery of punishers such as hurtful sarcasm, rudeness, or ridicule. In contrast, avoidance and escape almost always produce the removal of the feared stimulus and the resulting decrease in anxiety. As a result, the uncertainty of reinforcement may play a crucial role in the occurrence of escape and avoidance, thus further increasing the likelihood of future instances of such behavior. Although delay and certainty often are discussed independently, several researchers have suggested that these two processes are highly related (e.g., Mischel & Grusec, 1967). For example, as the delay to a reinforcer increases, the likelihood that the reinforcer will actually be presented is decreased. When considered together, these variables provide powerful clues to understanding impulsive and self-controlled behavior.

Although often considered solely as basic research phenomena, delay and certainty of reinforcement and punishment clearly are applicable to the understanding and treatment of social anxiety and phobia. Via systematic exposure to social situations, the individual may begin to notice particular cues that signal future reinforcer and punisher delivery. For example, a heterosexual phobic individual interacting with a member of the opposite sex that he finds interesting may notice particular facial gestures (e.g., smiling) or posturing (e.g., leaning closer) that are associated with a positive interaction. As such, the occurrence of these behaviors from women may signal that a positive evaluation will follow. Thus, actually targeting these social cues from others in treatment might produce beneficial results in terms of increased awareness of delay and certainty of reinforcers.

Although such an approach may provide insight into the etiology and treatment of SAD, it nevertheless remains somewhat of mystery what variables control the discrimination and interpretation of subtle social cues. In the following section, signal detection theory will be reviewed as a potential explanation.

Signal Detection

Several theories have been proposed suggesting that individuals diagnosed with an anxiety disorder are better at detecting panic attack-related changes in physiological responding than individuals without such anxiety difficulties

(Margraf & Ehlers, 1989; Rapee, 1987). Although mixed results have been provided, Ehlers and Breuer (1992) found that individuals diagnosed with PD were better able to detect their own heart rate than controls. A similar hypothesis could be proposed regarding individuals with SAD and their sensitivity to evaluative cues from others. Specifically, individuals with social concerns often are more sensitive to potential criticism than other individuals, and it may be this greater attention to cues from others that leads to avoidance and other SAD behaviors (Rapee & Heimberg, 1997). "Attentional bias" has been extensively studied in SAD. Recent data suggest that individuals with GSAD, relative to controls, are more vigilant to angry faces relative to neutral faces in the first 500 ms of a 5000 ms exposure, but this difference disappears thereafter (Gamble & Rapee, 2010).

Alternatively, it has been hypothesized that these individuals often are inattentive to social cues. Given the previously mentioned data, it may be that social cues capture attention early on but then are relatively ignored if there is no immediate social threat. Beidel and Turner (1998) suggest that, when in a group of people, an individual with SAD may focus so much on his own behavior and what he might say that he is oblivious to what is being said by others around him. As a result, these individuals appear uninterested in what others are saying or doing and miss important social cues. Considering these two hypotheses, two questions emerge for individuals with SAD during or after social interactions: (1) "Did an evaluative cue occur?" and, if so, (2) "Was the evaluative cue negative?"

To provide a more quantitative analysis of cue recognition and interpretation, an analysis based on signal detection theory may be used. The specifics of a signal detection analysis are beyond the scope of this chapter, but, in brief, it provides a mathematical method for determining both an individual's accuracy at interpreting social cues (i.e., sensitivity) and the bias she or he may have towards over- or under-assuming that a particular cue is positive or negative. Once this information is determined, the underlying principles maintaining SAD for an individual may become clearer.

In general, a signal detection analysis poses the question: "Did something happen or not?" Specific to SAD, the first question would be "Did an evaluation occur?" Answers to this question can be placed into one of four categories. When an evaluation has occurred, the correct identification of its occurrence is labeled a hit, whereas a failure to identify its occurrence is labeled a miss. When an evaluation has not occurred, the correct identification that no evaluation has occurred is labeled a correct rejection, whereas the incorrect identification of its occurrence is labeled a false alarm. In cases in which an evaluation is correctly (hit) or incorrectly (false alarm) identified, a second question becomes: "Was the evaluation negative?" Answers to this question also can be placed into one of four categories. If the evaluation was negative, the correct interpretation is labeled a hit, whereas interpreting it as neutral or positive is labeled a miss. When the evaluation is not negative, the correct interpretation (i.e., interpreting a cue as neutral or positive) is labeled a correct rejection, whereas the incorrect interpretation of a neutral or positive cue as negative is labeled a false alarm.

Regarding the identification and interpretation of evaluative cues, some research has been conducted within a signal detection framework, in addition to the study by Gamble and Rapee (2010) mentioned earlier. Winton, Clark, and Edelmann (1995) found that high scorers on the FNE, compared to low scorers, showed a response bias towards interpreting facial expressions as negative despite no greater ability to detect negative facial cues (i.e., no difference in sensitivity). In a similar study, however, Veljaca and Rapee (1998) found that individuals reporting high social anxiety showed both a response bias towards interpreting facial expressions as negative and a greater ability to detect negative facial cues. Additionally, low anxious subjects showed a greater ability to detect positive facial expressions. According to Veljaca and Rapee, these results support cognitive models of SAD that postulate a biased allocation of attentional resources to negative evaluation. Although these results can be taken as support for such an explanation, a simpler behavioral explanation also is possible. Specifically, individuals with SAD likely have a history of negative social experiences. As such, the consequences of negative social evaluation may be more salient. Thus, these individuals may be more vigilant to social cues. Additionally, these individuals also may be more likely to interpret cues as negative because the consequences of incorrectly interpreting a cue as negative and then avoiding or escaping the situation may be less aversive (especially in the short term) than incorrectly interpreting a negative cue as positive, and remaining in the situation and experiencing further negative evaluation.

Regardless of interpretation, the mathematical precision of such an analysis might be helpful for determining whether a particular individual's phobic difficulties are due to an inability to identify the occurrence of evaluative cues, or bias towards assuming particular cues are indicative of a negative evaluation (see Winton et al., 1995). Along the same lines, a signal detection analysis might be useful for treatment planning. If an individual is shown to be highly sensitive to the presentation of negative social cues, anxiety reduction techniques could be used to ameliorate the individual's anxiety-related vigilance. Furthermore, if an individual is found to be insensitive to social cues, a form of skills training can be used to help the individual improve his/her ability to identify social cues (see Gambrill, 1995). Alternatively, anxiety reduction techniques might be necessary to limit "interference" that prevents the identification of these cues. In contrast, if an individual is shown to have a bias towards interpreting most or all social cues negatively, exposure with response prevention to social situations may be sufficient to allow the individual the opportunity to continue in a situation in which cues were incorrectly interpreted as negative and then experience that negative consequences do not occur. Similarly, the person who consistently avoids social encounters due to the negative thoughts and physiological responses that are evoked during them, and thus is engaging in experiential avoidance, also may benefit from exposure approaches. A signal detection analysis also can be used to distinguish the individual with a bias towards negative evaluation and the individual with poor social skills who receives and correctly identifies frequent negative evaluations. For the latter individual, anxiety may develop, but, as social skills deficits are the primary concern, social skills training should be the principal treatment intervention.

SUMMARY AND CONCLUSIONS

This chapter reviewed current behavioral theorizing relating to social anxieties and fears, and their related disorders. One advantage of a behavioral theory of SAD consists of the wealth of both basic and applied research establishing principles that may be applicable to the understanding and treatment of this syndrome. Although the current behavioral theories of SAD are theoretically consistent and highly effective when applied to its treatment, many of the underlying principles of these theories have not been developed nor highlighted adequately. The learning principles discussed here are underutilized in terms of problem conceptualization and treatment. For example, behavioral theories of SAD most always focus upon reinforcers available for phobic and nonphobic behavior, yet few place this conceptualization within a matching law framework. As a result, the principles have heretofore been used only within a loose approximation, thus limiting their potential precision.

Presently, from a behavioral perspective, exposure and skills training are standard treatment components, yet there has not been much theoretical guidance provided as to the situations in which these treatments work and what to do in cases in which they do not work. For example, both a signal detection analysis and the matching law have been implicated in the treatment of several psychological disorders and would be useful to guide treatment when more basic approaches such as exposure and removing negative reinforcement do not reduce the behavior to the desired levels. In such a case, the matching law might guide treatment to additionally focus on increasing available reinforcement for nonphobic behavior.

Although basic behavioral principles have received relatively little attention within the SAD literature, principles such as equivalence and impulsivity have begun to be incorporated and tested within other disorders via general packages applicable to psychopathology in general, such as acceptance and commitment therapy (ACT) (Hayes, Strosahl, & Wilson, 1999), and functional analytic psychotherapy (Kohlenberg & Tsai, 1991; Tsai et al., 2009), as well as more specific treatment packages for problems such as substance use disorders (Azrin, 1976; Higgins et al., 1995). It is our hope that future theories and treatments will begin to incorporate these principles, thereby providing a firm theoretical and empirical basis.

Behavioral formulations of psychopathology often are thought to be both oversimplified and unable to capture the richness of human experience. Related to SAD, exclusion of cognitive variables limits the potential usefulness of a behavioral approach. It is our opinion, however, that such a view is applicable to behavioral theories that acknowledge only basic conditioning as the process that influences the development and maintenance of SAD. As such, we have attempted to provide a variety of more complex behavioral principles that should be useful in developing a comprehensive understanding of the disorder. Furthermore, although cognitive variables are not recognized as causal agents, their existence and importance is acknowledged. In sum, we believe that a behavioral conceptualization of SAD can be comprehensive, and also may provide information on the etiology and treatment of the disorder that may not be possible from other theoretical perspectives.

ACKNOWLEDGMENTS

Preparation of this revised chapter was supported in part by a Fulbright New Zealand Senior Scholar Fellowship to the first author.

Cynthia L. Turk provided helpful comments on an earlier version of this chapter.

REFERENCES

Ainslie, G. (1975). Specious reward: A behavioral theory of impulsiveness and impulse control. *Psychological Bulletin*, *82*, 463–496.

Anderson, C. M., Hawkins, R. P., & Scotti, J. R. (1997). Private events in behavior analysis: Conceptual basis and clinical relevance. *Behavior Therapy*, *28*, 157–179.

Augustson, E. M., & Dougher, M. J. (1997). The transfer of avoidance evoking functions through stimulus equivalence classes. *Journal of Behavior Therapy and Experimental Psychiatry*, *28*, 181–191.

Azrin, N. H. (1976). Improvements in the community reinforcement approach to alcoholism. *Behaviour Research and Therapy*, *14*, 339–348.

Barlow, D. G. (2002). *Anxiety and its disorders: The nature and treatment of anxiety and panic* (2nd ed.). New York: Guilford.

Barnes, D. (1994). Stimulus equivalence and relational frame theory. *Psychological Record*, *44*, 91–124.

Barrett, P. M., Rapee, R. M., Dadds, M. M., & Ryan, S. M. (1996). Family enhancement of cognitive style in anxious and aggressive children. *Journal of Abnormal Child Psychology*, *24*, 187–203.

Beck, A. T., & Emery, G. (1985). *Anxiety disorders and phobias: A cognitive perspective*. New York: Basic Books.

Beidel, D. C., Morris, T. L., & Turner, M. W. (2004). Social phobia. In T. L. Morris & J. S. March (Eds.), *Anxiety disorders in children and adolescents* (2nd ed.) (pp. 141–163). New York: Guilford.

Beidel, D. C., & Turner, S. M. (1998). *Shy children, phobic adults: Nature and treatment of social anxiety disorder*. Washington, DC: American Psychological Association.

Bjorkman, M. (1984). Decision making, risk taking, and psychological time: Review of empirical findings and psychological theory. *Scandinavian Journal of Psychology*, *25*, 31–49.

Bögels, S. M., Alden, L., Beidel, D. C., Clark, L. A., Pine, D. S., Stein, M. B., et al. (2010). Social anxiety disorder: Questions and answers for the DSM-V. *Depression and Anxiety*, *27*, 168–189.

Catania, A. C., Matthews, B. A., & Shimoff, E. (1982). Instructed versus shaped human verbal behavior. *Journal of the Experimental Analysis of Behavior*, *38*, 233–248.

Clark, D. M., & Wells, A. (1995). A cognitive model of social anxiety disorder. In R. G. Heimberg, M. R. Liebowitz, D. A. Hope, & F. R. Schneier (Eds.), *Social anxiety disorder: Diagnosis and treatment* (pp. 69–93). New York: Guilford.

Conger, R., & Killeen, P. (1974). Use of concurrent operants in small group research: A demonstration. *Pacific Sociological Review*, *17*, 399–416.

Deluty, M. Z. (1978). Self-control and impulsiveness involving aversive events. *Journal of Experimental Psychology: Animal Behavior Processes*, *4*, 250–266.

Dougher, M. J., & Markham, M. (1994). Stimulus equivalence, functional equivalence and the transfer of function. In S. C. Hayes, L. H. Hayes, M. Sato, & K. Ono (Eds.), *Cognitive and verbal events: A behavior analytic view.* Reno, NV: Context Press.

Eelen, P., & Vervliet, B. (2006). Fear conditioning and clinical implications: What can we learn from the past? In M. G. Craske, D. Hermans, & D. Vansteenwegen (Eds.), *Fear and learning: From basic processes to clinical implications* (pp. 17–35). Washington, DC: American Psychological Association.

Ehlers, A., & Breuer, P. (1992). Increased cardiac awareness in panic disorder. *Journal of Abnormal Psychology*, *101*, 371–382.

Eifert, G. H., & Plaud, J. J. (1998). From behavior theory to behavior therapy: An overview. In G. H. Eifert & J. J. Plaud (Eds.), *From behavior theory to behavior therapy* (pp. 1–14). Needham Heights, MA: Allyn & Bacon.

Eifert, G. H., Schulte, D., Zvolensky, M. J., Lejuez, C. W., & Lau, A. M. (1997). Manualized behavior therapy: Merits and challenges. *Behavior Therapy*, *28*, 499–510.

Emmelkamp, P. M. G., & Mersch, P. P. (1982). Cognition and exposure *in vivo* in the treatment of agoraphobia: Short term and delayed effects. *Cognitive Therapy and Research*, *6*, 77–90.

Feske, U., & Chambless, D. L. (1995). Cognitive-behavioral versus exposure treatment for social anxiety disorder: A meta-analysis. *Behavior Therapy*, *26*, 695–720.

Fields, L., Reeve, K. F., Adams, B. J., & Verhave, T. (1991). Stimulus generalization and equivalence classes: A model for natural categories. *Journal of the Experimental Analysis of Behavior*, *55*, 305–312.

Forsyth, J. P., Eifert, G. H., & Barrios, V. (2006). Fear conditioning in an emotion regulation context: A fresh perspective on the origins of anxiety disorders. In M. G. Craske, D. Hermans, & D. Vansteenwegen (Eds.), *Fear and learning: From basic processes to clinical implications.* (pp. 133–153). Washington, DC: American Psychological Association.

Galizio, M. (1979). Contingency-shaped and rule-governed behavior: Instructional control of human loss avoidance. *Journal of the Experimental Analysis of Behavior*, *31*, 53–70.

Gamble, A. L., & Rapee, R. M. (2010). The time-course of attention to emotional faces in social phobia. *Journal of Behavior Therapy and Experimental Psychiatry*, *41*, 39–44.

Gambrill, E. (1995). Helping shy, socially anxious, and lonely adults: A skill-based contextual approach. In W. O'Donohue & L. Krasner (Eds.), *Handbook of psychological skills training: Clinical techniques and application* (pp. 247–268). Needham Heights, MA: Allyn & Bacon.

Greco, L. A., & Morris, T. L. (2002). Parental child-rearing style and child social anxiety: Investigation of child perceptions and actual father behavior. *Journal of Psychopathology and Behavioral Assessment*, *24*, 259–267.

Grusec, J. E. (1968). Waiting for rewards and punishments: Effects of reinforcement value on choice. *Journal of Personality and Social Psychology*, *9*, 85–89.

Guerin, B. (1994). *Analyzing social behavior: Behavior analysis and the social sciences*. Reno, NV: Context Press.

Hayes, S. C., Kohlenberg, B. S., & Hayes, L. J. (1991). The transfer of specific function and general consequential functions through simple and conditional equivalence relations. *Journal of the Experimental Analysis of Behavior, 56*, 119–137.

Hayes, S. C., Strosahl, K. D., & Wilson, K. G. (1999). *Acceptance and commitment therapy: An experiential approach to behavior change*. New York: Guilford.

Hayes, S. C, Zettle, R. D., & Rosenfarb, I. (1989). Rule-following. In S. C. Hayes (Ed.), *Rule-governed behavior* (pp. 191–220). New York: Plenum.

Herrnstein, R. J. (1961). Relative and absolute strength of a response as a function of frequency of reinforcement. *Journal of the Experimental Analysis of Behavior, 4*, 267–272.

Herrnstein, R. J. (1970). On the law of effect. *Journal of the Experimental Analysis of Behavior, 13*, 243–266.

Higgins, S. T., Budney, A. J., Bickel, W. K., Badger, G. J., Foerg, F. E., & Ogden, D. (1995). Outpatient behavioral treatment for cocaine dependence: One year outcome. *Experimental and Clinical Psychopharmacology, 3*, 205–212.

Hofmann, S. G., Ehlers, A., & Roth, W. T. (1995). Conditioning theory: A model for the etiology of public speaking anxiety? *Behaviour Research and Therapy, 33*, 567–571.

Hofmann, S. G. (2007). Cognitive factors that maintain social anxiety disorder: A comprehensive model and its treatment implications. *Cognitive Behaviour Therapy, 36*, 193–207.

Hofmann, S. G., & Barlow, D. G. (2002). Social phobia (social anxiety disorder). In D. G. Barlow (Ed.), *Anxiety and its disorders: The nature and treatment of anxiety and panic* (2nd ed.) (pp. 454–476). New York: Guilford.

Hofmann, S. G., Heinrichs, N., & Moscovitch, D. A. (2004). The nature and expression of social phobia: Toward a new classification. *Clinical Psychology Review, 24*, 769–797.

Holt, C. S., Heimberg, R. G., Hope, D. A., & Liebowitz, M. R. (1992). Situational domains of social phobia. *Journal of Anxiety Disorders, 6*, 63–77.

Honig, W. K., & Urcuioli, P. J. (1981). The legacy of Guttman and Kalish (1956): 25 years of research on stimulus generalization. *Journal of the Experimental Analysis of Behavior, 36*, 405–445.

Hope, D. A., Heimberg, R. G., & Bruch, M. A. (1995). Dismantling cognitive-behavioral group therapy for social anxiety disorder. *Behaviour Research and Therapy, 33*, 637–650.

Hopko, D., McNeil, D. W., Zvolensky, M. J., & Eifert, G. E. (2001). The relation between anxiety and skill in performance-based anxiety disorders: A behavioral formulation of social phobia. *Behavior Therapy, 32*, 185–207.

Kohlenberg, R. J., & Tsai, M. (1991). *Functional analytic psychotherapy: Creating intense and curative therapeutic relationships*. New York: Plenum.

Lejuez, C. W., Schaal, D. W., & O'Donnell, J. (1998). Behavioral pharmacology and the treatment of substance abuse. In J. J. Plaud & G. H. Eifert (Eds.), *From behavior theory to behavior therapy* (pp. 116–131). Needham Heights, MA: Allyn & Bacon.

Lewinsohn, P. M. (1974). A behavioral approach to depression. In R. J. Friedman & M. M. Katz (Eds.), *The psychology of depression: Contemporary theory and research* (pp. 157–178). Oxford, UK: Wiley.

Liebowitz, M. R., Gorman, J. M., Fyer, A. J., & Klein, D. F. (1985). Social anxiety disorder: Review of a neglected anxiety disorder. *Archives of General Psychiatry, 42*, 729–736.

MacCorquodale, K., & Meehl, P. E. (1948). Hypothetical constructs and intervening variables. *Psychological Review, 55*, 596–611.

Margraf, J., & Ehlers, A. (1989). Etiological models of panic: Psychophysiological and cognitive aspects. In R. Baker (Ed.), *Panic disorder: Theory, research and therapy* (pp. 205–231). Oxford, UK: Wiley.

Marks, I. M. (1969). *Fears and phobias*. New York: Academic Press.

Marks, I. M. (1970). The classification of phobic disorders. *British Journal of Psychiatry*, *116*, 377–386.

Marks, I. M. (1985). Behavioral treatment of social anxiety disorder. *Psychopharmacology Bulletin*, *21*, 615–618.

Marks, I. M. (1987). *Fears, phobias, and rituals: Panic, anxiety, and their disorders*. New York: Oxford.

Marks, I. M., & Gelder, M. G. (1966). Different ages of onset in varieties of phobia. *American Journal of Psychiatry*, *123*, 218–221.

Masia, C., McNeil, D. W., Cohn, L. G., & Hope, D. A. (1999). Exposure to social anxiety words: Treatment for social phobia based on the Stroop paradigm. *Cognitive and Behavioral Practice*, *6*, 248–258.

Masia, C. L., & Morris, T. L. (1998). Parental factors associated with social anxiety: Methodological limitations and suggestions for integrated behavioral research. *Clinical Psychology: Science and Practice*, *5*, 211–228.

McDowell, J. J. (1982). The importance of Herrnstein's mathematical statement of the law of effect for behavior therapy. *American Psychologist*, *37*, 771–779.

McNeil, D. W., & Kyle, B. N. (2009). Exposure-based strategies. In S. Cormier, P. S. Nurius, & C. J. Osborn (Eds.), *Interviewing and change strategies for helpers* (6th ed.) (pp. 486–516). Belmont, CA: Brooks/Cole.

Miller, N. E. (1977). The effects of learning on visceral functions. *New England Journal of Medicine*, *296*, 1274–1278.

Mineka., S., & Öhman, A. (2002). Born to fear: Non-associative versus associative factors in the etiology of phobias. *Behaviour Research and Therapy*, *40*, 173–184.

Mineka, S., & Sutton, J. (2006). Contemporary learning theory perspectives on the etiology of fears and phobias. In M. G. Craske, D. Hermans, & D. Vansteenwegen (Eds.), *Fear and learning: From basic processes to clinical implications* (pp. 75–97). Washington, DC: American Psychological Association.

Mineka, S., & Zinbarg, R. (1995). Conditioning and ethological models of social anxiety disorder. In R. G. Heimberg, M. R. Liebowitz, D. A. Hope, & F. R. Schneier (Eds.), *Social anxiety disorder: Diagnosis, assessment, and treatment* (pp. 134–162). New York: Guilford.

Mineka, S., & Zinbarg, R. (1996). Conditioning and ethological models of anxiety disorders: Stress-in-dynamic-context anxiety models. In D. A. Hope (Ed.), *Nebraska symposium on motivation* (pp. 135–210). Lincoln, NB: University of Nebraska Press.

Mischel, W., & Grusec, J. (1967). Waiting for rewards and punishments: Effects of time and probability on choice. *Journal of Personality and Social Psychology*, *5*, 24–31.

Moscovitch, D. A. (2009). What is the core fear in social phobia? A new model to facilitate individualized case conceptualization and treatment. *Cognitive and Behavioral Practice*, *16*, 123–134.

Mowrer, O. H. (1947). On the dual nature of learning - a re-interpretation of "conditioning" and "problem-solving." *Harvard Educational Review*, *17*, 102–148.

Newman, M. G., Hofmann, S. G., Trabert, W., Roth, W. T., & Taylor, C. B. (1994). Does behavioral treatment of social anxiety disorder lead to cognitive changes? *Behavior Therapy*, *25*, 503–517.

Ohman, A., Dimberg, U., & Ost, L.-G. (1985). Animal and social anxiety disorders: Biological constraints on learned fear responses. In S. Reiss & R. R. Bootzin (Eds.), *Theoretical issues in behavior therapy* (pp. 123–178). Orlando, FL: Academic Press.

Öhman, A., & Mineka, S. (2001). Fears, phobias, and preparedness: Toward an evolved model of fear. *Current Directions in Psychological Science*, *12*, 5–9.

Öst, L.-G., & Hugdahl, K. (1981). Acquisition of phobias and anxiety response patterns in clinical patients. *Behaviour Resarch and Therapy*, *16*, 439–447.

Pavlov, I. (1927). *Conditioned reflexes*. London: Oxford University Press.

Rachlin, H., & Baum, W. M. (1972). Effects of alternative reinforcement: Does the source matter? *Journal of the Experimental Analysis of Behavior, 18*, 231–241.

Rachlin, H., & Green, L. (1972). Commitment, choice, and self-control. *Journal of the Experimental Analysis of Behavior, 17*, 15–22.

Rachman, S. J. (1976). The passing of the two-stage theory of fear and avoidance: Fresh possibilities. *Behaviour Research and Therapy, 14*, 125–131.

Rachman, S. J. (1977). The conditioning theory of fear acquistion: A critical examination. *Behaviour Research and Therapy, 15*, 375–387.

Rapee, R. M. (1987). The psychological treatment of panic attacks: Theoretical conceptualizations and review of evidence. *Clinical Psychology Review, 7*, 427–438.

Rapee, R. M., & Heimberg, R. G. (1997). A cognitive-behavioral model of anxiety in social anxiety disorder. *Behaviour Research and Therapy, 35*, 741–756.

Renner, K. E. (1964). Delay of reinforcement: A historical overview. *Psychological Bulletin, 61*, 341–361.

Schaal, D. W., & Branch, M. N. (1990). Responding of pigeons under variable-interval schedules of signaled–delayed reinforcement: Effects of delay–signal duration. *Journal of the Experimental Analysis of Behavior, 53*, 103–121.

Schaal, D. W., Schuh, K. J., & Branch, M. N. (1992). Key pecking of pigeons under variable–interval schedules of briefly signaled delayed reinforcement: Effects of variable–interval value. *Journal of the Experimental Analysis of Behavior, 58*, 277–286.

Schneier, F., & Welkowitz, L. (1996). *The hidden face of shyness: Understanding and overcoming social anxiety*. New York: Avon.

Scholing, A., & Emmelkamp, P. M. G. (1996). Treatment of generalized social anxiety disorder: Results at long-term follow-up. *Behaviour Research and Therapy, 34*, 447–452.

Schwartz, C., Snidman, N., & Kagan, J. (1999). Adolescent social anxiety as an outcome of inhibited temperament in childhood. *Journal of the American Academy of Child and Adolescent Psychiatry, 38*, 1008–1015.

Sidman, M., Wynne, C. K., Maguire, R. W., & Barnes, T. (1989). Functional classes and equivalence relations. *Journal of the Experimental Analysis of Behavior, 52*, 261–274.

Skinner, B. F. (1953). *Science and human behavior*. New York: The Free Press.

Stemberger, R. T., Turner, S. M., Beidel, D. C., & Calhoun, K. S. (1995). Social anxiety disorder: An analysis of possible developmental factors. *Journal of Abnormal Psychology, 104*, 526–531.

Strahan, E., & Conger, A. J. (1998). Social anxiety and its effect on performance and perception. *Journal of Anxiety Disorders, 12*, 293–305.

Tancer, M., Lewis, M. H., & Stein, M. B. (1995). Biological aspects. In M. B. Stein (Ed.), *Social anxiety disorder: Clinical and research perspectives* (pp. 229–257). Washington, DC: American Psychiatric Press.

Tarpy, R. M., & Sawabini, F. L. (1974). Reinforcement delay: A selective review of the last decade. *Psychological Review, 81*, 984–997.

Trower, P., & Gilbert, P. (1989). New theoretical conceptions of social anxiety and social anxiety disorder. *Clinical Psychology Review, 9*, 19–35.

Trower, P., Gilbert, P., & Sherling, G. (1990). Social anxiety, evolution, and self-presentation. In H. Leitenberg (Ed.), *Handbook of social and evaluation anxiety* (pp. 11–45). New York: Plenum.

Trower, P., & Turland, D. (1984). Social anxiety disorder. In S. M. Turner (Ed.), *Behavioral theories and treatment of anxiety* (pp. 321–365). New York: Plenum.

Tsai, M., Kohlenberg, R. J., Kanter, J. W., Kohlenberg, B., Follette, W. C., & Callaghan, G. M. (Eds.), (2009). *A guide to functional analytic psychotherapy: Awareness, courage, love, and behaviorism*. New York: Springer.

Vaughan, W., Jr. (1988). Formation of equivalence sets in pigeons. *Journal of Experimental Psychology: Animal Behavior Processes, 14*, 36–42.

Veljaca, K. A., & Rapee, R. M. (1998). Detection of negative and positive audience behaviors by socially anxious subjects. *Behaviour Research and Therapy, 36*, 311–321.

Watson, J. B., & Rayner, R. (1920). Conditioned emotional reactions. *Journal of Experimental Psychology, 3*, 1–14.

Weeks, J. W., Rodebaugh, T. L., Heimberg, R. G., Norton, P. J., & Jakatdar, T. A. (2009). "To avoid evaluation, withdraw:" Fears of evaluation and depressive cognitions lead to social anxiety and submissive withdrawal. *Cognitive Therapy and Research, 33*, 375–389.

Winton, E. C., Clark, D. M., & Edelmann, R. J. (1995). Social anxiety, fear of negative evaluation, and the detection of negative emotions in others. *Behaviour Research and Therapy, 33*, 193–196.

Wolpe, J. (1958). *Psychotherapy by reciprocal inhibition*. Stanford, CA: Stanford University Press.

Chapter 14

Cognitive Biases in Social Anxiety Disorder

Nader Amir and Jessica Bomyea
Joint Doctoral Program, San Diego State University/University of California, San Diego, CA, USA

INTRODUCTION

Psychopathologists have been greatly influenced by information processing models of emotional disorders, suggesting that preferential processing of threat-relevant information (i.e., information processing biases) underlies these disorders (Beck, Emery, & Greenberg, 1985; Williams, Watts, MacLeod, & Mathews, 1988, 1997). Information processing biases are thought to influence attending to, remembering, and interpreting threat-relevant information leading to the maintenance of anxiety. Although it is likely that such biases may play a role in the development of anxiety, most studies of information processing bias in anxious individuals have been descriptive and correlational in nature. However, since the first edition of this book, researchers in this area have begun utilizing experimental approaches to modifying information processing biases. Based on a number of these studies, it appears that observed information processing biases may be causally implicated in anxiety.

A large number of studies now show that information processing biases do characterize anxious individuals. Experimental psychopathologists have divided information processing into three distinct categories: attention, memory, and interpretation. Although different experiments usually address one of these areas, these domains are clearly related. In this chapter we summarize the evidence for information processing biases that may characterize SAIs. With few exceptions (e.g., McNeil, Reis, Taylor, & Boone, 1995; described below), the literature does not report many studies on experimental psychopathology that directly compare subgroups of specific versus GSAD. Therefore, we report those results based on the presence of social anxiety (SA). For each domain, we will provide a review of the literature, including updated information from the previous edition, summarize the findings, and suggest areas of future research.

Social Anxiety: Clinical, Developmental, and Social Perspectives. DOI: 10.1016/B978-0-12-375096-9.00014-6

ATTENTION

The limited capacity of the human attentional system dictates that some information in the environment will be attended to while other information will be ignored. This suggests that incoming information must be prioritized. A bias in this prioritization can lead to increased availability of threat, causing anxiety. To examine attentional bias for threat-relevant information in individuals with SAI, researchers have used the emotional Stroop task (Williams, Mathews, & MacLeod, 1996). In this task, participants are asked to name the color in which emotional words are written while ignoring the meaning of these words. SAIs are slower at color-naming socially relevant threat words than neutral words, whereas nonanxious controls are not (Amir, Freshman, & Foa, 2002; Amir et al., 1996; Hope, Rapee, Heimberg, & Dombeck, 1990; Mattia, Heimberg, & Hope, 1993; Spector, Pecknold, & Libman, 2003). This finding suggests that the activation of threat meaning of the words may interfere with the color-naming task in SAIs to a greater extent than it does in controls. Moreover, several studies have indicated that this Stroop effect is specific to GSAD and not specific speech phobia (McNeil et al., 1995) or depression with or without SA (Grant & Beck, 2006). However, the Stroop task is considered an impure measure of attention because some versions of the paradigm (i.e., presenting a block of words on one card) may involve post-attentional processing of the stimuli (Fox, 1994), and because attention is measured while responding to threat material. Therefore, the Stroop paradigm may involve both biased attention to threat and attempts at inhibition of word meaning.

Partly in response to the above criticism, researchers have used more direct measures of attention for examining attentional biases for threat-relevant material in SA, such as the probe detection paradigm (MacLeod, Mathews, & Tata, 1986). In the probe detection task, subjects are presented with a threat and a nonthreat word simultaneously, one on top of the other. Subjects then see a probe that is located in place of either the top or bottom word and are instructed to identify the location of the probe by pressing one of two buttons. Attentional bias in this task is revealed by shorter reaction times for the probe when it replaces the location of the previously presented threat stimulus. Asmundson and Stein (1994) found that SAIs were faster to respond to probes that replaced a social threat word. A more recent study by Musa, Lépine, Clark, Mansell, & Ehlers (2003) has replicated this finding of attentional bias toward threat words in patients with SAD. Their findings were also consistent with studies using the emotional Stroop task, namely that individuals with comorbid depression did not demonstrate the attentional bias characteristic of SAIs. Similar modifications of the probe detection task have indicated that attentional bias in SA may be the result of difficulty disengaging attention from threat-relevant stimuli (Amir, Elias, Klumpp, & Przeworski, 2003).

The studies described above have used words as stimuli. However, facial expressions of emotions may constitute a more ecologically valid set of stimuli than words when studying cognitive biases in social anxiety. First, facial expressions of approval or disapproval are related to social evaluations. In contrast, words are only indirect representations of these social signals. Second, facial expressions of emotions are prototypic, biologically significant social stimuli (Mineka & Zinbarg, 1996). Indeed, attention to facial features (facial perception) appears very early in the developmental sequence, is extremely efficient, and tends to operate at a pre-attentive level (e.g., Ekman, 1992; Hansen & Hansen, 1994; Öhman, 1986).

With these considerations in mind, Yuen (1994) modified the dot-probe paradigm, using neutral and negative facial expressions rather than words. Subjects were presented with two faces for one second, one above the other, after which one of the faces was replaced by a dot. SAIs showed longer response latency for detecting the dot when it appeared on a spatial location of the previously presented negative face than when the dot replaced the neutral face. No such differences were obtained for nonanxious individuals. This finding suggests that anxious individuals may show an attentional bias away from threatening faces, and has been replicated in more recent studies (e.g., Chen, Ehlers, Clark, & Mansell, 2002; Mansell, Clark, Ehlers, & Chen, 1999). However, other recent studies have also provided evidence that individuals with social anxiety preferentially attend *toward* threat faces (Mogg & Bradley, 2002; Mogg, Philippot, & Bradley, 2004; Pishyar, Harris, & Menzies, 2004; Sposari & Rapee, 2007). For example, Pishyar, Harris, and Menzies (2004) administered a probe detection task with threat faces presented both in front view (Study 1) and in profile view (Study 2). Results revealed that individuals with social anxiety demonstrated attentional bias toward threat faces in both studies. Similarly, Sposari and Rapee (2007) demonstrated that patients with GSAD preferentially attended to faces, regardless of expression, relative to household objects. Although there is some inconsistency in this body of literature, Amir, Weber, Beard, Bomyea, and Taylor (2008) concluded that the average effect size of studies demonstrating attentional bias toward threatening faces is large and significantly different from zero under the following conditions (outlined by Bögels & Mansell, 2004): two faces are shown in each trial of the paradigm (vs. one face and one household item) and the stimulus presentation is brief (i.e., 500 ms).

Researchers have also used other paradigms to assess attentional bias in SA. For example, in the face-in-the-crowd task (Byrne & Eysenck, 1995), participants are presented with an array (e.g., 8 or 12) of faces (Hansen & Hansen, 1988). On some trials all faces are of identical emotional expressions, whereas on other trials one face ("target") displays a different emotion from the rest ("crowd"). Subjects are asked to detect the presence of a target face (e.g., an angry face in a happy crowd, or a happy face in an angry crowd). Hansen and Hansen (1988) found that angry faces were detected faster than were happy faces by undergraduate students. These investigators also found that crowds of angry faces were processed slower than were crowds of happy faces. Gilboa-Schechtman, Foa, and

Amir (1999) presented SAIs and nonanxious controls (NACs) with arrays of 12 faces (i.e., crowd) of the same individual. On some trials all faces were identical (no discrepancy), while on other trials one face displayed a different emotional expression. There were three types of "crowds" – neutral, happy, and angry – and four types of targets – neutral, happy, angry, and disgust. Subjects were asked to detect the presence of a discrepant face in a crowd by pressing a computer key and to press a different key if no faces were discrepant. These authors found that, compared to NACs, individuals with SA showed a greater attentional bias for angry faces in a neutral crowd. Furthermore, SAIs demonstrated slower performance for happy and angry vs. neutral distracters, relative to the NACs. Finally, SAIs were faster to detect angry than disgust expressions; NACs detected both types of faces equally quickly. These authors concluded that attentional bias to detecting negative emotional expression in individuals with SA is particularly pronounced for angry expressions. This finding has been subsequently replicated (Gilboa-Schechtman, Presburger, Marom, & Hermesh, 2005), and extended to a more ecologically valid "face in the audience" paradigm (Perowne & Mansell, 2002). Other forms of attentional bias assessment that have been utilized in recent empirical studies of social anxiety include the rapid serial visual presentation task (de Jong & Martens, 2007) and eye tracking paradigms (Horley, Williams, Gonsalvez, & Gordon, 2003). In general, these studies support the conclusion that social anxiety is characterized by aberrant attentional processing of socially relevant stimuli and hypervigilance to threatening information.

Although the aforementioned studies indicate that social anxiety is associated with biased attention, they do not speak to the issue of causality. Indirect evidence for the causal role of attentional bias to threat in SAD has been evaluated in the context of treatment outcome studies. That is, if attentional bias to threat is a necessary condition for SAD, then amelioration of the disorder should be associated with a reduction of attentional bias to threat. Empirical investigations of this question have generally supported this hypothesis in SAIs using both the emotional Stroop paradigm (Lundh & Öst, 2001; Mattia et al., 1993) and the dot probe paradigm (Pishyar, Harris, & Menzies, 2008; Hofmann, 2000). Thus, there is evidence that successful treatment for SAD is associated with a normalization of attentional bias for threat. This finding is consistent with the view that attentional bias to threat-relevant information plays a role in the maintenance of SAD.

Researchers have also examined the causal relationship between attentional bias and social anxiety using experimental methods that manipulate attention to examine the effect on anxiety. For example, Amir and colleagues (2008) administered a single-session attention training program to individuals with high levels of social anxiety. The authors modified the dot probe procedures used by Mathews and MacLeod (2002) to encourage participants to disengage their attention from threat stimuli. Specifically, the paradigm created a contingency between the location of the nonthreat stimuli (i.e., neutral face) and the probe in one group (attention modification program, or AMP) and not in the other (attention control condition, or ACC). Attentional, bias was assessed before and after training, and participants were also asked to give a speech to determine the effect of the manipulation on anxiety. Results revealed that the procedure effectively modified attention disengagement. Moreover, participants in the AMP condition experienced less anxiety reactivity as a result of the speech, and were judged as having superior speech performance relative to control participants by independent raters. Moreover, Amir et al. (2009) utilized this training in patients with GSAD in a randomized controlled trial delivered over eight bi-weekly sessions. Results from this study indicated that the AMP group experienced significantly less social anxiety at the conclusion of the study relative to individuals in the control group. These results have been replicated in another sample of socially anxious students (Li, Tan, Qian, & Liu, 2008) and in individuals with GSAD (Schmidt, Richey, Buckner, & Timpano, 2009). These studies provide initial but convincing evidence for the causal role of attentional bias to threat in the maintenance of social anxiety and indicate that attention modification procedures may have clinical utility.

In summary, studies using diverse methodologies have demonstrated that individuals with social anxiety are characterized by an attentional bias for threat-relevant information. Moreover, this bias appears to be causally implicated in the maintenance of anxiety. However, some unanswered questions remain. For example, although prior studies indicate that there is an attentional bias toward threat cues in SAIs, not all studies have found consistent results. This may be due to subcomponents of attention associated with emotional information processing (e.g., Fan, McCandliss, Sommer, Raz, & Posner, 2002; Weierich, Treat, & Hollingworth, 2008). Weierich et al. (2008) proposed that variations in findings in the extant literature on anxiety and spatial orientation of attention may result from methodological issues in the attention paradigms used. They argued that attention assessments such as the dot probe that use time scales allowing overt eye movements and present multiple competing stimuli support the hypothesis that anxious individuals are hypervigilant toward threatening stimuli. In contrast, in tasks in which covert attention is measured and there is no competition among stimuli (e.g., modified Posner cueing task; Posner, 1980), anxiety appears to hinder attention disengagement from threatening stimuli (e.g., Amir, Elias et al., 2003; Fox, Russo, Bowles, & Dutton, 2001). In conjunction with other studies demonstrating that the relationship between social anxiety and attentional bias depends on level of social evaluative threat (e.g., Amir et al., 1996; Helfinstein, White, Bar-Haim, & Fox, 2008), it is safe to assume that a simple relation between attentional bias and anxiety does not fully account for the obtained results. These questions should be addressed in future research.

INTERPRETATION

Studies of interpretation bias in social anxiety are informative because social interactions are often ambiguous. Thus, to the extent that SAIs interpret ambiguous social events as threatening, they would be more likely to experience social interactions as negative. The inherent ambiguity of social feedback means that one needs to judge the adequacy of one's performance and judge the approval or disapproval of others. This judgment is often based on limited and incomplete information, so that levels of uncertainty are high. A stern look from a friend, an unenthusiastic response to a greeting, or a temporary disagreement with a friend can all be interpreted in a neutral or negative (i.e., critical or sarcastic) way. Given identical ambiguous cues in a scripted social encounter, such as an interview for a job, SAIs habitually make more negative inferences about their performance than do nonanxious individuals (Hirsch & Mathews, 1997).

Researchers have used a number of paradigms to examine interpretation bias in anxiety using semantic, verbal stimuli. These methods include the interpretation of ambiguous scenarios (e.g., Eysenck, Mogg, May, Richards, & Mathews, 1991; Foa, Franklin, Perry & Herbert, 1996; Stopa & Clark, 2000), interpretation of homophones (i.e. words with similar pronunciation but different meanings)/(Richards, Reynolds, & French, 1993), and interpretation of homographs (i.e. words with similar spelling but different meaning)/(Amir, Foa, & Coles, 1998a). In general, these studies suggest that SAIs are characterized by a bias toward negative interpretations, as well as a lack of benign and positive interpretations.

For example, Eysenck et al. (1991) had anxious patients and controls listen to sentences that could lead to negative or neutral interpretations, such as "Everyone giggled at Sandy's speech." A subsequent recognition test included alternate versions of these sentences that were either unambiguously threatening or emotionally neutral (e.g. "Everyone laughed at Sandy's awful/witty speech"). Patients were instructed to rate these sentences for similarity of meaning to the originals. In two experiments, controls rated the benign versions as being more similar in meaning to the ambiguous sentences they had heard previously. The anxious patients, however, endorsed the negative and benign versions as being equally similar in meaning to the original sentences. Recovered patients resembled the controls, strongly favoring the nonthreatening version. Although this study also relied to some extent on memory processes, other studies have found similar results. That is, SAIs display negative interpretation biases when asked to rate experimenter-provided interpretations (e.g., Amir, Foa, & Coles, 1998b; Voncken, Bögels, & Peeters, 2007; Wilson & Rapee, 2005). Moreover, Huppert, Foa, Furr, Filip, and Mathews (2003) demonstrated that negative interpretations of social situations were positively associated with social anxiety, while presence of a positive social interpretation bias was negatively related to social anxiety (as well as general negative affect). Positive and negative interpretation bias were only moderately related in this study, suggesting they may lie on two separate continuums, rather than being opposite ends of a single dimension. However, both forms of bias may be associated with social anxiety. In a second study, Huppert, Pasupuleti, Foa, and Mathews (2007) provided participants with ambiguous social sentences and asked participants to (1) generate multiple responses to complete the sentence and (2) indicate which of these responses best completed the sentence. SAIs generated and endorsed more negative or anxious responses and fewer positive and neutral responses than individuals low in social anxiety. These studies suggest that, in addition to generating more negative interpretations than NACs, SAIs also appear to lack a positive bias characteristic of NACs.

More ecologically valid ambiguous stimuli have also been used to evaluate interpretation bias in SAIs. For example, Amir, Beard, and Przeworski (2005) assessed interpretation bias using ambiguous videos rather than sentences. In each video, an actress approached the viewer and made a comment (either ambiguous, positive, or negative) about the viewer. Participants rated the emotional valance of each video as to how they would feel in that situation. Results from this study revealed that SAIs rated ambiguous social interactions more negatively than did nonanxious individuals, high trait anxious individuals, and dysphoric individuals. Similarly, studies using face stimuli also indicate that SAIs may be more sensitive to detecting negative face cues in ambiguous pictures relative to nonanxious individuals. For example, Richards et al. (2002) presented SAIs and individuals low in social anxiety with pictures of faces containing two emotional expressions (happiness, surprise, anger, fear, disgust, and sadness) blended at varying gradations using digital facial morphing software. Thus, each participant was shown five faces representing different proportions of an angry face and a happy face (i.e., 90/10, 70/30, 50/50, 30/70, 10/90). Participants were then asked to classify the emotion. Results from this study indicated that SAIs categorized significantly more faces as expressing fear, thus suggesting a tendency to be sensitive to the presence of fear-relevant cues in ambiguous faces relative to controls.

However, not all studies find interpretation bias in SAIs using negative face stimuli; at least two studies using face-morphing paradigms similar to Richards et al. (2002) did not find between-group differences in SAIs and nonanxious individuals (Philippot & Douilliez, 2005; Schofield, Coles, & Gibb, 2007). Methodological differences may explain these discrepant findings. For example, Philippot and Douilliez (2005) blended negative emotional prototypes with neutral faces, rather than blending two valenced emotions (e.g., anger and happiness). Schofield et al. (2007) did combine two types of valenced face stimuli but did not include fearful faces. Although in these studies SAIs did not differ in their ability to correctly categorize the emotion, Shofield et al. demonstrated that these individuals rated the cost of interacting with individuals with negative emotional expressions as worse than did nonanxious controls. Thus, interpretive biases demonstrated by SAIs may be detected specifically when the ambiguity in a facial expression is a combination of fear and another valenced expression (e.g., happy). Furthermore, interpretive biases may be more pronounced when participants are asked to evaluate the costs associated with information that is negatively valenced.

Consistent with this hypothesis, research has demonstrated that SAIs differ from nonanxious individuals in their reactions to unambiguously negative stimuli. Foa et al. (1996) asked SAIs and nonanxious controls to estimate the probability of mildly negative situations and their cost. SAIs estimated both the probability and cost of negative social events to be greater than did (NACs). Foa et al. also showed that social phobics judged the probability of negative social outcomes as more likely and costly than other nonsocial outcomes (before, but not after, treatment), compared to NACs. Reduction in perceived social costs was the best predictor of post-treatment social anxiety (partial correlation controlling for pretreatment anxiety was 0.76). Similarly, Stopa and Clark (2000) found that SAIs rated mildly negative sentences as more negative than did low SAIs. The authors conclude that social anxiety may be associated with a tendency to catastrophize negative information and events. Increased sensitivity to negative information has also been demonstrated in SAIs using face stimuli. Coles, Heimberg, and Schofield (2008) asked participants who were high or low in social anxiety to rate schematic faces on dimensions of negative valence, potency, and activity. Results indicated that SAIs made judgments about negative valence based on the presence of threatening eyebrow expression, while those with low social anxiety levels utilized both eyebrow and mouth expressions. Thus, SAIs appeared to evaluate faces as negative based on fewer pieces of information compared to those without social anxiety.

Although most studies have examined the relationship between social anxiety and interpretations or judgments about ambiguous or *negative* information, other studies suggest that SAIs may possess an interpretation bias in relation to *positive* information as well. Relative to nonanxious individuals, SAIs tend to interpret positive social situations negatively (Alden, Taylor, Mellings, & Laposa, 2008; Vassilopoulos, 2006) and to interpret positive facial expressions as less approachable (Campbell et al., 2009). Moreover, research has also demonstrated that SAIs experience fear surrounding *positive* evaluation, as well as negative (e.g., Weeks, Heimberg, Rodebaugh, & Norton, 2008).

The studies presented thus far have primarily used self-report of semantic interpretations or face judgments. Several studies reported similar results using objective measures, such as the time taken to read a word or sentence consistent with a negative or positive interpretation (e.g. Calvo, Eysenck, & Estevez, 1994; Richards et al., 1993). Other studies evaluating interpretation bias using reaction time measures have used paradigms such as a modified emotional card-sorting task (Mohlman, Carmin, & Price, 2007), an incidental learning paradigm (Yoon & Zinbarg, 2008), homograph decision tasks (Amir et al., 2005; Amir et al., 1998a), and an emotional priming paradigm (Yoon &

Zinbarg, 2007). Although these studies have used diverse methodologies (e.g., face vs. word stimuli, including a social stressor vs. not), in general, findings suggest that SAIs are more likely than nonanxious individuals to interpret ambiguous information negatively. For example, Hirsch and Mathews (1997) asked SAIs and controls to read a realistically ambiguous description of themselves being interviewed for a job, presented line by line on a computer. At unpredictable intervals, they had to make a speeded decision about a probe word that matched possible negative or positive inferences. For example, immediately after reading the (incomplete) sentence, "As the interviewer asks you the first question, you realize that all your preparation has been . . .". one of two probe words could be presented. In this example, the probe word could be "forgotten" (matching a negative inference) or "useful" (matching a positive inference). Speed of deciding whether the probe word could logically complete the sentence was used to operationalize the extent to which these different inferences had been made by the individual. SAIs were relatively faster to endorse threatening probes whereas controls were faster to endorse the words matching positive or nonthreatening inferences. Thus, controls demonstrated a positive interpretative bias, likely to protect their self-image, whereas those fearing interviews demonstrated negative bias. Hirsch and Mathews (1997) suggested that such a reversal of a normally protective bias leaves SAIs more vulnerable to anxiety disorders.

In summary, results have shown that SAIs are characterized by a tendency to interpret ambiguous information negatively. Moreover, SAIs have more negative interpretations of mildly negative information and also tend to interpret positive information in a more negative way relative to nonanxious individuals. These types of biases appear to be present in processing of both semantic and facial expression stimuli, although results from studies using facial expressions are somewhat mixed. Future research in this area is needed to delineate the parameters of interpretation bias for face and other ecologically valid stimuli.

Similarly to the body of research on attention, recent empirical work suggests that interpretive biases in social anxiety may be malleable (e.g., Beard & Amir, 2008; Hirsch, Mathews, & Clark, 2007; Murphy, Hirsch, Mathews, Smith, & Clark, 2007, Voncken & Bögels, 2006). In these studies, interpretation biases are modified by requiring participants to repeatedly access benign meanings of ambiguous events. For example, in Beard and Amir (2008), participants viewed either a benign or negative word, followed by an ambiguous sentence. Participants were asked to decide whether or not the word and sentence were related. To modify interpretations, participants were given feedback about their relatedness judgments. Participants in the training group were given positive feedback (i.e., "You are correct!") for endorsing a benign interpretation or rejecting a threat interpretation, and negative feedback (i.e., "You are incorrect") for rejecting a benign interpretation or endorsing a threat interpretation. Feedback for participants in the control condition was not contingent upon response type. Studies using this and similar methodologies indicate that effectively modifying interpretations can decrease anxiety (Beard & Amir, 2008; Murphy et al., 2007). Thus, these studies support the causal relationship between interpretation bias and social anxiety outlined in theories of the disorder.

MEMORY

Compared to studies of attentional bias, studies of memory bias in social anxiety are less conclusive. While some studies have found enhanced memory for threat-relevant information in SAI (e.g., Foa, Gilboa-Schechtman, Amir, & Freshman, 2000), at least one study has found decreased memory for threat-relevant information (Wenzel & Holt, 2002) and others have found no memory biases (e.g., Rapee, McCallum, Melville, Ravenscroft, & Rodney, 1993; Rinck & Becker, 2005; Wenzel, Jackson, & Holt, 2002). For example, Claeys (1989) found that individuals high in social anxiety exhibited better recall of negative self-descriptive adjectives than did individuals low in social anxiety. On the other hand, in a series of four studies using a variety of memory tasks and stimuli, Rapee et al. (1993) did not find a memory bias for negatively valenced stimuli in individuals with SAD.

These divergent results may be in part due to different memory processes examined in different studies. Cognitive psychologists distinguish between explicit and implicit memory (Roediger, 1990; Schacter, 1992). According to Schacter (1992), "Implicit memory is revealed when previous experiences facilitate performance on a task that does not require conscious or intentional recollection of those experiences; explicit memory is revealed when performance on a task requires conscious recollection of previous experiences" (p. 501). Implicit memory is measured by tasks such as stem-completion and perceptual identification, which reveal the effects of prior exposure to information without requiring that subjects consciously remember this information. Explicit memory tasks involve subjects retrieving previously presented information.

In a typical experiment, subjects are first presented with a list of words for encoding (e.g., HONEY). Memory is then measured by presenting subjects with a set of word stems (e.g., HON_ _). Explicit memory is measured by asking subjects to complete the stems with the words they had seen earlier in the experiment. Implicit memory, on the other hand, is measured by asking subjects to complete the stems with the first word that comes to mind. Although instructions to subjects differ, the subjects' tasks are identical.

Although research suggests that anxious patients may be characterized by aberrant implicit (unconscious, capacity-free, automatic) memory for threat-related information more so than explicit (conscious, effortful, strategic) memory, studies of implicit and explicit memory bias in social anxiety have produced inconsistent results. Using cued recall and stem completion tasks, Rapee et al. (1993) failed to find support for either an implicit or explicit bias in SAIs. However, Lundh and Öst (1997) found that individuals with non-generalized SAD showed an implicit bias for social threat words.

The studies discussed above have relied on stem-completion as the measure of implicit memory. However, stem-completion, the most commonly used measure of implicit memory, has at least two limitations. First, it is strongly influenced by orthographic, perceptual aspects of the material rather than by their conceptual, semantic aspects (e.g., Roediger, 1990; Schacter, 1992). For example, if subjects are first exposed to words written in upper case letters during the study phase and later shown stems in lower case letters during the test phase, priming effects diminish (Roediger & Blaxton, 1987). Because of their relative insensitivity to semantics, word–stem procedures have limited relevance for the study of automatic access to meaningful emotional memories (McNally, 1994, p. 132). Second, performance on the stem-completion task may be contaminated by explicit memory processes because subjects may use their explicit memory of the previously seen items to complete the task (Nugent & Mineka, 1994). However, a number of other paradigms have subsequently been used in memory research with SAIs.

One implicit memory paradigm that addresses the above concerns is Jacoby, Allan, Collins, and Larwill's (1988) noise judgment paradigm. In this paradigm, participants first hear a set of sentences and repeat them aloud. Next, participants hear these "old" sentences intermixed with a new set of sentences against a background of noise. Participants are asked to repeat the sentences and to rate the volume of the background noise. Jacoby et al. found that noise accompanying "old" sentences was rated as less loud than noise accompanying "new" sentences. This differential noise rating for the "old" and "new" sentences was interpreted as reflecting implicit memory for the former. Interestingly, priming effects in the noise judgment paradigm seem to persist even when participants are fully informed about how the paradigm works and are instructed to resist its effects (Jacoby, Roth, Lindsay, & Debner, 1992).

Amir, Foa, and Coles (2000) examined implicit and explicit memory bias for threat-relevant information in SAIs. They hypothesized that if SAIs are characterized by an implicit memory bias for social-threat information, they should rate the noise accompanying old social-threat sentences as less loud than the noise accompanying new social-threat sentences, whereas control subjects should not. If SAIs are characterized by an explicit memory bias for threat, they should show better recognition of these sentences. Consistent with their prediction, these authors found that individuals with GSAD are characterized by an implicit, but not an explicit, memory bias of threat-relevant information.

The studies described above used words and sentences as stimuli for social threat. As described earlier, there are a number of reasons to believe that more ecologically valid stimuli, such as faces, may constitute more appropriate material for studying cognitive biases in social anxiety. Accordingly, a number of studies have adapted implicit memory paradigms for use with nonverbal material. For example, Amir, Bower, Briks, & Freshman (2003) subsequently modified the noise judgment paradigm to make the stimuli more ecologically valid. Instead of rating clarity of auditory stimuli, participants were asked to provide a visual clarity rating with videos of positive or negative social scenarios. Results from this study revealed that this type of task effectively indexed implicit memory and that individuals with SA demonstrated a bias in implicit memory favoring negative scenarios relative to nonanxious individuals and depressed individuals.

Similarly, implicit memory bias in SAIs has also been examined using face stimuli. To assess recognition memory for facial expressions, Lundh and Öst (1996) presented 20 photographs to SAIs and to controls and asked them to rate whether the face was critical or accepting. Following a distracter task, participants were presented with 20 photographs of individuals encountered in the initial task and 60 distracter photographs. Subjects were asked to identify the faces they had seen in the initial task. SAIs recognized more faces they had rated as "critical" than faces they had rated as "accepting," whereas controls exhibited the opposite pattern.

The design of the study made it impossible to determine whether a response bias or a memory bias underlies SAIs' preference for critical faces. Moreover, it did not address whether this bias was specific to expressions conveying different types of negative emotion (e.g., anger, disgust). Foa and colleagues (2000) examined these questions in two experiments. In the first experiment, SAIs and NACs were shown 12 pictures of faces with each individual depicting a specific emotional expression (e.g., surprise, disgust, fear, sadness; Phase I). They were asked to remember the names of the individuals being shown. Next, they were shown pictures of each individual in three different emotional expressions (happy, angry, neutral) and asked to name the individual and label his/her emotional expression (Phase II). Participants were then asked to write down the names of the individuals they had seen in Phase II and their corresponding emotional expression. Participants then completed a cued recall task, where they were provided with a list of the names of the 12 individuals presented in Phases I and II. Participants were asked to write down the emotional expression each individual expressed in Phase II (i.e., the emotional encoding phase). The results revealed that individuals with social anxiety have enhanced recall for facial expressions compared to nonanxious controls. However, SAIs were not characterized by specific enhanced memory for angry expressions. This experiment involved memory for verbal information (i.e., names) as well as memory for facial expressions and it is possible that the use of verbal information in this experiment attenuated the memory bias for facial expressions in SAIs. In addition, the results of the cued recall may have been influenced by the preceding free recall task. To correct for these possible confounds, these authors modified the experimental method and used only visual information and a single memory task. In the second experiment, subjects were first presented with images of individuals with neutral, happy, angry, and disgust expressions. Later, they were presented with the same ("old") images interspersed with images of the same individuals with different emotional expressions ("new") and were asked to label each image as either "old" or "new." Dependent measures were percent of correct versus incorrect recognition and latencies for making recognition decisions. The results of this experiment revealed that SAIs, but not NACs, exhibit enhanced recognition of negative compared to nonnegative facial expressions. Thus, the findings from Foa et al. (2000) suggest that an enhanced memory for negative emotional expression (in Experiment 2) is present even when SAIs encode information in a situation that does not explicitly refer to social threat or to negative evaluation.

Additionally, these investigators found that, while SAIs did not exhibit better recognition for anger versus disgust expressions, they had longer latencies for identifying angry (compared to disgust) expressions as unfamiliar. This finding suggests that they engage in more extensive processing of such expressions. It seems that individuals with SAD have a tendency to perceive all angry faces as familiar and, in order to overcome this tendency, they study such faces more carefully than they do faces expressing other emotions. Such a tendency is yet another factor that may play a role in the maintenance of social anxiety. The procedure of Foa et al.'s Experiment 2 allowed individuals with social anxiety to use compensatory strategies to overcome this tendency and to correctly identify angry expressions as unfamiliar. That is, using enhanced processing resources, SAIs may have been able to perform the recognition task. However, under the pressure of an ongoing social situation, such strategies may not be readily available, resulting in a negatively skewed memory of social interactions.

An additional method for examining memory bias in SAIs is to evaluate memory functioning in the context of learning information. The retrieval-induced forgetting paradigm (Amir, Coles, Brigidi, & Foa, 2001; Anderson & Spellman, 1995) is one such method. In this task, individuals are shown category-plus-exemplar pairs (e.g., fruit–orange). They are then asked to practice remembering half of the items from half of the categories. After a delay, a cued-recall test is used to examine how retrieval practice impacts memory. In general, results from these paradigms reveal that practicing half of the items negatively impacts recall of the second half of items. Amir et al. (2001) modified this paradigm by creating four nonsocial categories and four social categories, both with positively and negatively associated words. In this study, individuals with GSAD showed the same memory patterns as nonanxious controls for practiced categories for positive social and nonsocial words. For negative social words, however, individuals with GSAD benefited less from practice relative to the nonanxious individuals. Their performance was also decreased less from the effect of practicing competing negative social information, relative to NACs. The authors conclude that type of biased cognitive processing might play a role in learning and habituation processes related to social information in these individuals.

Further evidence suggesting that SAIs may have dysfunctional memory processes associated with learning comes from Garner, Mogg, and Bradley (2006). The authors administered an illusory correlation/covariation bias paradigm developed by Tomarken, Mineka, and Cook (1989) to individuals high and low in social anxiety. In this study, pictures of facial expressions (i.e., angry, happy, neutral) were paired with one of four outcomes over eight trial blocks: aversive images (i.e., physical injuries), positive images (i.e., butterflies), neutral images (i.e., mushrooms), or no image. At the end of each block of trials, participants were asked to estimate the association between each type of face stimuli and each type of outcome (e.g., "Given that you saw an angry face, on what percentage of trials was the angry face followed by an unpleasant picture?"). Results revealed that all participants showed an expectation of aversive outcomes following angry faces and positive outcomes following happy faces. However, over the course of the experiment, these expectations were diminished, with the exception of the positive expectancy in the low socially anxious group. That is, individuals in the low socially anxious group continued to expect positive outcomes to follow positive faces. Moreover, high SAIs overestimated the number of angry faces that were presented during the task. Thus, individuals high in social anxiety appeared to be lacking a bias toward positive information that is characteristic of nonanxious individuals when learning this type of contingency.

Although this study evaluated a memory process by asking participants to reflect on a past association between feared stimuli and emotionally valenced outcomes, the authors note that task performance may also be closely associated with other forms of information processing, such as interpretation bias. Indeed, recent studies evaluating the presence of memory biases have begun to examine the interaction of memory and other forms of information processing, including interpretation bias (Brendle & Wenzel, 2004; Hertel, Brozovich, Joorman, & Gotlib, 2008; Wenzel, Finstrom, Jordan, & Brendle, 2005) PEP (Mellings & Alden, 2000; Morgan & Banerjee, 2008), and imagery (Stopa & Jenkins, 2007). In general, these studies suggest that memory biases apparent in SAIs may be the product of multiple interactive information processing biases that make threat-relevant information more salient at the time of information retrieval.

For example, Hertel et al. (2008) presented individuals with GSAD and nonanxious individuals with ambiguous social and nonsocial scenarios and asked them to complete the scenario (Experiment 1). After a brief distraction period, they then asked participants to recall the content of the scenarios. Trained raters determined whether any apparent memory errors were the product of intrusions of the participants' interpretations of the scenario. Results indicated that individuals with GSAD reported a larger percentage of memory intrusions that were consistent with negative, but not neutral or positive, interpretations made about the ambiguous social scenarios relative to nonanxious individuals. Similarly, in Experiment 2 of this study, the authors demonstrated that similar negative memory intrusions can also be induced in nonanxious individuals by providing instructions to imagine oneself in the given scenario and providing the negative resolutions of the scenarios. Thus, the authors conclude that errors in memory in GSAD may be related to interpretation biases of social information. This is consistent with prior studies indicating that memory biases in SAIs may reflect biased interpretation, rather than inability to recall factual detail (Brendle & Wenzel, 2004; Wenzel et al., 2005).

In summary, studies using diverse methodologies have demonstrated that individuals with social anxiety are characterized by a memory bias for threat-relevant information. However, these findings are not unequivocal. Moreover, because many of the studies that do demonstrate a memory bias or its absence have not been replicated, it is difficult to suggest a comprehensive role of memory bias for threat in social anxiety. At present, the role of memory bias for threat in social anxiety seems to be confined to certain memory systems and materials. Thus, the task for future researchers will be to delineate the role of various forms of memory bias in a comprehensive model of social anxiety, and to determine what types of negative emotional expressions elicit such biases (e.g., contempt). Future research might also continue to examine how different types of cognitive biases, such as interpretation biases, might lead to memory biases in the disorder.

CONCLUSIONS

While studies have concluded that individuals with SAI exhibit attentional bias, sporadic memory bias, and interpretation bias for threat-relevant information, no integrated explanation for the observed biases has been proposed. A preliminary model would have to account for the finding of attentional bias to threat as well as paradoxical effects (e.g., elimination of this bias under anxiety). Studies of interpretation have pointed out that this domain of bias may play a primary role in SA. Regarding the role of memory bias in SA, theories should address the lack of findings in some studies (i.e., those using words and explicit memory) and the presence of such biases in implicit memory and in studies using complex (e.g., faces) stimuli.

Some evidence suggests that, given sufficient time, social phobics are able to suppress threat meanings of ambiguous information that has been automatically activated. How can this "vigilance–avoidance" model of information processing account for the maintenance of social fears? Mogg, Bradley, Bono, and Painter (1997) suggested that this "vigilance–avoidance" pattern of processing may be a hallmark of clinical anxiety states because a faster detection of threat and a subsequent avoidance of strategic processing of such information would prevent habituation, or objective evaluation, of such material. Threat-relevant information would then retain its anxiety-provoking properties. This conceptualization of SA is consistent with models of emotional disorders that posit a lack of emotional processing as the cause of pathological anxiety (Foa & Kozak, 1986; Rachman, 1980).

The conviction that studies of information processing are useful in explaining pathological anxiety is based on the notion that these biases are the most proximal level of analysis for the phenomenon of interest; i.e., the identification of psychological vulnerability in anxious individuals. As such, these biases may serve as a better indicator of the underlying construct than self-report measures. Studying such biases may allow us to relate symptoms to cognitive vulnerabilities, i.e., information processing bias, and to use these measures of vulnerability to implement prevention, assess treatment efficacy, and predict relapse. Finally, we may be able to use these measures to pinpoint the specific mechanisms of successful treatment. This is because, unlike self-report measures, information processing measures are less reactive to assessment (Kazdin, 1986) and hence may allow for more frequent and sensitive longitudinal assessment.

In summary, it is likely that information processing biases that are responsible for the development and maintenance of social anxiety involve multiple stages of information processing. Research indicates that information processing biases may have utility as treatment targets. Studies examining information processing modification in both attention and interpretation domains indicate that these biases are malleable. Moreover, the manipulation of these biases leads to substantial reductions in anxiety symptoms and reactivity. In the present chapter we have summarized the extant literature and suggest that a "vigilance–avoidance" pattern of information processing of threat-relevant information may underlie the maintenance of social anxiety. Future studies should address the specificity of these biases by examining other anxious populations and including threatening stimuli of a nonsocial nature, in addition to continuing to examine the use of information processing training in the treatment of social anxiety.

REFERENCES

Alden, L. E., Taylor, C. T., Mellings, T. M. J. B., & Laposa, J. M. (2008). Social anxiety and the interpretation of positive social events. *Journal of Anxiety Disorders*, *22*, 577–590.

Amir, N., Beard, C., & Przeworski, A. (2005). Resolving ambiguity: The effect of experience on interpretation of ambiguous events in generalized social phobia. *Journal of Abnormal Psychology*, *114*, 402–408.

Amir, N., Beard, C., Taylor, C. T., Klumpp, H., Elias, J., Burns, M., et al. (2009). Attention training in individuals with generalized social phobia: A randomized controlled trial. *Journal of Consulting and Clinical Psychology*, *77*, 961–973.

Amir, N., Bower, E., Briks, J., & Freshman, M. (2003). Implicit memory for negative and positive social information in individuals with and without social anxiety. *Cognition and Emotion*, *17*, 567–583.

Amir, N., Coles, M. E., Brigidi, B., & Foa, E. B. (2001). The effect of practice on recall of emotional information in individuals with generalized social phobia. *Journal of Abnormal Psychology*, *110*, 76–82.

Amir, N., Elias, J., Klumpp, H., & Przeworski, A. (2003). Attentional bias to threat in social phobia: Facilitated processing of threat or difficulty disengaging attention from threat? *Behaviour Research and Therapy*, *41*, 1325–1335.

Amir, N., Foa, E. B., & Coles, M. (1998a). Automatic activation and strategic avoidance of threat-relevant information in Social Phobia. *Journal of Abnormal Psychology*, *107*, 285–290.

Amir, N., Foa, E. B., & Coles, M. (1998b). Social phobics' evaluation of ambiguous situations. *Behaviour Research and Therapy*, *36*, 945–957.

Amir, N., Foa, E. B., & Coles, M. E. (2000). Implicit memory bias for threat relevant information in individuals with generalized social phobia. *Journal of Abnormal Psychology*, *109*, 713–720.

Amir, N., Freshman, M., & Foa, E. (2002). Enhanced stroop interference for threat in social phobia. *Journal of Anxiety Disorders*, *16*, 1–9.

Amir, N., McNally, R. J., Riemann, B. C., Burns, J., Lorenz, M., & Mullen, J. T. (1996). Suppression of the emotional Stroop effect by increased anxiety in patients with social phobia. *Behaviour Research and Therapy*, *34*, 945–948.

Amir, N., Weber, G., Beard, C., Bomyea, J., & Taylor, C. T. (2008). The effect of a single-session attention modification program on response to a public-speaking challenge in socially anxious individuals. *Journal of Abnormal Psychology*, *117*, 860–868.

Anderson, M. C., & Spellman, B. A. (1995). On the status of inhibitory mechanisms in cognition: Memory retrieval as a model case. *Psychological Review*, *102*, 68–100.

Asmundson, G. J. G., & Stein, M. B. (1994). Selective processing of social threat in patients with generalized social phobia: Evaluation using a dot-probe paradigm. *Journal of Anxiety Disorders*, *8*, 107–117.

Beard, C., & Amir, N. (2008). A multi-session interpretation modification program: Changes in interpretation and social anxiety symptoms. *Behaviour Research and Therapy*, *46*, 1135–1141.

Beck, A. T., Emery, G., & Greenberg, R. L. (1985). *Anxiety disorders and phobias: A cognitive perspective*. New York: Basic books.

Bögels, S. M., & Mansell, W. (2004). Attention processes in the maintenance and treatment of social phobia: Hypervigilance, avoidance and self-focused attention. *Clinical Psychology Review. Special Issue: Social Phobia and Social Anxiety*, *24*, 827–856.

Brendle, J. R., & Wenzel, A. (2004). Differentiating between memory and interpretation biases in socially anxious and nonanxious individuals. *Behaviour Research and Therapy*, *42*, 155–171.

Byrne, A., & Eysenck, M. W. (1995). Trait anxiety, anxious mood, and threat detection. *Cognition and Emotion*, *9*, 549–562.

Calvo, M. G., Eysenck, M. W., & Estevez, A. (1994). Ego-threat interpretive bias in test anxiety: On-line inferences. *Cognition and Emotion*, *8*, 127–146.

Campbell, D. W., Sareen, J., Stein, M. B., Kravetsky, L. B., Paulus, M. P., Hassard, S. T., et al. (2009). Happy but not so approachable: The social judgments of individuals with generalized social phobia. *Depression and Anxiety*, *26*, 419–424.

Chen, Y. P., Ehlers, A., Clark, D. M., & Mansell, W. (2002). Patients with generalized social phobia direct their attention away from faces. *Behaviour Research and Therapy*, *40*, 677–687.

Claeys, W. (1989). Social anxiety, evaluative threat and incidental recall of trait words. *Anxiety Research*, *2*, 27–43.

Coles, M. E., Heimberg, R. G., & Schofield, C. A. (2008). Interpretation of facial expressions and social anxiety: Specificity and source of biases. *Cognition and Emotion*, *22*, 1159–1173.

de Jong, P. J., & Martens, S. (2007). Detection of emotional expressions in rapidly changing facial displays in high- and low-socially anxious women. *Behaviour Research and Therapy*, *45*, 1285–1294.

Ekman, P. (1992). An argument for basic emotions. *Cognition and Emotion*, *6*, 169–200.

Eysenck, M. W., Mogg, K., May, J., Richards, A., & Mathews, A. (1991). Bias in interpretation of ambiguous sentences related to threat in anxiety. *Journal of Abnormal Psychology*, *100*, 144–150.

Fan, J., McCandliss, B. D., Sommer, T., Raz, A., & Posner, M. I. (2002). Testing the efficiency and independence of attentional networks. *Journal of Cognitive Neuroscience, 14*, 340–347.

Foa, E. B., & Kozak, M. J. (1986). Emotional processing of fear: Exposure to corrective information. *Psychological Bulletin, 99*, 20–35.

Foa, E. B., Franklin, M. E., Perry, K. J., & Herbert, J. D. (1996). Cognitive biases in generalized social phobia. *Journal of Abnormal Psychology, 3*, 433–439.

Foa, E. B., Gilboa-Schechtman, E., Amir, N., & Freshman, M. (2000). Memory bias in generalized social phobia: Remembering negative emotional expressions. *Journal of Anxiety Disorders, 14*, 501–519.

Fox, E. (1994). Interference and negative priming from ignored distractors: The role of selection difficulty. *Perception and Psychophysics, 56*, 565–574.

Fox, E., Russo, R., Bowles, R., & Dutton, K. (2001). Do threatening stimuli draw or hold visual attention in subclinical anxiety? *Journal of Experimental Psychology: General, 130*, 681–700.

Garner, M., Mogg, K., & Bradley, B. P. (2006). Orienting and maintenance of gaze to facial expressions in social anxiety. *Journal of Abnormal Psychology, 115*, 760–770.

Gilboa-Schechtman, E., Foa, E. B., & Amir, N. (1999). Attentional biases for facial expressions in social phobia: The face-in-the-crowd paradigm. *Cognition & Emotion, 13*, 305–318.

Gilboa-Schechtman, E., Presburger, G., Marom, S., & Hermesh, H. (2005). The effects of social anxiety and depression on the evaluation of facial crowds. *Behaviour Research and Therapy, 43*, 467–474.

Grant, D. M., & Beck, J. G. (2006). Attentional biases in social anxiety and dysphoria: Does comorbidity make a difference? *Journal of Anxiety Disorders, 20*, 520–529.

Hansen, C. H., & Hansen, R. D. (1988). Finding the face in the crowd: An anger superiority effect. *Journal of Personality and Social Psychology, 54*, 917–924.

Hansen, C. H., & Hansen, R. D. (1994). Automatic emotion: Attention and facial efference. In P. M. Niedenthal & S. Kitayama (Eds.), *The heart's eye: Emotional influences in perception and attention* (pp. 217–243). New York: Academic Press.

Helfinstein, S. M., White, L. K., Bar-Haim, Y., & Fox, N. A. (2008). Affective primes suppress attention bias to threat in socially anxious individuals. *Behaviour Research and Therapy, 46*, 799–810.

Hertel, P. T., Brozovich, F., Joormann, J., & Gotlib, I. H. (2008). Biases in interpretation and memory in generalized social phobia. *Journal of Abnormal Psychology, 117*, 278–288.

Hirsch, C., & Mathews, A. (1997). Interpretative inferences when reading about emotional events. *Behaviour Research and Therapy, 35*, 1123–1132.

Hirsch, C. R., Mathews, A., & Clark, D. M. (2007). Inducing an interpretation bias changes self-imagery: A preliminary investigation. *Behaviour Research and Therapy, 45*, 2173–2181.

Hofmann, S. G. (2000). Self-focused attention before and after treatment of social phobia. *Behaviour Research and Therapy, 38*, 717–725.

Hope, D. A., Rapee, R. M., Heimberg, R. G., & Dombeck, M. J. (1990). Representations of self in social phobia: Vulnerability to social threat. *Cognitive Therapy and Research, 14*, 177–189.

Horley, K., Williams, L. M., Gonsalvez, C., & Gordon, E. (2003). Social phobics do not see eye to eye: A visual scanpath study of emotional expression processing. *Journal of Anxiety Disorders, 17*, 33–44.

Huppert, J. D., Foa, E. B., Furr, J. M., Filip, J. C., & Mathews, A. (2003). Interpretation bias in social anxiety: A dimensional perspective. *Cognitive Therapy and Research, 27*, 569–577.

Huppert, J. D., Pasupuleti, R. V., Foa, E. B., & Mathews, A. (2007). Interpretation biases in social anxiety: Response generation, response selection, and self appraisals. *Behaviour Research and Therapy*, *45*, 1505–1515.

Jacoby, L. L., Allan, L. G., Collins, J. C., & Larwill, L. K. (1988). Memory influences subjective experience: Noise judgment. *Journal of Experimental Psychology: Learning, Memory, and Cognition*, *14*, 240–247.

Jacoby, L. L., Roth, J. P., Lindsay, D. S., & Debner, J. A. (1992). Lectures for a layperson: Methods for revealing unconscious processes. In R. F. Bornstein & T. S. Pittman (Eds.), *Perception without awareness* (pp. 81–120). New York: Guilford Press.

Kazdin, A. (1986). Comparative outcome studies of psychotherapy: Methodological issues and strategies. *Journal of Consulting & Clinical Psychology, Special Issue: Psychotherapy Research*, *54*, 95–105.

Li, S., Tan, J., Qian, M., & Liu, X. (2008). Continual training of attentional bias in social anxiety. *Behaviour Research and Therapy*, *46*, 905–912.

Lundh, L. G., & Öst, L. G. (1996). Recognition bias for critical faces in social phobics. *Behavioral Research and Therapy*, *34*, 787–794.

Lundh, L. G., & Öst, L. G. (1997). Explicit and implicit memory bias in social phobia. The role of subdiagnostic type. *Behaviour Research and Therapy*, *35*, 305–317.

Lundh, L., & Öst, L. (2001). Attentional bias, self-consciousness and perfectionism in social phobia before and after cognitive-behaviour therapy. *Scandinavian Journal of Behaviour Therapy*, *30*, 4–16.

MacLeod, C., Mathews, A., & Tata, P. (1986). Attentional bias in emotional disorders. *Journal of Abnormal Psychology*, *95*(1), 15–20. doi:10.1037/0021-843X.95.1.15.

Mansell, W., Clark, D. M., Ehlers, A., & Chen, Y. (1999). Social anxiety and attention away from emotional faces. *Cognition and Emotion*, *13*, 673–690.

Mathews, A., & MacLeod, C. (2002). Induced processing biases have causal effects on anxiety. *Cognition and Emotion*, *16*, 331–354.

Mattia, J. L., Heimberg, R. G., & Hope, D. A. (1993). The revised Stroop color naming task in social phobics. *Behavioral Research and Therapy*, *3*, 305–313.

McNally, R. J. (1994). *Panic disorder: A critical analysis*. New York: Guilford Press.

McNeil, D., Reis, B. T., Taylor, L. J., & Boone, M. L. (1995). Comparison of social phobia subtypes using Stroop tests. *Journal of Anxiety Disorders*, *9*, 47–57.

Mellings, T. M. B., & Alden, L. E. (2000). Cognitive processes in social anxiety: The effects of self-focus, rumination and anticipatory processing. *Behaviour Research and Therapy*, *38*, 243–257.

Mineka, S., & Zinbarg, R. (1996). Conditioning and ethnological models of anxiety disorders: Stress-in-dynamic-context anxiety models. Perspectives on anxiety, panic, and fear. *Nebraska Symposium on Motivation*, *43*, 135–211.

Mogg, K., & Bradley, B. P. (2002). Selective orienting of attention to masked threat faces in social anxiety. *Behaviour Research and Therapy*, *40*, 1403–1414.

Mogg, K., Bradley, B. P., Bono, J. D., & Painter, M. (1997). Time course of attentional bias for threat information in non-clinical anxiety. *Behaviour Research and Therapy*, *35*, 297–303.

Mogg, K., Philippot, P., & Bradley, B. P. (2004). Selective attention to angry faces in clinical social phobia. *Journal of Abnormal Psychology*, *113*, 160–165.

Mohlman, J., Carmin, C. N., & Price, R. B. (2007). Jumping to interpretations: Social anxiety disorder and the identification of emotional facial expressions. *Behaviour Research and Therapy*, *45*, 591–599.

Morgan, J., & Banerjee, R. (2008). Post-event processing and autobiographical memory in social anxiety: The influence of negative feedback and rumination. *Journal of Anxiety Disorders*, *22*, 1190–1204.

Murphy, R., Hirsch, C. R., Mathews, A., Smith, K., & Clark, D. M. (2007). Facilitating a benign interpretation bias in a high socially anxious population. *Behaviour Research and Therapy*, *45*, 1517–1529.

Musa, C., Lépine, J., Clark, D. M., Mansell, W., & Ehlers, A. (2003). Selective attention in social phobia and the moderating effect of a concurrent depressive disorder. *Behaviour Research and Therapy*, *41*, 1043–1054.

Nugent, K., & Mineka, S. (1994). The effect of high and low trait anxiety on implicit and explicit memory tasks. *Cognition and Emotion*, *8*, 147–164.

Öhman, A. (1986). Face the beast and fear the face: Animal and social fears as prototypes for evolutionary analyses of emotion. *Psychophysiology*, *23*, 123–145.

Perowne, S., & Mansell, W. (2002). Social anxiety, self-focused attention, and the discrimination of negative, neutral and positive audience members by their non-verbal behaviours. *Behavioural and Cognitive Psychotherapy*, *30*, 11–23.

Philippot, P., & Douilliez, C. (2005). Social phobics do not misinterpret facial expression of emotion. *Behaviour Research and Therapy*, *43*, 639–652.

Pishyar, R., Harris, L. M., & Menzies, R. G. (2004). Attentional bias for words and faces in social anxiety. *Anxiety, Stress & Coping: An International Journal*, *17*, 23–36.

Pishyar, R., Harris, L. M., & Menzies, R. G. (2008). Responsiveness of measures of attentional bias to clinical change in social phobia. *Cognition and Emotion*, *22*, 1209–1227.

Posner, M. I. (1980). Orienting of attention. *Quarterly Journal of Experimental Psychology*, *32*(1), 3–25.

Rachman, S. (1980). Emotional processing. *Behaviour Research and Therapy*, *18*, 51–60.

Rapee, R. M., McCallum, S. L., Melville, L. F., Ravenscroft, H., & Rodney, J. M. (1993). Memory bias in social phobia. *Behavioral Research and Therapy*, *32*, 89–99.

Richards, A., French, C. C., Calder, A. J., Webb, B., Fox, R., & Young, A. W. (2002). Anxiety-related bias in the classification of emotionally ambiguous facial expressions. *Emotion*, *2*, 273–287.

Richards, A., Reynolds, A., & French, C. C. (1993). Anxiety and the spelling and use in sentences of threat/neutral homophones. *Current Psychology: Developmental, Learning, Personality, Social*, *12*, 18–25.

Rinck, M., & Becker, E. S. (2005). A comparison of attentional biases and memory biases in women with social phobia and major depression. *Journal of Abnormal Psychology*, *114*, 62–74.

Roediger, H. L. (1990). Implicit memory: Retention without remembering. *American Psychologist*, *45*, 1043–1056.

Roediger, H. L., & Blaxton, T. A. (1987). Effects of varying modality, surface features, and retention interval on priming in word fragment completion. *Memory and Cognition*, *15*, 379–388.

Schacter, D. L. (1992). Understanding implicit memory: A cognitive neuroscience approach. *American Psychologist*, *47*, 559–569.

Schmidt, N. B., Richey, J. A., Buckner, J. D., & Timpano, K. R. (2009). Attention training for generalized social anxiety disorder. *Journal of Abnormal Psychology*, *118*, 5–14.

Schofield, C. A., Coles, M. E., & Gibb, B. E. (2007). Social anxiety and interpretation biases for facial displays of emotion: Emotion detection and ratings of social cost. *Behaviour Research and Therapy*, *45*, 2950–2963.

Spector, I., Pecknold, J. C., & Libman, E. (2003). Selective attentional bias related to the noticeability aspect of anxiety symptoms in generalized social phobia. *Journal of Anxiety Disorders*, *17*, 517–531.

Sposari, J. A., & Rapee, R. M. (2007). Attentional bias toward facial stimuli under conditions of social threat in socially phobic and nonclinical participants. *Cognitive Therapy and Research, 31*, 23–37.

Stopa, L., & Clark, D. M. (2000). Social phobia and interpretation of social events. *Behaviour Research and Therapy, 38*, 273–283.

Stopa, L., & Jenkins, A. (2007). Images of the self in social anxiety: Effects on the retrieval of autobiographical memories. *Journal of Behavior Therapy and Experimental Psychiatry, 38*, 459–473.

Tomarken, A. J., Mineka, S., & Cook, M. (1989). Fear-relevant selective associations and covariation bias. *Journal of Abnormal Psychology, 98*, 381–394.

Vassilopoulos, S. (2006). Interpretation and judgment biases in socially anxious and nonanxious individuals. *Behavioural and Cognitive Psychotherapy, 34*, 243–254.

Voncken, M. J., & Bögels, S. M. (2006). Changing interpretation and judgmental bias in social phobia: A pilot study of a short, highly structured cognitive treatment. *Journal of Cognitive Psychotherapy. Special Issue: Recent Advances in the Treatment of Social Phobia, 20*, 59–73.

Voncken, M. J., Bögels, S. M., & Peeters, F. (2007). Specificity of interpretation and judgemental biases in social phobia versus depression. *Psychology and Psychotherapy: Theory, Research and Practice, 80*, 443–453.

Weeks, J. W., Heimberg, R. G., Rodebaugh, T. L., & Norton, P. J. (2008). Exploring the relationship between fear of positive evaluation and social anxiety. *Journal of Anxiety Disorders, 22*, 386–400.

Weierich, M. R., Treat, T. A., & Hollingworth, A. (2008). Theories and measurement of visual attentional processing in anxiety. *Cognition and Emotion, 22*, 985–1018.

Wenzel, A., Finstrom, N., Jordan, J., & Brendle, J. R. (2005). Memory and interpretation of visual representations of threat in socially anxious and nonanxious individuals. *Behaviour Research and Therapy, 43*, 1029–1044.

Wenzel, A., & Holt, C. S. (2002). Memory bias against threat in social phobia. *British Journal of Clinical Psychology, 41*, 73–79.

Wenzel, A., Jackson, L. C., & Holt, C. S. (2002). Social phobia and the recall of autobiographical memories. *Depression and Anxiety, 15*, 186–189.

Williams, J. M. G., Mathews, A., & MacLeod, C. (1996). The emotional Stroop task and psychopathology. *Psychological Bulletin, 120*, 3–24.

Williams, J. M. G., Watts, F. N., MacLeod, C., & Mathews, A. (1988). *Cognitive psychology and the emotional disorders*. Chichester: John Wiley.

Williams, J. M. G., Watts, F. N., MacLeod, C., & Mathews, A. (1997). *Cognitive psychology and emotional disorders* (2nd edition). New York: John Wiley and Sons.

Wilson, J. K., & Rapee, R. M. (2005). Interpretative biases in social phobia: Content specificity and the effects of depression. *Cognitive Therapy and Research, 29*, 315–331.

Yoon, K. L., & Zinbarg, R. E. (2007). Threat is in the eye of the beholder: Social anxiety and the interpretation of ambiguous facial expressions. *Behaviour Research and Therapy, 45*, 839–847.

Yoon, K. L., & Zinbarg, R. E. (2008). Interpreting neutral faces as threatening is a default mode for socially anxious individuals. *Journal of Abnormal Psychology, 117*, 680–685.

Yuen, P. K. (1994). Social anxiety and the allocation of attention: Evaluation using facial stimuli in a dot-probe paradigm. Unpublished research project, Department of Experimental Psychology, University of Oxford, UK.

Chapter 15

A Cognitive Behavioral Model of Social Anxiety Disorder: Update and Extension

Richard G. Heimberg[1], Faith A. Brozovich[1], and Ronald M. Rapee[2]
[1]Adult Anxiety Clinic of Temple University, Philadelphia, Pennsylvania, [2]Centre for Emotional Health, Macquarie University, Sydney, Australia

SAD is characterized by an intense fear of negative evaluation from others in social and/or performance situations according to the *Diagnostic and Statistical Manual of Mental Disorders*, fourth edition, text revision (DSM-IV-TR) (American Psychiatric Association, 2000). Since social anxiety was first recognized as a mental disorder with the publication of DSM-III (American Psychiatric Association, 1980), its prevalence (Kessler, Berglund et al., 2005; Kessler, Chiu, Demler, Merikangas, & Walters, 2005); chronicity (Bruce et al., 2005; Chartier, Hazen, & Stein, 1998; Reich, Goldenberg, Vasile, Goisman, & Keller, 1994); associated personal, economic, and societal costs (Acarturk, de Graaf, van Straten, ten Have, & Cuijpers, 2008; Acarturk et al., 2009; Rodebaugh, 2009; Safren, Heimberg, Brown, & Holle, 1997; Schneier, Johnson, Hornig, Liebowitz, & Weissman, 1992; Schneier et al., 1994; Tolman et al., 2009; Whisman, Sheldon, & Goering, 2000); and comorbidity with other disorders (Magee, Eaton, Wittchen, McGonagle, & Kessler, 1996; Ruscio et al., 2008) have been well documented. To move our understanding of the nature and treatment of SAD forward, several researchers have proposed explanatory models over the past three decades, dating back to the early work of Schlenker and Leary (1982). The most widely cited and applied of these models have been those of Clark and Wells (1995; see also Clark, 2001) and Rapee and Heimberg (1997), although several potentially fruitful models have been more recently proposed (e.g., Hofmann, 2007; Kimbrel, 2008; Moscovitch, 2009). In this chapter, we focus on our original 1997 cognitive behavioral model for SAD, which delineates the processes by which SAIs are affected by their fear of negative evaluation in potentially social-evaluative situations.

Social Anxiety: Clinical, Developmental, and Social Perspectives. DOI: 10.1016/B978-0-12-375096-9.00015-8

The original model has provided a solid framework for understanding the factors that comprise and maintain SAD. Since the publication of Rapee and Heimberg (1997), we have provided updates in the form of reviews of the literature that support various aspects of the model (Roth & Heimberg, 2001; Turk, Lerner, Heimberg, & Rapee, 2001), applied the model to a case study of a person with SAD (Heimberg, Rapee, & Turk, 2002), and conducted a comparison between our model and the very influential and productive model proposed by Clark and Wells (Schultz & Heimberg, 2008). Given that there has been over a decade of intervening research, however, there are areas in the model that warrant expansion, as well as additional factors that necessitate inclusion in the model. The present chapter presents a revised cognitive behavioral model of SAD and the research supporting these modifications. Five areas will be the primary foci of the following discussion: the important role of imagery (and imagery perspective), PEP, the combined cognitive biases hypothesis, fear of positive evaluation (FPE), and the potential role of difficulties in the regulation of emotional responses, including but not limited to anxiety. First, we present a summary of the model as originally proposed. Research support appears in the other papers cited above.

THE ORIGINAL MODEL

The Rapee–Heimberg model (see Figure 15.1) attempts to explain the generation and maintenance of anxiety in affected persons upon entry into or anticipation of a social situation. We define social situations broadly, suggesting that the presence of a perceived audience may constitute significant threat. When these situations are encountered, individuals with SAD experience fear because they assume that others are naturally critical and that negative evaluation will logically follow. Also, individuals with SAD consider being liked and regarded with high esteem as fundamentally important. In the presence of threat (i.e., after the detection of an audience), SAIs become increasingly vigilant for cues that would signal the realization of their feared outcomes, and they attend to several sources for possible information on the proximity of these outcomes, including environmental cues, a mental representation of how they believe they appear to others, and cognitive, behavioral, and affective cues related to the severity of their anxiety in the moment.

Perceived Audience

For the SAI, the perceived audience not only includes the members of the audience when one is giving a formal public speech or a person who conducts an evaluative job interview but may also include others with whom the individual interacts in dating or casual social interactions, or even those individuals who could pose a seemingly more distant potential threat that the person might be negatively evaluated. Thus, someone walking down the street who might view

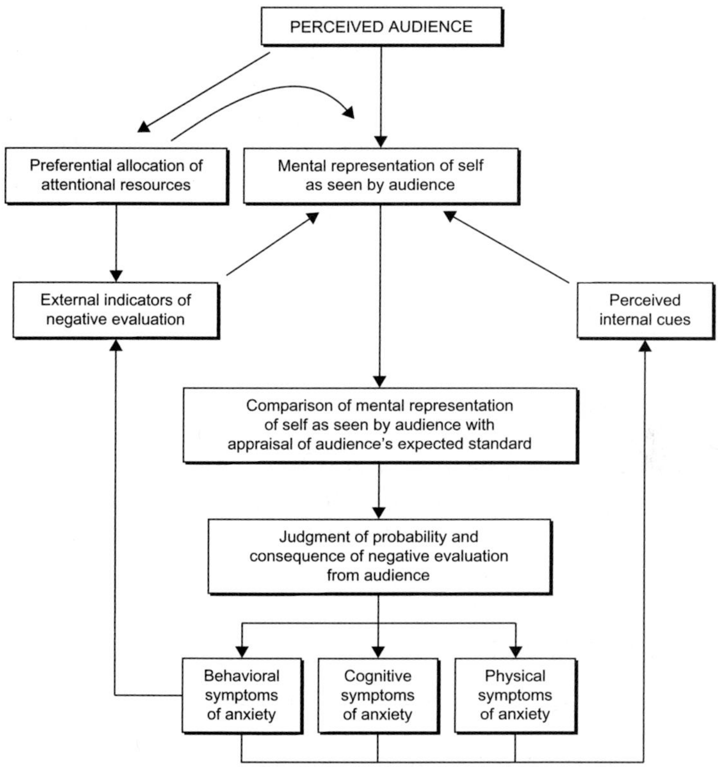

FIGURE 15.1 Rapee and Heimberg's (1997) cognitive behavioral model of social anxiety's generation and maintenance. *(From Behaviour Research and Therapy, 35, R. M. Rapee & R. G. Heimberg, A cognitive-behavioral model of anxiety in social phobia, page 743. Copyright 1997, with kind permission from Elsevier.)*

the socially anxious person and think poorly of how he or she looks, a person sitting on a facing bench when waiting for a train, or a person seated at another table at a restaurant may (unwittingly) become the perceived audience in the mind of the SAI. Characteristics of the audience (e.g., importance, attractiveness) as well as features of the situation (e.g., degree of anonymity of the SAI) influence the level of anxiety experienced.

Mental Representation of the Self as Seen by the Audience

In response to the perception of the audience, the SAI forms (or accesses) an internal mental representation of how he or she is perceived by the audience. This representation may be an image or a vague sense of how one appears to others, which likely involves seeing oneself as if through the eyes of the audience (they are, after all, the source of potential negative evaluation and, therefore, there is considerable survival value in "modeling" how they think). The mental representation of the self as perceived by the audience is a composite formed from a number of different sources, and it is very likely to be distorted among persons with SAD. For instance, this image may be informed by a sense of how one generally appears to others (information obtained in mirrors, photographs, etc.) and past difficult experiences in social situations that are consistent with negative core beliefs and self-schema. These inputs may constitute a "baseline image" (Rapee & Heimberg, 1997, p. 745) that is modified by external and internal inputs during distressing social situations. The mental representation of the self should be influenced by autonomic symptoms of anxiety, particularly those that may be visible to others, such as blushing and sweating. The SAI may also monitor his or her behavior (e.g., fidgeting, wiping one's brow) and exaggerate how it must appear to audience members as well as what it must mean about his or her competence. Furthermore, socially anxious persons may perceive that they have social performance deficits, such as stuttering or freezing or not knowing what to say, as well as a sense that they might be coming across as "boring" or "quiet," that would also be exaggerated in the mental representation of the self. Moment-to-moment modifications of the mental representation occur based on (over-)interpretations of internal feedback (e.g., feeling warm means "I'm visibly sweating"), observations of one's own behavior (e.g., standing on the edge of a group means "I look out of place"), and the reactions of others (e.g., another person's expression means "I look stupid").

Preferential Allocation of Attentional Resources

SAIs will preferentially allocate attentional resources toward detecting social threat in the environment; in fact, there are compelling evolutionary reasons why this should be the case. However, it is hypothesized that SAIs also allocate attentional resources toward monitoring and adjusting their mental representation of how they are perceived by the audience. In effect, SAIs attempt to simultaneously monitor the environment for evidence of negative evaluation, monitor their appearance and behavior for flaws that might elicit negative evaluation from others, *and* attend to and engage in the social tasks at hand. In effect, socially anxious persons operate within the equivalent of a "multiple task paradigm," which increases the probability of disrupted social performance (MacLeod & Mathews, 1991). Therefore, complex social tasks are more likely to result in poorer performance, due to limited processing resources, than less complex tasks.

Comparison of One's Mental Representation of the Self as Seen by the Audience with One's Appraisal of the Audience's Expected Standard

In addition to monitoring their mental representation of how they are perceived by the audience, persons with SAD also project the performance standard expected by the audience. SAIs typically believe that the perceived audience members have extremely high standards for their performance, and the more they believe their behavior and appearance fall short of their estimate of the audience's expectations, the more likely negative evaluation and its accompanying painful consequences are predicted to be. The degree to which SAIs believe their behavior meets the expectation of the audience can fluctuate based on changing perceptions of the audience, the demands of the social situation, and their own behavior. Thus, it is not uncommon for the level of social anxiety to vary while in a social situation.

Judgment of the Probability and Consequences of Negative Evaluation from the Audience

The culmination of the preceding stages of the model suggests that socially anxious persons will judge the probability and cost of negative evaluation by the audience to be high. Enhanced memory for past social "failures" may also make it more likely that SAIs will anticipate that current or future social interactions will go poorly. Stated otherwise, socially anxious persons focus on the discrepancy between their own mental representation of self as seen by the audience and their perception of the audience's unachievable standards for their performance. This seemingly insurmountable difference leads them to overestimate the social costs of the event. Often these judgments and expectations of negative outcomes contribute to behavioral, cognitive, and physical symptoms of anxiety.

The Anxiety Response Among Persons with Social Anxiety Disorder

Cognitive Symptoms

The socially anxious person will react with situation-specific thoughts of negative evaluation in response to social stimuli (e.g., "They think I don't know what I'm talking about"). In anxiety-provoking social situations, SAIs engage in a predominantly negative internal dialogue in which they may berate themselves ("I'm such a jerk") or catastrophize about what other people are thinking about them ("She is not interested in me; nobody ever will be"). SAIs typically accept these thoughts as facts and may become increasingly focused upon them as the interaction progresses. Focus on these thoughts may interfere with attention to the task at hand. For example, SAIs may have difficulty maintaining a conversation because they are quick to judge things they could say as "stupid" or "uninteresting."

Behavioral Symptoms

An appraisal that negative evaluation is a likely and costly outcome may produce overt avoidance of or escape from the social situation. Even if SAIs persist in the feared social situation, they may engage in a variety of subtle behaviors that are aimed at avoiding negative evaluation from others (Wells et al., 1995). These behaviors, referred to as "safety behaviors" in common parlance (e.g., Clark, 2001), may include avoiding eye contact, standing on the outside of a crowd, or minimizing participation in a conversation. Unfortunately, these avoidant behaviors may frequently have the effect of reducing effective social performance. Consequently, SAIs may receive verbal and nonverbal feedback from the audience that their performance is inferior. Furthermore, safety behaviors may undermine the person's opportunity to learn that he or she may have handled the situation just fine without reliance on these apparent safety cues.

Physical Symptoms

Many studies have demonstrated that SAIs exhibit physiological arousal when exposed to feared social situations. Compared to individuals with other anxiety disorders, socially anxious persons are more likely to endorse physical symptoms that may be observed by others such as blushing, muscle twitching, and sweating. SAIs tend to overestimate the visibility of their anxiety, catastrophize about how negatively others will react to their anxiety, and become focused on those symptoms that they believe hold a high potential for eliciting negative evaluation from others.

Perceived Internal Cues

Internal anxiety cues are then used as a source of information that feeds back into the mental representation of the self as seen by the audience. For example, feeling shaky may be taken to mean that others can observe the person visibly trembling or that the person may be about to lose control of his or her behavior, which may result in further negative evaluation from others. In addition to feedback from the ANS, the individual will also receive proprioceptive information that may funnel into his or her judgment regarding the possibility of negative evaluation. For example, proprioceptive cues may provide information that the individual is not sitting up straight during a job interview. The individual then alters the mental representation of the self as seen by the audience to reflect a (probably exaggerated) slumping posture. This mental representation of having a slumping posture is likely to compare unfavorably with the interviewer's projected standard of behavior. The possibility of negative evaluation will be judged to be more likely, which should result in increased anxiety and predictions that the interview will turn out badly.

External Indicators of Negative Evaluation

Anxiety and, in perhaps some cases, poor social skills may function to reduce effective social performance and result in negative verbal or nonverbal feedback from the audience. Importantly, social feedback is often indirect and ambiguous. Given an information processing bias toward detecting and possibly remembering threatening social information, SAIs will readily incorporate possible external indications of negative evaluation into their ongoing and long-term mental representation of themselves.

The Vicious Cycle

The socially anxious person's focus on external threat cues and the mental representation of the self as seen by the audience is informed by internal anxiety symptoms (i.e., physiological, behavioral, and cognitive), exacerbates state anxiety, and maintains SAD. However, these processes do not operate in isolation; each component interacts with the others in the form of a positive feedback loop. For instance, the biased detection of negative audience behaviors (e.g., frowning, yawning) would likely result in greater focus on the mental representation of the self (e.g., increased frequency of cognitions regarding how uninteresting one is). Focus on the mental representation of the self should not only exacerbate anxiety but should also increase the detection of negative audience behaviors. As individuals with SAD look to their mental representations for information about how they come across, they necessarily see a negatively biased caricature informed by anxious feelings and assumptions about others' evaluations when, realistically, the data needed to support such self-assessment cannot be obtained in ambiguous social situations. This person may then look to the audience to confirm his or her fears and is likely to find information consistent with his self-appraisals. These appraisals feed back into the mental representation of the self and result in its readjustment in a negative direction, which is a cycle likely to be repeated multiple times over the course of an ongoing social situation.

IMAGERY IN SOCIAL ANXIETY DISORDER

SAIs are overly concerned about being humiliated or embarrassed in social situations. This fear is often demonstrated in their mental images of themselves in social situations and represented in Rapee and Heimberg's model in the concept of the mental representation of the self as seen by the audience. Researchers studying imagery and emotion have asserted that affective imagery activates a network that evokes a fearful physiological, behavioral, and conceptual response, the same network that is activated when confronted with a threatening stimulus (Lang, 1979). The response to affective imagery is apparent in all individuals; however, it is intensified among anxious individuals (McTeague et al., 2009). Several studies have demonstrated that imagery elicits stronger emotional responses than verbal processing (e.g., Acosta & Vila, 1990; Holmes & Mathews, 2005; Holmes, Mathews, Dalgleish, & Mackintosh, 2006; Lang, Levin, Miller, & Kozak, 1983; Vrana, Cuthbert, & Lang, 1986).

Therefore, it is likely that, when SAIs engage in imagery, it intensifies their emotional experience, and it may have disruptive effects on their social performance as well. In the current context, there are three questions that seem to be important for the study of SAD and for the fuller explication of the mental representation of the self as seen by the audience. These are: (1) Do socially anxious persons spontaneously engage in imagery that may have a negative effect on the mental representation? (2) Do they preferentially recall social situations from the perspective of the audience (referred to in the literature as the observer perspective) and is this perspective associated with negative outcomes? and (3) Does holding a negative image of oneself in mind while performing various social tasks adversely affect performance?

Do Socially Anxious Persons Spontaneously Engage in Imagery that May Have a Negative Effect on the Mental Representation of the Self as Seen by the Audience?

In fact, it appears they do, as demonstrated in two clinical studies by Hackmann and colleagues (Hackmann, Clark, & McManus, 2000; Hackmann, Surawy, & Clark, 1998). Hackmann and colleagues (1998) examined whether socially anxious persons were more likely than nonanxious controls to spontaneously recall images of past social situations when they were feeling their most anxious in a recent social situation and whether these spontaneously recalled images had any specific characteristics. SAIs reported a higher frequency of mental images before, during, and after social situations, and their images were more negative and distorted. They also reported images significantly more from an observer perspective than a field perspective compared to the images reported by the nonanxious participants (more on the observer perspective to follow). Seventy-seven percent of socially anxious participants, compared to only 10% of controls, reported a spontaneously occurring image that was rated as negative, distorted, and coming from the observer perspective.

In their follow-up study (Hackmann et al., 2000), all 22 interviewed participants with SAD were able to identify a spontaneously occurring image that occurred to them in social situations, and the image had a number of important characteristics. First, it was recurrent, stable over time, and had been experienced for a number of years. Second, the imaged events clustered in time around the time of onset of the person's social anxiety. Hackmann et al. speculate that these events may have been involved in the development of the person's SAD or the exacerbation of social anxiety symptoms. Third, the recurrent image was experienced in multiple sensory modalities. Fourth, the negative and distorted qualities of the image did not appear to have been moderated by positive or neutral social experiences that intervened between the imaged event and the event that provided the later context for the image.

Erwin, Heimberg, Marx, and Franklin (2006) approached the issue from a different vantage point but came to similar conclusions. Forty-five socially anxious clients and 30 nonanxious controls were asked to describe the worst "socially stressful event" that they had ever experienced. By design, these were events that may have been quite unpleasant, but none met Criterion A for a diagnosis of PTSD: "actual or threatened death or serious injury, or a threat to the physical integrity of self or others . . . [and responded to with] intense fear, helplessness, or horror" (American Psychiatric Association, 1994, pp. 427–428). However, compared to controls, clients responded to memories of these events with significantly more hyperarousal and avoidance symptoms, although they did not report more re-experiencing symptoms. The clients did, on average, endorse sufficient symptoms in all clusters to have met criteria for PTSD if these symptoms had been in response to a Criterion A event. For those clients who also had a history of comorbid PTSD, there was no difference in the pattern of their responses to the socially stressful and Criterion A events. Anecdotally, several reported that they suffered more with the memory of the socially stressful event than the Criterion A event.

Do Socially Anxious Persons Preferentially Recall Social Situations from the Perspective of the Audience and Is This Perspective Associated with Negative Outcomes?

One aspect of imagery that has been studied more thoroughly among SAIs is the perspective from which individuals recall or visualize social situations. The observer perspective entails seeing a situation from a third party's point of view; in other words, through the eyes of the audience. The field perspective entails viewing a situation as if from one's own eyes. From this perspective, individuals would not see themselves in the image but rather would see the audience or whatever might be before them. These perspectives have their roots in social psychology (e.g., Duval & Wicklund's, theory of self-awareness (1972)). In fact, the results of one early study (Ickes, Wicklund, & Ferris, 1973) suggested that taking an observer perspective may heighten levels of self-criticism and negative emotion. It is important to study SAI's perspective in social situations because it may inform how they encode, process, and remember potentially socially threatening events.

Following the Hackmann et al. (1998) study described above, Wells, Clark, and Ahmad (1998) examined the differences in perspective-taking during recalled (rather than spontaneously generated) images of social versus nonsocial situations. Individuals with SAD and controls recalled recent social and nonsocial situations in which they were feeling nervous and anxious and rated the degree to which they remembered the event from an observer-versus-field perspective. SAIs took a much more observer perspective for social situations, whereas nonanxious controls took more of a field perspective. For nonsocial situations, both socially anxious and control participants took more of a field perspective. The difference between observer and field perspectives was only significant among the socially anxious participants.

Next, Wells and Papageorgiou (1999) tested whether an observer perspective was evident in persons with social-evaluative anxiety disorders on a broader scope (including agoraphobia as well as SAD), compared to persons with an anxiety disorder not related to social evaluation (i.e., blood/injury phobia). Similarly to Wells et al. (1998), participants were asked to remember and image a recent anxiety-provoking social situation and a recent non-anxiety-provoking nonsocial situation and rate the extent to which their image was from an observer perspective or a field perspective. Both socially anxious and agoraphobic individuals reported an observer perspective when imaging a social situation; blood/injury phobics and controls reported a field perspective. However, only the socially anxious participants showed a shift between perspectives as a function of the type of situation.

These studies illustrate that social situations elicit an observer perspective among SAIs. Coles, Turk, Heimberg, and Fresco (2001) examined the effects of varying levels of anxiety on perspective-taking. First, participants with GSAD thought of social situations that evoked low anxiety, moderate anxiety, and high anxiety and then completed a memory interview in which they were asked to recall these situations and any associated images. Participants then rated the degree of observer/field perspective. Differences in perspective-taking among SAIs depended upon the level of anxiety experienced. Specifically, SAIs rated high anxiety-provoking social situations more from an observer perspective than low and moderate anxiety-provoking social situations. Nonanxious control participants tended to perceive all social situations from a field perspective. Thus, it is not simply that SAIs automatically recall images of all social situations from an observer perspective, but rather that this pattern is specific to highly anxiety-evoking social situations.

Coles, Turk, and Heimberg (2002) examined perspective in anxiety-provoking social situations in the laboratory and over time. It is well documented that there is an increasing chance an individual will recall a situation from an observer perspective as more time passes since the index event (Frank & Gilovich, 1989; Nigro & Neisser, 1983). To study the effects of imagery in real time, they asked participants to complete two four-minute role-played social situations: an impromptu speech and a party situation. Participants were asked to think about the image they had of themselves during each situation and to rate the degree to which the image was from a field or an observer perspective. Participants made these ratings after the role-plays and again three weeks later. As predicted, socially anxious participants recalled the social situations from more of an observer perspective after the situation occurred and three weeks later, compared to nonanxious controls. Over the three-week interval, SAI's memories shifted more toward an observer perspective, but the perspective of the nonanxious participants did not change.

Researchers have also been interested in manipulating participants' perspectives during behavioral tasks. Vassilopoulos (2005) examined the effects of perspective-taking during a speech task. Undergraduates scoring high or low on the FNE (Watson & Friend, 1969) were randomly assigned to negative or positive imagery conditions. Participants were given one minute to plan a short speech they would be giving to a video camera. Those in the negative imagery condition were asked to imagine a recent anxiety-provoking situation and remember it from an observer perspective, whereas those in the positive image condition were asked to imagine a recent situation in which they felt confident and relaxed. They were not instructed to take an observer perspective. After imaging the situation for a brief time, participants were instructed to give their two-minute speech while holding the image they had generated in mind. SAIs in the negative imagery condition reported more physical sensations during the speech and rated their performance more negatively, whereas this was not true for SAIs in the positive imagery condition. Low anxious participants did not differ on anxiety or ratings of performance regardless of their assigned imagery condition. It should be noted that instructions to adopt an observer perspective were included in the negative but not the positive imagery condition. Thus, we cannot be certain that the results were due to differences in perspective-taking.

Spurr and Stopa (2003) experimentally manipulated high and low anxious students' perspective-taking when they gave two speeches (one while holding in mind an observer-perspective image of themselves giving the speech, the other while holding a field-perspective image). Overall, participants reported more negative frequent thoughts, more safety behaviors, and poorer self-evaluation of performance when taking an observer perspective. However, high SAIs rated their speeches more poorly than low SAIs, regardless of perspective.

Although a full review of the observer perspective is beyond the scope of this chapter, the studies described here converge to suggest that observer-perspective imagery is more common among socially anxious persons, especially likely to occur when recalling highly anxiety-evoking situations, becomes more pronounced with the passage of time, and (although these studies have their flaws) is associated with more frequent negative thoughts, more negative self-evaluation of performance, more physical sensations, and more frequent use of safety behaviors.

Does Holding a Negative Image of Oneself in Mind While Performing Social Tasks Adversely Affect Performance?

Rapee and Heimberg's (1997) model asserts that one's mental representation (image) of oneself as seen by the audience is activated in social situations. Several studies by Hirsch and others have provided information concerning the effects of holding positive or negative images in mind.

Hirsch, Clark, Mathews, and Williams (2003) asked individuals with SAD to generate negative and control self-images in a counterbalanced design. Participants were asked to hold the first image in mind while having a conversation with someone they had never met. They then rated aspects of the image, such as vividness and the amount of time they held the image in mind, and made various symptom and behavioral ratings. Afterwards, they were asked to hold the second image in mind while having another conversation with the same person and completed similar ratings. When holding a negative image in mind, socially anxious participants judged that they were more anxious and performed less well in the conversation than they were rated by independent assessors. They also judged their own performance and anxiety worse in the negative image condition than in the control image condition. Interestingly, even though the assessors did not rate the SAI's performance in the negative image condition as poorly as these participants rated themselves, they still rated them less well than the socially anxious participants in the control condition. Thus, holding a negative image in mind can strongly affect how an individual experiences anxiety and how others perceive him in a social situation. It also affects how well individuals perform based on their own and others' perceptions.

A follow-up study with socially anxious undergraduates and nonanxious conversation partners was conducted to further test the impact of negative imagery (Hirsch, Meynen, & Clark, 2004). The socially anxious participants had two conversations with their non-socially anxious partners in which they visualized either a negative or a control image. After each conversation, participants completed measures concerning the conversation and behaviors of the SAI. Socially anxious participants also completed ratings about their anxiety and use of safety behaviors. Once again, holding a negative image in mind impeded SAI's performance. Specifically, the socially anxious participants, while in the negative image condition, reported more anxiety and worse perception of their performance in the conversation than when they held a control image in mind. Conversation partners also rated socially anxious participants' performance in the negative imagery condition as worse and perceived more anxiety symptoms. The SAIs, when in the negative imagery condition, also provided evidence that they used more safety behaviors in the conversation compared to the control imagery condition.

As reported earlier, Vassilopoulos (2005) found results consistent with Hirsch, Clark, Mathews, and Williams (2003) and Hirsch et al. (2004). The socially anxious participants in the negative imagery condition rated their speech performance more poorly and endorsed more physical symptoms during the speech. It is unclear whether differences could be attributed to the observer-perspective focus of the negative imagery or simply the valence of the image. Still, it points to disadvantageous effects on performance of holding a negative image in mind.

To see whether negative imagery affected social performance in non-socially anxious individuals, Hirsch, Mathews, Clark, Williams, and Morrison (2006) investigated this phenomenon in self-assured public speakers. Participants were randomly assigned to positive, negative, or control imagery conditions. In the positive imagery condition, participants were asked to recall a speech they had given that went particularly well. In the negative imagery condition, they were asked to recall a speech that went poorly or to imagine what it would have been like if the speech had gone poorly. In the control condition, participants were simply asked to think about a shopping trip. Next, they gave a 4 min speech about the costs and benefits of living in London. Afterwards, they completed a series of questionnaires measuring thoughts, behaviors, anxiety, and depression. Consistent with the other studies, the participants in the negative imagery condition felt more anxious during the speech and rated their performance more poorly than individuals in the positive imagery condition. Possibly because of the nature of the sample, the assessors' ratings of speech performances in the various imagery conditions did not differ.

Stopa and Jenkins (2007) examined the relationship of imagery to anxiety, and speech performance among 20 socially anxious undergraduates. This study employed a within-subjects design to examine the effects of eliciting positive and negative images. Participants imagined a positive or negative image of themselves in a mirror, depending on the condition to which they were assigned. Then they were asked to hold that image in mind while giving a brief impromptu speech. This sequence was repeated for the other image. Similarly to the other studies reviewed here, participants experienced more anxiety and rated their performance more poorly during the speech in the negative imagery condition.

These studies provide compelling evidence from experimental manipulations of negative imagery; however, it should be noted that there are limitations to the methods employed. Asking someone to actively hold an image in mind requires a certain amount of effort. When we think of imagery coming to mind in a natural context, the process is likely much more habitual and passive. This raises the issue of automaticity versus effortfulness of thoughts (McNally, 1995). Simply asking individuals to effortfully think of an image presents a certain amount of cognitive load in a performance task that potentially could alter one's performance. Also, holding a negative image in mind likely elicits negative emotions and memories, which may be more impairing and distracting than the emotions and memories elicited by a positive image. This may be particularly difficult for those individuals who have difficulty regulating their negative emotions and/or who have higher levels of depression.

POST-EVENT PROCESSING

SAIs heightened concerns about their performance in social situations leads them to brood about the specifics of social events, a self-focused thought process often referred to as PEP (Brozovich & Heimberg, 2008) or post-event rumination (Abbott & Rapee, 2004). SAIs may engage in PEP following a social event or when they anticipate a similar upcoming event. The individual reviews his or her actions and behavior in the situation as well as the reactions and behaviors of the other individuals or audience members. It is likely that individuals engage in this analysis of situations to better understand their behavior, to examine it closely for potentially embarrassing moments that may require some degree of "damage control," or to prepare themselves for the upcoming event (likely in an attempt to avert a perceived negative outcome). PEP has played a role in other models of SAD (Clark & Wells, 1995; Hofmann, 2007). Several studies have examined PEP among SAIs using self-report questionnaires (Fehm, Schneider, & Hoyer, 2007; Fehm, Hoyer, Schneider, Lindemann, & Klusmann, 2008; McEvoy & Kingsep, 2006; Rachman, Grüter-Andrew, & Shafran, 2000), diary recordings (Lundh & Sperling, 2002), examination of responses to giving a speech or participating in a role-played social interaction (Abbott & Rapee, 2004; Brozovich & Heimberg, 2010; Dannahy & Stopa, 2007; Edwards, Rapee, & Franklin, 2003; Kashdan & Roberts, 2007; Mellings & Alden, 2000; Perini, Abbott, & Rapee, 2006; Rapee & Abbott, 2007), or experimental manipulations of the type of PEP (Field & Morgan, 2004; Kocovski, Endler, Rector, & Flett, 2005).

Diary recordings suggest that socially anxious persons are most likely to engage in PEP after situations that hold the potential for negative evaluation (Lundh & Sperling, 2002). An examination of a sampling of studies of reactions to these situations in the laboratory highlights the nature of this maladaptive and pernicious process.

Abbott and Rapee (2004) examined PEP following a speech task in a clinical sample of individuals seeking treatment for social anxiety disorder and nonanxious controls. After completing several anxiety and mood questionnaires, participants gave a three-minute impromptu speech. They were told that recordings of the speech would be evaluated by an independent judge. Following the speech, participants evaluated their performance. One week later, participants completed a PEP questionnaire and re-evaluated their performance. SAIs evaluated their speech performance more negatively than the controls immediately after, and their appraisals remained negative over the one-week interval. Control participants, on the other hand, showed significant improvement in their evaluations of their performance over the week. Furthermore, SAIs engaged in more negative PEP over the week than the nonanxious individuals, and the relationship between social anxiety and later PEP was mediated by their perception of performance immediately after the speech. These results were replicated by Perini et al. (2006).

In a subsequent study in the same line, Rapee and Abbott (2007) demonstrated another mediational relationship of note – that PEP during the one-week interval after a speech task mediated the relationship between social anxiety and negative bias in the recollection of speech performance among clients with SAD. In addition, Brozovich and Heimberg (2010) conducted a study with high and low socially anxious students. Participants engaged in a 12-minute conversation with a confederate and completed several questionnaires (including a measure of typical levels of PEP) and evaluated their performance in the conversation. They also re-evaluated their performance during a one-week follow-up phone call. Typical levels of PEP reported in the initial session moderated the relationship between social anxiety and individuals' evaluation of their performance at the one-week follow-up. These two studies demonstrate that PEP among SAIs, whether it is assessed as a state variable or a trait variable, has a significant relationship to later performance evaluations.

Dannahy and Stopa (2007) examined undergraduates scoring high or low on the FNE. Participants rated their own performance in a social interaction as well as the frequency of their PEP. At a second session a week later, participants were instructed that they would be having another social interaction, completed additional measures of PEP, and predicted how well they would do in the second interaction. In a pattern slightly different from that reported by Abbott and Rapee (2004), socially anxious participants' ratings of their performance in the first interaction became more negative over time, whereas the ratings of control participants did not change. Socially anxious participants also reported more negative PEP at both assessments. Significantly, socially anxious participants expected to do more poorly than control participants in the second interaction, and the tendency to predict a poorer performance in the second interaction was predicted by negatively valenced PEP.

Although a fuller review of PEP is beyond our scope (for a review see Brozovich & Heimberg, 2008), it appears to be an important maintaining factor in social anxiety. It leads to biases in one's memory of past events and predictions about success in future situations. By taking apart and putting together the elements of the situation and placing his or her own interpretations on them each time, the person develops a more distorted view of the situation, its outcome, and his or her responsibility for it. The more iterations of PEP in which someone engages, the further and further from an accurate memory of the event he or she is likely to move, but the reconstructed memory may be more easily accessible. Thus, SAIs memory for events becomes increasingly negative over time (Dannahy & Stopa, 2007; Mellings & Alden, 2000). PEP likely becomes more negative over time and may contribute to increases in anticipatory anxiety about upcoming events. Thus, it serves to connect one social situation to another and perpetuates social anxiety across time and situations.

PEP may also impede progress in CBT. Successful experiences confronting feared situations may be turned into perceived failures by the process of microexamination of the event, which is the essence of PEP. Thus, it may be particularly important to include cognitive exercises after exposures are completed to stem the tide of this maladaptive process. Nevertheless, the propensity to engage in PEP of social events does appear to be reduced after a course of CBT (Abbott & Rapee, 2004; McEvoy, Mahoney, Perini, & Kingsep, 2009).

THE COMBINED COGNITIVE BIASES HYPOTHESIS

Earlier in this chapter, we noted that imagery and PEP may influence or interact with other cognitive processes. Rapee and Heimberg (1997), as well as other models for SAD (e.g., Clark & Wells, 1995), posit a system of cognitive biases that interact to maintain the disorder. However, Hirsch, Clark, and Mathews (2006) more explicitly laid out these interconnections when they introduced the combined cognitive biases hypothesis. This hypothesis simply states that cognitive biases do not operate in isolation, but rather are one part of a set of processes. The combined cognitive biases hypothesis points out to researchers that we are limiting our knowledge of SAD (and other disorders) by only investigating one process at a time. It will be more useful to examine how potentially biased cognitive processes affect other cognitive biases as well.

The frequency of negative self-imagery in SAD is well documented in this chapter, and support for biased interpretation of ambiguous social stimuli in SAD is abundant (e.g., Amir, Foa, & Coles, 1998; Hertel, Brozovich, Joorman, & Gotlib, 2008; Hirsch & Mathews, 1997, 2000; Huppert, Pasupuleti, Foa, & Mathews, 2007; Roth, Antony, & Swinson, 2001; Stopa & Clark, 2000). Hirsh, Clark, and Mathews (2006) describe how negatively biased self-imagery and interpretation biases may affect each other and also interact with each other to maintain SAD. Hirsch and Mathews (1997) originally made a distinction between on-line (i.e., in real time as a situation unfolds) and off-line (i.e., on reflection or in anticipation of a situation) interpretation bias. The literature strongly supports an off-line negative interpretation bias in SAD. However, Hirsch and Mathews (2000) demonstrated that this is not the case on-line (when having to make snap decisions about ambiguous passages of text in a lexical decision task). In fact, nonanxious persons demonstrated a bias toward positive resolutions, and socially anxious persons demonstrated no on-line bias at all. Hirsch, Mathews, Clark, Williams, and Morrison (2003) demonstrated that imagery could replicate the same pattern of group differences. Low anxious participants read the same passages about job interviewing as used in the previous studies, either while holding a negative self-image in mind or without any specific instruction about images. The no-instruction group showed the expected positive bias, whereas the low anxious participants instructed to hold a negative image in mind showed no on-line bias, as had been demonstrated for socially anxious persons in the previous studies.

Interpretation also influences imagery, as demonstrated by Hirsch, Mathews, and Clark (2007). Low anxious participants were allocated to one of two training conditions designed to induce either a benign or a negative interpretation bias (reading ambiguous scenarios that were routinely resolved in either a benign or negative manner). They then read additional ambiguous scenarios and generated images of themselves in those situations. Those previously exposed to the negative resolutions generated significantly more unpleasant imagery than those exposed to the benign resolutions, and this was the case in terms of ratings conducted both by the participants and by objective observers. This group also rated their anxiety as higher and their performance as poorer in a hypothetical social situation (leading a seminar discussion) than the group exposed to the benign resolutions.

As demonstrated by the latter two studies, imagery and interpretation biases can each influence the other. As Hirsch, Clark, and Mathews (2006) point out, it is not a great leap to suggest that this influence is reciprocal and that this reciprocal effect may play a role in the maintenance of SAD. If we think back to the description of the images reported by participants with SAD in Hackmann et al. (1998, 2000), these were extreme and quite distorted. It is likely that the original event was interpreted in a negatively exaggerated manner and that this was incorporated into the reported image with the exaggeration intact. To the extent that these images are recurrent, they are analogous to the negative images held in mind in many of the studies described in this chapter, and they may have acted to over-ride any positive inferential bias or to block the receipt of positive information from the social environment. Of course, this latter piece is speculative and awaits further research.

Another cognitive process that has been hypothesized to be influenced by imagery is memory. Stopa and Jenkins (2007), in a study described in part above, strove to test the relationship between imagery and autobiographical memory bias in a socially anxious undergraduate sample. Participants imagined they had a mirror, pictured a positive or negative image of themselves in the mirror, in a within-subjects design, and held that image in mind while giving a brief impromptu speech. Following the speech, the participants were asked to recall a specific memory for 15 positive, negative, and neutral words. The participants completed the procedure twice, in counterbalanced order on two different days, separated by a week. The valence of imagery influenced the valence of one's autobiographical memories. Individuals were quicker to retrieve negative memories when they had previously held a negative image of themselves in mind and they were quicker to retrieve a positive memory when they had held a positive image in mind. They also showed a delayed response in retrieving positive memories when holding a negative image in mind. Activation of a negative cognitive image facilitated retrieval of congruent memories and slowed retrieval of incongruent memories. Again, it is not hard to imagine that this pattern would support an anxious response to an upcoming social event.

In a study by Hertel et al. (2008, Experiment 1), participants with SAD were presented with a number of social and nonsocial scenarios and asked to provide endings to these stories (termed "continuations" by the authors). Continuations were more likely to be negatively biased among socially anxious participants compared to controls. Furthermore, and most importantly here, participants were asked to recall these scenarios, and the frequency and type of intrusions were examined. Socially anxious participants were more likely than controls to demonstrate intrusions that were consistent with the biased interpretations that they had made at the earlier point in the study. That is, biased interpretations provided by the participants had become part of their memories for the scenarios themselves. This is an important finding that embodies the potential clinical significance of the combined cognitive biases hypothesis, as the socially anxious participants' "memory" was, in fact, a troubled mix of memory of the scenario and of the socially anxious or negative continuations they had provided. One could easily envision other source-monitoring errors in social situations, arising from the effects of one cognitive bias on another; e.g., an attentional bias toward threat may stimulate an increased frequency of threat detection as well as a greater likelihood of interpretation of ambiguous social events as threatening, resulting in memory for these events as more threatening than was actually the case and contributing to greater anxiety in anticipation of the next social situation that occurs in the individual's life.

FEAR OF POSITIVE EVALUATION

Over the past few years, our research group has examined a phenomenon we have referred to as the FPE and have developed the Fear of Positive Evaluation Scale (FPES) for its measurement (Weeks, Heimberg, & Rodebaugh, 2008; Weeks, Heimberg, Rodebaugh, & Norton, 2008; Weeks, Norton, & Heimberg, 2009; Weeks, Rodebaugh, Heimberg, Norton, & Jakatdar, 2009; Weeks, Jakatdar, & Heimberg, 2010). Fear of negative evaluation is typically thought of as a core feature of SAD, but our research suggests that it may be any type of evaluation that is feared by persons with SAD.

FPE can occur through a number of pathways, one of which is that successful social performance may activate the belief that others will expect continued success in future social interactions, but the person may doubt his or her ability to meet these increased expectations. For example, Wallace and Alden (1997) demonstrated that a manipulation designed to give participants the sense that they had succeeded in a social interaction actually led to predictions of reduced success in a future interaction among socially anxious participants. This outcome appeared to be related to their judgments that others' expectations for them would go up but that their ability to perform successfully had not changed. However, FPE, as we have conceptualized it, derives from a psycho-evolutionary perspective on SAD. Gilbert (2001) proposed that social anxiety is an evolutionary mechanism that facilitates nonviolent interactions between individuals and suggested that SAIs may fear increases in status that could lead to conflict with more powerful others. Gilbert further suggested that SAIs may fear that they will not be able to maintain or defend social gains in the future and dubbed this concept the "fear of doing well" (p. 742).

FPE is correlated with fear of negative evaluation (FNE), but confirmatory factor analyses of the combined FPES–FNE item pool have yielded separate factors (Weeks, Heimberg, & Rodebaugh, 2008; Weeks et al., 2010). FPE also contributes unique variance to the prediction of social anxiety, after accounting for the variance contributed by FNE (Weeks, Heimberg, & Rodebaugh, 2008; Weeks, Heimberg, Rodebaugh, & Norton, 2008). Furthermore, FPE predicted response to a bogus personality test. Participants were asked to write an open-ended paragraph on a subject of their choosing and were informed that expert raters trained in the personality assessment technique would examine their paragraphs and provide them with personality profiles based on their responses. They were later provided with a profile consisting of 10 identical feedback statements that were positively oriented and pertained to a wide range of social-evaluative contexts. Participants high in FPE expressed greater discomfort in receiving this positive feedback and less certainty about its accuracy (Weeks, Heimberg, Rodebaugh, & Norton, 2008); FNE did not predict these responses. Importantly, the FPES has shown strong psychometric characteristics in all of our studies, and treatment-seeking individuals with SAD score higher on the FPES than individuals with other anxiety disorders (Fergus et al., 2009).

EMOTION DYSREGULATION IN SOCIAL ANXIETY DISORDER

Difficulties in emotion regulation have been related to a number of different emotional disorders (Campbell-Sills & Barlow, 2007; Kring & Sloan, 2010). As of yet, there is little research on this topic as it relates to SAD. However, the studies that have been conducted suggest that this may be a fruitful area for continued research and investigation.

In one of our studies on emotion dysregulation in GAD, socially anxious participants served as a comparison group (Turk, Heimberg, Luterek, Mennin, & Fresco, 2005). Individuals with GAD reported greater intensity of felt emotion and fear of the experience of depression than socially anxious persons and nonanxious controls. More importantly in this context, SAIs indicated being less expressive of positive emotions, paying less attention to their emotions, and having more difficulty describing their emotions than either persons with GAD or controls.

The finding that SAIs were less expressive of positive emotions suggests that their attempts to regulate their emotions may have interpersonal effects. In fact, Meleshko and Alden (1993) demonstrated that socially anxious persons were less likely than nonanxious participants to reciprocate the self-disclosures of interaction partners. The self-protective behaviors of the socially anxious participants were associated with less liking and more discomfort on the part of their partners.

Socially anxious persons may also be less expressive of negative emotions, such as anger (Erwin, Heimberg, Schneier, & Liebowitz, 2003). Compared to nonanxious controls, treatment-seeking persons with SAD demonstrated higher scores on a number of anger scales (e.g., intensity of situationally experienced anger and disposition to experience anger in a wide range of situations). However, when it came to expression of those angry feelings, persons with SAD were more likely than controls to suppress them or direct them toward themselves. Interestingly, greater anger suppression predicted poorer response to CBT.

In another study (Spokas, Luterek, & Heimberg, 2009), socially anxious undergraduates reported greater use of emotional suppression than their non-socially anxious peers. They also reported greater ambivalence about emotional expression, more difficulties in emotional responding, more fears of emotional experiences, and more negative beliefs about emotional expression. The belief that emotional expression must be kept in control and is a sign of weakness partially mediated the association between social anxiety and emotional suppression. These beliefs may play a role in the inhibition of self-disclosure reported by Meleshko and Alden (1993) and of anger reported by Erwin et al. (2003).

Werner, Goldin, Ball, Heimberg, and Gross (2010) examined the responses of individuals with SAD and nonanxious controls to an interview based on Gross' (1998) model of emotion regulation. Participants were interviewed about their emotional reactivity and regulation during a laboratory speech task and two social anxiety-evoking situations that had occurred during the past month. Compared to controls, clients with SAD reported greater use of avoidance and expressive suppression. They also reported less success in implementing cognitive reappraisal and expressive suppression strategies. These regulation deficits were not accounted for by differences in emotional reactivity.

Studies are beginning that attempt to map emotion regulation deficits onto specific brain regions using fMRI (e.g., Goldin, Manber, Hakimi, Canli, & Gross, 2009; Goldin, Manber-Ball, Werner, Heimberg, & Gross, 2009), but space limitations preclude a review of these preliminary studies. The studies reviewed here, however, build a case that persons with SAD inhibit the expression of a range of emotions in an attempt to control the potentially negative social consequences of that expression (e.g., rejection, negative evaluation), although they may not believe they do so very effectively, and these attempts at suppression may interfere with their interpersonal functioning. This line of thinking suggests that expressive suppression may be considered a form of safety behavior, as described by Wells et al. (1995) and Clark (2001), and that safety behaviors may serve an emotion regulatory function.

IMPLICATIONS FOR THE RAPEE–HEIMBERG MODEL OF SOCIAL ANXIETY DISORDER

After reviewing Rapee and Heimberg's (1997) model of SAD, we have examined the literatures on imagery and imagery perspective in socially anxious persons, those persons' tendency to engage in PEP, the ways in which one cognitive bias may affect another or the ways in which two cognitive biases may interact to maintain SAD, FPE, and emotion dysregulation and suppression among persons with SAD. What are the implications of these diverse literatures for our thinking about SAD?

Imagery can be very powerful among anxious persons; in fact, anxiety disorders in general could be easily characterized as disorders of imagination. Now, however, it is clear that imagery in SAD is intense and negatively biased. It is likely to be experienced from the observer perspective, especially in high-anxiety situations, and the likelihood of taking this perspective increases over time. Persons with SAD may carry images of social events with unfortunate outcomes with them into new situations. These images may predispose them toward anticipatory anxiety or, to the extent that they persist, heightened anxiety and expectations of negative outcomes throughout these situations. Negative images held in mind during social interactions or speeches are causally related to heightened anxiety, reduced ratings of performance, and increased physical sensations. It is unlikely that such negatively biased imagery could have anything but a deflating effect on the mental representation of the self as seen by the audience. This effect and others are reflected in Figure 15.2, which updates the original figure in some respects.

PEP is similar to the apocryphal story of the child who takes a clock apart but, in putting it back together again, ends up with two clocks rather than one. The point here is that PEP is a reconstructive event. The memory of the original event changes each time it is taken apart and put back together again, and it is likely that it is more horrific than it was in its previous iteration. What was once a perceived unpleasant event becomes a nightmarish memory, and, with continued rehearsal, a virtual certainty to repeat itself when the next situation occurs – in a sense, it is no longer a memory but rather a feared outcome. It is likely that this process is tied into the imagery of the socially anxious person as described above, and it may well be involved in many instances of combined cognitive bias described below. As regards the Rapee–Heimberg model, which was put forth as an attempt to explain the psychological experience of the person with SAD *within a situation*, the most important aspect of PEP would appear to be that it not only occurs in response to situations past, but also can be activated in response to situations in the future, as the person reviews past mis-steps so as to avoid future ones. This process would appear to be very important in explaining how social anxiety maintains over time – PEP provides the bridge from the socially anxious past to the socially anxious future. Although we consider this a very important aspect of the updated model, it is not reflected in Figure 15.2.

The combined cognitive biases hypothesis put forth by Hirsch, Clark, and Mathews (2006) is a very important hypothesis for continued research. The several studies reviewed in that section show well how negative imagery and interpretation biases may influence each other and how each may affect memory bias. Although it has not yet been systematically studied, it is also very likely that biased attention toward threat is influenced by interpretation bias (there will be more threat to find!) and that this combination will have an influence on memory. Memory bias should then increase the likelihood of biased attention toward threat as the person moves into the future.

Research on the FPE is in its earliest stages. We are still learning about its basic nature, its correlates, and its ultimate role in social anxiety. Conclusions about FPE are limited by the early stage in the research and also by the fact that there is currently only a single instrument for its assessment. However,

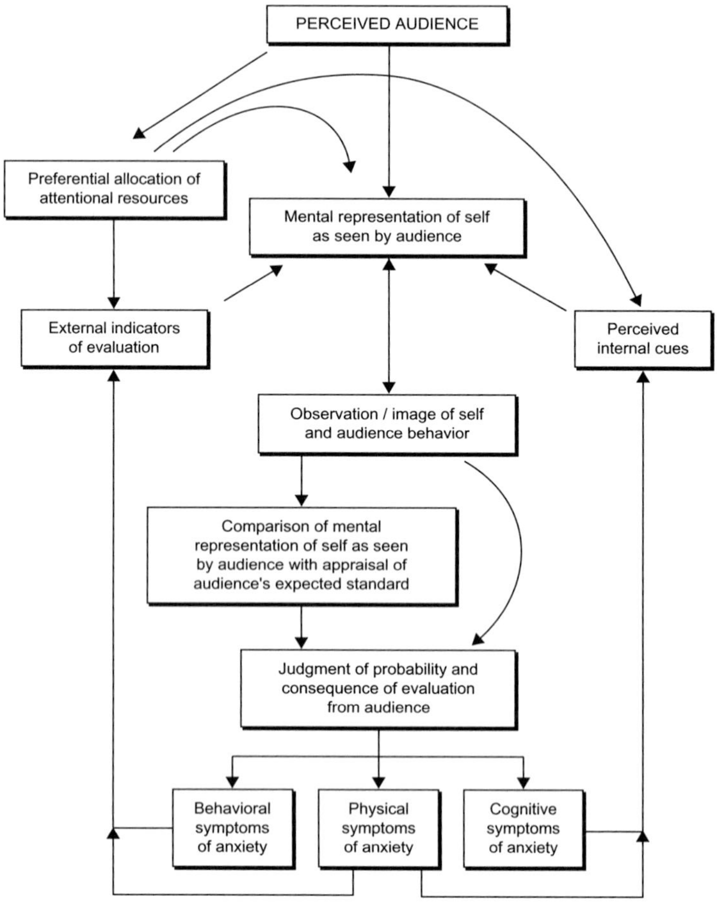

FIGURE 15.2 An updated cognitive behavioral model of social anxiety disorder. *(Adapted from Behaviour Research and Therapy, 35, R. M. Rapee & R. G. Heimberg, A cognitive-behavioral model of anxiety in social phobia, page 743. Copyright 1997, with kind permission from Elsevier.)*

the research to date on FPE makes one thing quite clear. It is not only negative evaluation that is feared by persons with SAD. Positive evaluation is also feared, because it may predict later negative evaluation, because it may predict an evolutionarily determined need to protect one's resources or status, because it may put the person in conflict with others, or for other reasons yet to be determined. FPE is correlated with, but distinct from, FNE, and it contributes unique variance to the prediction of social anxiety. SAD may be better characterized as a fear of evaluation than as a fear of negative evaluation.

Emotion regulation is an essential part of normal human functioning, but it can go wrong in myriad ways and it appears to do so in SAD. Again, this is a relatively new area of inquiry, but it appears that an important means of emotion regulation in SAD is expressive suppression; that is, actively deciding not to express an emotion (not at all limited to anxiety) in an interpersonal context as a means of warding off unwanted consequences (e.g., potential rejection pursuant to self-disclosure of positive emotions or possible angry retaliation or negative evaluation pursuant to expressed anger). Persons with SAD believe that expression is dangerous and therefore suppression is wise, although they do not believe they do it very well. These choices are made to minimize negative outcomes, but there is some evidence to suggest that they bring on other negative consequences (the person may be less liked by others, who themselves may feel less comfortable interacting with the socially anxious person; Meleshko & Alden, 1993; see also Butler et al., 2003). Like other safety behaviors, expressive suppression may rob the person of the opportunity to observe that feared consequences may not occur or, if they do occur, they may do so in a manner less extreme than imagined – which brings us full circle back to imagery.

Each of the five areas reviewed in this chapter inform the model of SAD put forth by Rapee and Heimberg (1997). It will be important to evaluate changes to the model in future research with well delineated hypotheses that test the specific actions and interactions posed herein.

REFERENCES

Abbott, M. J., & Rapee, R. M. (2004). Post-event rumination and negative self-appraisal in social phobia before and after treatment. *Journal of Abnormal Psychology*, *113*, 136–144.

Acarturk, C., de Graaf, R., van Straten, A., ten Have, M., & Cuijpers, P. (2008). Social phobia and number of social fears, and their association with comorbidity, health-related quality of life and help seeking: A population-based study. *Social Psychiatry and Psychiatric Epidemiology*, *43*, 273–279.

Acarturk, C., Smit, F., de Graaf, R., van Straten, A., ten Have, M., & Cuijpers, P. (2009). Economic costs of social phobia: A population-based study. *Journal of Affective Disorders*, *115*, 421–429.

Acosta, A., & Vila, J. (1990). Emotional imagery: Effect of autonomic response information on physiological arousal. *Cognition and Emotion*, *4*, 145–160.

American Psychiatric Association. (1980). *Diagnostic and statistical manual of mental disorders* (3rd ed.) (DSM-III). Washington, DC: Author.

American Psychiatric Association. (1994). *Diagnostic and statistical manual of mental disorders* (4th ed.) (DSM-IV). Washington, DC: Author.

American Psychiatric Association. (2000). *Diagnostic and statistical manual of mental disorders* (4th ed., text revision) (DSM-IV-TR). Washington, DC: Author.

Amir, N., Foa, E. B., & Coles, M. E. (1998). Negative interpretation bias in social phobia. *Behaviour Research and Therapy*, *36*, 959–970.

Brozovich, F., & Heimberg, R. G. (2008). An analysis of post-event processing in social anxiety disorder. *Clinical Psychology Review*, *28*, 891–903.

Brozovich, F., & Heimberg, R. G. (2010). The relationship of post-event processing to self-evaluation of performance in social anxiety. Manuscript submitted for publication.

Bruce, S. E., Yonkers, K. A., Otto, M. W., Eisen, J. L., Weisberg, R. B., Pagano, M., et al. (2005). Influence of psychiatric comorbidity on recovery and recurrence in generalized anxiety disorder, social phobia, and panic disorder: A 12-year prospective study. *American Journal of Psychiatry*, *162*, 1179–1187.

Butler, E. A., Egloff, B., Wilhelm, F. H., Smith, N., Erickson, E. A., & Gross, J. J. (2003). The social consequences of expressive suppression. *Emotion*, *3*, 48–67.

Campbell-Sills, L., & Barlow, D. H. (2007). Incorporating emotion regulation into conceptualizations and treatments of anxiety and mood disorders. In J. J. Gross (Ed.), *Handbook of emotion regulation* (pp. 542–559). New York: Guilford Press.

Chartier, M. J., Hazen, A. L., & Stein, M. B. (1998). Lifetime patterns of social phobia: A retrospective study of the course of social phobia in a nonclinical population. *Depression and Anxiety*, *7*, 113–121.

Clark, D. M. (2001). A cognitive perspective on social phobia. In W. R. Crozier & L. E. Alden (Eds.), *International handbook of social anxiety: Concepts, research, and interventions relating to the self and shyness* (pp. 405–430). New York: John Wiley & Sons.

Clark, D. M., & Wells, A. (1995). A cognitive model of social phobia. In R. G. Heimberg, M. R. Liebowitz, D. A. Hope, & F. R. Schneier (Eds.), *Social phobia: Diagnosis, assessment, and treatment* (pp. 69–93). New York: Guilford Press.

Coles, M. E., Turk, C. L., & Heimberg, R. G. (2002). The role of memory perspective in social phobia: Immediate and delayed memories for role-played situations. *Behavioural and Cognitive Psychotherapy*, *30*, 415–425.

Coles, M. E., Turk, C. L., Heimberg, R. G., & Fresco, D. M. (2001). Effects of varying levels of anxiety within social situations: Relationship to memory perspective and attributions in social phobia. *Behaviour Research and Therapy*, *39*, 651–665.

Dannahy, L., & Stopa, L. (2007). Post-event processing in social anxiety. *Behaviour Research and Therapy*, *45*, 1207–1219.

Duval, S., & Wicklund, R. A. (1972). *A theory of objective self-awareness*. Oxford: Academic Press.

Edwards, S. L., Rapee, R., & Franklin, J. (2003). Post-event rumination and recall bias for social performance event in high and low socially anxious individuals. *Cognitive Therapy and Research*, *27*, 603–617.

Erwin, B. A., Heimberg, R. G., Marx, B. P., & Franklin, M. E. (2006). Traumatic and socially stressful life events among persons with social anxiety disorder. *Journal of Anxiety Disorders*, *20*, 896–914.

Erwin, B. A., Heimberg, R. G., Schneier, F. R., & Liebowitz, M. R. (2003). Anger experience and expression in social anxiety disorder: Pretreatment profile and predictors of attrition and response to cognitive-behavioral treatment. *Behavior Therapy*, *34*, 331–350.

Fehm, L., Hoyer, J., Schneider, G., Lindemann, C., & Klusmann, U. (2008). Assessing post-event processing after social situations: A measure based on the cognitive model for social phobia. *Anxiety, Stress, and Coping*, *21*, 129–142.

Fehm, L., Schneider, G., & Hoyer, J. (2007). Is post-event processing specific for social anxiety? *Journal of Behavior Therapy and Experimental Psychiatry*, *38*, 11–22.

Fergus, T. A., Valentiner, D. P., McGrath, P. B., Stephenson, K., Stephanie Gier, S., & Jencius, S. (2009). The Fear of Positive Evaluation Scale: Psychometric properties in a clinical sample. *Journal of Anxiety Disorders*, *23*, 1177–1183.

Field, A. P., & Morgan, J. (2004). Post-event processing and the retrieval of autobiographical memories in socially anxious individuals. *Journal of Anxiety Disorders*, *18*, 647–663.

Frank, M. G., & Gilovich, T. (1989). The effect of memory perspective on retrospective causal attributions. *Journal of Personality and Social Psychology*, *57*, 399–403.

Gilbert, P. (2001). Evolution and social anxiety: The role of attraction, social competition, and social hierarchies. *Psychiatric Clinics of North America*, *24*, 723–751.

Goldin, P. R., Manber, T., Hakimi, S., Canli, T., & Gross, J. J. (2009). Neural bases of social anxiety disorder: Emotional reactivity and cognitive regulation during social and physical threat. *Archives of General Psychiatry*, *66*, 170–180.

Goldin, P. R., Manber-Ball, T., Werner, K., Heimberg, R., & Gross, J. J. (2009). Neural mechanisms of cognitive reappraisal of negative self-beliefs in social anxiety disorder. *Biological Psychiatry*, *66*, 1091–1099.

Gross, J. J. (1998). The emerging field of emotion regulation: An integrative review. *Review of General Psychology*, *2*, 271–299.

Hackmann, A., Clark, D. M., & McManus, F. (2000). Recurrent images and early memories in social phobia. *Behaviour Research and Therapy*, *38*, 601–610.

Hackmann, A., Surawy, C., & Clark, D. M. (1998). Seeing yourself through others' eyes: A study of spontaneously occurring images in social phobia. *Behavioural and Cognitive Psychotherapy*, *26*, 3–12.

Heimberg, R. G., Rapee, R. M., & Turk, C. L. (2002). A cognitive-behavioral formulation of social phobia. In R. G. Heimberg & R. E. Becker (Eds.), *Cognitive-behavioral group therapy for social phobia: Basic mechanisms and clinical strategies* (pp. 93–106). New York: Guilford Press.

Hertel, P. T., Brozovich, F., Joormann, J., & Gotlib, I. H. (2008). Biases in interpretation and memory in generalized social phobia. *Journal of Abnormal Psychology*, *117*, 278–288.

Hirsch, C. R., Clark, D. M., & Mathews, A. (2006). Imagery and interpretations in social phobia: Support for the combined cognitive biases hypothesis. *Behavior Therapy*, *37*, 223–236.

Hirsch, C. R., Clark, D. M., Mathews, A., & Williams, R. (2003). Self-images play a causal role in social phobia. *Behaviour Research and Therapy*, *41*, 909–921.

Hirsch, C. R., & Mathews, A. (1997). Interpretative inferences when reading about emotional events. *Behaviour Research and Therapy*, *35*, 1123–1132.

Hirsch, C. R., & Mathews, A. (2000). Impaired positive inferential bias in social phobia. *Journal of Abnormal Psychology*, *109*, 705–712.

Hirsch, C. R., Mathews, A., & Clark, D. M. (2007). Inducing an interpretation bias changes self-imagery: A preliminary investigation. *Behaviour Research and Therapy*, *45*, 2173–2181.

Hirsch, C. R., Mathews, A., Clark, D. M., Williams, R., & Morrison, J. (2003). Negative self-imagery blocks inferences. *Behaviour Research and Therapy*, *41*, 1383–1396.

Hirsch, C. R., Mathews, A., Clark, D. M., Williams, R., & Morrison, J. A. (2006). The causal role of negative imagery in social anxiety: A test in confident public speakers. *Journal of Behaviour Therapy and Experimental Psychiatry*, *37*, 159–170.

Hirsch, C. R., Meynen, T., & Clark, D. M. (2004). Negative self-imagery in social anxiety contaminates social interactions. *Memory*, *12*, 496–506.

Hofmann, S. G. (2007). Cognitive factors that maintain social anxiety disorder: A comprehensive model and its treatment implications. *Cognitive Behaviour Therapy*, *36*, 193–209.

Holmes, E. A., & Mathews, A. (2005). Mental imagery and emotion: A special relationship? *Emotion*, *5*, 489–497.

Holmes, E. A., Mathews, A., Dalgleish, T., & Mackintosh, B. (2006). Positive interpretation training: Effects of mental imagery versus verbal training on positive mood. *Behavior Therapy*, *37*, 297–305.

Huppert, J. D., Pasupuleti, R. V., Foa, E. B., & Mathews, A. (2007). Interpretation biases in social anxiety: Response generation, response selection, and self-appraisals. *Behaviour Research and Therapy*, *45*, 1505–1515.

Ickes, W. J., Wicklund, R. A., & Ferris, C. B. (1973). Objective self-awareness and self-esteem. *Journal of Experimental and Social Psychology*, *9*, 202–219.

Kashdan, T. B., & Roberts, J. E. (2007). Social anxiety, depressive symptoms, and post-event rumination: Affective consequences and social contextual influences. *Journal of Anxiety Disorders*, *21*, 284–301.

Kessler, R. C., Berglund, P., Demler, O., Jin, R., Merikangas, K. R., & Walters, E. E. (2005). Lifetime prevalence and age-of-onset distributions of DSM-IV disorders in the National Comorbidity Survey Replication. *Archives of General Psychiatry*, *62*, 593–768.

Kessler, R. C., Chiu, W. T., Demler, O., Merikangas, K., & Walters, E. E. (2005). Prevalence, severity, and comorbidity of 12-month DSM-IV disorders in the National Comorbidity Survey Replication. *Archives of General Psychiatry*, *62*, 617–627.

Kimbrel, N. A. (2008). A model of the development and maintenance of generalized social phobia. *Clinical Psychology Review*, *28*, 592–612.

Kocovski, N. L., Endler, N. S., Rector, N. A., & Flett, G. L. (2005). Ruminative coping and post-event processing in social anxiety. *Behaviour Research and Therapy*, *43*, 971–984.

Kring, A. M., & Sloan, D. M. (Eds.), (2010). *Emotion regulation and psychopathology: A transdiagnostic approach to etiology and treatment*. New York: Guilford Press.

Lang, P. J. (1979). A bio-informational theory of emotional imagery. *Psychophysiology*, *16*, 495–512.

Lang, P. J., Levin, D. N., Miller, G. A., & Kozak, M. J. (1983). Fear imagery and the psychophysiology of emotion: The problem of affective response integration. *Journal of Abnormal Psychology*, *92*, 276–306.

Lundh, L., & Sperling, M. (2002). Social anxiety and post-event processing of socially distressing events. *Cognitive Behaviour Therapy*, *31*, 129–134.

MacLeod, C., & Mathews, A. (1991). Biased cognitive operations in anxiety: Accessibility of information or assignment of processing priorities? *Behaviour Research and Therapy*, *29*, 599–610.

Magee, W. J., Eaton, W. W., Wittchen, H.-U., McGonagle, K. A., & Kessler, R. C. (1996). Agoraphobia, simple phobia, and social phobia in the National Comorbidity Survey. *Archives of General Psychiatry*, *53*, 159–168.

McEvoy, P. M., & Kingsep, P. (2006). The Post-Event Processing Questionnaire in a clinical sample with social phobia. *Behaviour Research and Therapy*, *44*, 1689–1697.

McEvoy, P. M., Mahoney, A., Perini, S. J., & Kingsep, P. (2009). Changes in post-event processing and metacognitions during cognitive behavioral group therapy for social phobia. *Journal of Anxiety Disorders*, *23*, 617–623.

McNally, R. J. (1995). Automaticity and the anxiety disorders. *Behaviour Research and Therapy*, *33*, 747–754.

McTeague, L. M., Lang, P. J., Laplante, M., Cuthbert, B. N., Strauss, C. C., & Bradley, M. M. (2009). Fearful imagery in social phobia: Generalization, comorbidity, and physiological reactivity. *Biological Psychiatry*, *65*, 374–382.

Meleshko, K. G. A., & Alden, L. E. (1993). Anxiety and self-disclosure: Toward a motivational model. *Journal of Personality and Social Psychology*, *64*, 1000–1009.

Mellings, T. M. B, & Alden, L. E. (2000). Cognitive processes in social anxiety: The effects of self-focus, rumination and anticipatory processing. *Behaviour Research and Therapy*, *38*, 243–257.

Moscovitch, D. A. (2009). What is the core fear in social phobia?: A new model to facilitate individualized case conceptualization and treatment. *Cognitive and Behavioral Practice*, *16*, 123–134.

Nigro, G., & Neisser, U. (1983). Point of view in personal memories. *Cognitive Psychology*, *15*, 467–482.

Perini, S. J., Abbott, M. J., & Rapee, R. M. (2006). Perception of performance as a mediator in the relationship between social anxiety and negative post-event rumination. *Cognitive Therapy and Research*, *30*, 645–659.

Rachman, S., Grüter-Andrew, J., & Shafran, R. (2000). Post-event processing in social anxiety. *Behaviour Research and Therapy*, *38*, 611–617.

Rapee, R. M., & Abbott, M. J. (2007). Modelling relationships between cognitive variables during and following public speaking in participants with social phobia. *Behaviour Research and Therapy*, *45*, 2977–2989.

Rapee, R. M., & Heimberg, R. G. (1997). A cognitive-behavioral model of anxiety in social phobia. *Behaviour Research and Therapy*, *35*, 741–756.

Reich, J., Goldenberg, I., Vasile, R., Goisman, R., & Keller, M. (1994). A prospective follow-along study of the course of social phobia. *Psychiatry Research*, *54*, 249–258.

Rodebaugh, T. L. (2009). Social phobia and perceived friendship quality. *Journal of Anxiety Disorders*, *23*, 872–878.

Roth, D. A., Antony, M. M., & Swinson, R. P. (2001). Interpretations for anxiety symptoms in social phobia. *Behaviour Research and Therapy*, *39*, 129–138.

Roth, D. A., & Heimberg, R. G. (2001). Cognitive-behavioral models of social anxiety disorder. In F. R. Schneier (Ed.), *Psychiatric Clinics of North America: Vol. 24. Social anxiety disorder* (pp. 753–771). New York: W. B. Saunders Company.

Ruscio, A. M., Brown, T. A., Chiu, W. T., Sareen, J., Stein, M. B., & Kessler, R. C. (2008). Social fears and social phobia in the USA: Results from the National Comorbidity Survey Replication. *Psychological Medicine*, *38*, 15–28.

Safren, S. A., Heimberg, R. G., Brown, E. J., & Holle, C. (1997). Quality of life in social phobia. *Depression and Anxiety*, *4*, 126–133.

Schlenker, B. R., & Leary, M. R. (1982). Social anxiety and self-presentation: A conceptualization and model. *Psychological Bulletin*, *92*, 641–669.

Schneier, F. R., Heckelman, L. R., Garfinkel, R., Campeas, R., Fallon, B. A., Gitow, A., et al. (1994). Functional impairment in social phobia. *Journal of Clinical Psychiatry*, *55*, 322–331.

Schneier, F. R., Johnson, J., Hornig, C. D., Liebowitz, M. R., & Weissman, M. M. (1992). Social phobia: Comorbidity and morbidity in an epidemiologic sample. *Archives of General Psychiatry*, *49*, 282–288.

Schultz, L. T., & Heimberg, R. G. (2008). Attentional focus in social anxiety disorder: Potential for interactive processes. *Clinical Psychology Review*, *28*, 1206–1221.

Spokas, M., Luterek, J. A., & Heimberg, R. G. (2009). Social anxiety and emotional inhibition: The mediating role of beliefs. *Journal of Behavior Therapy and Experimental Psychiatry*, *40*, 283–291.

Spurr, J. M., & Stopa, L. (2003). The observer perspective: Effects on social anxiety and performance. *Behaviour Research and Therapy*, *41*, 1009–1028.

Stopa, L., & Clark, D. M. (2000). Social phobia and interpretation of social events. *Behaviour Research and Therapy*, *38*, 273–283.

Stopa, L., & Jenkins, A. (2007). Images of the self in social anxiety: Effects on the retrieval of autobiographical memories. *Journal of Behavior Therapy and Experimental Psychiatry*, *38*, 459–473.

Tolman, R. M., Himle, J., Bybee, D., Abelson, J. L., Hoffman, J., & Van Etten-Lee, M. (2009). Impact of social anxiety disorder on employment among women receiving welfare benefits. *Psychiatric Services*, *60*, 61–66.

Turk, C. L., Heimberg, R. G., Luterek, J. A., Mennin, D. S., & Fresco, D. M. (2005). Emotion dysregulation in generalized anxiety disorder: A comparison with social anxiety disorder. *Cognitive Therapy and Research*, *29*, 89–106.

Turk, C. L., Lerner, J., Heimberg, R. G., & Rapee, R. M. (2001). An integrated cognitive-behavioral model of social anxiety. In S. G. Hofmann & P. M. DiBartolo (Eds.), *From social anxiety to social phobia: Multiple perspectives* (pp. 281–303). Needham Heights, MA: Allyn & Bacon.

Vassilopoulos, S. (2005). Social anxiety and the effects of engaging in mental imagery. *Cognitive Therapy and Research*, *29*, 261–277.

Vrana, S. R., Cuthbert, B. N., & Lang, P. J. (1986). Fear imagery and text processing. *Psychophysiology*, *23*, 247–253.

Wallace, S. T., & Alden, L. E. (1997). Social phobia and positive social events: The price of success. *Journal of Abnormal Psychology*, *106*, 416–424.

Watson, D., & Friend, R. (1969). Measurement of social-evaluative anxiety. *Journal of Consulting and Clinical Psychology*, *33*, 448–457.

Weeks, J. W., Heimberg, R. G., & Rodebaugh, T. L. (2008). The Fear of Positive Evaluation Scale: Assessing a proposed cognitive component of social anxiety disorder. *Journal of Anxiety Disorders*, *22*, 44–55.

Weeks, J. W., Heimberg, R. G., Rodebaugh, T. L., & Norton, P. J. (2008). Exploring the relationship between fear of positive evaluation and social anxiety. *Journal of Anxiety Disorders*, *22*, 386–400.

Weeks, J. W., Jakatdar, T. A., & Heimberg, R. G. (2010). Comparing and contrasting fears of positive and negative evaluation as facets of social anxiety. *Journal of Social and Clinical Psychology*, *29*, 68–94.

Weeks, J. W., Norton, P. J., & Heimberg, R. G. (2009). Exploring the latent structure of two cognitive components of social anxiety: Taxometric analyses of fears of negative and positive evaluation. *Depression and Anxiety*, *26*, E40–E48.

Weeks, J. W., Rodebaugh, T. L., Heimberg, R. G., Norton, P. J., & Jakatdar, T. A. (2009). "To avoid evaluation, withdraw": Fears of evaluation and depressive cognitions lead to social anxiety and submissive withdrawal. *Cognitive Therapy and Research*, *33*, 375–389.

Wells, A., Clark, D. M., & Ahmad, S. (1998). How do I look with my mind's eye: Perspective taking in social phobic imagery. *Behaviour Research and Therapy*, *36*, 631–634.

Wells, A., Clark, D. M., Salkovskis, P., Ludgate, J., Hackmann, A., & Gelder, M. (1995). Social phobia: The role of in-situation safety behaviors in maintaining anxiety and negative beliefs. *Behavior Therapy*, *26*, 153–161.

Wells, A., & Papageorgiou, C. (1999). The observer perspective: Biased imagery in social phobia, agoraphobia, and blood/injury phobia. *Behaviour Research and Therapy*, *37*, 653–658.

Werner, K. H., Goldin, P. R., Ball, T. M., Heimberg, R. G., & Gross, J. J. (2010). Emotion regulation in social anxiety disorder. Manuscript submitted for publication.

Whisman, M., Sheldon, C., & Goering, P. (2000). Psychiatric disorders and dissatisfaction with social relationships: Does type of relationship matter? *Journal of Abnormal Psychology*, *109*, 803–808.

Chapter 16

Social Anxiety, Social Anxiety Disorder, and the Self

Lynn E. Alden and Marci J. Regambal
Department of Psychology, University of British Columbia, Vancouver, BC, Canada

Knowing others is wisdom.
Knowing the self is enlightenment.
Lao Tzu

THE SELF

What is the self? This question has been pondered by the foremost scholars in philosophy, sociology, religion, and anthropology, as well as psychology. The self has been variously viewed as a unified being that is the source of consciousness (Locke, reprinted in 1997). Conversely, the self has been dismissed as an abstraction, a "convenient fiction," nothing more (or less) than a character in the stories we tell ourselves to make sense of our world (Dennett, 1992). In some mystical and eastern meditative traditions, the self is viewed as an illusion that must be dissolved through becoming aware of one's true nature. Interestingly, Buddhist thinking does not deny the existence of an "empirical self," i.e., thoughts and feelings, but rather the notion of a permanent, distinct entity; "self-control" is viewed as a quality of the enlightened mind or "great self" (e.g., Harvey, 1995). In contrast, Erik Ericksen (1968), working in the psychodynamic tradition, viewed the development of self-identity as essential to psychological adjustment and well-being. Those who fail to achieve a sense of personal identity remain in a state of identity diffusion, fated to stumble through life pursing goals not of their own choosing while caught up in hollow relationships. The neuroscientist Joseph LeDoux suggested that the self is the molecular changes in CNS synaptic receptor sites that occur in response to life experiences (LeDoux, 2002). Whether the self is viewed as an illusion, an essential goal in psychological development, a narrative character, or a molecular change, philosophers, scholars, scientists, and spiritual leaders have all felt compelled to address the nature of the self. If the self is a fiction, it appears to

Social Anxiety: Clinical, Developmental, and Social Perspectives. DOI: 10.1016/B978-0-12-375096-9.00016-X

be a fiction that humans feel the need to grapple with. That is also our task in the current chapter.

OVERVIEW

Self-related concepts figure prominently in contemporary clinical models of social anxiety disorder (Clark & Wells, 1995; Hofmann, 2007; Rapee & Heimberg, 1997). Among these are negative self-beliefs, self-focused attention, biased self-judgments, and negative self-images. While there is a growing body of clinical research on these concepts and the way in which they enter into SAD, we as clinical researchers have devoted relatively little attention to defining what we mean by "self" and articulating clear models of the nature of the "self" that is at the center of these processes. In contrast, writers in cognitive, social, and personality psychology have produced a burgeoning "self" literature in which they propose well-defined models of self and identify a number of critical unresolved questions about nature and core features of the self. Some of these writers have gone on to discuss how the self enters into social anxiety. In the following pages, we examine how the construct of self has been treated in theories of social anxiety and SAD.

To guide our efforts, we begin with a brief discussion of the notion of the self-schema presented in the social cognition literature. This literature underscores several core questions about the nature of self, which will form the framework within which we compare views of self arising from social-personality theories to those found in clinical theories of SAD. We end the chapter with a brief consideration of how these diverse views might inform each other to provide potential leads for future research.

A SOCIAL-COGNITIVE PERSPECTIVE

Contemporary views of the self are heavily influenced by self research in social cognition (e.g., Bargh, 1982; Markus, 1977). These writers view the self as an organized knowledge structure, or cognitive schema, that contains all known information about oneself (Markus, 1977). The self-schema includes information about our past experiences, current knowledge, feelings, beliefs, and self-related evaluations, as well as imaginary elements, such as our notions of the possible selves that we could become (Markus & Nurius, 1986). One of the enduring contributions made by these researchers is the recognition that information related to the self-schema is more readily processed and remembered: the so-called "self-reference effect" (e.g., Bargh, 1982; Higgins & Bargh, 1987; Klein & Loftus, 1988; Markus, 1977). Thus, the self-schema guides the way in which the person samples, processes, and evaluates information, which in turn influence decisions about future courses of action and the behavioral strategies necessary to achieve them, and tends to perpetuate existing views of self (see review by Ellemers, Spears, & Doosje, 2002).

Because the self-schema is viewed as an important determinant of human cognition and behavior, these writers have devoted attention to questions about its nature and structure. The first concerns whether information about the self is contained in a unified, cohesive schema or whether different types of self-knowledge are stored in separate, albeit interconnected, structures. Put another way, are we talking about a single self or multiple selves? Although the notion that self-knowledge is organized in multiple, context-specific structures is more widely accepted, unitary models also have their proponents (see Baumeister, 1999, for a discussion). Katzko (2003) suggested that the multiplicity–unitary debate arises from the reification of cognitive processes and experiences. He argues that proponents of the "multiple selves" perspective are actually referring to *objective* properties of the self (e.g., one's abilities, appearance), whereas the "unitary self" adherents are referring to the subjective sense of consciousness, continuity, and self-agency that characterizes the human experience. Following that distinction, we will define "multiple selves" to mean "multiple aspects" (facets) of the self-schema.

A second question pertains to the relationship between different facets of the self-schema. Some writers have argued that the harmony between various types of self-knowledge, or self-structures, is as important as their content. For example, incongruence between different self sub-structures, particularly the discrepancy between one's experienced self and internalized standards, has been found to increase susceptibility to negative emotional states (e.g., Carver & Scheier, 1986; Higgins, 1987).

Social cognitive researchers have also been interested in the paradox of how the self can be both stable and malleable. On one hand, self-concepts have been shown to be stable over time and context (e.g., Kihlstom & Cantor, 1984; Markus, 1977). On the other, social cognitivists generally believe that one's experience of self changes as situational cues and motivational factors activate different aspects of self-knowledge (e.g., McGuire, 1984). Nevertheless, most writers agree that some types of self-knowledge are chronically accessible; that is, more readily brought into consciousness or working memory due to frequent long-term use and therefore more likely to influence one's sense of self (e.g., Markus, 1977; Srull & Wyer, 1979).

A question of critical importance pertains to the type of information that is most central to an individual's sense of self. A body of research indicates that individuals differ in terms of how they construe themselves in relation to others. Some individuals construe themselves as independent or separate from others. When they self-reflect, they focus on their unique attributes; for example, their personal feelings and goals. Other individuals base their self-identity more on their social roles and relationships with other people; that is to say, they have a *relational* or *interdependent* sense of self (e.g., Cheek, 1989; Cross, Bacon & Morris, 2000; Cross, Morris & Gore, 2002; Greenwald & Pratkanis, 1984; Marcus & Kitayama, 1991). Among other things, people's predominant self-construal has been found to affect how they encode and organize information, interpret others' behavior, and select careers (e.g., Cross et al., 2002; Seta, Schmidt, & Bookhout, 2006; Seta, Seta & Hundt, 2001). Just as independent or relational information is more salient to different individuals, so too do different theories treat the self in an independent or relational manner. Writers who take a relational perspective assume that information about self and others is inherently connected and that consideration of the self requires consideration of the person's historical and current social context. In contrast, theorists who adopt an independent perspective emphasize other types of self-information; for example, personal beliefs, goals, and self-conscious emotions, such as pride and shame.

The issues raised in the social cognitive literature suggest several dimensions on which to compare social-personality theories of social anxiety with clinical theories of SAD. Is the self treated as a unitary or multidimensional entity? How does the theory deal with issues related to the organization of the self-schema? To what extent is the self viewed as stable or malleable? What types of self-related information are important in the theory; more specifically, does the theory take a relational or independent view of the self? We begin by considering the social anxiety literature, opening with a brief review of the intellectual tradition that gave rise to this body of work and then analyzing the role of the self, drawing on the questions identified above.

THEORETICAL AND RESEARCH PERSPECTIVES ON SOCIAL ANXIETY

Social anxiety theories integrate concepts from social cognition with the earlier writings of personality and dynamic theorists. The seminal writings of William James have been particularly influential (James, 1890). Among other contributions, James distinguished the "me" self – i.e., what is known about the self – from the "I" self – i.e., the "knower." He also introduced the notion of the private versus the social (public) self, and recognized that social situations can elicit different self-features.

> *[A man] has as many different social selves as there are distinct groups of persons about whose opinion he cares. He generally shows a different side of himself to each of these different groups.*
>
> James, 1890, chapter 10

These writings inspired generations of social and personality theorists to examine the motivational and behavioral ramifications of the social self (Baumeister, 1986; Leary, 2007).

Dynamic writers, from Freud onward, devoted considerable effort to explaining how the self develops within the context of familial and peer relationships. Interpersonal writers, such as Harry Stack Sullivan, argued that self is nothing other than the distillation of one's relationships with significant others (e.g., Sullivan, 1953). Contemporary object-relations and interpersonal dynamic theorists have continued this tradition in their depictions of the self as a psychic entity built around internalized representations of relationships with significant others. These internalized structures guide the way in which individuals perceive and behave in interpersonal encounters (e.g., Benjamin, 1996; Kernberg, 1976). The notion that the self contains internalized representations of significant others is also reflected in contemporary theories of social anxiety. We now consider three such theories, each of which describes the role of the self in social anxiety.

Social Anxiety Theories

The Strategic Self (Leary, 1995)

Leary's self-presentation model arises from James's distinction between the personal (private) and social (public) selves (Leary, 1995; Schlenker & Leary, 1982). The private self is defined as one's private subjective state of consciousness, including personal values, goals, thoughts, and feelings. The public self is less consistently defined, but is generally interpreted as one's perceptions of other people's impressions of oneself. Social anxiety arises when people are motivated to make a certain impression on others but doubt their ability to do so (Leary, 1995; Schlenker & Leary, 1982). When internal or external cues indicate a threat to the success of the person's social performance, the likelihood of conveying the desired image is evaluated. If this assessment process indicates that the desired impression is unlikely to be achieved, the person experiences social anxiety and either withdraws from the situation or adopts a cautious, innocuous, or noncommittal presentation to avoid disapproval. Thus, social anxiety triggers a switch from a socially acquisitive strategy, in which the person directs their efforts to garner approval, to a self-protective strategy, in which the person adopts behavior designed to avoid disapproval. The experience of social anxiety is thus envisioned as a secondary reaction, one that arises from situations (e.g., salient evaluation) or characteristics (e.g., inadequate social skills, need for approval, high standards) that heighten people's self-presentation concerns or activate doubts about success.

Research Focus

The research that flows from this model is unique in its emphasis on impression-management and social acceptance. Various studies have demonstrated that manipulations that increase such concerns affect social anxiety and social behavior (e.g., Depaulo, Epstein & LeMay, 1990; Leary, 1986; Leary & Kowalski, 1995; Maddux, Norton, & Leary, 1988). Another important contribution is the observation that the socially anxious individual can adopt a variety of behavioral strategies, not just social withdrawal or avoidance. For example, socially anxious people can engage in displays of innocuous sociability or even acquisitive behavior, such as initiating social interactions or disclosing personal information, if the circumstances are correct (e.g., Alden & Bieling, 1998; Arkin, 1981; Arkin, Lake & Baumgardner, 1986; Shepperd & Arkin, 1990). These findings support the idea that the person strategically selects various public behaviors to avoid social rejection and exclusion. A third theme that arises from this and related personality perspectives is that there are individual differences that predispose the person to social anxiety. Some of these relate to the self; for example, dispositional public self-consciousness (e.g., Buss, 1980) and the relative importance of the private and public selves (e.g., Cheek & Briggs, 1982; Seta et al., 2006). Overall, the notion of a bilateral (public/private) self directs research efforts toward studying when and how the public self becomes salient and the effects of this on social anxiety and interpersonal behavior.

The Discrepant Self (Strauman & Higgins, 1987)

Higgins and Strauman addressed social anxiety within the framework of their self-discrepancy theory, a variant of the self-regulation perspective on human behavior. According to these writers, the self consists of a number of different knowledge structures, most notably the "actual-self," the "ideal-self," and the "ought-self," each of which can be considered from the perspective of oneself or the perceived perspectives of others. The ideal and ought selves are viewed as standards, or self-guides, for the regulation of the actual-self. Self-regulation is a function of the dynamic relationships between various self-state representations. When the person perceives a significant discrepancy between the actual-self and these guides, he or she experiences emotional distress and attempts to reduce the discrepancy (Higgins, 1987). The "ought-other" self-representation is central to the experience of social anxiety. This sub-structure is based on parental expectations and represents the self one believes others think one ought to be. Social anxiety arises when the person becomes aware of a discrepancy between the actual and ought-other self-representations. This sense of incongruence triggers cognitive and behavioral processes designed to realign the two self-states.

Research Focus

Self-state researchers have been particularly interested in establishing that specific discrepancies evoke different types of emotional reactions. For example, Higgins and Strauman demonstrated that priming procedures that increased awareness of discrepancies between the actual-self and the ought-other self were uniquely predictive of arousal as opposed to depression (e.g., Higgins, Klein, & Strauman, 1985). They also found that actual–ought-other discrepancies distinguished patients with social phobia from those with depression (Strauman, 1989, 1992).

The Relational Self (Baldwin, 1992)

Baldwin's theory of social anxiety integrates concepts from social cognition with those drawn from dynamic interpersonal approaches. The focal point of this model is the notion of relational schemas, cognitive structures that represent regularities in past interactions with others. These relational schemas consist not only of representations of self and others but, more importantly, an interpersonal script, which represents "a sequence of actions and events that defines a stereotyped relational pattern" (Baldwin, 1992, p. 468). Part of the interpersonal script involves expectations about the thoughts, feelings, goals, and likely behaviors of the self and the other, as well as procedural knowledge, a set of rules about how to reach relevant goals. This procedural knowledge can be viewed as a set of "if–then" stipulations, such as "If I get close to others, then I will be hurt." A relational schema is activated by cues associated with the initial interpersonal episodes that led to schema formation. Consistent with the general concept of schematic processing, activation of a particular relational schema increases sensitivity to and efficiency in processing schema-consistent social information, which facilitates recall of this information, and bias interpretation of ambiguous information. Moreover, because the interpersonal script includes goals and proscribes specific actions, schema activation directly guides interpersonal behavior.

Baldwin proposed that negative social expectancies arise as the result of the activation of relational schemas involving social evaluation and disapproval. Individuals who have more extensive experience with disapproving others develop better-elaborated relational schema related to negative social outcomes, which are easily activated by cues associated with those early experiences. Once activated, these schemas lead to negative expectancies and subsequent social anxiety.

Research Focus

Baldwin's research has focused on studying priming strategies that activate different relational schemas and on showing that self and social information are inherently connected, an idea that supports the notion of a relational schema. Baldwin and colleagues found that procedures that prime social relationships, such as pictures, names, or visualization of significant others, lead to alterations in affect, self-esteem, and self-evaluation (e.g., Baldwin, 1994; Baldwin & Holmes, 1987; Baldwin, Carrell, & Lopez, 1990). Priming relational knowledge has also been shown to influence interpretation of social information and partner preference (Baldwin, Keelan, Fehr, Enns, & Koh-Rangarajoo, 1996). Directly relevant to social anxiety is a study demonstrating that even short-term disapproval established a negative relational schema that persisted across situations (Baldwin & Main, 2001). Consistent with Leary's theory, this effect was found only for individuals with high dispositional public self-consciousness.

Analysis

Social-personality theories are built on clearly delineated models of the self. Indeed, these theorists begin with a model of the self and then consider the way in which social anxiety fits into that model. Within all three perspectives, the self is envisioned as a multifaceted structure. Leary describes two distinct components, private and public, each of which contains various pieces of information. Higgins and Strauman view the self as a structured, multifaceted cognitive entity, the most critical aspect of which is the congruency of information contained within the various self-structures (Higgins, Klein, & Strauman, 1985). Baldwin envisions the person as having multiple "selves" that arise from the activation of various relational schemas.

Within all three theories, the self is viewed as malleable, with various self-features increasing or decreasing in salience depending on environmental circumstances. According to Leary, situational cues or dispositional tendencies shift the person's awareness to various private or public aspects of the self. As one's sense of self is altered, so too is one's affect, cognition, and behavior. In the Higgins–Strauman framework, one's subjective sense of self varies depending on which self-structures are most salient. Situational cues can also increase awareness of discrepancies between these structures. According to Baldwin, fluctuations in the cognitive accessibility of various relational schemas will lead to fluctuations in one's momentary sense of self. Thus, the self-schema consists of substructures containing different types of self-knowledge that can be activated by different internal and external cues resulting in changes in the person's experience and evaluation of self.

Perhaps the most striking aspect of the entire social-personality perspective is the importance of relational information to social anxiety and the emphasis on the contribution of social relationships to the development and content of the individual's sense of self. There is some variability in how the various writers envision relational information in the self-schema. Leary depicts the public self as incorporating information about others' expected reactions. This information is pivotal to the experience of social anxiety because it is when the public self becomes salient that social anxiety can emerge. Moreover, one of the primary goals of social anxiety is to maintain social connectedness, even at the expense of personal objectives. Self-discrepancy writers view the ought–other self as an internalized representation of the self that significant others want one to be, and it is the activation of this information that can evoke social anxiety. Baldwin envisions relational schemas as distillations of episodic memories of past relationships. Thus, one's sense of self is socially embedded, and one's experience of self and self-esteem derive from "who I am in this relationship." However depicted, all of these frameworks reflect the idea that information about the self is intertwined with information about others.

Recent social-personality writings provide a persuasive rationale for the evolutionary value of incorporating relational information in the self-schema (Leary, 2007; Leary & Baumeister, 2000). According to these writers, the desire for social acceptance, or, more accurately, the desire to avoid social exclusion, is one of the most powerful motives that drives human behavior, and people strategically manage their behavior in order to accomplish this end. A growing body of research underscores the emotional and physical consequences of social rejection. Social exclusion has been found to lower the individual's sense of emotional well-being, sense of life meaning, purpose, self-efficacy, and self-worth (Stillman et al., 2009; Zadro, Boland, & Richardson, 2006). Threats to the social self, for example, criticism, have been found to increase cortisol and proinflammatory cytokine activity (Dickerson, Gruenewald, & Kemeny, 2009; Gruenewald, Kemeny, Aziz, & Fahey, 2004) and thus may affect physical as well as emotional well-being. Moreover, socially anxious people appear to be particularly sensitive to social exclusion (e.g., Oaten, Williams, Jones, & Zadro, 2008; Zadro et al., 2006).

Leary proposed that self-esteem acts as a monitor of one's acceptability to the group: a "sociometer." A drop in self-esteem serves to warn the individual of potential social exclusion, so that the person can alter behavior or take other steps to avoid rejection (e.g., Leary, 2007; Leary, Tambor, Terdal, & Downs, 1995). Recent studies support these speculations in that social acceptability, as measured by others' liking or conversely by interpersonal conflict, was found to be a causal determinant of self-esteem; the reverse was also true (e.g., Denissen, Penke, Schmitt, & van Aken, 2008; Srivastava & Beer, 2005). Indeed, Leary argues that what are commonly labeled *self*-processes (e.g., self-enhancement, the tendency to over-value features associated with the self), as well as self-conscious emotions (e.g., shame, embarrassment, and pride) do not exist for the sake of the individual himself. Rather, they evolved to promote the individual's social connection to and acceptance by other people (e.g., Leary, 2007).

Finally, a distinctive feature of this viewpoint is that social anxiety serves the positive function of alerting the individual to possible threats to their social relationships and inhibits ongoing behavior to prevent further social damage. Self-protective behavioral strategies serve to maintain the person's contact with others while reducing the likelihood of disapproval. The desire to make a good impression arises in the service of the larger, more basic drive to avoid social exclusion.

The primary goal of these researchers has been to study how social events affect the development and experience of the self, the structure and content of the self-schema, and how activation of different self-elements affects behavior and emotions. They devote less attention to the clinical applications of these ideas. Leary (1995) proposed that clinicians should identify the specific personality or situational factors that create negative expectancies and impression concerns and tailor therapy to address them. Baldwin suggested that it may be possible to develop strategies that could be used to activate more positive types of relational information prior to social situations. He also noted that increasing patient awareness of chronically accessible relational schema may allow them to compensate for their effects (Baldwin, 1994). For example, if a patient becomes aware that he is prone to adopting the role of a criticized child even when this is unwarranted, he can learn to respond to such feelings with assertive behavior, rather than the anxious withdrawal that characterized his early relationships. Self-structure researchers have not addressed how self-discrepancies might be resolved and, therefore, the application of these ideas to treatment remains to be developed.

We turn now to the clinical domain, which has been explicitly driven by the search for clinical applications.

THEORETICAL AND RESEARCH PERSPECTIVES ON SOCIAL ANXIETY DISORDER

The behavioral revolution of the 1950s and 60s rejected the study of cognitive constructs and phenomena, such as self-identity and consciousness. The nadir of the construct was radical behaviorist attempts to operationalize the self as the set of verbal behaviors that contain the term "self" (Staats & Staats, 1964). The earliest modern-day theories of SAD were based on learning theory, and social fears were viewed as the result of conditioned anxiety or deficient social skills. The self, being a cognitive entity, played little role in these models, except perhaps as a passive observer of personal deficiencies.

Subsequent research revealed that people with SAD are not veridical observers of social events. Their social expectations and self-evaluations display biases that stem from the way in which they process social information, and these biases contribute to their social problems. Moreover, treatment studies indicated that behavioral treatments for SAD were enhanced by cognitive procedures (see Taylor, 1996). Accordingly, current theories of SAD incorporate cognitive factors, many of which are related to the self, and draw on basic cognitive research regarding selective attention and retrieval of information. Each theory has expanded the degree to which these processes relate to the self, and thus the self has received increasingly more attention. The theories began with the seminal work of A. T. Beck (Beck & Emery, 1985), which was followed, and expanded on, by D. M. Clark (Clark & Wells, 1995) and by Rapee and Heimberg (1997). Each perspective is reviewed below.

The Vulnerable Self (Beck, 1996; Beck & Emery, 1985)

Beck (1996) contends that different psychological disorders stem from the activation of different "personality modes," which comprise a series of structured cognitive schema. The anxiety disorders are hypothesized to stem from the activation of the vulnerability mode, which prepares the organism to cope with danger and enhances safety (Beck, 1996, p. 7). The specific thematic content of the danger schema, or what is feared, is postulated to be unique for each anxiety disorder.

For people with SAD, schemas used for processing social danger are hypervalent and readily activated by social scrutiny (Beck & Emery, 1985, chapter 9). The cognitive system comprises two levels. At the deepest level are core (i.e., unconditional) beliefs about the self (e.g., "I am inept") and primitive views of others (e.g., "Other people are evaluators who look for weakness"; Beck & Emery, 1985, p. 163). Closer to surface awareness are conditional rules (e.g., "If I mingle with others, I will be rejected"). Activation of the vulnerability mode also leads to behavioral inhibition and heightened anxiety, which interfere with effective social performance. Overall, a vicious cognitive-emotional cycle is created; schematic activation results in preferential processing of negative self and social information, which leads anxious people to perceive themselves and social events to be more negative than they actually are. In turn, ineffective social behavior and anxiety are interpreted as signs that the person is not meeting the social rules, which further increases the sense of vulnerability.

Cognitive behavioral treatment strategies stemming from this model are designed to modify inaccurate conditional rules and core beliefs, many of which focus on the self schema. Attention is devoted to first identifying the conditional rules that guide behavior and then working down to the underlying core beliefs (e.g., 1995) with an overall goal of modifying existing schema through the systematic collection of new information (e.g., behavioral experiments). The result is a more accurate schematic representation of oneself and other people. In turn, schematic modification is expected to correct biases in processing social information, thereby reducing social anxiety and avoidance.

Research Focus

It is not surprising that the research that flows from this model is directed toward establishing the thematic specificity of the relevant schema. Studies using the Stroop task revealed that patients with social phobia displayed greater interference when naming colors of words whose content reflected social threat rather than physical threat (e.g., Becker, Rinck, Margraf, & Roth, 2001; Mattia, Heimberg, & Hope, 1993; see, however, Amir et al., 1996), the opposite pattern of that found for panic disordered patients (e.g., Hope, Rapee, Heimberg, & Dombeck, 1990). Other studies have found that socially anxious and depressed people differ in the thematic content of their thoughts (Cho & Telch, 2005), but not in underlying beliefs or cognitive processes, such as self-focused attention (Sanz & Avia, 1994). Thus, specificity emerged more clearly in the content of surface cognitions rather than underlying cognitive features. It is notable that neither type of research distinguished self-related beliefs and processes.

The Distorted Self (Clark & Wells, 1995)

Clark and Wells's (1995) cognitive model of SAD is based on the notion of biased information processing. According to these writers, people with SAD hold negative assumptions (e.g., failure is likely and costly) and beliefs (e.g., "I'm inadequate") that lead to anxious apprehension prior to entering the social situation. These beliefs automatically activate an "anxiety program" designed to protect the person from harm. Once the program is activated, people with SAD direct attention to a detailed monitoring of themselves, particularly their anxiety-related internal sensations, thoughts, and behaviors. Another element in the model is the notion that people with SAD construct negative self-images, based in part on past events. They assume these images are veridical reflections of how they appear to other people. A key aspect of the model is the role of self-focused attention, which is postulated to increase the salience of negative self-related information at the expense of external information about the social situation. This process not only exacerbates anxiety, but also leads to negative biases in the person's social judgments both during and after the situation, particularly about the person's own performance. The adoption of safety behaviors, designed to avoid negative outcomes, contributes to this process by increasing anxiety and self-focused attention and preventing the disconfirmation of negative beliefs. Following social situations, individuals with SAD ruminate about the interaction, which results in further processing of negative self-related information, fixing it more permanently in memory. Finally, anxious apprehension prior to the next situation activates memories of previous failures, causing the cycle to begin again.

This theory leads directly to a number of specific treatment strategies. In particular, patients with SAD are encouraged to increase their exposure to feared situations, reduce their use of safety behaviors, and focus their attention outwardly to observe whether feared outcomes actually occur (e.g., Wells et al., 1995). The overall goal of this process is to disconfirm dysfunctional assumptions and misinterpretations of social events, thereby eliminating the negative self-beliefs and cognitive biases that perpetuate social fears.

Research Focus

Research arising from the model has been directed toward examining the cognitive behavioral processes involved in SAD, and establishing that these processes create or maintain biases in attention and social judgment. This work reveals that self-focus is initiated under conditions of social scrutiny (e.g., Alden, Teshuck, & Tee, 1992; Buss, 1980; see, however, Bögels & Lamers, 2002) and that under social threat these individuals direct their attention away from external stimuli (e.g., Chen, Ehlers, Clark, & Mansell, 2002; Mansell, Clark, Ehlers, & Chen, 1999; Mellings & Alden, 2000). Consistent with the model, when individuals are given feedback about increased physiological changes during a social interaction, whether true or not, they display increased self-focus and negative thoughts (Wells & Papageorgiou, 2001). Research further supports the existence of negative biases in their self and social judgments (e.g., Alden & Wallace, 1995; Lucock & Salkovskis, 1988; McEwan & Devins, 1983; Rapee & Lim, 1992; Stopa & Clark, 1993, 2000; Taylor & Alden, 2005; Voncken, Bögels, & Peeters, 2007).

Research on Clark and Wells's assertion that the individual creates an impression of self has been tested in the realm of self-imagery. Accordingly, individuals who are socially anxious are more likely to take an observer perspective than nonanxious individuals when recalling social events (Coles, Turk, Heimberg, & Fresco, 2001; Wells, Clark, & Ahmad, 1998; Wells & Papageorgiou, 1999). Furthermore, focusing on a negative self-image during social interactions plays a causal role in perceiving one's anxiety as more visible, rating one's own performance as poor, and observers rating the performance of the socially anxious person more negatively (Hirsch, Clark, Mathews, & Williams, 2003; Hirsch, Meynen, & Clark, 2004; Stopa & Jenkins, 2007). Interestingly, individuals high on social anxiety rate the negative image as more accurate of themselves than a positive image (Vassilopoulos, 2005).

The Threatened Self (Rapee & Heimberg, 1997)

According to Rapee and Heimberg (1997), people with SAD place a high value on being positively appraised by others, but at the same time assume that other people are inherently critical. When socially anxious individuals detect the presence of a perceived audience, they form a prediction of the standard the audience has for an acceptable performance. This standard will vary based on the particular audience (e.g., boss, friend) and situation (e.g., informal or formal setting). At the same time, they create a mental representation of their self, which is representative of what they think the audience perceives about them. However, this representation also takes into account external cues from the audience (e.g., yawning), and attention is allocated to *both* the self (e.g., appearance and behavior) and social environment for on-going social threat cues. The constant monitoring of both internal and external cues creates a feedback loop. For example, seeing an audience yawning could create an internal representation of the self as "boring" (Schultz & Heimberg, 2008), which would increase anxiety symptoms. Rapee and Heimberg's emphasis on externally focused attention, and the influence of external cues on the self, represents a major diversion from Clark and Wells's (1995) emphasis on interoceptive cues in forming an impression of the self.

Notably, the self-image is likely not objective. Attention is skewed to the negative aspects of the individual's self and to threatening audience behavior. This negative bias is problematic as it creates a gap between the individual's perception of the audience's standards for that situation and his or her perception of the audience's appraisal of their performance. It is from this discrepancy that the individual makes a prediction of the likelihood of negative evaluation and the social consequences of that evaluation.

Rapee and Heimberg (1997) make a number of treatment suggestions with the ultimate goal of incorporating new, more accurate information into the individual's self representation. These strategies include attention-training techniques that shift attention away from the self, and cognitive restructuring with a specific focus on a realistic appraisal of how the audience sees the individual (e.g., other people think I am boring) and their perceived expectations.

Notably, this is different from restructuring beliefs about how the individual sees themselves (e.g., I am a boring person), as outlined in the Beck and Emery (1985) model.

Research Focus

Because the Rapee–Heimberg model shares many features with the Clark–Wells model, the research findings reviewed above (e.g., self-focused attention, negative self-images) also support the Rapee–Heimberg model. The model has also led to research efforts to evaluate whether people with SAD do indeed display heightened vigilance to and processing of external threat cues. Indirect evidence for attention to external stimuli comes from studies that show an attentional bias for words describing anxiety symptoms that could be observed (e.g., blushing) versus those that could not (e.g., breathing; Spector, Pecknold, & Libman, 2003). Individuals with SAD were also found to display processing biases when asked to detect an angry face in pictures of neutral crowds, compared to a happy face in neutral crowds (e.g., Gilboa-Schechtman, Foa, & Amir, 1999; Gilboa-Schectman, Presburger, Marom, & Hermesh, 2005; Joorman & Gotlib, 2006). In addition, highly socially anxious individuals who gave a speech were found to selectively attend to negative, and ignore positive, behaviors from a real-life audience, even when both were present in equal numbers (e.g., Veljaca & Rapee, 1998; see, however, Perowne & Mansell, 2002).

Another unique research focus has been to examine the role of social developmental experiences in the development of SAD (see review by Rapee & Spence, 2004). This work points to the interpersonal learning experiences that result in heightened concern with social acceptability and negative beliefs about self and others. Finally, recent studies by Rapee have dealt more directly with the self. Wilson and Rapee (2005a) found that social anxiety was associated with the tendency to view negative social outcomes as indicative of negative self-characteristics and that change in such interpretations predicted treatment outcomes (Wilson & Rapee, 2005b). These writers also found that individuals with SAD displayed reduced subjective confidence and longer reaction times when rating the self-descriptiveness of personality characteristics, a pattern that pointed to them having less clarity about their self-concepts (Wilson & Rapee, 2006).

Analysis

Each of the models reviewed differs in the emphasis placed on constructs of the self (e.g., self-schema, self impressions) and how cognitive and behavioral processes influence the self, or vice versa. For Beck and Emery, the concept of self takes second place to the thematic content of the schema activated. In the case of SAD, the socially inept self-schema is a sub-unit of the vulnerability mode. Furthermore, when the vulnerability mode is activated, attention is directed to social danger cues from any source (e.g., speech problems, other people's facial expressions, large lecture room). Thus, the self-schema is apparently only one of the cognitive schema whose activation might trigger social anxiety.

In contrast to Beck, self-related processes are at the core of SAD in the models proposed by Clark and Wells (1995) and Rapee and Heimberg (1997). Clark and Wells emphasize self-focused attention, which leads to an exaggeration of negative aspects of the self, based mainly on interoceptive cues. Rapee and Heimberg, on the other hand, emphasize a feedback loop where a negative self-impression is formed and the attention to negative cues in the environment further reinforces this negative impression.

The theoretical emphasis on cognitive processes is reflected in clinical research activities. Empirical efforts focus on delineating how self-related cognitive processes perpetuate SAD, and on how these processes can be corrected. Cognitive behavioral strategies such as attention-training to overcome self-focused attention (Bögels, 2006) and behavioral experiments to collect objective information are implemented with the ultimate goal of correcting negatively biased self-judgments and negative self beliefs. Research findings support the assumption that cognitive behavioral strategies alter these processes and that changes in self-related cognitions mediate treatment response (e.g., Hofmann, Moscovitch, Kim, & Taylor, 2004; Schulz, Alpers, & Hofmann, 2008; Wilson & Rapee, 2005b).

Comparison of Domains

There are many similarities between social-personality theories of social anxiety and clinical theories of SAD. All refer to the self, whether conceptualized in terms of self-schema, self-concept, self-representation, or self-related beliefs. Individuals become socially anxious in large part because they are prone to view themselves as inadequate and unacceptable to others. The theories also agree that these individuals have had negative interpersonal experiences that are cognitively represented in some form and that social events can increase the salience of this stored knowledge. As a result, the person's perceptions of, and reactions to, current situations are altered, often in a negative direction, and lead to social anxiety.

As we consider each of the specific questions raised at the beginning of this chapter, some differences also emerge between the two domains. As noted earlier, social-personality theorists devote considerable attention to the structure of the self, whereas clinical theories historically have not. Within the social-personality literature, the self-schema is envisioned as consisting of sub-structures containing different types of self-information, the activation of which impact self-esteem and social behavior. Clinical theories do not explicitly address the structure of the self or a self-schema in a way that would give someone an overarching sense of self. The self is conceptualized as largely unidimensional in that the SAD theories focus on the negative aspects of oneself in social situations. Thus, there is little focus on the positive elements of self, or the self outside of social threat.

In regards to malleability, in social-personality theories, the person's sense of self is envisioned as complex and subject to changes in response to situational factors. Although clinical theories also discuss how social cues activate negative self-information, they direct greater attention to the subsequent cognitive and behavioral processes that operate to *maintain* this negative self-information and related social fears. Compared to other clinical models, Rapee and Heimberg conceptualize a more malleable self in social situations. They hypothesize that stored in long-term memory is a "baseline" image of the self derived from past experiences. However, this baseline image can be altered during social situations based on information from external cues. Moreover, the alteration can be positive if attention is redirected to positive cues or away from negative cues. Notably, all clinical models assert that one's self-schema can be changed through cognitive behavioral techniques.

Overall, social-personality theorists place greater emphasize on the role of relational information within the self-schema. Information (e.g., beliefs, evaluations) about the self is inherently entwined with information (e.g., expectations) about others. It is the activation of this self-in-relationship knowledge that triggers social anxiety, whether in the form of awareness of the public self, actual-ought–other discrepancies, or negative relational schema. Theories of SAD also contain some interpersonal elements, Beck and Emery (1985) in the form of core social schema; Clark and Wells (1995) in the form of assumptions about others; and Rapee and Heimberg (1997) with their emphasis on the social development of SAD and hypervigilance to threat cues in others' behavior. Nonetheless, these relational concepts have received less attention in the clinical realm.

An additional, albeit more subtle, difference emerges in the function of schematic activation. Both sets of writers agree that the central function of social anxiety is to motivate efforts to protect oneself from impending danger. However, theories of social anxiety posit that schematic activation has an overarching positive function, such as avoiding social exclusion (Leary) or motivating behavior to meet the perceived expectations for oneself (Higgins and Strauman). Theories of SAD are more apt to emphasize the dysfunctional aspects of schema activation such as the preferential processing of negative information or the activation of behaviors that hinder social interactions. This is perhaps a reflection of the dysfunctional (i.e., diffuse, restricted, stable, negative) self depicted in these theories.

There are many reasons why differences should have emerged between these two domains. The two sets of theories developed from intellectual traditions that placed different emphases on the role of the self. Moreover, the goal of social/personality researchers has been the scientific study of a phenomenon, the self as a cognitive schema, whereas the goal of clinical researchers is, in large part, to understand and devise treatment strategies for patients with chronic social anxiety. Social-personality researchers seek to develop theories and findings that generalize to the whole spectrum of people, whereas clinical researchers want to generalize to other patients with the same disorder.

In the same vein, the way in which the self-schema is depicted may follow from the selves researchers actually observe in their subjects. As clinicians studying patients seeking treatment for SAD, we often find that these individuals behave as though they have a diffuse, restricted, negative sense of themselves that is resistant to change. It may be that clinical researchers place less emphasis on studying the conditions under which other types of self-information become salient precisely because negative self-information is chronically activated in these patients. In support of that idea, people with SAD were found to engage in self-criticism in nonsocial situations, which indicates that SAD may be associated with a more pervasive disturbance about self-worth that should be addressed in treatment (e.g., Cox, Walker, Enns, & Karpinski, 2002). In contrast, social and personality researchers generally study university students, who are more likely to have clear and complex views of themselves. These individuals are also more likely to have had positive interpersonal experiences, resulting in positive relational information within the self-schema. Thus, the "anxious self" may constitute only one of many facets of self-identity in these people, whereas for individuals with SAD it is the entire show.

FUTURE DIRECTIONS

An examination of the literature from a "self" perspective points to ways that social-personality and clinical research might each enhance the other. Examining social-personality models of self in clinical samples might provide information about the boundaries of those models. Consider the following examples. While public self-consciousness is often viewed by social-personality theorists as a prerequisite for social anxiety, research in clinical populations reveals that patients with SAD display considerable individual variation in this characteristic, which argues against its causal role in social anxiety of clinical severity (e.g., Makris & Heimberg, 1995). Additionally, an attempt to replicate the specificity of the actual-ought–other self discrepancy in a clinical SAD sample revealed that these patients were characterized by actual–ideal discrepancies as well, and, further, that both of these self-discrepancies were shared with patients with dysthymia (Weilage & Hope, 1999). These findings indicate that, while individuals with clinical disorders are indeed characterized by incongruence between various self-structures, these discrepancy are less specific than previously thought.

In a similar vein, social-personality self perspectives suggest intriguing questions for clinical research. To take some examples: Although SAD patients often appear to have a diffuse, negative, stable sense of self, it may be valuable to determine whether there are positive facets to the self. If, as suggested by the Cox et al. (2002) study, this is not the case, would it be useful to address this deficiency in treatment? Another potential direction is suggested by research indicating that individual differences in complexity and clarity of the self-schema influence emotional wellbeing (e.g., Campbell, 1990; Linville, 1985, 1987). One potential question is whether self-concept complexity or clarity predicts symptom severity or treatment response. If so, do strategies to increase the complexity or clarity of patients' self-concepts lead to improvements? Another potential direction is to consider how relational views of the self might be extended to SAD. Among the questions that might be addressed is whether, as suggested by Baldwin, increasing patients' awareness of negative relational scripts, and how they developed, allows them to more effectively disengage from self-defeating interpersonal patterns.

In summary, theories of social anxiety and of SAD contain differing views of the nature of self. We suggest that these diverse views might be used to identify potentially fruitful leads for future research.

REFERENCES

Alden, L. E., & Bieling, P. J. (1998). Interpersonal consequences of the pursuit of safety. *Behaviour Research and Therapy*, *36*, 53–64.

Alden, L. E, Teshuck, M., & Tee, K. (1992). Public self-awareness and withdrawal from social interactions. *Cognitive Therapy and Research*, *16*, 249–267.

Alden, L. E., & Wallace, S. T. (1995). Social phobia and social appraisal in successful and unsuccessful interactions. *Behaviour Research and Therapy*, *33*, 497–506.

Amir, N., McNally, R. J., Riemann, B. C., Burns, J., Lorenz, M., & Mullen, J. T. (1996). Suppression of the emotional Stroop effect by increased anxiety in patients with social phobia. *Behaviour Research and Therapy*, *34*, 945–948.

Arkin, R. M. (1981). Self-presentation styles. In J. T. Tedeschi (Ed.), *Impression management theory and social psychological research* (pp. 311–333). New York: Academic Press.

Arkin, R. M., Lake, E., & Baumgardner, A. H. (1986). Shyness and self-presentation. In W. Jones, J. Cheek, & S. R. Briggs (Eds.), *Shyness: Perspectives on research and treatment* (pp. 189–204). New York: Plenum.

Baldwin, M. W. (1992). Relational schemas and the processing of social information. *Psychological Bulletin*, *112*, 461–484.

Baldwin, M. W. (1994). Primed relational schemas as a source of self-evaluative reactions. *Journal of Social and Clinical Psychology*, *13*, 380–403.

Baldwin, M. W., Carrell, S. E., & Lopez, D. F. (1990). Priming relationship schemas: My advisor and the Pope are watching me from the back of my mind. *Journal of Experimental Social Psychology*, *26*, 435–454.

Baldwin, M. W., & Holmes, J. G. (1987). Salient private audiences and awareness of the self. *Journal of Personality and Social Psychology*, *52*, 1087–1098.

Baldwin, M. W., Keelan, J. P. R., Fehr, F., Enns, V., & Koh-Rangarajoo, E. (1996). Social-cognitive conceptualization of attachment working models: Availability and accessibility, effects. *Journal of Personality and Social Psychology*, *71*, 94–109.

Baldwin, M. W., & Main, K. T. (2001). Social anxiety and the cued activation of relational knowledge. *Personality and Social Psychology Bulletin*, *27*, 1637–1647.

Bargh, J. A. (1982). Attention and automaticity in the processing of self-relevant information. *Journal of Personality and Social Psychology*, *43*, 425–436.

Baumeister, R. F. (1999). The self. In D. T. Gilbert, S. T. Fiske, & G. Lindzey (Eds.), *The handbook of social psychology* (pp. 680–740). New York: Oxford University Press.

Baumeister, R. F. (Ed.). (1986). *Public self and private self.* New York: Springer.

Beck, A. T. (1996). Beyond belief: A theory of modes, personality, and psychopathology. In P. M. Salkovskis (Ed.), *Frontiers of cognitive therapy* (pp. 1–25). New York: Guilford Press.

Beck, A. T., & Emery, G. (1985). *Anxiety disorders and phobias: A cognitive perspective* (Chapter 9). New York: Basic Books.

Beck, J. S. (1995). *Cognitive therapy: Basics and beyond.* New York: Guilford.

Becker, E. S., Rinck, M., Margraf, J., & Roth, W. T. (2001). The emotional Stroop effect in anxiety disorders: General emotionality or disorder specificity. *Journal of Anxiety Disorders, 15,* 147–159.

Benjamin, L. S. (1996). *Interpersonal diagnosis and treatment of personality disorders* (2nd ed.). New York: Guilford Press.

Bögels, S. M. (2006). Task concentration training versus applied relaxation, in combination with cognitive therapy, for social phobia patients with fear of blushing, trembling, and sweating. *Behaviour Research and Therapy, 44,* 1199–1210.

Bögels, S. M., & Lamers, C. T. J. (2002). The causal role of self-awareness in blushing-anxious, socially-anxious and social phobic individuals. *Behaviour Research and Therapy, 40,* 1367–1384.

Buss, A. H. (1980). *Self-consciousness and social anxiety.* San Francisco, CA: Freeman & Company.

Campbell, J. D. (1990). Self-esteem and clarity of the self-concept. *Journal of Personality and Social Psychology, 59,* 538–549.

Carver, C. S., & Scheier, M. F. (1986). Self and the control of behavior. In M. L. Hartman & K. R. Blankstein (Eds.), *Perception of self in emotional disorder and psychotherapy. Advances in the study of communication and affect* (pp. 5–35). New York: Plenum.

Cheek, J. M. (1989). Identity orientations and self-interpretation. In D. M. Buss & N. Canton (Eds.), *Personality psychology* (pp. 275–285). New York: Springer-Verlag.

Cheek, J. M., & Briggs, S. R. (1982). Self-consciousness and aspects of identity. *Journal of Research in Personality, 16,* 401–408.

Chen, Y. P., Ehlers, A., Clark, D. M., & Mansell, W. (2002). Patients with generalized social phobia direct their attention away from faces. *Behaviour Research and Therapy, 40,* 677–687.

Cho, Y., & Telch, M. J. (2005). Testing the cognitive content-specificity hypothesis of social anxiety and depression: An application of structural equation modeling. *Cognitive Therapy and Research, 29,* 399–416.

Clark, D. M., & Wells, A. (1995). A cognitive model of social phobia. In R. G. Heimberg, M. R. Liebowitz, D. A. Hope, & F. R. Schneier (Eds.), *Social phobia: Diagnosis, assessment and treatment.* New York: Guilford Press.

Coles, M. E., Turk, C. L., Heimberg, R. G., & Fresco, D. M. (2001). Effects of varying levels of anxiety within social situations: Relationships to memory perspective and attributions in social phobia. *Behaviour Research and Therapy, 39,* 651–665.

Cox, B. J., Walker, J. R., Enns, M. W., & Karpinski, D. C. (2002). Self-criticism in generalized social phobia and response to cognitive-behavioral treatment. *Behavior Therapy, 33,* 479–491.

Cross, S. E., Bacon, P. L., & Morris, M. L. (2000). The relational-interdependent self-construal and relationships. *Journal of Personality and Social Psychology, 78,* 791–808.

Cross, S. E., Morris, M. L., & Gore, J. S. (2002). Thinking about oneself and others: The relational-interdependent self-construal and social cognition. *Journal of Personality and Social Psychology, 82,* 399–418.

Denissen, J. J., Penke, L., Schmitt, D. P., & van Aken, M. A. G. (2008). Self-esteem reactions to social interactions: Evidence for sociometer mechanisms across days, people, and nations. *Journal of Personality and Social Psychology*, *95*, 181–196.

Dennett, Daniel C. (1992). The self as a center of narrative gravity. In F. Kessel, P. Cole, & D. Johnson (Eds.), *Self and consciousness: Multiple perspectives*. Hillsdale, NJ: Erlbaum.

DePaulo, B. M., Epstein, J. A., & LeMay, C. S. (1990). Responses of the socially anxious to the prospect of interpersonal evaluation. *Journal of Personality*, *58*, 623–640.

Dickerson, S. S., Gruenewald, T. L., & Kemeny, M. E. (2009). Psychobiological responses to social self threat: Functional or detrimental? *Self and Identity*, *8*, 270–285.

Ellemers, N., Spears, R., & Doosje, B. (2002). Self and social identity. *Annual Review of Psychology*, *53*, 161–186.

Eriksen, E. H. (1968). *Identity: Youth and crisis*. New York: Norton.

Gilboa-Schechtman, E., Foa, E. B., & Amir, N. (1999). Attentional biases for facial expressions in social phobia: The face-in-the-crowd paradigm. *Cognition and Emotion*, *13*, 305–318.

Gilboa-Schechtman, E., Presburger, G., Marom, S., & Hermesh, H. (2005). The effects of social anxiety and depression on the evaluation of facial crowds. *Behaviour Research and Therapy*, *43*, 467–474.

Greenwald, A. G., & Pratkanis, A. R. (1984). The self. In R. S. Wyer & T. K. Srull (Eds.), *Handbook of social cognition: Vol. 3* (pp. 129–178). Hillsdale, NJ: Erlbaum.

Gruenewald, T. L., Kemeny, M. E., Aziz, N., & Fahey, J. L. (2004). Acute threat to the social self: Shame, social self-esteem and cortisol activity. *Psychosomatic Medicine*, *66*, 915–924.

Harvey, P. (1995). *The selfless mind: Personality, consciousness and Nirvana in early Buddhism*. Richmond, UK: Curzon Press.

Higgins, E. T. (1987). Self-discrepancy: A theory relating self and affect. *Psychological Review*, *94*, 319–340.

Higgins, E. T., & Bargh, J. A. (1987). Social cognition and social perception. In M. R. Rosenweig, & L. W. Porter (Eds.), *Annual review of psychology: 38* (pp. 369–425). Palo Alto, CA: Annual Reviews.

Higgins, E. T., Klein, R., & Strauman, T. (1985). Self-concept discrepancy theory: A psychological model for distinguishing among different aspects of depression and anxiety. *Social Cognition*, *3*, 51–76.

Hirsch, C. R., Clark, D. M., Mathews, A., & Williams, R. (2003). Self-images play a causal role in social phobia. *Behaviour Research and Therapy*, *41*, 909–921.

Hirsch, C. R., Meynen, T., & Clark, D. M. (2004). Negative self-imagery in social anxiety contaminates social interactions. *Memory*, *12*, 496–506.

Hofmann, S. G. (2007). Cognitive factors that maintain social anxiety disorder: A comprehensive model and its treatment implications. *Cognitive Behaviour Therapy*, *36*, 193–209.

Hofmann, S. G., Moscovitch, D. A., Kim, H. J., & Taylor, A. N. (2004). Changes in self-perception during treatment of social phobia. *Journal of Consulting and Clinical Psychology*, *72*, 588–596.

Hope, D. A., Rapee, R. M., Heimberg, R. G., & Dombeck, M. J. (1990). Representations of the self in social phobia: Vulnerability to social threat. *Cognitive Therapy and Research*, *14*, 177–189.

James, W. (1890). *The principles of psychology*. New York: Holt.

Joormann, J., & Gotlib, I. H. (2006). Is this happiness I see? Biases in the identification of emotional facial expressions in depression and social phobia. *Journal of Abnormal Psychology*, *115*, 705–714.

Katzko, M. W. (2003). Unity versus multiplicity: A conceptual analysis of the term "self" and its use in personality theories. *Journal of Personality*, *71*, 83–110.

Kernberg, O. F. (1976). *Object relations theory and clinical psychoanalysis*. New York: Aronson.
Kihlstrom, J. F., & Cantor, N. (1984). Mental representations of the self. In L. Berkowitz (Ed.), *Advances in experimental social psychology: Vol. 17* (pp. 1–47). New York: Academic Press.
Klein, S. B., & Loftus, J. (1988). The nature of self-referent encoding: the contributions of elaborative and organizational processes. *Journal of Personality and Social Psychology*, *55*, 5–11.
LeDoux, J. (2002). *Synaptic self: How our brains become who we are*. New York: Viking Press.
Leary, M. R. (1986). The impact of interactional impediments on social anxiety and self-presentation. *Journal of Experimental Social Psychology*, *22*, 122–135.
Leary, M. R. (1995). *Self-presentation: Impression management and interpersonal behavior*. Milwaukee, WI: Brown & Benchmark.
Leary, M. R. (2007). Motivational and emotional aspects of the self. *Annual Review of Psychology*, *58*, 317–344.
Leary, M. R., & Baumeister, R. F. (2000). The nature and function of self-esteem: Sociometer theory. In M. P. Zanna (Ed.), *Advances in experimental social psychology, 32* (pp. 1–62). San Diego, CA: Academic Press.
Leary, M. R., & Kowalski, R. M. (1995). *Social anxiety*. New York: Guilford.
Leary, M. R., Tambor, E. S., Terdal, S. K., & Downs, D. L. (1995). Self-esteem as an interpersonal monitor: The sociometer hypothesis. *Journal of Personality and Social Psychology*, *68*, 518–530.
Linville, P. W. (1985). Self-complexity and affective extremity: Don't put all your eggs in one cognitive basket. *Social Cognition*, *3*, 94–120.
Linville, P. W. (1987). Self-complexity as a cognitive buffer against stress-related illness and depression. *Journal of Personality and Social Psychology*, *52*, 663–676.
Locke, John. (1997). *An essay concerning human understanding*. New York: Penguin Classics.
Lucock, M. P., & Salkovskis, P. M. (1988). Cognitive factors in social anxiety and its treatment. *Behaviour Research and Therapy*, *26*, 297–302.
Maddux, J. E., Norton, L. W., & Leary, M. R. (1988). Cognitive components of social anxiety: An investigation of the integration of self-presentation theory and self-efficacy theory. *Journal of Social and Clinical Psychology*, *6*, 180–190.
Makris, G. S., & Heimberg, T. G. (1995). The Scale of Maladaptive Self-Consciousness: A valid and useful measure in the study of social phobia. *Personality and Individual Differences*, *19*, 731–740.
Mansell, W., Clark, D. M., Ehlers, A., & Chen, Y. P. (1999). Social anxiety and attention away from emotional faces. *Cognition and Emotion*, *13*, 673–690.
Markus, H. (1977). Self-schemata and processing information about the self. *Journal of Personality and Social Psychology*, *35*, 63–78.
Markus, H., & Kitayama, S. (1991). Culture and the self: Implications for cognition, emotion, and motivation. *Psychological Review*, *98*, 224–253.
Markus, H., & Nurius, P. (1986). Possible selves. *American Psychologist*, *41*, 954–969.
Mattia, J. I., Heimberg, R. G., & Hope, D. A. (1993). The revised Stroop color-naming task in social phobics. *Behaviour Research and Therapy*, *31*, 305–315.
McEwan, K. L., & Devins, G. M. (1983). Is increased arousal in social anxiety noticed by others? *Journal of Abnormal Psychology*, *92*, 417–421.
McGuire, W. J. (1984). Search for the self: Going beyond self-esteem and the reactive self. In R. A. Zucker, J. Aronoff, & A. I. Rabin (Eds.), *Personality and the prediction of behavior.* New York: Academic Press.
Mellings, T. M. B., & Alden, L. E. (2000). Cognitive processes in social anxiety: The effects of self-focused attention, rumination, and anticipatory processing. *Behaviour Research and Therapy*, *38*, 243–257.

Oaten, M., Williams, K. D., Jones, A., & Zadro, L. (2008). The effects of ostracism on self-regulation in the socially anxious. *Journal of Social & Clinical Psychology*, *27*, 471–504.

Perowne, S., & Mansell, S. (2002). Social anxiety, self-focused attention, and the discrimination of negative, neutral and positive audience members by their non-verbal behaviours. *Behavioural and Cognitive Psychotherapy*, *30*, 11–23.

Rapee, R. M., & Heimberg, R. G. (1997). A cognitive-behavioral model of anxiety in social phobia. *Behaviour Research and Therapy*, *35*, 741–756.

Rapee, R. M., & Lim, L. (1992). Discrepancy between self and observer ratings of performance in social phobics. *Journal of Abnormal Psychology*, *101*, 728–731.

Rapee, R. M., & Spence, S. H. (2004). The etiology of social phobia: Empirical evidence and an initial model. *Clinical Psychology Review*, *24*, 737–767.

Sanz, J., & Avia, M. D. (1994). Cognitive specificity in social anxiety and depression: Self-statements, self-focused attention, and dysfunctional attitudes. *Journal of Social and Clinical Psychology*, *13*, 105–137.

Schlenker, B., & Leary, M. R. (1982). Social anxiety and self-presentation: A conceptualization and model. *Psychological Bulletin*, *92*, 641–669.

Schultz, L. T., & Heimberg, R. G. (2008). Attentional focus in social anxiety disorder: Potential for interactive processes. *Clinical Psychology Review*, *28*, 1206–1221.

Schultz, S. M., Alpers, G. W., & Hofmann, S. G. (2008). Negative self-focused cognitions mediate the effect of trait social anxiety on state anxiety. *Behaviour Research and Therapy*, *46*, 438–449.

Seta, C. E., Schmidt, S., & Bookhout, C. M. (2006). Social identity orientation and social role attributions: Explaining behavior through the lens of the self. *Self and Identity*, *5*, 355–364.

Seta, C. E., Seta, J. J., & Hundt, G. (2001). Exaggerating the differences between relatively successful and unsuccessful groups: Identity orientation as a perceptual lens. *Group Dynamics*, *5*, 19–32.

Shepperd, J. A., & Arkin, R. M. (1990). Shyness and self-presentation. In W. R. Crozier (Ed.), *Shyness and embarrassment* (pp. 286–314). New York: Cambridge University Press.

Spector, I., Pecknold, J. C., & Libman, E. (2003). Selective attentional bias related to the noticeable aspect of anxiety symptoms in generalized social phobia. *Journal of Anxiety Disorders*, *17*, 517–531.

Srivastava, S., & Beer, J. S. (2005). How self-evaluations related to being liked by others: Integrating sociometer and attachment perspectives. *Journal of Personality and Social Psychology*, *89*, 966–977.

Srull, T. K., & Wyer, R. S. (1979). The role of category accessibility in the interpretation of information about persons: Some determinants and implications. *Journal of Personality and Social Psychology*, *37*, 1660–1672.

Staats, A. W., & Staats, C. K. (1964). *Complex human behavior*. New York: Holt, Rinehart & Winston.

Stillman, T. F., Baumeister, R. F., Lambert, N. M., Crescioni, A. W., DeWall, C. N., & Fincham, F. D. (2009). Alone and without purpose: Life loses meaning following social exclusion. *Journal of Experimental Social Psychology*, *45*, 686–694.

Stopa, L., & Clark, D. M. (1993). Cognitive processes in social phobia. *Behaviour Research and Therapy*, *31*, 255–267.

Stopa, L., & Clark, D. M. (2000). Social phobia and interpretation of social events. *Behaviour Research and Therapy*, *38*, 273–283.

Stopa, L., & Jenkins, A. (2007). Images of the self in social anxiety: Effects on the retrieval of autobiographical memories. *Journal of Behavior Therapy and Experimental Psychiatry*, *38*, 459–473.

Strauman, T. J. (1989). Self-discrepancies in clinical depression and social phobia: Cognitive structures that underlie emotional disorders? *Journal of Abnormal Psychology*, *98*, 14–22.

Strauman, T. J. (1992). Self-guides, autobiographical memory, and anxiety and dysphoria: Toward a cognitive model of vulnerability to emotional distress. *Journal of Abnormal Psychology*, *101*, 87–95.

Strauman, T. J., & Higgins, E. T. (1987). Automatic activation of self-discrepancies and emotional syndromes: When cognitive structures influence affect. *Journal of Personality and Social Psychology*, *53*, 1004–1014.

Sullivan, H. S. (1953). *The interpersonal theory of psychiatry*. New York: Norton.

Taylor, C. T., & Alden, L. E. (2005). Social interpretation bias and generalized social phobia: The influence of developmental experiences. *Behaviour Research and Therapy*, *43*, 759–777.

Taylor, S. (1996). Meta-analysis of cognitive-behavioral treatment for social phobia. *Journal of Behavior Therapy & Experimental Psychiatry*, *27*, 1–9.

Vassilopoulos, S. (2005). Social anxiety and the effects of engaging in mental imagery. *Cognitive Therapy and Research*, *29*, 261–277.

Veljaca, K. A., & Rapee, R. M. (1998). Detection of negative and positive audience behaviours by socially anxious subjects. *Behaviour Research and Therapy*, *36*, 311–321.

Voncken, M. J., Bögels, S. M., & Peeters, F. (2007). Specificity of interpretation and judgmental biases in social phobia versus depression. *Psychology and Psychotherapy: Theory, Research and Practice*, *80*, 443–453.

Weilage, M., & Hope, D. A. (1999). Self-discrepancy in social phobia and dysthymia. *Cognitive Therapy and Research*, *23*, 637–650.

Wells, A., Clark, D. M., & Ahmad, S. (1998). How do I look with my mind's eye: Perspective taking in social phobic imagery. *Behaviour Research and Therapy*, *36*, 631–634.

Wells, A., & Papageorgiou, C. (1999). The observer perspective: Biased imagery in social phobia, agoraphobia, and blood/injury phobia. *Behavioural Research and Therapy*, *37*, 653–658.

Wells, A., & Papageorgiou, C. (2001). Social phobic interoception: Effects of bodily information on anxiety, beliefs and self-processing. *Behaviour Research and Therapy*, *39*, 1–11.

Wells, A., Clark, D. M., Salkovskis, P., Ludgate, J., Hackmann, A., & Gelder, M. G. (1995). Social phobia: The role of in-situation safety behaviors in maintaining anxiety and negative beliefs. *Behavior Therapy*, *26*, 153–161.

Wilson, J. K., & Rapee, R. M. (2005a). The interpretation of negative social events in social phobia with versus without comorbid mood disorder. *Journal of Anxiety Disorders*, *19*, 245–274.

Wilson, J. K., & Rapee, R. M. (2005b). The interpretation of negative social events in social phobia: Changes during treatment and relationship to outcome. *Behaviour Research and Therapy*, *43*, 373–389.

Wilson, J. K., & Rapee, R. M. (2006). Self-concept certainty in social phobia. *Behaviour Research and Therapy*, *44*, 113–136.

Zadro, L., Boland, C., & Richardson, R. (2006). How long does it last? The persistence of the effects of ostracism in the socially anxious. *Journal of Experimental Social Psychology*, *42*, 692–697.

Chapter 17

Social Anxiety, Positive Experiences, and Positive Events

Todd B. Kashdan[1] and Justin W. Weeks[2]
[1]Department of Psychology, George Mason University, Fairfax, VA 22030, [2]Department of Psychology, Ohio University, Athens, OH 45701

By definition, people with emotional disturbances experience significant distress and impairment. Thus, when there is an opportunity to engage in an activity that can generate positive experiences, people with emotional disturbances might be expected to be less successful than other people. Despite the appeal of this formulation, there is reason to believe that attenuated positive experiences are only relevant to a selective number of disturbances. In this chapter, we discuss recent advances in the phenomenology of social anxiety. This includes data showing that social anxiety is associated with low intensity, short-lived positive experiences, infrequent positive events, and distinct cognitive biases that restrict the quality of life.

For decades, psychologists have advocated a single, bipolar continuum with positive emotions and approach behavior at one endpoint and negative emotions and avoidance behavior as the other endpoint. However, recent research in personality, motivation, and social neuroscience suggests that there are two separate biobehavioral systems that reflect very different purposes (Carver, Sutton, & Scheier, 2000; Gray & McNaughton, 1996). Specifically, on the one hand, there is an avoidance system whose purpose is to prevent people from being exposed to danger. To meet this aim, behavior that might lead to pain, punishment, or other undesirable outcomes is inhibited. As an early warning system of possible danger, this system activates negative emotions which, in turn, increase the likelihood of avoidance or escape. On the one hand, independent from the avoidance system, there is an approach system whose purpose is to guide people toward situations that might offer rewards. To meet this aim, attention and energy are mobilized to pursue activities that can generate resources such as food, the cooperation of others, sexual partners, and knowledge that provides an evolutionary advantage for survival and reproduction.

Social Anxiety: Clinical, Developmental, and Social Perspectives. DOI: 10.1016/B978-0-12-375096-9.00017-1

Whereas the onset of negative emotions operates to narrow our options, there is evidence that the experience of positive emotions, a component of the approach system, widens the array of thoughts, behaviors, and executive functioning capacities at our disposal (Fredrickson, 1998). That is, positive emotions ensure that we remain attentive and open to rewarding opportunities with the possession of sufficient stamina to exploit them.

Given the relatively independent roles of these systems, it is not surprising that positive and negative emotions show only a small relation to each other and each is associated with distinct experiential, cognitive, physiological, and behavioral processes. This means that, in the absence of additional information, the degree to which people are sensitive to pain and punishment offers little insight about the pleasure, engagement, and meaning in their lives. However, there are meaningful exceptions to this rule. The emotional disturbances that have received the most attention for deficient positive experiences and events are depression and schizophrenia (e.g., Berenbaum & Oltmanns, 1992; Blanchard, Mueser, & Bellack, 1998; Rottenberg, 2005). Less attention has been given to social anxiety and the pathological variant, SAD, as possible impediments to the elements of a positive, enriching existence. For decades, researchers characterized attenuated positive experiences as being part of the structure of depression, but not anxiety (Brown, Chorpita, & Barlow, 1998; Clark, Steer, & Beck, 1994; Clark & Watson, 1991). One problem with this premature declaration was that studies examining how the anxiety and mood disorders relate to positive affect systematically failed to include people with social anxiety problems.

A SELF-REGULATION PERSPECTIVE ON SOCIAL ANXIETY

Any psychological condition that directly interferes with social relationships has the potential to disrupt a primary source of positive events and experiences. Socially anxious people are hyper-focused on making a good impression on other people but either doubt that they can do so (Schlenker & Leary, 1982) or fear the consequences of doing so. Part of the doubt of being able to make a good impression stems from the belief that their anxiety and extreme self-awareness will disrupt their social performance (Rapee & Heimberg, 1997). In response, socially anxious people devote considerable attentional and cognitive resources to fearing, controlling, and avoiding anxious thoughts, feelings, and behaviors. This includes engaging in "safety behaviors" such as talking very little, nodding obsequiously, and deflecting attention by asking questions of other people to minimize the possibility of rejection (Clark & Wells, 1995). Regular, intense efforts to control anxiety and the probability of being rejected put socially anxious people in prevention mode, where the avoidance of threat and failure take precedence. Unfortunately, being in prevention mode is liable to disrupt people's ability to be mindfully aware in the present moment and open to environmental reward cues.

People who inefficiently allocate resources to impression management and the regulation of anxious symptoms tend to show impairments in other goal-directed behaviors that require effort and intention (Vohs, Baumeister, & Ciarocco, 2005). This is because people have a limited amount of physical stamina, attention, and self-control at any given point of time and over-exertion can essentially drain this pool of resources (Muraven & Baumeister, 2000).

The enormous effort and energy devoted to emotion regulation diminishes contact with present experiences, interferes with progress toward valued goals, and yields impairments in the frequency and quality of positive events (Hayes, Luoma, Bond, Masuda, & Lillis, 2006; Kashdan, Breen, & Julian, 2010). The paradox is that excessive attempts to make a positive impression, be less anxious, and avoid rejection lead to a depletion of the necessary self-regulatory resources to effectively attend to and extract rewards from the social environment (such as laughter, intimacy, cooperation, and compassion). All else being equal, less socially anxious people, without this resource drain, should be better at pursuing aspirational goals involving rewards.

SOCIAL ANXIETY AND POSITIVE EXPERIENCES

The question of whether diminished positive experiences are a distinct feature of the social anxiety spectrum, from subclinical symptoms to SAD, has implications for etiology, phenomenology, maintenance, prevention, and treatment. The earliest indication that social anxiety might be an "exception to the rule" that diminished positive affect is relevant to depression but not anxiety was a study by Watson, Clark, and Carey (1988). Based on 21 people with SAD out of 150 outpatients with various anxiety and mood diagnoses, these researchers found a -0.23 correlation with a global trait measure of positive affect that failed to hold after accounting for the presence of comorbid depression ($pr = -0.12$). Although intriguing, the small magnitude of the relationship, small sample, and relatively crude measurement approach (cross-sectional general surveys) failed to inspire changes to the social anxiety landscape.

In the past several years, a proliferation of research has emerged on how social anxiety is related to positive experiences, with an emphasis on positive emotions and curiosity. Without a systematic quantitative review of isolated findings, the general strength of these relationships would remain unclear. A meta-analysis would provide guidance to clinical researchers by answering a few vital questions. Is social anxiety related to positive emotions and curiosity and, if so, with what magnitude? Are these relationships specific to social anxiety or are they a function of the presence and severity of depressive symptoms? Which variables – with respect to both the characteristics of participants and methodologies used – might moderate any existing relationships?

With these questions at the forefront, one of the authors conducted a meta-analysis of published and unpublished studies on this topic from 1950 onward (Kashdan, 2007). Based on 19 studies and 2976 participants, results supported a stable, moderate, inverse relationship between social anxiety and positive affect ($r = -0.36$; 95% CI: -0.31 to -0.40); based on 15 studies and 2091 participants, results also supported a similar relationship to curiosity and exploratory behavior patterns ($r = -0.24$; 95% CI: -0.20 to -0.28). Of course, this leaves the possibility that these relationships might be a function of the comorbidity between social anxiety and depression. This can be handled with tests of construct specificity where the shared variance among these emotional disturbances is removed. The problem is that, by removing the conceptual overlap between these conditions, we remove part of the social anxiety construct (i.e., co-occurrence cannot be conceived narrowly as an artifact or "noise"). In addition, anhedonia, or the inability to experience pleasure from previously enjoyable events, is a component of depression, overlapping with positive affect or the outcome of interest. Despite caveats about interpreting any chimerical, residual variance, the unique links between social anxiety and dampened positive affect ($r = -0.21$; 95% CI: -0.16 to -0.26) and curiosity ($r = -0.21$; 95% CI: -0.08 to -0.32) could not be explained by the presence or severity of depression.

With the availability of a large pool of studies, variables that strengthen or weaken the relation between social anxiety and positive experiences could be uncovered. Importantly, the strategy for assessing social anxiety mattered. The magnitude of dampened positive affect was strongest when researchers used the Anxiety Disorder Interview Schedule (Brown, DiNardo, & Barlow, 1994) or SIAS (Mattick & Clarke, 1998) (arguably the gold standards for interview and self-report methodologies, respectively); instruments that are relevant to other emotional disturbances, such as the FNE (Watson & Friend, 1969), led to the weakest relationships with positive affect. The only other variable that changed the magnitude of social anxiety effects was the population being studied, with the largest effects being found with clinical samples, followed by college students, and then combat veterans and other adults in the community without SAD. These findings suggest that seemingly inconsequential decisions about research design are important and should be carefully considered prior to conducting research on this topic.

Although the evidence is promising, most of these studies relied on crude methods. Nearly all of the studies used a single global questionnaire to measure how often people experienced positive emotions – a retrospective approach that cannot disentangle the information processing biases associated with social anxiety from actual positive responses to events. At the time of this meta-analysis, only two studies used a social interaction experiment where changes in positive emotions were assessed (Kashdan & Roberts, 2004; Wallace & Alden, 1997). Only four studies used a daily diary approach to evaluate the presence of positive emotions in the naturalistic, everyday environment of people with elevated social anxiety (Kashdan & Collins, 2010; Kashdan, Julian, Merritt, & Uswatte, 2006; Kashdan & Steger, 2006; Vittengl & Holt, 1998). Of these, only one ensured that entries recorded by people with varying levels of social anxiety were on the appropriate day (via computerized time-and-date stamping) (Kashdan & Collins, 2010). This particular study had participants carry around palm pilots to report on their experiences in-the-moment during four random assessments per day in their normal environment for two weeks. Interestingly, not only was social anxiety associated with less intense positive emotions during these random assessments throughout the day, but being around other people (versus being alone) did not significantly alter these effects. That is, socially anxious people showed a general dampening of positive experiences, and, in fact, other work shows that this relationship holds regardless of being in a conversation with familiar or unfamiliar partners (Brown, Silvia, Myin-Germeys, & Kwapil, 2007; Vittengl & Holt, 1998); that being said, socially anxious people do report greater negative self-focused attention and preference for being alone when socializing with unfamiliar people.

Benefits of daily diary designs include maximizing ecological validity, minimizing retrospective biases, and modeling situational parameters that might moderate relationships. With over 20 studies on the topic, it might be time to move beyond context-free studies of positive experiences in the lives of socially anxious people (i.e., asking people how often they feel particular positive emotions over their lifetime with questionnaires such as the trait version of the Positive and Negative Affect Schedule; Watson, Clark, & Tellegen, 1988). There is a need for precise studies of how and when social anxiety alters the presence, intensity, and longevity of positive emotions and other rewarding experiences such as curiosity and exploratory behavior.

Testing a Self-Regulatory Model

Whereas social anxiety is commonly associated with negative emotions and BI, there is evidence to suggest that, at least for some people, social anxiety is related to diminished positive affect and curiosity. Yet, it might be overly simplistic to focus on bivariate relationships between social anxiety and positive experiences and events. Fitting with a self-regulatory perspective (Leary, 2000; Vohs et al., 2005), these relationships might vary as a function of how much energy and effort are devoted to managing anxiety, thereby exhausting the attention and stamina that would otherwise be available for exploiting rewarding opportunities.

One study tested this nuanced model by examining whether levels of social anxiety and the manner in which emotions are regulated might operate together to predict positive emotions and events in people's natural environment over a 21-day assessment period (Kashdan & Steger, 2006). Beginning with simple effects, results showed that people at the high end of social anxiety (1 standard deviation above the mean) reported 39% fewer positive events in a given day than people at the lower end of social anxiety (−1 standard deviation from the mean). This line of research clarifies how social anxiety influences the number of rewarding opportunities available.

These initial findings set the framework for a more complex model. Few studies have explicitly tested whether socially anxious people are more reactive to being socially anxious on a given day in their lives. Furthermore, the presence of social anxiety on a given day might only be important if people are focused on avoiding, hiding, or suppressing their negative emotions. Upon combining these separate vulnerability factors, there was evidence for a synergistic relationship among trait social anxiety, the amount of social anxiety on a given day, and the dominant strategy used to regulate daily negative emotions. Of people at the high end of social anxiety, those reporting the most daily social anxiety and the greatest tendencies to suppress their emotions on a given day reported 24% fewer positive events than other people classified as high in social anxiety. These findings point to conditions when socially anxious people are most vulnerable to a loss of rewards. At the opposite end of functioning, the evidence suggested that people at the lower end of social anxiety with greater tendencies to be open and expressive of their emotions reported the most frequent positive events. People are not passive vehicles that experience emotions; people form relationships with their emotions and attempt to manage them with varying degrees of success. If scientists are going to understand when people with excessive social anxiety are more or less responsive to everyday positive events, they will have to continue studying social anxiety and self-regulatory strategies in tandem.

POSITIVE COGNITIONS RELEVANT TO THE SOCIAL ANXIETY SPECTRUM

Besides positive emotion, mood, and events, there is a large body of research on whether positive cognitions in response to social situations are relevant to social anxiety. The past 15 years have witnessed an emerging reform of SAD models that initially focused on anticipation of negative outcomes as the core of social fear (Clark & Wells, 1995; Hofmann, 2007; Rapee & Heimberg, 1997). The overall findings pertaining to positive cognitions can be broadly encapsulated within two separate principles: social anxiety is characterized both by (1) an *absence* of a normative, positive interpretation bias with regard to *ambiguous* social outcomes; and (2) *increased* apprehension and anxiety in response to *overtly* positive social outcomes.

Absence of a Normative Positive Interpretation Bias

There is evidence that, in the general population, positive and negative evaluative responses are governed by distinct underlying motivational systems, with the positive motivational system characterized by a "positivity offset." Essentially, for the average person, when impending threat is weak or absent, people show a slight motivational trend toward actively seeking and engaging with various environmental rewards. This general approach or exploratory system ensures that energies are directed toward learning and accruing knowledge of the world (Cacioppo, Gardner, & Berntson, 1997; Ito & Cacioppo, 2005; Panksepp, 1998). It has been suggested that survival depends on the ability to continually be exposed to novelty, learn, and grow. Thus, evaluating and embracing beneficial stimuli is rewarding for its own sake and as a means to other positive endstates.

It was long held that the cognitions of people with SAD were primarily the outcome of negative interpretations of ambiguous social information, which served to maintain and/or increase social anxiety (Rapee & Heimberg, 1997). However, available evidence (Boucher & Osgood, 1969; Cacioppo et al., 1997) suggests that, even in the absence of threats to social or physical survival, socially anxious people might *lack* this *normative* and *potentially protective* positive outlook about the world (Hirsch & Mathews, 2000). More specifically, Hirsch and Mathews suggested that people with SAD do not routinely make "online" inferences, or, assess and process ambiguous information offered in the present moment. Instead, people with SAD judge their own performance by *looking back* – determining their course of action from pre-existing negative self-appraisals and expectations, and ruminations on prior mistakes and failures. All of these cognitive activities prevent people with SAD from modifying global negative beliefs and adopting positive beliefs. In support of this concept, clients with SAD take longer in a lexical decision task to choose endings for ambiguous passages pertaining to social situations in a positive (or negative) manner; matched controls do not exhibit this deficit, and, thus, it truly appears normal to engage a positive bias within social contexts (Hirsch & Mathews, 2000).

High and low socially anxious people were presented with a random series of angry, happy, and neutral faces, followed by one of four outcomes: aversive, pleasant, or neutral emotional pictures, or nothing at all. Although high socially anxious people initially overestimated the occurrence of pleasant outcomes following happy faces, this positive interpretative bias decreased over time, whereas low anxious people continued to overestimate the occurrence of pleasant outcomes following happy faces. Furthermore, although high socially anxious people initially reported that aversive outcomes were unlikely to follow happy faces (consistent with a positive expectancy bias), this expectancy also decreased over time (Garner, Mogg, & Bradley, 2006). These findings further support the notion that social anxiety is about believing that positive social cues fail to predict pleasant outcomes along with beliefs that negative social cues predict aversive outcomes.

At the neurobiological level, when given ambiguous social situations and asked to choose positive or negative endings, socially anxious people show a particular pattern of ERP. Specifically, socially anxious people fail to show a difference in the strength of event-related brain potentials (P600) when choosing between positive and negative endings (Moser, Hajcak, Huppert, Foa, & Simons, 2008). Increases in the P600 indicate that an outcome was unexpected; thus, positive and negative endings are equally expected by high socially anxious people. In contrast, low socially anxious people exhibit larger P600s to negative than to positive endings, suggesting that they have a greater tendency to expect positive endings (Moser et al., 2008). These neurobiological data converge with other research showing that the average person shows a tendency toward positive emotions and approach behavior in the absence of impending threat (Cacioppo et al., 1997) and people with greater social anxiety lack this positive inferential bias.

A recent set of studies (de Jong, de Graaf-Peters, van Hout, & van Wees, 2009) sought to further understand whether women with greater social anxiety show a reduced tendency to pair social cues with positive outcomes. Participants were presented with descriptions of ambiguous social events or comparison descriptions of animals or nature scenes, which were randomly paired with images of either happy (approval), disgusted (rejection), or neutral faces. "Online" ratings during the task indicated that people with greater social anxiety felt that happy faces and social events often fail to co-occur. The absence of a positive bias was more extreme in the context of *overtly negative* social situations, suggesting that people with greater social anxiety have low expectations that unpleasant events will eventually resolve. These findings by de Jong and colleagues provide additional support for a deficient positive bias in social anxiety.

The function of positive interpretation biases over time has also been examined. Socially anxious and non-socially anxious individuals read passages that were either positive social, negative social, or neutral, and were assessed for factual memory and interpretation immediately post-task and at a 48-hour follow-up. High and low socially anxious people showed similar accuracy in the memory of details from the passages. However, socially anxious people made less positive (and more negative) interpretations of details included in the positive passages following the 48-hour delay, and this positive bias effect remained even after controlling for depression, and state and trait anxiety (Brendle & Wenzel, 2004). Thus, socially anxious people appear to appropriately encode memories of threatening social events, but have a tendency to interpret their memories of social events in a less positive (and more negative) manner, with this bias emerging even stronger over time.

So, we know that highly socially anxious people tend to lack a positive social bias. This is important because this positive bias provides psychological benefits for the majority of the general population. Essentially, in the absence of threat, people are biased to explore and engage their environment in search of rewarding opportunities (Cacioppo et al., 1997). This begs the question of whether highly socially anxious people can be trained to acquire and use a protective social bias to their advantage. Based on initial findings, highly socially anxious people are able to adopt a *benign* interpretation bias, thereby facilitating *either positive or non-negative* interpretations when presented with threatening social scenarios. Following training, these individuals show less negative interpretations of new ambiguous social situations, and predict that they would be less anxious in future social situations, in comparison to an untrained high social anxiety control group (Murphy, Hirsch, Mathews, Smith, & Clark, 2007). The fact that interpretative biases are malleable for high socially anxious people, and that the facilitation of a benign positive bias served to reduce anxiety about future social situations, provides some support for the concept that positive interpretation biases might serve as a protective buffer against the development of high social anxiety.

However, findings on positive interpretation biases within either *ambiguous* or *overtly negative* social contexts represent only one broad domain of positive cognitive factors when studying or treating social anxiety. We now turn to the area of *increased* apprehension and anxiety in response to *overtly positive* social outcomes.

Fear of Positive Evaluation

Cognitive behavioral models have long labeled fear of negative evaluation a core cognitive feature of social anxiety (Clark & Wells, 1995; Rapee & Heimberg, 1997), and extensive evidence supports this (e.g., Coles, Turk, Heimberg, & Fresco, 2001; Hackmann, Surawy, & Clark, 1998; Horley, Williams, Gonsalvez, & Gordon, 2004; Mansell & Clark, 1999). However, converging with prior findings that suggest that social anxiety is linked to dysfunctional cognitions about positive social events, researchers hypothesized that a *general* fear of evaluation is important in social anxiety, including fears of both positive and negative evaluation (e.g., Weeks, Heimberg, & Rodebaugh, 2008; Weeks, Heimberg, Rodebaugh, & Norton, 2008).

FPE is a construct distinct from, albeit strongly related to, the construct of fear of negative evaluation (FNE). Specifically, FPE pertains to the sense of dread associated with being evaluated *favorably* and *publicly*, which begs a direct social comparison of the self to others and therefore causes a person to feel conspicuous and "in the spotlight" (Weeks, Heimberg, & Rodebaugh, 2008). In contrast, FNE pertains to the sense of dread associated with being evaluated *unfavorably* while anticipating or participating in a social situation. Both socio-evaluative fears independently contribute to social anxiety (Fergus et al., 2009; Weeks, Heimberg, & Rodebaugh, 2008; Weeks, Heimberg, Rodebaugh, & Norton, 2008).

FPE is consistent with theory proposing that social anxiety is an evolutionary mechanism that facilitates group cohesion, in part by preventing conflict between members of varying levels of social ranking (Gilbert, 2001). People who perceive themselves as ranking lower on a social hierarchy are proposed to experience anxiety when interacting with higher-ranking group members, prompting the expression of submissive gestures. These submissive gestures serve to appease the higher-ranking people of a group, thus minimizing potential conflict over group resources. With respect to FNE, Gilbert proposes that avoiding negative evaluation would have been adaptive in demonstrating to others that one is worthy of social investments, as well as in avoiding conflict with people who ranked higher on a social hierarchy. Consistent with the construct of FPE, Gilbert suggested that socially anxious people might also fear *increases in social status* that could lead to conflict with more powerful others. Gilbert further suggested that socially anxious people may fear they will be unable to maintain or defend social gains in the future; a concept dubbed the "fear of doing well" (p. 742).

To evaluate this expanded conceptualization of fear, researchers developed a 10-item self-report measure, the FPES, with strong psychometric properties in both undergraduate (e.g., Weeks, Heimberg, & Rodebaugh, 2008; Weeks, Heimberg, Rodebaugh, & Norton, 2008) and clinical (Fergus et al., 2009) samples. In support of Gilbert's (2001) psycho-evolutionary model, self-reported submissive behavior and lower perceived social status were associated both with greater social anxiety and disability in clients with SAD as well as healthy controls (Schneier, Heimberg, Belzer, & Liebowitz, 2006). Similarly, FPE and FNE both relate positively to submissive behaviors and negatively to social self-rankings (Weeks, Jakatdar, & Heimberg, 2010). In addition, FPE relates more strongly to self-reported concerns of unwanted social consequences (e.g., envy from people of higher social status) following interpersonal successes and accomplishments than either FNE or trait social anxiety (Weeks, 2009).

In terms of specificity, FPE shows stronger relationships with social anxiety compared with worry, anxiety sensitivity, and depression in both undergraduate (Weeks, Heimberg, & Rodebaugh, 2008; Weeks, Heimberg, Rodebaugh, & Norton, 2008) and clinical (Fergus et al., 2009) samples; clients with SAD exhibit elevated FPE in comparison to people meeting criteria for other anxiety disorders (Fergus et al., 2009); and FPE has been shown to be sensitive to CBT for SAD, decreasing from pre- to post-treatment (Fergus et al., 2009). In further support of the separation between fears of positive and negative evaluation, FPE (but not FNE) relates positively to discomfort after receiving positive social feedback and negatively to perceived accuracy of this feedback (Weeks, Heimberg, Rodebaugh, & Norton, 2008). Social anxiety may be characterized by a self-image simultaneously biased by indicators of not only negative (e.g., Coles et al., 2001; Hackmann et al., 1998), but also positive (Weeks, Heimberg, & Rodebaugh, 2008; Weeks, Heimberg, Rodebaugh, & Norton, 2008), aspects of the self. But in contrast to the bias involved in negative aspects of the self-image (i.e., FNE), which are magnified in the mental representation, FPE may lead to a *minimization* of positive aspects of the self. Thus, SAIs may possess a self-image that specifies that they *are* nervous-looking and *are not* fun to be around (Weeks, Heimberg, Rodebaugh, & Norton, 2008). In essence, social threat could be perceived in *any* situation in which the person might receive either positive or negative evaluation (see Weeks, Heimberg, Rodebaugh, 2008). Indeed, the severity of state anxiety experienced during a social role-play has been found to vary as discrete functions of the interactions between FPE/FNE and exposure to specific social cues. For example, for people who engage in a semi-structured role-play with experimental confederates trained to respond to them in a standard positive manner (e.g., smiling, agreeing, nodding one's head often), higher FPE was associated with *maintained/elevated* state anxiety during the role-play in response to positive social signals; FNE, in contrast, was associated with *decreased* state anxiety in response to positive signals (Weeks, Jakatdar, & Heimberg, 2009).

Converging with data showing that SAD is characterized by less frequent positive affect (Kashdan, 2007) and frequent negative affect (Brown et al., 1998), FPE and FNE are both associated with greater negative affect and lesser positive affect in typical social interactions (Weeks et al., 2010). In parallel, FPE and FNE each are related to (less) positive and (more) negative automatic thoughts during social interactions (Weeks, 2009). Taken together, FPE and FNE may best be characterized as hand-in-hand core cognitive features of social anxiety.

Interpreting Positive Events as Threats of Future Failure

The work of Alden and colleagues (Alden & Wallace, 1995; Alden, Mellings, & Laposa, 2004; Alden, Taylor, Mellings, & Laposa, 2008) has been highly influential in informing our understanding of the responses that people with SAD have to overtly positive social outcomes. For example, when clients with generalized SAD and matched nonclinical controls engage in a role-play with experimental assistants who respond with either standardized positive or negative behavior, the clients with SAD who received the positive feedback predicted that their partner would expect more from them in the next interaction. In turn, they feared they would fall short of these heightened expectations (Alden & Wallace, 1995). Thus, fear of *eventual* negative appraisal (i.e., a delayed form of FNE) accounts in part for acute fear of positive appraisal. In fact, following a social role-play, SAD clients presented with feedback highlighting the *positive* aspects of their performance predicted they would be *more anxious* in a second interaction than SAD clients provided with feedback framed to highlight the *absence of negative* performance qualities (Alden et al., 2004).

To better examine whether people with SAD indeed worry that they will eventually fall short of heightened expectations, researchers developed an 8-item self-report measure, the Interpretation of Positive Events Scale (IPES), with strong psychometric properties in both college and clinical samples (Alden et al., 2008; Laposa, Cassin, & Rector, 2010). It is worth noting that, consistent with Alden and colleagues' (1995, 2004) interpretation that acute concerns over positive social events pertain primarily to eventual fear of negative appraisal, the majority of IPES items specify concerns of future negative evaluation (e.g., "I will disappoint them in the future"). Social interaction anxiety has been shown to account for unique variance in interpreting positive events as threats of future failure (i.e., IPES scores) beyond general negative affect. In addition, these negative interpretations of positive events are elevated in clients with generalized SAD compared with healthy community controls during a positive social interaction task, even upon controlling for depressive symptoms (Alden et al., 2008). Interpretations of positive events as threats of future failure are also higher in treatment-seeking clients with SAD than in clients with GAD and PD (Laposa et al., 2010).

It has also been suggested that PEP, a post-mortem analysis that tends to follow social interactions and that is ruminative and negative in nature (Clark & Wells, 1995; Hofmann, 2007), may be linked to interpretations of positive events as threats of future failure (Laposa et al., in press). This makes intuitive sense, given that both PEP and interpretations of positive events as threats of future failure involve a negative focus on social interactions. Both cognitive events occur following a social event and both involve distal (i.e., past or future) rather than proximal (i.e., present) social processing.

Life Satisfaction and Quality of Life

Beyond fears of positive evaluation and particular positive beliefs, we can focus on a broader level of positive cognitions that includes life satisfaction and quality of life. Quality of life refers to "a person's subjective evaluation of the degree to which his or her most important needs, goals, and wishes have been fulfilled" in meaningful life domains (Frisch, 1994). Alongside positive and negative emotions, these cognitive evaluations about one's life can be considered a cornerstone of happiness (Diener, Suh, Lucas, & Smith, 1999). More fine-grained components of quality of life can include personal fulfillment in work and leisure, significant and satisfying social bonds, and an enriching neighborhood and community. Alternative conceptualizations of quality of life that address the ability to successfully perform physical activities and the continuum from illness to health are not addressed because they are beyond the scope of positive psychological functioning.

When generic measures of quality of life are used, clinic outpatients with SAD show marked deficits that are comparable to outpatients with depression or the presence of both SAD and depression (Wittchen, Fuetsch, Sonntag, Müller, & Liebowitz, 2000). Even upon accounting for the functionally impairing nature of social anxiety symptoms, people with SAD endorse a poor overall sense of well-being (Hambrick, Turk, Heimberg, Schneier, & Liebowitz, 2003), suggesting that quality of life is not synonymous with disability.

Inverse relations between quality of life and the social anxiety spectrum have been replicated with other sampling strategies. Using an epidemiological survey of more than 8000 Canadian residents, people with SAD endorsed less satisfaction and functioning in nearly every life domain compared to people without SAD (Stein & Kean, 2000). In fact, even after accounting for lifetime history of depression, age, gender, and socioeconomic status, people with SAD showed marked dissatisfaction with their family life, friendships, and leisure and recreation. In primary care settings, people diagnosed with SAD show a substantially increased risk of being markedly dissatisfied with their friendships and leisure activities (Stein, McQuaid, Laffaye, & McCahill, 1999).

When focusing on positive emotions, behaviors, cognitions, and events, questions arise as to whether current treatments require modification to address these novel targets. Two studies provide preliminary evidence that existing cognitive behavioral treatment protocols for clients with SAD can lead to improvements in quality of life (Eng, Coles, Heimberg, & Safren, 2001, 2004). Importantly, treatment affected more than just satisfaction with relationships; in fact, some of the greatest benefits arose in perceived playfulness, clarification of goals and values, being exposed to new knowledge and experiences, and creativity. These findings imply that the tools taught in cognitive behavioral treatment have broad effects beyond the scope of life domains that are explicitly addressed. However, it is important to note that additional improvements were not observed at the six-month follow-up assessment (Eng et al., 2001). Empirically supported adjunct modules that directly target positive emotions, the discovery and regular application of personal strengths, and fulfillment in various life domains should be explored for their potential in aiding people beyond merely achieving statistically significant improvements to high endstate functioning, to instead striving for levels similar to successful, psychologically healthy members of society.

BIOLOGICAL MARKERS OF DIMINISHED REWARDS IN SOCIAL ANXIETY

If social anxiety and SAD are characterized by attenuated positive experiences and fewer positive events, this effect should not be circumscribed to subjective and behavioral levels of analysis. Impairments in the neural circuitry linked to positive experiences and approach-oriented exploratory behavior should be observable. As might be expected, compared with research using self-report methodologies, there is less research on biobehavioral reward mechanisms. To understand these mechanisms, it is useful to distinguish between "wanting" and "liking" (Panksepp, 1998). Wanting reflects incentive motivation or the desire to recognize, seek, and exploit interesting and desirable rewards. Liking reflects the pleasurable experience of consuming rewards. For example, a little girl might crave a puppy, visiting pet stores, talking about it to friends and family, and spending time learning how to care for one and preparing her house in case she finally gets one; this is wanting. Liking is manifested by the subjective pleasure of getting a puppy, and behavioral reactions such as smiling at and hugging the puppy. Wanting is the motivation for reward: the creation, pursuit, and progress toward cognitive goals; curiosity and exploration are central, with dopaminergic neurotransmission as the biological underpinnings (e.g., Berridge, 2007; Depue & Collins, 1999; Ikemoto & Panksepp, 1999). Liking reactions reflect pleasure and satisfaction; positive emotions and cognitive evaluations are central, with opiate neurotransmission as the biological underpinnings (e.g., Pecina, 2008; Smith & Berridge, 2007). Of course, these neurotransmitters often operate together as rewarding situations unfold in dynamic, fluid, complex ways outside of static experimental settings (Panksepp, 1998).

Unfortunately, the literature is relatively devoid of research on measurements of opiate receptor activity in reference to SAD. Thus, we focus on links between SAD and dopaminergic activity. In general, at rest, people with SAD exhibit lower DA reuptake density in the ventral striatal region compared with nondisordered adults (Tiihonen et al., 1997). Similarly, people with SAD exhibit less DA receptor binding in the same striatal region compared with nondisordered adults (Schneier et al., 2000). Of course, SAD is defined by fearful reactions when exposed to potentially threatening information and, thus, it might be more informative to examine what happens during challenging tasks. In one study, while being observed during fMRI, people with SAD participated in a cognitively challenging learning task (Sareen et al., 2007). Despite an absence of group differences in behavioral performance, people with SAD exhibited less activity in the striatal brain regions – the largest repository of DA receptors in the brain. Taken together, existing data converges with self-report research demonstrating that socially anxious people experience fewer positive events and are less curious and approach-oriented in their daily lives. It will be important to broaden this small body of work by observing how people with SAD respond at the neurobiological level in dynamic social situations. To our knowledge, in the only study to address this, EEG activity was measured while people with SAD and nondisordered controls anticipated making a speech in front of strangers (Davidson, Marshall, Tomarken, & Henriques, 2000). For people with SAD, greater reactivity in the right anterior and lateral prefrontal cortex relative to the comparison group suggests greater motivation to escape and less approach-related motivation (which coincides with left prefrontal cortex activation). This is an important study that requires replication. Without exposure to feared situations, spanning the anticipation, engagement in, and recollection of social encounters, it is difficult to understand which neurotransmitter systems and brain regions are dysregulated and which are most amenable to change via psychological and pharmacological treatments.

MEANINGFUL HETEROGENEITY IN SOCIAL ANXIETY

Affective processes in psychopathology are often studied without an appreciation of heterogeneity. On average, people with social anxiety problems can be characterized by diminished positive emotions and curiosity and infrequent positive events (among other qualities referenced by the authors of other chapters). As reported above, some initial work suggests that this profile varies according to how people regulate their emotions. Other strategies for subtyping people with social anxiety are also relevant to understanding links to positive experiences and events.

To date, most of the work on social anxiety subtypes has focused on the number and types of feared and avoided social situations. In particular, generalized SAD refers to fearing most social situations involving direct interactions with others, whereas nongeneralized SAD refers to the fear of circumscribed social situations such as giving performances or being observed by others (American Psychiatric Association, 2000). There is evidence that diminished positive emotions and curiosity relate primarily to generalized social interaction fears, whereas small to near-zero relationships exist with social performance and observation fears (Hughes et al., 2006; Kashdan, 2002). Furthermore, compared to people with the nongeneralized (public speaking) SAD subtype, people in the community with generalized SAD had a seven times greater likelihood of being classified with severe impairment in quality of life (on indicators such as energy, interest in life, and satisfaction about relationships) (Stein & Kean, 2000); other studies also find that quality of life is only relevant to social interaction anxiety and the generalized subtype of SAD (and not performance and observational fears; Safren, Heimberg, Brown, & Holle, 1997). These findings fit with existing theory and research suggesting that connections with other people are the primary source of positive experiences in life, from pleasures to profound love and meaning (Reis, Collins, & Berscheid, 2000). Although successful performances in front of other people can be a source of pleasure and meaning, such an experience is often transitory and pales in comparison to the significant, lasting, energizing quality of fulfilling relationships.

Alternative strategies for classifying people suffering from social anxiety are also relevant to the current discussion of positive experiences and events. In fact, one of the more useful subtyping strategies accounts for variability in approach and avoidance processes. The motivation to avoid negative evaluation leads socially anxious people to avoid or escape social situations. Although most of the work on social anxiety has focused on over-regulated, risk-averse responses, there is reason to expect heterogeneity in the self-regulatory strategies used in an attempt to avoid rejection. At least a subset of socially anxious people use qualitatively different strategies that are best described as risk-prone approach behavior (Hofmann, Heinrichs, & Moscovitch, 2004; Kachin, Newman, & Pincus, 2001; Kashdan, Collins, & Elhai, 2006; Kashdan, Elhai, & Breen, 2008). For instance, a socially anxious person might argue with another person, ostracizing them, to gain a sense of dominance before the other person has a chance to even consider rejecting them. Another socially anxious person might have sex with a stranger or prostitute, thereby extracting immediate sensory pleasure and feelings of belonging. These seemingly atypical, uninhibited behaviors differ in form from the shyness and inhibition that is stereotypical of social anxiety in the literature. However, the functional goal of these risk-prone approach behaviors is proposed to be the same: to temporarily avoid the unwanted experience of anxiety or the likelihood of rejection.

In several studies, researchers sought to determine whether socially anxious people can be meaningfully differentiated by strategies that, at least on the surface, vary in approach and avoidance. In one study of outpatients with generalized SAD, a distinct subgroup endorsed high novelty seeking and exploratory tendencies in response to impulsive decision-making compared to a more stereotypical group with a near absence of novelty seeking (Kashdan & Hofmann, 2008). In another study with a non-clinical sample, researchers found two distinct subgroups of socially anxious people based on their appraisals for being aggressive, engaging in risky sex, and abusing alcohol and drugs (Kashdan et al., 2008). There was a stereotypically inhibited group characterized by the strongest beliefs that doing these activities would be personally threatening and would fail to enhance their social status, and there was a relative absence of curiosity about the potential experience. In stark contrast, there was an approach-oriented group characterized by strong curiosity for engaging in these risk-taking behaviors and beliefs that doing so would enhance their social status. As support for the separation between these two groups, over a three-month period, socially anxious people in the approach-oriented group reported more frequent aggression, risky sexual behavior, and substance use and abuse.

Taken together, these studies suggest self-regulatory strategies that have been omitted from most descriptions of social anxiety and thus fail to inform theory or treatment. It appears that at least a subset of people with elevated social anxiety are prone to behaviors that can generate opportunities for positive experiences in the short-term by inducing a sense of power and control (e.g., violence), serenity (e.g., substance abuse), orgasmic pleasure (e.g., sex with prostitutes), and/or curiosity and excitement (e.g., novelty and thrill-seeking). However, these same behaviors appear to detract from quality of life in the longer term (Kashdan & McKnight, 2010; Kashdan, McKnight, Richey, & Hofmann, 2009). People with deficient impulse control show less intelligent problem-solving skills, less persistence on demanding tasks, less satisfaction and commitment in social relationships, and poorer physical health (e.g., Baumeister, Gailliot, DeWall, & Oaten, 2006). The presence of meaningful subsets of socially anxious people provides one explanation for the often modest correlations with positive experiences and events. Nonsignificant and trivial relationships with positive outcomes might be a function of merging diverse sets of people into a single pool; studies with clinic samples or a neurobiological focus are notorious for smaller samples, and so might be particularly affected. Conclusions about the nature, course, and treatment of the positive spectrum of human functioning in social anxiety may be compromised by failing to account for heterogeneous regulatory styles.

SUMMARY

There is some evidence that social anxiety is associated with diminished positive experiences, infrequent positive events, an absence of positive inferential biases in social situations, and poor quality of life that cannot be explained by the co-occurrence or severity of depression. Existing research suggests that general social interaction anxiety appears more relevant to attenuated positive experiences than circumscribed social anxiety problems (e.g., performance and observation fears). Of note, these positive constructs serve to distinguish SAD and elevated social interaction anxiety from other anxiety conditions (Brown et al., 1998). Initial evidence suggests that the relationship between social anxiety and positive events might vary as a function of how people manage their emotions in everyday life (Kashdan & Steger, 2006; Vohs et al., 2005). It will be important to conduct additional studies to explore the intriguing notion that high social anxiety in conjunction with tendencies to conceal or hide emotions leads to the greatest vulnerability in terms of infrequent positive emotions, cognitions, behaviors, and events in daily life. Another promising mechanism that might explain these social anxiety effects is the depletion of finite cognitive resources and stamina as a result of hypervigilant efforts to regulate anxiety, manage social impressions, and avoid potential social threats (Hayes et al., 2006; Leary, 2000).

In the absence of impending threat or in ambiguous situations, the average person shows a tendency to be approach-oriented and exploratory (Cacioppo et al., 1997). However, this positive motivational bias appears to be deficient in people with excessive social anxiety, who often experience disruptions in the ability to process what is happening in the present moment (regardless of whether the situation is overtly negative, ambiguous, or slightly positive). Instead of being mindfully aware of what is happening, socially anxious people often find themselves trapped in a ruminative mindset. When evaluating events that one has taken part in, people with greater social anxiety focus on and recall less positive (and more negative) details (de Jong et al., 2009; Garner et al., 2006; Hirsch & Mathews, 2000). As time unfolds after an event, this lack of a positive bias only strengthens (Brendle & Wenzel, 2004). These inferential biases extend to the FPE and positive social outcomes. These fears are due in part to concerns of direct social comparison, social reprisal from people perceived to be of higher social status (Weeks, Heimberg, & Rodebaugh, 2008; Weeks, Heimberg, Rodebaugh, & Norton, 2008), and concerns of unintentionally setting social standards that will be unattainable in the future (Alden et al., 2008). Taken together, we gain a clearer picture of why people with excessive social anxiety tend to engage less in approach behaviors and are inclined toward BI. Although this profile might be prototypical of people with excessive social anxiety, evidence suggests the presence of meaningful alternative profiles.

A subset of high socially anxious people appears to engage in excitable, impulsive, and novelty-seeking behavior patterns. This combination of high social anxiety and behavioral disinhibition appears to characterize a particularly impaired subgroup. To be more specific, they report short-term pleasures such as increased sexual activity and socializing but this fails to translate into lasting satisfaction or well-being (Kashdan et al., 2008, 2009; Kashdan & McKnight, 2010). The neurotransmitters, cortical regions, and cortical activity relevant to novelty-seeking and approach behavior (e.g., dopaminergic agents, left prefrontal cortex activity) are distinct from those relevant to negative affect and avoidance activity. Thus, future studies are needed to examine the incremental validity of this new scheme for understanding how and when social anxiety is related to the generation of and sensitivity to rewarding events – beyond what is observed by assuming a homogenous group or distinguishing people by types of social fears (generalized v.s. nongeneralized). The research reviewed in this chapter suggests that subsets of people with excessive social anxiety differ in their experience of and sensitivity to rewarding events. It will be important to continue constructing the psychological, social, cultural, and biological factors that are most relevant to vulnerability and resilience.

Research on the developmental origins of attenuated positive experiences, cognitions, and events has lagged behind knowledge about phenomenology and maintenance. There is reason to suspect that dysfunctional early attachments and extensive peer rejection and ostracism in childhood might precipitate social anxiety problems and, in turn, lead to reduced reward responsiveness to social interactions (Vertue, 2003). That is, socially anxious children might learn to expect nonrewards when interacting with other people. As social creatures, losing out on the pleasures of anticipating, experiencing, and savoring contact with other people might dramatically alter the hedonistic tone of daily life. There is a need for fine-grained analyses of the types of parenting practices, peer relationships, romantic relationships, and stressors that differentially affect people with particular genetic and personality characteristics and social skills. As an addition to these diathesis-stress models, future work can examine the presence of critical developmental periods when social anxiety problems and diminished positive functioning show the greater probability of developing (under the right conditions). Of course, work on vulnerability should be tempered with an equal emphasis on factors that offer protective effects.

The integration of the positive spectrum of human functioning into the study and treatment of social anxiety is in its infancy. However, the current data suggest some new targets of intervention and early evidence suggests that positive cognitions can be altered by current forms of CBT (Eng et al., 2001, 2004; Murphy et al., 2007). As for increasing the frequency of positive events and the ability to extract pleasure and meaning from them, it remains to be seen whether current interventions that are efficacious at targeting social anxiety symptoms will suffice. Also, although there is some initial evidence that people with SAD can enhance their positive cognitions, by the end of treatment, their functioning is still far below the normative levels found in the general population. The goal of practitioners should be extended beyond the reduction of distress and disorder to helping people discover and maintain sustainable sources of positive emotions, engagement, and meaning. We can begin by expanding the repertoire of constructs studied in relation to social anxiety to include neglected elements of a good life, such as the development of strengths of character and devoting daily effort toward meaningful, approach-oriented strivings. With translational research, we can understand the conditions and intervention modules that best facilitate positive states and traits. The inclusion of adjunct modules that address positive elements of living might offer incremental benefit to existing therapies. We hope that the current chapter inspires clinical scientists interested in social anxiety and the related disorders to broaden their research and treatment efforts to the vast, rarely explored territory of the positive.

REFERENCES

Alden, L. E., Mellings, T. M. B., & Laposa, J. M. (2004). Framing social information and generalized social phobia. *Behaviour Research and Therapy*, *42*, 585–600.

Alden, L. E., Taylor, C. T., Mellings, T. M. B., & Laposa, J. M. (2008). Social anxiety and the interpretation of positive social events. *Journal of Anxiety Disorders*, *22*, 577–590.

Alden, L. E., & Wallace, S. T. (1995). Social phobia and social appraisal in successful and unsuccessful interactions. *Behaviour Research and Therapy*, *33*, 497–506.

American Psychiatric Association (2000). *Diagnostic and statistical manual of mental disorders* (4th ed.) (DSM-IV). Washington, DC: Author.

Baumeister, R. F., Gailliot, M., DeWall, C. N., & Oaten, M. (2006). Self-regulation and personality: How interventions increase regulatory success, and how depletion moderates the effects of traits on behavior. *Journal of Personality*, *74*, 1773–1801.

Berenbaum, H., & Oltmanns, T. F. (1992). Emotional experience and expression in schizophrenia and depression. *Journal of Abnormal Psychology*, *101*, 37–44.

Berridge, K. C. (2007). The debate over dopamine's role in reward: The case for incentive salience. *Psychopharmacology*, *191*, 391–431.

Blanchard, J. J., Mueser, K. T., & Bellack, A. S. (1998). Anhedonia, positive and negative affect, and social functioning in schizophrenia. *Schizophrenia Bulletin*, *24*, 413–424.

Boucher, J., & Osgood, C. E. (1969). The Pollyanna hypothesis. *Journal of Verbal Learning and Verbal Behavior*, *8*, 1–8.

Brendle, J. R., & Wenzel, A. (2004). Differentiating between memory and interpretation biases in socially anxious and nonanxious individuals. *Behaviour Research and Therapy*, *42*, 155–171.

Brown, L. H., Silvia, P. J., Myin-Germeys, I., & Kwapil, T. R. (2007). When the need to belong goes wrong: The expression of social anhedonia and social anxiety in daily life. *Psychological Science*, *18*, 778–782.

Brown, T. A., Chorpita, B. F., & Barlow, D. H. (1998). Structural relationships among dimensions of DSM-IV anxiety and mood disorders and dimensions of negative affect, positive affect, and autonomic arousal. *Journal of Abnormal Psychology*, *107*, 179–192.

Brown, T. A., DiNardo, P. A., & Barlow, D. H. (1994). *Anxiety Disorders Interview Schedule for DSM-IV.* (ADIS-IV). New York: Oxford University Press.

Cacioppo, J. T., Gardner, W. L., & Berntson, G. G. (1997). Beyond bipolar conceptualizations and measures: The case of attitudes and evaluative space. *Personality and Social Psychology Review*, *1*, 3–25.

Carver, C. S., Sutton, S. K., & Scheier, M. F. (2000). Action, emotion, and personality: Emerging conceptual integration. *Personality and Social Psychology Bulletin*, *26*, 741–751.

Clark, D. A., Steer, R. A., & Beck, A. T. (1994). Common and specific dimensions of self-reported anxiety and depression: Implications for the cognitive and tripartite models. *Journal of Abnormal Psychology*, *103*, 645–654.

Clark, D. M., & Wells, A. (1995). A cognitive model of social phobia. In R. G. Heimberg, M. R. Liebowitz, D. A. Hope, & F. R. Schneier (Eds.), *Social phobia: Diagnosis, assessment, and treatment* (pp. 69–94). New York: Guilford Press.

Clark, L. A., & Watson, D. (1991). Tripartite model of anxiety and depression: Psychometric evidence and taxonomic implications. *Journal of Abnormal Psychology, 100*, 316–336.

Coles, M. E., Turk, C. L., Heimberg, R. G., & Fresco, D. M. (2001). Effects of varying levels of anxiety within social situations: Relationship to memory perspective and attributions in social phobia. *Behaviour Research and Therapy, 39*, 651–665.

Davidson, R. J., Marshall, J. R., Tomarken, A. J., & Henriques, J. B. (2000). While a phobic waits: Regional brain electrical and autonomic activity in social phobics during anticipation of public speaking. *Biological Psychiatry, 47*, 85–95.

de Jong, P. J., de Graaf-Peters, V., van Hout, W. J. P. J., & van Wees, R. (2009). Covariation bias for social events and signs of (dis)approval in high and low socially anxious individuals. *Journal of Behavior Therapy and Experimental Psychiatry, 40*, 359–373.

Depue, R. A., & Collins, P. F. (1999). Neurobiology of the structure of personality: Dopamine, facilitation of incentive motivation, and extraversion. *Behavioral and Brain Sciences, 22*, 491–569.

Diener, E., Suh, E. M., Lucas, R. E., & Smith, H. L. (1999). Subjective well-being: Three decades of progress. *Psychological Bulletin, 125*, 276–302.

Eng, W., Coles, M. E., Heimberg, R. G., & Safren, S. A. (2001). Quality of life following cognitive behavioral treatment for social anxiety disorder: Preliminary findings. *Depression and Anxiety, 13*, 192–193.

Eng, W., Coles, M. E., Heimberg, R. G., & Safren, S. A. (2004). Domains of life satisfaction in social anxiety disorder: Relation to symptoms and response to cognitive behavioral therapy. *Journal of Anxiety Disorders, 19*, 143–156.

Fergus, T. A., Valentiner, D. P., McGrath, P. B., Stephenson, K., Gier, S., & Jencius, S. (2009). The Fear of Positive Evaluation Scale: Psychometric properties in a clinical sample. *Journal of Anxiety Disorders, 23*, 1177–1183.

Fredrickson, B. L. (1998). What good are positive emotions? *Review of General Psychology, 2*, 300–319.

Frisch, M. B. (1994). *Quality of Life Inventory: Manual and treatment guide*. Minneapolis, MN: National Computer Systems.

Garner, M., Mogg, K., & Bradley, B. P. (2006). Fear-relevant selective associations and social anxiety: Absence of a positive bias. *Behaviour Research and Therapy, 44*, 201–217.

Gilbert, P. (2001). Evolution and social anxiety: The role of attraction, social competition, and social hierarchies. *Psychiatric Clinics of North America, 24*, 723–751.

Gray, J. A., & McNaughton, N. (1996). The neuropsychology of anxiety: Reprise. In D. A. Hope (Ed.), *Perspectives on anxiety, panic, and fear: Vol. 43.* (pp. 61–134). Lincoln, NB: University of Nebraska Press.

Hackmann, A., Surawy, C., & Clark, D. M. (1998). Seeing yourself through others' eyes: A study of spontaneously occurring images in social phobia. *Behavioural and Cognitive Psychotherapy, 26*, 3–12.

Hambrick, J. P., Turk, C. L., Heimberg, R. G., Schneier, F. R., & Liebowitz, M. R. (2003). The experience of disability and quality of life in social anxiety disorder. *Depression and Anxiety, 18*, 46–50.

Hayes, S. C., Luoma, J. B., Bond, F. W., Masuda, A., & Lillis, J. (2006). Acceptance and commitment therapy: Model, processes and outcomes. *Behaviour Research and Therapy, 44*, 1–25.

Hirsch, C. R., & Mathews, A. (2000). Impaired positive inferential bias in social phobia. *Journal of Abnormal Psychology, 109*, 705–712.

Hofmann, S. G. (2007). Cognitive factors that maintain social anxiety disorder: A comprehensive model and its treatment implications. *Cognitive Behaviour Therapy*, *36*, 193–209.

Hofmann, S. G., Heinrichs, N., & Moscovitch, D. A. (2004). The nature and expression of social phobia: Toward a new classification. *Clinical Psychology Review*, *24*, 769–797.

Horley, K., Williams, L. M., Gonsalvez, C., & Gordon, E. (2004). Face to face: Visual scanpath evidence for abnormal processing of facial expressions in social phobia. *Psychiatry Research*, *127*, 43–53.

Hughes, A. A., Heimberg, R. G., Coles, M. E., Gibb, B. E., Liebowitz, M. R., & Schneier, F. R. (2006). Relations of the factors of the tripartite model of anxiety and depression to types of social anxiety. *Behaviour Research and Therapy*, *44*, 1629–1641.

Ikemoto, S., & Panksepp, J. (1999). The role of nucleus accumbens dopamine in motivated behavior: A unifying interpretation with special reference to reward-seeking. *Brain Research Reviews*, *31*, 6–41.

Ito, T. A., & Cacioppo, J. T. (2005). Variations on a human universal: Individual differences in positivity offset and negativity bias. *Cognition and Emotion*, *19*, 1–26.

Kachin, K. E., Newman, M. G., & Pincus, A. L. (2001). An interpersonal problem approach to the division of social phobia subtypes. *Behavior Therapy*, *32*, 479–501.

Kashdan, T. B. (2002). Social anxiety dimensions, neuroticism, and the contours of positive psychological functioning. *Cognitive Therapy and Research*, *26*, 789–810.

Kashdan, T. B. (2007). Social anxiety spectrum and diminished positive experiences: Theoretical synthesis and meta-analysis. *Clinical Psychology Review*, *27*, 348–365.

Kashdan, T. B., Breen, W. E., & Julian, T. (2010). Everyday strivings in combat veterans with posttraumatic stress disorder: Problems arise when avoidance and emotion regulation dominate. *Behavior Therapy*.

Kashdan, T. B., & Collins, R. L. (2010). Social anxiety and the experience of positive emotions and anger in everyday life: An ecological momentary assessment approach. *Anxiety, Stress, & Coping*, *23*, 259–272.

Kashdan, T. B., Collins, R. L., & Elhai, J. D. (2006). Social anxiety, positive outcome expectancies, and risk-taking behavioral intentions. *Cognitive Therapy and Research*, *30*, 749–761.

Kashdan, T. B., Elhai, J. D., & Breen, W. E. (2008). Social anxiety and disinhibition: An analysis of curiosity and social rank appraisals, approach-avoidance conflicts, and disruptive risk-taking behavior. *Journal of Anxiety Disorders*, *22*, 925–939.

Kashdan, T. B., & Hofmann, S. G. (2008). The high novelty seeking, impulsive subtype of generalized social anxiety disorder. *Depression and Anxiety*, *25*, 535–541.

Kashdan, T. B., Julian, T., Merritt, K., & Uswatte, G. (2006). Social anxiety and posttraumatic stress in combat veterans: Relations to well-being and human strengths. *Behaviour Research and Therapy*, *44*, 561–583.

Kashdan, T. B., & McKnight, P. E. (2010). The darker side of social anxiety: When aggressive impulsivity prevails over shy inhibition. *Current Directions in Psychological Science*, *19*, 47–50.

Kashdan, T. B., McKnight, P. E., Richey, J. A., & Hofmann, S. G. (2009). When social anxiety disorder co-exists with risk-prone, approach behavior: Investigating a neglected, meaningful subset of people in the National Comorbidity Survey-Replication. *Behaviour Research and Therapy*, *47*, 559–568.

Kashdan, T. B., & Roberts, J. E. (2004). Social anxiety's impact on affect, curiosity, and social self-efficacy during a high self-focus social threat situation. *Cognitive Therapy and Research*, *28*, 119–141.

Kashdan, T. B., & Steger, M. F. (2006). Expanding the topography of social anxiety: An experience sampling assessment of positive emotions and events, and emotion suppression. *Psychological Science*, *17*, 120–128.

Laposa, J. M., Cassin, S. E., & Rector, N. A. (2010). Interpretation of positive social events in social phobia: An examination of cognitive correlates and diagnostic distinction. *Journal of Anxiety Disorders*, *24*, 203–210.

Leary, M. R. (2000). Social anxiety as an early warning system: A refinement and extension of the self-presentational theory of social anxiety. In S. G. Hofman & P. M. DiBartolo (Eds.), *Social phobia and social anxiety: An integration* (pp. 321–334). New York: Allyn & Bacon.

Mansell, W., & Clark, D. M. (1999). How do I appear to others? Social anxiety and processing of the observable self. *Behaviour Research and Therapy*, *37*, 419–434.

Mattick, R. P., & Clarke, J. C. (1998). Development and validation of measures of social phobia scrutiny fear and social interaction anxiety. *Behaviour Research and Therapy*, *36*, 455–470.

Moser, J. S., Hajcak, G., Huppert, J. D., Foa, E. B., & Simons, R. F. (2008). Interpretation bias in social anxiety as detected by event-related brain potentials. *Emotion*, *8*, 693–700.

Muraven, M., & Baumeister, R. F. (2000). Self-regulation and depletion of limited resources: Does self-control resemble a muscle? *Psychological Bulletin*, *126*, 247–259.

Murphy, R., Hirsch, C. R., Mathews, A., Smith, K., & Clark, D. M. (2007). Facilitating a benign interpretation bias in a high socially anxious population. *Behaviour Research and Therapy*, *45*, 1517–1529.

Panksepp, J. (1998). *Affective neuroscience: The foundations of human and animal emotions*. New York: Oxford University Press.

Pecina, S. (2008). Opioid reward "liking" and "wanting" in the nucleus accumbens. *Physiology and Behavior*, *94*, 675–680.

Rapee, R. M., & Heimberg, R. G. (1997). A cognitive-behavioral model of anxiety in social phobia. *Behaviour Research and Therapy*, *35*, 741–756.

Reis, H. T., Collins, W. A., & Berscheid, E. (2000). The relationship context of human behavior and development. *Psychological Bulletin*, *126*, 844–872.

Rottenberg, J. (2005). Mood and emotion in major depression. *Current Directions in Psychological Science*, *14*, 167–170.

Safren, S. A., Heimberg, R. G., Brown, E. J., & Holle, C. (1997). Quality of life in social phobia. *Depression and Anxiety*, *4*, 126–133.

Sareen, J., Campbell, D. W., Leslie, W. D., Malisza, K. L., Stein, M. B., et al. (2007). Striatal function in generalized social phobia: A functional magnetic resonance imaging study. *Biological Psychiatry*, *61*, 396–404.

Schlenker, B. R., & Leary, M. R. (1982). Social anxiety and self-presentation: A conceptualization and model. *Psychological Bulletin*, *92*, 641–669.

Schneier, F. R., Heimberg, R. G., Belzer, K., & Liebowitz, M. R. (2006). Submissive behavior and social comparison in social anxiety disorder. Unpublished manuscript.

Schneier, F. R., Liebowitz, M. R., Abi-Dargham, A., Zea-Ponce, Y., Shu-Hsing, L., & Laruelle, M. (2000). Low dopamine D2 receptor binding potential in social phobia. *American Journal of Psychiatry*, *157*, 457–459.

Smith, K. S., & Berridge, K. C. (2007). Opioid limbic circuit for reward: Interaction between hedonic hotspots of nucleus accumbens and ventral pallidum. *Journal of Neuroscience*, *27*, 1594–1605.

Stein, M. B., & Kean, Y. M. (2000). Disability and quality of life in social phobia: Epidemiologic findings. *American Journal of Psychiatry*, *157*, 1606–1613.

Stein, M. B., McQuaid, J. R., Laffaye, C., & McCahill, M. E. (1999). Social phobia in the primary care setting. *Journal of Family Practice*, *48*, 514–519.

Tiihonen, J., Kuikka, J., Bergstrom, K., Lepola, U., Koponen, H., & Leinonen, E. (1997). Dopamine reuptake site densities in patients with social phobia. *American Journal of Psychiatry*, *154*, 239–242.

Vertue, F. M. (2003). From adaptive emotion to dysfunction: An attachment perspective on social anxiety disorder. *Personality and Social Psychology Review*, *7*, 170–191.

Vittengl, J. R., & Holt, C. S. (1998). Positive and negative affect in social interactions as a function of partner, familiarity, quality of communication, and social anxiety. *Journal of Social and Clinical Psychology*, *17*, 196–208.

Vohs, K. D., Baumeister, R. F., & Ciarocco, N. (2005). Self-regulation and self-presentation: Regulatory resource depletion impairs impression management and effortful self-presentation depletes regulatory resources. *Journal of Personality and Social Psychology*, *88*, 632–657.

Wallace, S. T., & Alden, L. E. (1997). Social phobia and positive social events: The price of success. *Journal of Abnormal Psychology*, *106*, 416–424.

Watson, D., Clark, L. A., & Carey, G. (1988). Positive and negative affect and their relation to anxiety and depressive disorders. *Journal of Abnormal Psychology*, *97*, 346–353.

Watson, D., Clark, L. A., & Tellegen, A. (1988). Development and validation of brief measures of positive and negative affect: The PANAS. *Journal of Personality and Social Psychology*, *54*, 1063–1070.

Watson, D., & Friend, R. (1969). Measurement of socio-evaluative anxiety. *Journal of Consulting and Clinical Psychology*, *33*, 448–457.

Weeks, J. W. (2009). Further integrating findings on fears of positive and negative evaluation: A bivalent fear of evaluation model of social anxiety. In J. W. Weeks (Chair), *Extending the exploration of fears of positive and negative evaluation: Integral cognitive components of social anxiety disorder?* Paper presented at the annual meeting of the Association for Behavioral and Cognitive Therapies, New York, NY.

Weeks, J. W., Heimberg, R. G., & Rodebaugh, T. L. (2008a). The Fear of Positive Evaluation Scale: Assessing a proposed cognitive component of social anxiety disorder. *Journal of Anxiety Disorders*, *22*, 44–55.

Weeks, J. W., Heimberg, R. G., Rodebaugh, T. L., & Norton, P. J., (2008b). Exploring the relationship between fear of positive evaluation and social anxiety. *Journal of Anxiety Disorders*, *22*, 386–400.

Weeks, J. W., Jakatdar, T. A., & Heimberg, R. G. (2009). Assessing state-based reactions associated with fears of positive and negative evaluation in social anxiety disorder: Parallel processing of distinct social cues. In E. A. Gordon (Chair), *Interpersonal processes in social anxiety disorder.* Paper presented at the annual meeting of the Association for Behavioral and Cognitive Therapies, New York, NY.

Weeks, J. W., Jakatdar, T. A., & Heimberg, R. G. (2010). Comparing and contrasting fears of positive and negative evaluation as facets of social anxiety. *Journal of Social and Clinical Psychology*, *29*, 68–94.

Wittchen, H. U., Fuetsch, M., Sonntag, H., Müller, N., & Liebowitz, M. (2000). Disability and quality of life in pure and comorbid social phobia: Findings from a controlled study. *European Psychiatry*, *15*, 46–58.

Chapter 18

Social Anxiety as an Early Warning System: A Refinement and Extension of the Self-Presentation Theory of Social Anxiety

Mark R. Leary
Department of Psychology, Duke University, Durham, NC 27708

Over the past 40 years, behavioral researchers have offered a variety of theoretical approaches for understanding social anxiety and its clinical manifestation, SAD. Although several explanations of social anxiety exist, most of them emphasize one of three sets of antecedents: biological mechanisms involving temperamental, genetic, psychophysiological, and evolutionary factors; cognitive patterns in how people think about themselves and their social worlds; and interpersonal processes that occur in the context of social interaction. These perspectives are not necessarily contradictory or mutually exclusive but rather approach the topic of social anxiety from different conceptual angles.

At its heart, the approach of the present chapter is decidedly social psychological in that it traces social anxiety to concerns that arise in the context of real, anticipated, and imagined interpersonal interactions. The chapter describes a refinement and extension of the self-presentational theory of social anxiety (Schlenker & Leary, 1982), a perspective that explains people's nervousness in social encounters in terms of their concerns about other people's perceptions of them. Although the self-presentation theory has fared well under the spotlight of empirical research, theoretical developments shed additional light on the self-presentational nature of social anxiety and provide a bridge by which our understanding of social anxiety may be linked to other phenomena involving interpersonal motives, social emotions, and the self. These theoretical refinements – which borrow from Baumeister and Leary's (1995) discussion of the need to belong, Baumeister and Tice's (1990) exclusion theory of anxiety, Leary and Downs's (1995) sociometer theory, and Leary's (2001)

Social Anxiety: Clinical, Developmental, and Social Perspectives. DOI: 10.1016/B978-0-12-375096-9.00018-3

conceptualization of relational value – do not contradict or refute self-presentation theory but rather take it to a deeper level, demonstrating precisely why it is that people worry so much about what other people think of them.

THE ORIGINAL SELF-PRESENTATION THEORY

The self-presentational theory of social anxiety has been described in detail elsewhere (Leary & Kowalski, 1995a, 1995b; Schlenker & Leary, 1982), so I will present it only briefly here. The theory's fundamental proposition is that people experience social anxiety before or during social encounters when they are motivated to make a desired impression on other people but doubt that they will successfully make the desired impression. Because the impressions that people make on others have important implications for how they are evaluated and treated in everyday life, people are understandably motivated to convey certain impressions of themselves and to avoid making certain other impressions (Leary, 1995; Schlenker, 2003). In most instances, the images that people want to convey of themselves are positive, socially desirable ones, but, under certain circumstances, people want to be perceived in a socially undesirable fashion. The theory predicts that, regardless of the kind of image that people wish to convey, the likelihood and intensity of social anxiety increases as people become more motivated to make a particular desired impression and less certain that they will successfully do so.

One virtue of the self-presentation theory is that it accounts for both the situational and dispositional antecedents of social anxiety – both the kinds of interpersonal situations that evoke anxiety as well as individual differences in the tendency to feel socially anxious. Presumably, any situational factor or dispositional trait that is associated with either high motivation to convey desired impressions to others or low confidence in one's ability to make the desired impression should increase social anxiety.

The self-presentational theory has received solid empirical support, both from studies that have taken an explicitly self-presentational perspective and those emerging from other theoretical traditions (see Leary & Kowalski, 1995a). For example, laboratory studies have shown that experimental manipulations that raise and lower participants' self-presentational concerns cause concomitant changes in their experience of social anxiety (DePaulo, Epstein, & LeMay, 1990; Leary, 1986; Sheffer, Penn, & Cassisi, 2001). Furthermore, people who are more concerned about their public images not only feel more anxious when they face an upcoming evaluation but also feel anxious earlier in the process of being evaluated (Skinner & Brewer, 1999). In addition, people's ratings of their self-presentational efficacy correlate negatively with how anxious they feel in both real and imagined encounters (Maddux, Norton, & Leary, 1988; Patterson & Ritts, 1997; Skinner & Brewer, 1999).

The personality characteristics that predict trait social anxiety most strongly are also variables that are associated with concern over others' impressions. People who are particularly attuned to and concerned about how they are perceived by others score higher on measures of trait social anxiety than those who are less concerned with how they are perceived and evaluated (Fenigstein, 1979; Goldfried & Sobocinski, 1975; Hope & Heimberg, 1988; Kashdan, 2007; Leary & Kowalski, 1993; Reno & Kenny, 1992; Watson & Friend, 1969). People who do not believe that they will make desired impressions – for example, because they think others will view them as physically unattractive, socially unskilled, or incompetent in a domain with implications for their public image (such as public speaking or athletic contests) – also tend to be particularly socially anxious (Curran, Wallander, & Fischetti, 1980; Hart, Leary, & Rejeski, 1989; Leary, Kowalski, & Campbell, 1988; Martin & Mack, 1996; Segrin, 1996). In brief, research supports the notion that self-presentational concerns are strongly associated with social anxiety.

Not surprisingly, then, socially anxious people benefit when they are released from the pressure to make a positive impression (Broome & Wegner, 1994; Leary, 1986). For example, Leary (1986) asked participants to have a casual conversation with another individual while loud noise was played to simulate the din of a large party. Participants were told either that the noise would interfere with their conversation, making it difficult for them to converse and to form accurate impressions of one another, or that the noise would have a minimal impact on their conversation. Results showed that participants who scored high in trait social anxiety expected to make as positive an impression as low socially anxious people when they thought that the noise was an impediment but expected to make a less positive impression than lows when the noise ostensibly had little effect. More importantly, participants were less anxiously aroused (as indicated by pulse rates) when they thought that the noise would interfere with the conversation than when they thought it would not, and this effect was more pronounced for low than high socially anxious participants early in the conversation. Ironically, then, the more difficult situation resulted in lower anxiety, presumably because participants believed that any interpersonal problems they experienced during the interaction, including self-presentational difficulties, would be attributed to the noise rather than to their personal deficiencies.

In linking social anxiety to people's self-presentational concerns, the theory encompasses other theoretical approaches to social anxiety. For example, research has demonstrated a modest relationship between trait social anxiety and social skills deficits and shown that social skills training reduces shyness and social anxiety (Curran, 1977; Greco & Morris, 2005; Patterson & Ricks, 1997; Segrin, 1996). According to the self-presentational perspective, the relationship between social skills and social anxiety is explained by the fact that people who have poor interpersonal skills doubt that they will make desired impressions on others. As a result, teaching them to interact more adeptly decreases their self-presentational concerns and lowers their anxiety in social encounters.

Other researchers and practitioners have advocated a cognitive approach to social anxiety, arguing that certain patterns of thought – for example, holding excessively high standards, having negatively biased views of oneself, and overemphasizing the importance of obtaining approval – lead to social anxiety (Cacioppo, Glass, & Merluzzi, 1979; Hirsch & Clark, 2004; Ledley & Heimberg, 2006; Lucock & Salkovskis, 1988; Pozo, Carver, Wellens, & Scheier, 1991; Sutton-Simon & Goldfried, 1979). In addition, people who overestimate interpersonal threats or underestimate how others perceive and value them tend to score higher in social anxiety (Foa, Franklin, Perry, & Herbert, 1996; Wallace & Alden, 1997). Consistent with the cognitive perspective, a great deal of research supports the notion that certain kinds of thoughts underlie social anxiety and that modifying people's cognitions about themselves and their social worlds reduces their social anxiety (Gould, Buckminster, Pollack, Otto, & Yap, 1997; Hartman, 1983; Hope, Gansler, & Heimberg, 1989; Lucock & Salkovskis, 1988). The self-presentation theory refines the cognitive approach by focusing attention on the fact that the cognitions that underlie social anxiety specifically involve or have implications for how people are perceived and evaluated by others.

Altogether, then, the evidence for the self-presentational theory is quite strong. The self-presentational perspective explains both situational and dispositional moderators of social anxiety, and provides a parsimonious account that can incorporate other theoretical approaches. Further, as we will explore later in the chapter, the self-presentational approach also offers insights regarding the most effective ways to treat social anxiety and SP.

EXTENDING THE SELF-PRESENTATION APPROACH: SOCIOMETER THEORY

Despite the theory's merits, it has been clear from the beginning that not every instance of self-presentational concern causes people to experience social anxiety. Although all episodes of social anxiety appear to involve self-presentational concerns, as the theory suggests, people do not feel socially anxious every time they think they will not make a particular desired impression. Self-presentational concern is a necessary but not always sufficient cause of social anxiety.

Imagine, for example, that a woman has had a very difficult week at work, full of problems, stresses, and disappointments. She wants very badly to conceal the fact that she is stressed-out, frustrated, and disappointed from the friends she will meet for drinks on Friday evening, both because she doesn't want to undermine their fun and because she wants to be seen as someone who faces work pressures with equanimity. Yet, she doubts that she'll be able to be her normal, happy self, and, in fact, once with her friends, she believes that her emotional turmoil is obvious and that everyone knows that she is coming unglued. Although she is highly motivated to make a desired impression and doubts that she can maintain it – the two conditions posited to cause social anxiety by the self-presentational perspective – I doubt that she would experience social anxiety.

If people do not always feel anxious about their self-presentational insecurities and failures, what variable allows us to account for the situations in which self-presentational difficulties do and do not cause people to feel anxious? One possibility is that self-presentational concerns result in social anxiety primarily when people's concerns about others' impressions of them have real or imagined negative implications for their "relational value." Relational value refers to the degree to which a person regards his or her relationship with another individual as valuable or important (Leary, 2001). Of course, the higher a person's relational value in the eyes of other people, the more likely they are to accept, support, and protect him or her, and the more they will provide a variety of positive social and tangible outcomes, so people are generally motivated to maintain a sufficiently high level of relational value to other people.

People feel socially anxious when they believe that the impressions they make will not lead others to value their relationships with them as much as they desire or, worse, may cause others to devalue, avoid, or reject them. The adolescent on a first date, the job applicant in an interview, the performer on stage, and the ill-at-ease party-goer are worried not merely about making undesired impressions but rather about making impressions that will diminish the degree to which other people value having relationships with them. In the previous example, the woman would probably not expect that her inability to appear relaxed and composed would affect the degree to which her friends valued their relationships with her, so her self-presentational concerns would not lead her to feel socially anxious.

Human beings appear to possess "a pervasive drive to form and maintain a minimum quantity of lasting, positive, and significant interpersonal relationships" (Baumeister and Leary, 1995, p. 497). Baumeister and Leary (1995) reviewed considerable evidence showing that people not only choose to spend most of their time with other people, but also that they form social attachments easily and strongly resist the dissolution of those relationships (even many seemingly insignificant ones). The universality and strength of the need for acceptance and belonging suggest that it likely evolved as a fundamental aspect of human nature because it conferred an adaptive advantage. If we consider the conditions under which *Homo sapiens* and their hominid ancestors lived during the vast majority of evolutionary history, the advantage of having interpersonal relationships is easy to see. Living in small groups of hunters and gatherers on the African savannah, early humans were likely to survive predators, starvation, injury, and illness only with the mutual support of the other individuals with whom they lived (Gilbert, 2001; Tooby & Cosmides, 1992). Prehistoric individuals who tried to live away from the clan – through choice, accident, or ostracism – were less likely to survive and reproduce than those who forged strong social bonds.

Given the vital importance of maintaining social bonds throughout prehistory, a motivational-affective system evolved that helped people to avoid jeopardizing their relationships with other people. This system allowed them to monitor, in an automatic and ongoing fashion, the degree to which they were being accepted and valued versus rejected and devalued by other people (Leary, 2006; Leary & Baumeister, 2000; Leary & Downs, 1995). Because people do not have the cognitive capacity to monitor constantly others' judgments of them on a conscious level, this system – the "sociometer" – typically operates in background mode, with little conscious awareness on the part of the individual. Although people sometimes consciously ponder how they are being perceived and evaluated by others, the sociometer typically monitors the social environment, including one's own behavior, at a preattentive level for indications of immediate or potential threats to relational value. Often, these cues are explicit – as when someone directly rejects us – but more often they are implicit, involving subtle verbal and nonverbal cues that convey others' disinterest or disapproval.

Social Anxiety as Output from the Sociometer

As long as the sociometer detects no impending threats to their relational value, people interact in a reasonably composed manner with a minimum of conscious self-reflection. Under such circumstances, people may not even be aware that they are monitoring others' reactions, although the ease with which potentially evaluative cues can evoke a response shows that the sociometer is active all along. The "cocktail party effect," in which a person who is engrossed in conversation nonetheless hears his or her name mentioned elsewhere in the hubbub of the party, demonstrates the system's ability to monitor the social environment for self-relevant cues in a nonconscious manner. Cooley (1902) made the same point when he suggested that people regularly live in the minds of others without knowing that they do so.

When the sociometer detects evidence of a potential problem in the individual's relational sphere, its presence becomes obvious. The system evokes a negative emotional response, causing the individual to feel uneasy if not downright distressed. Baumeister and Tice (1990) proposed that the typical response to perceived social exclusion is anxiety, which may be true, but many other negative social emotions also reflect responses to real, imagined, or potential low relational value. When people feel jealous, ashamed, embarrassed, lonely, hurt, or, most central to the present chapter, socially anxious, the precipitating cause appears to be perceived relational devaluation. These emotions differ from one another in terms of the cognitive appraisals that evoke them, their subjective feeling states, and their associated action tendencies (i.e., what they motivate the person to do), but they all involve real, potential, or imagined low relational value (Leary, Koch, & Hechenbleikner, 2001).

Unlike other emotional reactions to potential threats to relational value such as jealousy, hurt feelings, and embarrassment, social anxiety is inherently anticipatory. People feel socially anxious when they believe they *might* make an impression that *might* lower their relational value. In order to help people to avoid devaluation and rejection, the sociometer must not only detect actual instances of low relational value, but also must be sensitive to cues that indicate the mere possibility that one's acceptance by other people may be jeopardized. Forewarned of the possibility, people can behave in ways that lower the likelihood of devaluation. In fact, many of the behaviors that are associated with social anxiety – reticence, smiling, agreement with other people, and head-nodding, for example – may reflect ways of conveying a minimally acceptable image of innocuous sociability when people expect that their efforts to make specific desired impressions will fail. And even when they cannot avoid relational devaluation entirely, they will be motivated to take preemptive actions to buttress their relationships before the anticipated damage occurs. Viewed in this way, social anxiety may be regarded as an early warning signal for events that may lead to insufficiently low relational value, a warning that not only alerts people to possible relational difficulties but also motivates remedial self-presentations.

As an early warning system, the sociometer is inherently biased toward "false positives," sometimes detecting potential threats to relational value that may, in fact, turn out to be nothing. Just as a detection system for enemy missiles or for tornadoes will occasionally provoke false alarms because it is calibrated to maximize detection of all real threats, the sociometer may cause people to feel anxious regarding imagined, potential threats that never come to pass. Failing to detect a real threat to one's relational value is far more serious than occasionally interpreting benign cues as threatening. Thus, other people sometimes view an individual's social anxiety as unnecessary or overblown, even though the anxious individual experiences the threat as quite real.

In addition to serving as a warning signal that alerts people to threats to their relational value, social anxiety interrupts ongoing behavior and induces a conscious assessment of the potential threat and the individual's ability to deal with it. Strong emotions serve to interrupt behavior, thereby stopping organisms from continuing to behave in ways that might have disastrous consequences (Frijda, 1986; Simon, 1967). As suggested earlier, as long as the sociometer is quietly operating below the level of awareness, people may interact with little conscious thought or self-awareness, but activation of the sociometer's early warning system causes people to stop what they are doing and take stock of their situation. Research shows that people who feel socially anxious are acutely self-aware (Patterson & Ritts, 1997). They think about how others are perceiving and evaluating them and about their ability (or, often, inability) to cope with the situation, and they often have difficulty devoting their full attention to other things (Amir, Freshman, & Foa, 2002; Hartman, 1983; Hope et al., 1989). Self-preoccupation can be troubling to the self-focused individual, but it is an essential feature of social anxiety. If people are to protect the quality of their interpersonal relationships, they must consciously assess any challenges to relational value that arise.

The subjective experience of social anxiety serves one additional function. Because anxiety is inherently aversive, people try to avoid doing things that will make them anxious and they take action to reduce anxiety when it occurs. As a result, anxiety motivates behavior that helps people to maintain desired public images, prodding people to take preemptive or remediative steps to protect their social bonds.

Conceptualizing social anxiety from the standpoint of relational value makes it clear that, within bounds, social anxiety is not only functional but essential to interpersonal relations. Although the experience of anxiety is inherently unpleasant, people's interpersonal interests are protected by their capacity to experience social anxiety. People who are never socially anxious do not work to regulate others' perceptions and evaluations of them and, as a result, tend to behave in ways that offend and alienate others.

The Link to Self-Presentation

Sociometer theory views social anxiety as the subjective output of a psychological system that helps people manage their interpersonal relationships. Although the role of self-presentational concerns is less obvious in this conceptualization than in the original self-presentation theory (Schlenker & Leary, 1982), in fact, self-presentation is fundamentally involved.

People devalue and reject one another primarily on the basis of the impressions that they have formed (Leary, 1995). Whether accurate or inaccurate, certain impressions lead us to like, value, and accept an individual, whereas other impressions lead to disliking, devaluation, and rejection. Thus, the proximal cause of low relational value is that one person holds an undesirable impression of another. People know this, of course, which is precisely why they are frequently concerned with the impressions that other people form of them and why they feel anxious when they do not believe they can make desired impressions.

Most instances in which people are ignored, shunned, excluded, or otherwise devalued center around four themes. Stated differently, people are most likely to devalue their relationships with those who make one of four general kinds of impressions on them. First, people are devalued when they appear to be inept, incompetent, or unskilled. Competence is particularly important when one's value to other people depends on being able to perform certain tasks. The primitive hunter who misses the kill, the athlete who misses the shot, and the stockbroker who misses the financial projection are less likely to be valued as members of their respective groups (as well as by the constituents of those groups) than a more highly skilled hunter, athlete, or financial analyst. Although we do not necessarily reject people who are incompetent, all other things being equal, people value their relationships with reasonably competent individuals more highly than their relationships with incompetent ones.

Second, relational value is often influenced by a person's physical appearance. Physically attractive people are liked better than unattractive ones, and people tend to devalue relationships with unattractive individuals (Feingold, 1992). Knowing this, most people work to meet the minimum standards of attractiveness in their social groups (through grooming, keeping their weight within acceptable bounds, and so on), and, of course, many individuals strive to present a highly attractive image.

Third, people's acceptance may be jeopardized when they violate important group rules or standards. Minor violations of social norms lead people to be seen as inconsiderate or unsocialized; violations of important ethical guidelines result in being seen as immoral. In either case, people who deviate from group standards are typically devalued, and extreme deviants may even be ostracized (Schachter, 1951).

Finally, people may be ignored, avoided, or rejected when they are simply unappealing as social interactants. We do not value our relationships with people whom we view as disagreeable, abrasive, boring, or otherwise unpleasant as much as our relationships with people with whom it is more pleasant to interact (Jensen-Campbell et al., 2002).

Given the role that competence, attractiveness, adherence to group norms, and social desirability play in acceptance and rejection, people are understandably motivated to be perceived as competent, physically attractive, norm-abiding, and otherwise socially desirable. Most of the impressions that people try to convey of themselves can be subsumed within one of these four categories. Because these domains have the greatest implications for relational appreciation and devaluation, self-presentational doubts regarding whether one can successfully convey these kinds of images are most often associated with social anxiety. People appear to worry most about projecting images of being incompetent, unattractive, normatively deviant, and socially undesirable.

Although no research has examined the effects of people's self-presentational concerns across these different domains on social anxiety, we might expect that the kinds of impressions that people most want to convey and, thus, the specific self-presentational predicaments that are likely to arouse social anxiety, vary across contexts and individuals. For example, one person may be quite anxious when she thinks others see her as incompetent but relatively unfazed if others regard her as nonconforming or unattractive. Another person may become socially anxious when others regard him as physically unappealing but worry little about maintaining appearances of being particularly competent. Counselors and psychotherapists dealing with a socially anxious client may wish to consider whether the client's self-presentations involve his or her global image or only particular kinds of impressions.

SOCIAL ANXIETY AND INTERPERSONAL BEHAVIOR

When people feel socially anxious, they generally become inhibited and reticent, more concerned with protecting their social images than with promoting themselves, and likely to interact with others in an innocuously sociable manner (engaging, for example, in greater polite smiling, agreeableness, and increased head-nodding; see Patterson & Ritts, 1997, for a review and meta-analysis). In earlier discussions (e.g., Leary & Kowalski, 1995a; Schlenker & Leary, 1982), we interpreted these behaviors primarily in terms of their self-presentational functions. Innocuously sociable behaviors minimize the likelihood of making blatantly undesired impressions on other people when the person does not expect to make desired impressions. Although disaffiliation, quietness, protective self-presentations, and innocuous sociability are unlikely to make precisely the sort of impression the individual desires to convey, these behaviors may prevent full-blown self-presentational disasters.

This self-presentational interpretation of socially anxious behavior is accurate as far as it goes, but sociometer theory sheds additional light on the functions of these behaviors. Specifically, the behaviors that tend to accompany episodes of social anxiety may provide some degree of protection against relational devaluation and, ultimately, interpersonal rejection. A person who behaves in a quiet, unassuming, innocuously sociable manner is unlikely to be rejected by other people. In fact, if the anxious individual demonstrates quiet interest in other interactants and an attitude of agreeableness, he or she may be viewed as a valued social participant. Of course, in cases of SAD, inhibition and disaffiliation create interpersonal problems in their own right, but, even then, people may sometimes believe that they are better off in terms of protecting their relational value if they withdraw from social contact rather than remain engaged and risk rejection.

IMPLICATIONS FOR TREATMENT

Much of the empirical interest in social anxiety has focused on people who experience high levels of social anxiety – those who score high on measures of trait social anxiety or are diagnosed as having SAD. The sociometer approach provides a novel perspective on the sources of trait social anxiety, as well as suggestions for its treatment.

Antecedents of Trait Social Anxiety

The sociometer theory of social anxiety suggests that individual differences in social anxiety should be related to the degree to which people desire to be valued and accepted, as well as to the degree to which they perceive that others do, in fact, value and accept them. Scattered evidence supports this notion. For example, Inderbitzen, Walters, and Bukowski (1997) found that adolescents who were identified as "neglected" and "rejected" by their peers scored significantly higher in social anxiety than "average" and "popular" adolescents. Because people who exist on the periphery of social life are likely to perceive that they have lower relational value to others than more central individuals, they are more prone to social anxiety.

More direct evidence regarding the link between perceived acceptance and social anxiety was provided by Spivey (1990), who examined the relationship between trait social anxiety and both inclusionary status (generalized beliefs in the degree to which one is valued, accepted, and included by others) and exclusion motivation (the motive to avoid rejection and exclusion). As expected, trait social anxiety correlated negatively with inclusionary status (indicating that participants who felt less accepted were more prone to social anxiety) and positively with exclusion motivation (the more motivated participants were to avoid rejection, the more socially anxious they tended to be). Furthermore, people with high exclusion motivation *and* low inclusionary status were particularly prone to social anxiety, as the theory predicts.

As noted, people who are worried about others' perceptions and evaluations of them tend to be socially anxious, as are those who doubt that others perceive them as they desire (see Leary & Kowalski, 1995a). Given the effects of one's public image on the degree to which one is accepted versus rejected, these findings are easily subsumed under a model that attributes social anxiety to concerns with relational value.

Treating Trait Social Anxiety and Social Phobia

Various approaches have been proposed for the treatment of trait social anxiety and SAD: cognitive therapies that focus on changing clients' beliefs about themselves and their social interactions, social skills training that teaches socially unskilled clients more adroit ways of interacting with other people, practice interactions in which clients are given experience dealing with threatening social encounters, relaxation-based techniques such as systematic desensitization, and so on. All of these approaches have been demonstrated to be effective in lowering social anxiety in at least some instances (see Gould et al., 1997; Leary & Kowalski, 1995b; Rapee, Gaston, & Abbott, 2009).

For our purposes, the important point is that sociometer theory suggests that treatments for trait social anxiety and SAD will be maximally effective if they focus on clients' concerns regarding their relational value to other people. Indeed, we may hypothesize that, relaxation-based approaches aside, existing psychological treatments for social anxiety have their effects by influencing clients' perceptions of and reactions to their relational value. For example, cognitive therapies either lower clients' desire for acceptance or enhance their personal sense of social acceptability, and behavioral treatments (such as skills training) increase clients' ability to behave in ways that lead to affirming, accepting reactions from other people.

Viewing social anxiety as a response to potentially low relational value suggests ways of enhancing the effectiveness of these treatments. First, the treatments should focus on clients' concerns regarding their acceptability to other people rather than on self-acceptance. As we have seen, people feel socially anxious because they are worried about how other people value them, so bolstering their private self-images, although possibly effective, is at best an indirect way to lower social anxiety. On the other hand, convincing socially anxious clients that other people value them should be effective (Haemmerlie & Montgomery, 1982, 1984).

Second, counselors and psychotherapists should make an effort to determine whether a particular client's social anxiety is reasonable given their circumstances. Although many people are excessively concerned with being accepted and underestimate the degree to which they are valued, some individuals are anxious because they accurately detect that they have low relational value in many domains of their lives. For example, socially inept, disagreeable, or abrasive individuals may be socially anxious, assuming that their sociometers are working properly, because they behave in ways that undermine relational value and acceptance (Greco & Morris, 2005). Even well-adjusted, socially desirable people may become highly socially anxious when they find themselves in unsupportive social environments in which they feel inadequately valued. In the first instance, therapeutic efforts should be directed toward improving clients' relational acceptability as opposed to trying to convince them of their inherent worth as people or persuading them not to be concerned with other people's reactions. In the second instance, the client may be assured by the simple knowledge that his or her anxiety is a reasonable, functional reaction to the social context, accurately reflecting the absence of regular contact with people who value their relationships with him or her.

In either case, the counselor or psychotherapist may wish to consider whether a particular client's anxiety arises from concerns with his or her relationships with people in general or with a select few individuals. Although this issue has not been previously addressed, it seems likely that some SAIs are concerned about their social acceptability to other people in general, whereas other individuals are concerned primarily about being accepted by certain people or categories of people (e.g., members of the other sex, other professionals, customers).

Third, given that the proximal cause of people's concerns with their relational value involves the impressions that they think others are forming of them, treatments might fruitfully focus on the client's self-presentational concerns. Elsewhere, I have discussed different kinds of self-presentational concerns that may lead people to feel socially anxious and I have recommended different treatment approaches depending on the precise nature of the client's self-presentational difficulties (Leary, 1987). For example, a close analysis of two clients' idiosyncratic difficulties may show that one holds unrealistic expectations regarding how positively she should be regarded in order to feel valued and accepted, whereas another client has realistic self-presentational expectations but is excessively motivated to make favorable impressions and to be accepted. The first case may require efforts to create more realistic expectations regarding the client's social image, and the second case could profitably focus on reducing the client's excessive approval motivation. Specific kinds of self-presentational concerns may underlie specific cases of social anxiety and possible treatment approaches for each (Leary, 1987; Leary & Kowalski, 1995a, 1995b).

CONCLUSIONS

People appear to be innately prepared to detect and respond to threats involving their acceptance by other people (Baumeister & Leary, 1995; Leary et al., 2001). According to sociometer theory, social anxiety may be conceptualized as the emotional output of an early warning system that is designed to detect low relational value well in advance of actual rejection so that the individual may take steps to protect relationships that may be in jeopardy. Because the degree to which others value their relationships with the individual depends primarily on their impressions of him or her, indications that the individual is unable to make desired impressions raise the specter of relational devaluation and evoke social anxiety.

The advantages of this refinement and extension of the self-presentational theory over the original formulation are two-fold. First, as noted at the outset, people do not always experience social anxiety when they are worried about others' impressions of them, and tying social anxiety to the sociometer allows us to specify more precisely when social anxiety will and will not arise. Specifically, social anxiety should occur primarily when people believe that the impressions that others may form of them have undesired implications for their relational value.

Second, consideration of the adaptive significance of social anxiety as a means of avoiding rejection permits us to incorporate the construct within a broader theoretical framework that links it to the fundamental motivation to be accepted (Baumeister & Leary, 1995), the self (Leary & Downs, 1995), and other emotions that are involved in negotiating social life (Leary et al., 2001). To date, research on people's concerns with others' impressions, evaluations, and acceptance of them has been scattered among a number of disparate topics, such as self-presentation, evaluation apprehension, social anxiety, embarrassment, interpersonal rejection, stigmatization, ostracism, approval motivation, hurt feelings, and betrayal (Smart Richman & Leary, 2009). Recognizing that each of these phenomena involve people's concerns with relational value may provide an overarching framework for integrating research across these topics.

REFERENCES

Amir, N., Freshman, M., & Foa, E. B. (2002). Enhanced Stroop interference for threat in social phobia. *Journal of Anxiety Disorders*, *16*, 1–9.

Baumeister, R. F., & Leary, M. R. (1995). The need to belong: Desire for interpersonal attachments as a fundamental human motivation. *Psychological Bulletin*, *117*, 497–529.

Baumeister, R. F., & Tice, D. M. (1990). Anxiety and social exclusion. *Journal of Social and Clinical Psychology*, *9*, 165–195.

Broome, A., & Wegner, D. M. (1994, July). *Some positive effects of releasing socially anxious people from the need to please.* Paper presented at the meeting of the American Psychological Society, Washington, DC.

Cacioppo, J. T., Glass, C. R., & Merluzzi, T. V. (1979). Self-statements and self-evaluations: A cognitive response analysis of heterosocial anxiety. *Cognitive Therapy and Research, 3*, 249–262.

Cooley, C. H. (1902). *Human nature and the social order.* New York: Scribner.

Curran, J. P. (1977). Skills training as an approach to the treatment of heterosexual-social anxiety. *Psychological Bulletin, 84*, 140–157.

Curran, J. P., Wallander, J. L., & Fischetti, M. (1980). The importance of behavioral and cognitive factors in heterosexual-social anxiety. *Journal of Personality, 48*, 285–292.

DePaulo, B. M., Epstein, J. A., & LeMay, C. S. (1990). Responses of the socially anxious to the prospect of interpersonal evaluation. *Journal of Personality, 58*, 623–640.

Feingold, A. (1992). Good-looking people are not what we think. *Psychological Bulletin, 111*, 304–341.

Fenigstein, A. (1979). Self-consciousness, self-attention, and social interaction. *Journal of Personality and Social Psychology, 37*, 75–86.

Foa, E. B., Franklin, M. E., Perry, K. J., & Herbert, J. D. (1996). Cognitive biases in generalized social phobia. *Journal of Abnormal Psychology, 105*, 433–439.

Frijda, N. (1986). *The emotions.* Cambridge, UK: Cambridge University Press.

Gilbert, P. (2001). Evolution and social anxiety: The role of attraction, social competition, and social hierarchies. *Psychiatric Clinics of North America, 24*, 723–751.

Goldfried, M. R., & Sobocinski, D. (1975). Effect of irrational beliefs on emotional arousal. *Journal of Consulting and Clinical Psychology, 43*, 504–510.

Gould, R. A., Buckminster, S., Pollack, M. H., Otto, M. W., & Yap, L. (1997). Cognitive-behavioral and pharmacological treatment for social phobia: A meta-analysis. *Clinical Psychology: Science and Practice, 4*, 291–306.

Greco, L. A., & Morris, T. L. (2005). Factors influencing the link between social anxiety and peer acceptance: Contributions of social skills and close friendships during middle childhood. *Behavior Therapy, 36*, 197–205.

Haemmerlie, F. M., & Montgomery, R. L. (1982). Self-perception theory and unobtrusively biased interactions: A treatment for heterosocial anxiety. *Journal of Counseling Psychology, 29*, 362–370.

Haemmerlie, F. M., & Montgomery, R. L. (1984). Purposefully biased interactions: Reducing heterosocial anxiety through self-perception theory. *Journal of Personality and Social Psychology, 47*, 900–908.

Hart, E. A., Leary, M. R., & Rejeski, W. J. (1989). The measurement of social physique anxiety. *Journal of Sport and Exercise Psychology, 11*, 94–104.

Hartman, L. M. (1983). A metacognitive model of social anxiety: Implications for treatment. *Clinical Psychology Review, 3*, 435–456.

Hirsch, C. R., & Clark, D. M. (2004). Information-processing bias in social phobia. *Clinical Psychology Review, 24*, 799–825.

Hope, D. A., Gansler, D. A., & Heimberg, R. G. (1989). Attentional focus and causal attributions in social phobia: Implications from social psychology. *Clinical Psychology Review, 9*, 49–60.

Hope, D. A., & Heimberg, R. G. (1988). Public and private self-consciousness and social phobia. *Journal of Personality Assessment, 52*, 626–639.

Inderbitzen, H. M., Walters, K. G., & Bukowski, A. L. (1997). The role of social anxiety in adolescent peer relations: Differences among sociometric status groups and rejected subgroups. *Journal of Clinical Child Psychology, 26*, 338–348.

Jensen-Campbell, L. A., Adams, R., Perry, D. G., Workman, K. A., Furdella, J. Q., & Egan, S. K. (2002). Agreeableness, extraversion, and peer relations in early adolescence: Winning friends and deflecting aggression. *Journal of Research in Personality*, *36*, 224–251.

Kashdan, T. B. (2007). Social anxiety spectrum and diminished positive experiences. *Clinical Psychology Review*, *27*, 348–365.

Leary, M. R. (1986). The impact of interactional impediments on social anxiety and self-presentation. *Journal of Experimental Social Psychology*, *22*, 122–135.

Leary, M. R. (1987). A self-presentational model for the treatment of social anxieties. In J. E. Maddux, C. D. Stoltenberg, & R. Rosenwein (Eds.), *Social processes in clinical and counseling psychology* (pp. 126–138). New York: Springer-Verlag.

Leary, M. R. (1995). *Self-presentation: Impression management and interpersonal behavior*. Boulder, CO: Westview Press.

Leary, M. R. (2001). Towards a conceptualization of interpersonal rejection. In M. R. Leary (Ed.), *Interpersonal rejection* (pp. 3–20). New York: Oxford University Press.

Leary, M. R. (2006). Sociometer theory and the pursuit of relational value: Getting to the root of self-esteem. *European Review of Social Psychology*, *16*, 75–111.

Leary, M. R., & Baumeister, R. F. (2000). The nature and function of self-esteem: Sociometer theory. In M. P. Zanna (Ed.), *Advances in experimental social psychology, Vol. 32* (pp. 1–62). San Diego: Academic Press.

Leary, M. R., & Downs, D. L. (1995). Interpersonal functions of the self-esteem motive: The self-esteem system as a sociometer. In M. Kernis (Ed.), *Efficacy, agency, and self-esteem* (pp. 123–144). New York: Plenum.

Leary, M. R., Koch, E., & Hechenbleikner, N. (2001). Emotional responses to interpersonal rejection. In M. R. Leary (Ed.), *Interpersonal rejection* (pp. 145–166). New York: Oxford University Press.

Leary, M. R., & Kowalski, R. M. (1993). The Interaction Anxiousness Scale: Construct and criterion-related validity. *Journal of Personality Assessment*, *61*, 136–146.

Leary, M. R., & Kowalski, R. M. (1995a). *Social anxiety*. New York: Guilford.

Leary, M. R., & Kowalski, R. M. (1995b). The self-presentational model of social phobia. In R. G. Heimberg, M. R. Liebowitz, D. A. Hope, & F. R. Schneier (Eds.), *Social phobia: Diagnosis, assessment, and treatment*. New York: Guilford.

Leary, M. R., Kowalski, R. M., & Campbell, C. (1988). Self-presentational concerns and social anxiety: The role of generalized impression expectancies. *Journal of Research in Personality*, *22*, 308–321.

Ledley, D. R., & Heimberg, R. G. (2006). Cognitive vulnerability to social anxiety. *Journal of Social and Clinical Psychology*, *25*, 755–778.

Lucock, M. P., & Salkovskis, P. M. (1988). Cognitive factors in social anxiety and its treatment. *Behaviour Research and Therapy*, *26*, 297–302.

Maddux, J. E., Norton, L. W., & Leary, M. R. (1988). Cognitive components of social anxiety: An investigation of the integration of self-presentation theory and self-efficacy theory. *Journal of Social and Clinical Psychology*, *6*, 180–190.

Martin, K. A., & Mack, D. (1996). Relationships between physical self-presentation and sport competition trait anxiety: A preliminary study. *Journal of Sport and Exercise Psychology*, *18*, 75–82.

Patterson, M. L., & Ritts, V. (1997). Social and communicative anxiety: A review and meta-analysis. In B. R. Burleson (Ed.), *Communication yearbook 20* (pp. 263–303). Thousand Oaks, CA: Sage.

Pozo, C., Carver, C. S., Wellens, A. R., & Scheier, M. F. (1991). Social anxiety and social perception: Construing others' reactions to the self. *Personality and Social Psychology Bulletin*, *17*, 355–362.

Rapee, R. M., Gaston, J. E., & Abbott, M. J. (2009). Testing the efficacy of theoretically derived improvements in the treatment of social phobia. *Journal of Consulting and Clinical Psychology*, *77*, 317–327.

Reno, R. R., & Kenny, D. A. (1992). Effects of self-consciousness and social anxiety on self-disclosure among unacquainted individuals: An application of the social relations model. *Journal of Personality*, *60*, 79–94.

Schachter, S. (1951). Deviance, rejection, and communication. *Journal of Abnormal and Social Psychology*, *46*, 190–207.

Schlenker, B. R. (2003). Self-presentation. In M. R. Leary & J. P. Tangney (Eds.), *Handbook of self and identity* (pp. 492–518). New York: Guilford Publications.

Schlenker, B. R., & Leary, M. R. (1982). Social anxiety and self-presentation: A conceptualization and model. *Psychological Bulletin*, *92*, 641–669.

Segrin, C. (1996). The relationship between social skills deficits and psychosocial problems: A test of a vulnerability model. *Communication Research*, *23*, 425–450.

Sheffer, C. E., Penn, D. L., & Cassisi, J. E. (2001). The effects of impression management demands on heart rate, self-reported social anxiety, and social competence in undergraduate males. *Journal of Anxiety Disorders*, *15*, 171–182.

Simon, H. A. (1967). Motivational and emotional controls of cognition. *Psychological Review*, *74*, 29–39.

Skinner, N., & Brewer, N. (1999). Temporal characteristics of evaluation anxiety. *Journal of Anxiety Disorders*, *13*, 293–314.

Smart Richman, L., & Leary, M. R. (2009). Reactions to discrimination, stigmatization, ostracism, and other forms of interpersonal rejection: A dynamic, multi-motive model. *Psychological Review*, *116*, 365–383.

Spivey, E. (1990). Social exclusion as a common factor in social anxiety, loneliness, jealousy, and social depression: Testing an integrative model. Unpublished Master's thesis, Wake Forest University, Winston-Salem, NC.

Sutton-Simon, K., & Goldfried, M. R. (1979). Faulty thinking patterns in two kinds of anxiety. *Cognitive Therapy and Research*, *3*, 193–203.

Tooby, J., & Cosmides, L. (1992). The psychological foundations of culture. In J. H. Barkow, L. Cosmides, & J. Tooby (Eds.), *The adapted mind* (pp. 3–136). New York: Oxford University Press.

Wallace, S. T., & Alden, L. E. (1997). Social phobia and positive social events: The price of success. *Journal of Abnormal Psychology*, *106*, 416–424.

Watson, D., & Friend, R. (1969). Measurement of social-evaluative anxiety. *Journal of Consulting and Clinical Psychology*, *33*, 448–457.

Part III

Treatment Approaches

Chapter 19

Psychopharmacology for Social Anxiety Disorder

Carlos Blanco, Franklin R. Schneier, Mayumi Okuda, and Michael R. Liebowitz
Department of Psychiatry, Columbia University, New York, NY 10032

Established treatments for SAD include psychotherapy and pharmacotherapy. Although some patients may be surprised by the idea of taking medication for a problem that they see as a long-standing personality trait, pharmacotherapy is a reasonable option for most individuals with SAD, given the degree of associated impairment and the efficacy of established medication treatments for the disorder. Pharmacological approaches to SAD have been shown to substantially reduce avoidance and psychological distress. Furthermore, both cognitive and physical symptoms of anxiety can interfere with optimal performance and ultimately lead to avoidance of feared situations; thus, medications that can directly decrease anxiety and physical symptoms typical of the disorder may help improve performance in social or professional situations. Finally, tendencies toward shyness and excessive concerns about social comparisons are likely to be strongly biologically based, given the early onset of behaviorally inhibited temperament, evidence of a significant genetic contribution from twin and family studies, and the biological salience of social hierarchies in the evolution of humans as a group-living species. These findings support the use of biologically based treatments.

A number of medications have been studied for the treatment of SAD. Early reports suggested the potential value of MAOI, reversible inhibitors of MAO-A (RIMAs), and benzodiazepines. Over the past decade, research has focused on the effects of SSRIs and 5-HT norepinephrine reuptake inhibitors (SNRIs). Most clinical trials have included predominantly or exclusively patients with the generalized type of SAD. We present a review of the research progress on pharmacotherapy for SAD over time, focused mainly on controlled trials.

Social Anxiety: Clinical, Developmental, and Social Perspectives. DOI: 10.1016/B978-0-12-375096-9.00019-5

MEDICATION TREATMENTS

Irreversible, Nonselective Monoamine Oxidase Inhibitors

MAOIs were the first antidepressants to be widely studied as a treatment for SAD. The suggestion that MAOIs might have efficacy in the treatment of SAD came from two different sources. One line of evidence came from studies of the use of phenelzine in atypical depression, whereas the second line consisted of four placebo-controlled studies of phenelzine on mixed phobic populations.

Five double-blind, placebo-controlled trials have studied the efficacy of phenelzine in SAD. Liebowitz, Schneier, Campeas, Hollander, Hatterer, and colleagues (1992) randomized 85 patients to an eight-week trial of phenelzine, atenolol, or placebo. Mean doses of medication used were: phenelzine, 75.7 mg/day (*SD* = 16; range = 45–90 mg/day); and atenolol, 97.6 mg/day (*SD* = 10.9; range = 50–100 mg/day). Response rates, defined as a Clinical Global Impression Clinic Improvement (CGI-I) Scale score ≤2, were: phenelzine, 64%; atenolol, 30%; and placebo, 23%. Both social and performance anxiety were reduced, and social and work function improved on phenelzine.

Gelernter, Uhde, Cimbolic, Arnkoff, and Vitonne (1991) randomly assigned 65 patients to one of four groups: (1) CBT; (2) phenelzine (range = 30–90 mg/day; mean = 55 mg/day); (3) alprazolam (range = 2.1–6.3 mg/day; mean = 4.2 mg/day); or (4) placebo. Duration of the trial was 12 weeks for all treatments. All pharmacotherapy patients also were given exposure instructions. Medication dosages were increased until all symptoms of social anxiety had disappeared, until the maximum medication dosage was reached, or until side effects precluded further increases, as is customary in flexible-dose studies. Patients were considered responders if their final FQ; (Marks & Matthews, 1979) SAD scores were equal to or below a cut-off score based upon normative samples. According to that criterion, 69% of the patients taking phenelzine were responders, compared with 38% of those taking alprazolam, 24% of those receiving CBT, and 20% of those taking placebo.

In the third study, Versiani, Nardi, Mundim, Alves, Liebowitz et al. (1992) treated 78 patients with SAD with phenelzine, moclobemide, or placebo. The trial included three eight-week phases. In the acute phase, patients given phenelzine were titrated up to 90 mg/day or the highest tolerated dose (mean = 67.5 mg/day; *SD* = 15.0), and those given moclobemide were titrated up to 600 mg/day or the highest tolerated dose (mean = 570.7 mg/day; *SD* = 55.6). At week 8, phenelzine was superior to placebo on all global and SAD measures. After the first eight weeks, nonresponders, defined as those whose CGI did not change or worsened from baseline, were withdrawn from the study. All other patients entered the second eight-week phase, in which they continued with the same treatment. At the end of phase II, participants responding to placebo and those who relapsed on any of the groups were withdrawn from the study. Ninety-one percent and 82% of patients completing 16 weeks of treatment with phenelzine and moclobemide, respectively, were considered responders.

For patients who continued to respond to active drugs, half continued on active treatment in phase III and the other half were blindly switched to placebo. Patients in the active treatment group that were switched to placebo in the third phase of the study had an increase in the mean scores of all parameters at week 24, indicating that some patients relapse when treatment is discontinued. Moclobemide was also superior to placebo in this study (see section on reversible inhibitors of monoamine oxidase-A, below).

In the fourth study, Heimberg, Liebowitz, Schneier, Hope, Davies et al. (1998) compared phenelzine, placebo, an educational supportive group, or group CBT for 12 weeks ($n = 133$). Phenelzine and CBT were superior to the other groups, and phenelzine also was superior to CBT on some measures.

In the most recent study, Blanco, Heimberg, Schneier, Fresco, Chen et al. (2010) randomized 128 patients to phenelzine, CBT, combined CBT plus phenelzine, or placebo. There was a specific order of effects across treatments, with the largest reductions in social anxiety symptoms for the combined group, followed by each monotherapy, and the least reduction in the placebo group. Response rates followed the same pattern.

Two open trials studying the effect of the MAOI tranylcypromine on SAD have also been published. In the first one, Versiani, Mundim, Nardi, and Liebowitz (1988) treated 32 patients with SAD for up to one year. Of the 29 patients who completed at least one month of treatment, 62% showed marked improvement, 17% showed moderate improvement, and 21% showed no improvement. In all responders, improvement was maintained throughout the year. When tranylcypromine was discontinued, 62% of the patients relapsed to baseline within three months and an additional 22% had a partial return of their symptoms. In a second study, an eight-week open trial including 81 patients, Versiani, Nardi, and Mundim (1989) found statistically significant reductions in both CGI Scale severity and Liebowitz Social Anxiety Scale (LSAS) scores. Mean CGI Scale severity scores went from 5.2 ($SD = 0.9$) to 1.5 ($SD = 1.0$). LSAS scores changed from 90.4 ($SD = 18.7$) to 28.2 ($SD = 17.9$).

An open trial has examined the efficacy of selegiline, a selective MAO-B inhibitor. Simpson, Schneier, Marshall, Campeas, and Vermes (1998) administered 10 mg of selegiline divided into two oral doses of 5 mg a day to 16 individuals with SAD. The group showed an average improvement of 33% in the LSAS total score. Less than 20% (3 out of 16) were considered respondents. Further research is needed to establish whether selegiline is more efficacious at higher, nonselective doses, and to determine the efficacy of its newer transdermal formulation.

Overall, substantial evidence shows that phenelzine and probably other irreversible, nonselective MAOIs are highly effective in the treatment of many patients with SAD. However, the MAOI side-effect profile, particularly the risk of hypertensive crisis if a low-tyramine diet and related precautions are not strictly followed, led researchers to focus their attention and research efforts into other medications, including RIMAs, SSRIs, and SNRIs.

Reversible Inhibitors of Monoamine Oxidase-A (RIMAs)

The limitations of nonreversible MAOIs stimulated the development of the RIMAs. RIMAs have a significantly lower ability to potentiate the depressor effect of tyramine, which allows for relaxation or total elimination of dietary restrictions. Other side effects of MAOIs such as fatigue and hypotension also seem to be much less common when RIMAs are used. Unfortunately, RIMAs appear to be less effective than MAOIs and are not available in the United States. Moclobemide and brofaromine (which is an SSRI in addition to a RIMA) are the only RIMAs that have been studied in the treatment of SAD.

Moclobemide

Four double-blind, placebo-controlled studies of moclobemide have produced mixed results. In the aforementioned study by Versiani and colleagues (1992), moclobemide was superior to placebo on a number of measures at the end of week 8. Fourteen (67%) of the 21 responders at week 8 who entered a continuation phase were classified as responders at the end (week 16). Moclobemide was equally effective as phenelzine on all measures, except on the social avoidance subscale of the LSAS, and showed similar rates of side effects to those of placebo, especially in the second phase of the study.

In a much larger multicenter study, Katschnig, Stein, and Buller (1997) compared two doses of moclobemide (300 and 600 mg) with placebo using a double-blind design over a 12-week period. The 600 mg moclobemide group was superior to the placebo group on all measures, whereas the 300 mg moclobemide group was superior to placebo on the LSAS and Patient Impression of Change–Social Phobia scale; however, effect sizes were much smaller than those initially found by Versiani. In another large multicenter study, Noyes, Moroz, Davidson, Liebowitz, Davidson et al. (1997) found no significant improvement with five doses of moclobemide (75, 150, 300, 600, and 900 mg/day) compared to placebo in a 12-week double-blind study.

In a double-blind, flexible-dose study, Schneier, Goetz, Campeas, Fallon, Marshall et al. (1998) administered moclobemide (mean dose = 728 mg) or placebo to 77 patients with SAD. At week 8, 7 of the 40 (18%) moclobemide patients and 5 of the 37 (14%) placebo patients were considered responders. Moclobemide was superior to placebo on only 2 of 10 outcome measures. Patients at least minimally improved on the CGI Scale after the eight weeks ($n = 21$) were offered eight additional weeks of the same treatment. Although some further improvement occurred on the CGI Scale in the moclobemide group, neither group showed significant changes on any continuous measures.

More recently, Stein, Cameron, Amrein, and Moclobemide Social Phobia Clinical Study Group (2002) randomized 309 subjects with SAD to moclobemide or placebo for 12 weeks. At week 12, 43% of patients in the moclobemide group and 31% in the placebo group were considered responders, a statistically significant difference. Subjects were offered the option of participating in a continuation phase. Fifty patients on moclobemide and 40 on placebo continued with the same treatment for an additional six months. Moclobemide-treated patients continued to improve, whereas some placebo-treated patients relapsed. At the ninth month, in the moclobemide group 86% were considered responders, compared to 58% in the placebo group.

In summary, placebo-controlled studies of moclobemide have shown mixed results. Moclobemide appears better tolerated, but it is clearly less efficacious than phenelzine in the treatment of SAD.

Brofaromine

Despite its classification as a reversible and selective type-A MAOI, brofaromine also has 5-HT reuptake inhibitory properties. Three studies on brofaromine have been conducted. In the first trial, Van Vliet et al. (1992) studied the effect of brofaromine in a 12-week placebo-controlled study and a follow-up phase of 12 additional weeks with 30 patients. The study found higher response rates in patients taking brofaromine. Three patients relapsed after four months of brofaromine discontinuation. Fahlen, Nilsson, Borg, Humble, and Pauli (1995), in a second double-blind trial, randomized 77 patients to brofaromine ($n = 37$) or placebo ($n = 40$) for 12 weeks. Seventy-eight percent of the patients taking brofaromine and 23% of those on placebo were classified as responders, according to CGI criteria. Furthermore, changes in LSAS scores were significantly greater among those taking brofaromine than placebo. Whereas the brofaromine group achieved further improvement during the nine-month follow-up period, 60% of the placebo responders who continued long-term treatment relapsed. In the third study, Lott, Greist, Jefferson, Kobak, and Katzelnick (1997) administered brofaromine (mean dose = 107.2 mg/day; $SD = 27.9$) to 52 patients and placebo to 50 patients for 10 weeks. Those in the brofaromine group had a significantly greater change from baseline on the LSAS than did patients in the placebo group. However, the superiority was modest as endpoint LSAS score was still in the clinical range. A significantly greater percentage of the brofaromine patients than the placebo patients were considered responders according the CGI Scale (50% vs. 19%). The development of brofaromine was stopped for reasons unrelated to its efficacy in SAD and it is not available for clinical purposes.

Selective Serotonin Reuptake Inhibitors (SSRIs) and Serotonin Norepinephrine, Reuptake Inhibitors (SNRIs)

SSRIs and SNRIs have been studied widely in recent years because of their efficacy, safety, and tolerability compared with other medications studied in earlier years. More than a dozen placebo-controlled trials have shown that SSRIs are highly efficacious in the treatment of SAD and six meta-analyses have supported their efficacy (Blanco, Schneier, Schmidt, Blanco-Jerez, & Marshall, 2003;

Federoff & Taylor, 2001; Gould, Buckminster, Pollack, Otto, & Yap, 1997; Hedges, Brown, Schwalb, Godfrey, & Larcher, 2007; Stein, Ipser, & Balkom 2004; van der Linden, Stein, & van der Balkom, 2000). In conjunction with their favorable side-effect profile and their ability to treat comorbid depression, these findings have established them as a first-line medication for SAD.

Although most patients can tolerate regular antidepressant starting doses, medication is frequently initiated at half the usual effective dose, as seeking a rapid response is rarely a priority in this chronic condition, with further dose increases after the first week of treatment. Since some patients appear to benefit from higher doses, it is a common practice to increase the dose as tolerated in those who have no response after four weeks of treatment.

Although controlled trials have been reported for all the SSRIs except citalopram, at present, paroxetine (immediate release and controlled release (CR)), sertraline, venlafaxine ER (extended-release), and fluvoxamine (controlled-release) are the SSRIs and the SNRI approved by the Food and Drug Administration (FDA) for the treatment of SAD. Trials comparing SSRIs with one another have not demonstrated that any one medication is superior to the others in the treatment of SAD.

Paroxetine

Stein, Liebowitz, Lydiard, Pitts, and Bushnell (1998) randomized 187 patients with GSAD to paroxetine or placebo for 12 weeks. The initial dose of paroxetine was 20 mg/day, with weekly increases of 10 mg permitted after the second week of treatment, up to a maximum of 50 mg/day. A higher number of patients receiving paroxetine were classified as responders than those receiving placebo (55% vs. 24%) as determined by a CGI score of 1 or 2. Furthermore, patients taking paroxetine ($n = 94$) had greater mean improvement from baseline than did those taking placebo ($n = 93$) on secondary outcome measures.

Similar results were obtained by another large multicenter 12-week trial. Baldwin, Bobes, Stein, Scharwachter, and Faure (1999), in a double-blind, placebo-controlled study ($n = 290$), found a response rate of 66% in the paroxetine group and 32% in the placebo group.

In Sweden, Allgulander (1999) conducted the third randomized controlled study of paroxetine. Ninety-two patients were randomized to paroxetine or placebo for 12 weeks. Patients were started at 20 mg/day of paroxetine or placebo, and the dosage was increased by 10 mg/day every week. At the end of the study, 70% of the patients on paroxetine and 8% of the patients on placebo were considered respondents based on CGI scores.

In order to better determine the effectiveness and safety of various daily dosages of paroxetine, Liebowitz, Stein, Tancer, Carpenter, Oakes, and colleagues (2002) conducted a 12-week double-blind, placebo-controlled trial. They randomly assigned 384 patients to receive either 20 mg/day, 40 mg/day, or 60 mg/day of paroxetine, or placebo. Although Liebowitz and colleagues, adopting a very conservative statistical approach, only considered the 20 mg/day dose to be superior to placebo, patients treated with paroxetine at any dosage showed significantly greater improvement compared with those receiving placebo on LSAS scores.

An additional study examined the long-term effects of paroxetine. Stein, Versiani, Hair, and Kumar (2002) conducted a placebo-controlled study comprising an initial 12-week single-blind acute treatment phase and a subsequent 24-week randomized, double-blind maintenance treatment phase for respondents in the initial phase. Four hundred thirty-seven adult patients with SAD entered the acute phase, and 323 continued into the maintenance phase (162 paroxetine and 161 placebo). Significantly fewer patients relapsed in the paroxetine group than in the placebo group. Paroxetine treatment significantly improved symptomatology according to the LSAS, SPI, SDS, Symptom Checklist-90 score, and EuroQol visual analogue scale, indicating decreased disability and increased well-being.

Furthermore, Seedat & Stein (2004) randomized 28 patients to receive clonazepam or placebo along with open-label paroxetine, 20 to 40 mg/day, for 10 weeks. More clonazepam/paroxetine patients (79%) than placebo/paroxetine patients (43%) were classified as CGI responders, but the effect was only significant at $p = 0.06$. The clonazepam group also showed greater change on dimensional measures, including the LSAS; however, these differences also failed to reach significance, possibly due to the limited power of the study.

In a reanalysis of three randomized controlled trials, Stein, Pitts, Kumar, and Hunter (2002) studied the time course of response (ratings of much or very much improvement on the CGI) to paroxetine. Among responders by week 4 in the paroxetine group, 84% remained responders at week 12. Of those considered responders at week 4 in the placebo group, 71% remained that way at week 12. Moreover, out of 166 patients classified as nonresponders at week 8, 28% became responders at week 12 after continuing treatment with paroxetine. Among nonresponders at week 8 in the placebo group, only 8.2% of subjects became responders at week 12, suggesting that an initial trial should last 12 weeks.

Additionally, Lepola, Bergtholdt, St Lambert, and Davy (2004) conducted a 12-week double-blind, placebo-controlled randomized trial comparing the controlled-release (CR) formulation of paroxetine (flexible dose of 12.5–37.5 mg/day) ($n = 186$) with placebo ($n = 184$). Statistically significant differences in favor of paroxetine CR compared with placebo were observed in the change from baseline to week 12 last-observation-carried-forward (LOCF) in LSAS total score and response rates (CGI ≤ 2).

In addition to these, two trials compared paroxetine with venlafaxine (Allgulander, Mangano, Zhang, Dahl, Lepola, et al., 2004; Liebowitz, Gelenberg, & Munjack 2005), one trial compared paroxetine with escitalopram (Lader, Stender, Burger, & Nil, 2004), and one trial was conducted in children and adolescents (Wagner, Berard, Stein, Wetherhold, Carpenter, et al., 2004). These trials are described below in the venlafaxine, escitalopram, and children and adolescent sections.

Sertraline

Katzelnick, Kobak, Greist, Jefferson, and Mantle (1995) conducted the first controlled trial of sertraline for SAD. Twelve patients were randomized to sertraline (dose range = 50–200 mg/day; mean dose = 133.5 mg/day; *SD* = 68.5) or placebo using a crossover design. Patients were assigned to receive a flexible dose of sertraline or placebo for 10 weeks, followed by taper and no treatment for 2 weeks, and finally crossed over to the other treatment for another 10 weeks. A statistically significant improvement on the LSAS was found in the sertraline group only.

In a larger, double-blind placebo-controlled trial, van Ameringen, Lane, Walker, Bowen, Chokka et al. (2001) randomized 204 patients to sertraline (mean dose = 146.7 mg/day; *SD* = 57) or placebo for a period of 20 weeks. At the end of the 20-week period, 53% of sertraline-treated patients versus 29% of the placebo-treated patients were considered respondents as determined by the CGI-I score.

In order to examine the ability of sertraline to prevent relapse, the study included a continuation phase (Walker, van Ameringen, & Swinson, 2000). Among sertraline-treated patients, those considered responders at the end of week 20 were randomly assigned again in a double-blind fashion to either continue sertraline or switch to placebo, whereas responders in the placebo group continued to receive double-blind placebo for 24 additional weeks. Significantly fewer patients in the sertraline-continuation group than in the placebo-switch group relapsed at study endpoint (4% vs. 36%). Overall, the risk for relapse on placebo was nine-fold the risk for relapse on sertraline.

In a general-practice setting, Blomhoff, Haug, Hellstrom, Holme, Humble et al. (2001) compared the efficacy of sertraline (dose range = 50–150 mg), exposure therapy, or their combination administered alone or combined for 24 weeks. Patients were further randomized to either exposure therapy or general medical care. The combined treatment and sertraline alone were significantly superior to placebo. A recent reanalysis of those data (Blanco et al., 2010) suggested a gradation of increasing response from placebo, to exposure therapy alone, sertraline alone, and combined treatment.

In the most recent study, Liebowitz, DeMartinis, Weihs, Longbord, Smith et al. (2003) randomly assigned 211 patients to sertraline (flexible dose up to 200 mg/day) or placebo. The authors reported a significant decrease in LSAS scores and higher response rates in the sertraline group compared to placebo at week 12 as determined by CGI criteria (47% vs. 26%).

Escitalopram and Citalopram

Lader et al. (2004) conducted a randomized, double-blind, placebo-controlled, fixed-dose trial that compared placebo, escitalopram 5 mg, 10 mg, 20 mg, and paroxetine 20 mg for 24 weeks. At week 12, both 5 and 20 mg doses of escitalopram and paroxetine were significantly more efficacious compared to placebo.

At week 24, escitalopram was superior to placebo at all doses, and 20 mg escitalopram was significantly superior to paroxetine from week 16 onwards.

Kasper, Stein, Loft, and Nil (2005) conducted a 12-week placebo-controlled trial in 358 patients with GSAD. Patients were randomized to receive 10–20 mg escitalopram (mean dose of 17.6 mg/day at week 12) or placebo. By the end of week 12, significantly higher response rate (54% vs. 39%) and greater decrease on LSAS total scores in the escitalopram group were observed. Escitalopram was well tolerated in general, with headaches as the most common side effect.

A study conducted by Montgomery, Nil, Durr-Pal, Loft, and Boulenger (2005) examined the ability of maintenance treatment with escitalopram to decrease rates of relapse among responders to acute escitalopram treatment of SAD. In the first phase of the study, 517 patients entered a open-label, flexible-dose trial of escitalopram (10–20 mg/day) for 12 weeks. Patients who responded were then randomly allocated to 24 weeks of either escitalopram, continuing the dose level administered at the end of the open trial, or placebo. There was a 22% relapse rate in the escitalopram group versus a 50% rate in the placebo group, a statistically significant difference. Results of this study showed that patients treated with placebo were more than two-fold more likely to relapse than those treated with escitalopram.

Pallanti and Quercioli (2006) conducted a study of subjects with at least one previously unsuccessful course of treatment with paroxetine (≥60 mg/day for ≥12 weeks). Patients meeting criteria for other Axis I diagnosis, including concurrent major depressive episode and marked depressive symptoms, were excluded. Twenty-nine patients received open-label escitalopram (mean dose = 18.5 mg/day) for 12 weeks. Low-dose benzodiazepines for insomnia were permitted. At the end of week 12, 48.3% of the patients were considered responders on the basis of the CGI-I score and reduction of >35% compared to baseline on the LSAS.

Some of these studies (Kasper et al., 2005; Lader et al., 2004; Montgomery et al., 2005) were used for further analyses on the effect of escitalopram on different patient subgroups and symptom dimensions. Stein, Kasper, Andersen, Nil, and Lader (2004) did an exploratory factor analysis of the LSAS and found that escitalopram was significantly superior to placebo in all six factors of the LSAS: social interaction, eating/drinking in public, speaking in public, assertiveness, observation fear, and partying. The analysis also found escitalopram to be effective regardless of gender, severity and chronicity of the disorder, and the presence of comorbid depressive symptoms.

In contrast to the amount of information available on escitalopram, to date, only one small, open-label trial of citalopram (mean dose = 55 mg; *SD* = 12.7 mg/day) for the treatment of SAD has been published. It included 10 patients with GSAD, of whom six had failed to respond or had not tolerated a prior medication treatment. Citalopram was well tolerated and patients improved significantly on all outcome measures (Simon, Korbly, Worthington, Kinrys, & Pollack, 2002).

Fluvoxamine

In a 12-week placebo-controlled study of fluvoxamine in 30 patients with SAD, van Vliet, den Boer, & Westenberg (1994) found that fluvoxamine (50–150 mg/day) was superior to placebo. Forty-seven percent of patients taking fluvoxamine and 7% of those taking placebo were classified as responders to treatment (as determined by a 50% reduction in the LSAS). Among those taking fluvoxamine, 93% chose to enter an additional 12-week continuation phase in which further improvement was observed.

In a multicenter randomized trial, Stein, Fyer, Davidson, Pollack, and Wiita (1999) found that fluvoxamine (dose range = 50–300 mg/day; mean dose = 202 mg/day; *SD* = 86) was superior to placebo in the treatment of SAD. From week 8 onward, fluvoxamine was superior to placebo on all SAD rating scales, and at week 12 a higher number of patients in the fluvoxamine group were considered as respondents than in the placebo group (43% vs. 23%)

The CR form of fluvoxamine has also been investigated in a randomized controlled trial lasting 12 weeks (Westenberg, Stein, Yang, Li, & Barbato, 2004). Fluvoxamine CR at flexible doses (dose range = 100–300 mg/day; mean dose = 209 mg/day) was significantly superior to placebo in almost all outcome measures. In a second, 12-week randomized control trial of fluvoxetine CR, Davidson, Yaryura-Tobias, DuPont, Stallings, Barbato et al. (2004) confirmed the superiority of fluvoxamine (dose range = 100–300 mg/d) over placebo in a sample of 279 patients with SAD. Treatment with fluvoxamine CR resulted in significant improvements in symptoms associated with GSAD as early as week 4.

Fluoxetine

Early uncontrolled studies of fluoxetine also suggested that it could be efficacious in the treatment of SAD (Black, Uhde, & Tancer, 1992; Schneier, Chin, Hollander, & Liebowitz, 1992; Sternbach, 1990; van Ameringen, Mancini, & Streitner, 1993). However, in a randomized study, Kobak, Greist, Jefferson, and Katzelnick (2002) found no significant difference between those receiving 14 weeks of fluoxetine (20–60 mg/day) or placebo. In a second study, Clark, Ehlers, McManus, Hackmann, Fennell et al. (2003) randomly assigned 60 patients to fluoxetine plus self-exposure, placebo plus self-exposure, or cognitive therapy in a 16-week trial. All three treatments resulted in significant improvement. Cognitive therapy was superior to fluoxetine plus self-exposure and placebo plus self-exposure from mid-treatment to the end of the booster period and at 12-month follow-up. There were no differences between fluoxetine plus self-exposure and placebo plus self-exposure.

In a third study, Davidson, Foa, et al. (2004) examined the efficacy of fluoxetine in a 14-week randomized, double-blind, placebo-controlled trial. In this two-site study, patients were randomized to fluoxetine alone, comprehensive cognitive-behavioral therapy (CCBT) alone, placebo alone, fluoxetine plus CCBT, or placebo plus CCBT. All active treatments were significantly better than placebo, but did not differ from each other. In the fluoxetine group, 50.9% were considered responders, 51.7% in the CCBT group, 52.4% in the fluoxetine plus CCBT group, 50.8% in the CCBT plus placebo group, and 31.7% in the placebo group. Overall, these findings suggest that fluoxetine may have some efficacy in the treatment of SAD, but the results appear less robust that those of other SSRIs.

Venlafaxine

Large randomized controlled trials have supported the efficacy of venlafaxine, an SRNI, on SAD. Rickels, Mangano, & Khan (2004) randomized 272 patients to venlafaxine ER at flexible doses (75–225 mg/day) or placebo for a 12-week period. As early as week 4, venlafaxine ER was superior to placebo on total LSAS scores and additional outcome measures. Subsequently, Liebowitz, Mangano, Bradwejn, and Asnis (2005) also found significantly greater rates of response (44% vs. 30%) and remission (20% vs. 7%) in the venlafaxine ER than in the placebo group. Venlafaxine was well tolerated, with no serious adverse events.

Stein, Pollack, Bystritsky, Kelsey, and Mangano (2005) conducted a 28-week multicenter randomized double-blind controlled trial. Three hundred ninety-five subjects with GSAD were randomized to either venlafaxine ER in a fixed low dose (75 mg/day), venlafaxine ER flexible higher dose (150–225 mg/day), or placebo. A greater and sustained improvement (58% vs. 33%) and higher rates of remission (31% vs. 16%) were observed in the venlafaxine ER groups (both 75 mg/day and 150–225 mg/day) compared to placebo. There were no significant differences in response and remission rates between the low and higher venlafaxine ER dosage groups.

As described before, two randomized trials of venlafaxine ER have included paroxetine as an active comparator in addition to placebo. In the first trial, Allgulander et al. (2004) randomly assigned patients to venlafaxine ER (75–225 mg/day), paroxetine (20–50 mg/day), or placebo for a 12-week period. Response rates of the venlafaxine ER and paroxetine groups were both significantly greater than those of the placebo group as early as week 3. However, a significant difference in remission rates emerged earlier in the venlafaxine group (week 4) than in the paroxetine group (week 8).

In the second trial, Liebowitz, Gelenberg et al. (2005) randomized a total of 440 patients with GSAD to receive either venlafaxine ER, paroxetine, or placebo for 12 weeks. Significantly greater reduction in LSAS mean score was observed for both venlafaxine and paroxetine groups when compared to placebo. Moreover, response rates for both the venlafaxine ER (58.6%) and the paroxetine group (62.5%) were significantly greater than those for the placebo group (36.1%).

Duloxetine

Duloxetine, at doses of 60 mg/day to 120 mg/day, has been shown to be efficacious in the treatment of depression and GAD. Recently, Crippa, Filho, Freitas, and Zuardi (2007) published two case reports on patients with GSAD and no Axis I comorbidity treated with duloxetine. A six-month follow-up on both duloxetine-treated patients showed no relapse of the symptoms. Further evaluations of duloxetine efficacy in the short- and long-term treatment of SAD are currently under way.

In conclusion, a large number of randomized controlled trials have established the efficacy of both SSRIs and SNRIs in the treatment of GSAD, although they have not been shown in direct comparisons to be superior to other medications or psychotherapy alone. Since, at doses typically prescribed, SSRIs and SNRIs have similar pharmacological properties and safety profiles, they share the established role in the treatment of SAD as the first-line pharmacological agents. No SSRI and SNRI has been established as superior in efficacy or acceptability to the others, although the published data on fluoxetine (Clark et al., 2003; Davidson, Foa, Huppert, Keefe, Franklin, et al., 2004; Kobak et al., 2002) probably make it the less preferred medication in this class.

Other Antidepressants

Mirtazapine

Mirtazapine is a presynaptic adrenoceptor antagonist. In an early open-label trial, van Veen, van Vliet, and Westenberg (2002) treated 14 patients with GSAD and no comorbid depression with mirtazapine 30 mg/day for 12 weeks. There was a 41.7% rate of response to mirtazapine and significant reductions on secondary outcome measures. Mirtazapine was generally well tolerated. Subsequently, Muehlbacher, Nickel, Kettler, Lahmann et al. (2005) randomly assigned 66 female patients to mirtazapine (fixed dose of 30 mg/day) or placebo in a 10-week placebo-controlled study. Mirtazapine was significantly superior to placebo on primary and secondary outcome measures and was relatively well tolerated by all patients.

Bupropion

Bupropion is a weak DA and norepinephrine reuptake inhibitor that has generated mixed results in two small open trials. Emmanuel, Brawman-Mintzer, Morton, Book, Johnson et al. (2000) administered bupropion sustained-release (SR) (dose range = 200 and 400 mg/day) to 10 patients with GSAD in a 12-week open-label trial. Five patients (50%) were considered to be responders. Bupropion was generally well tolerated in this study. However, others have reported negative results in a limited number of patients (Potts & Davidson, 1995).

Nefazodone

Nefazodone has been reported to have both 5-HT reuptake and 5-HT_{2A} receptor blockade properties. To date, only one randomized, placebo-controlled trial on the efficacy of nefazodone for SAD has been published, with negative results. Van Ameringen, Mancini, Oakman, Walker, Kjernisted et al. (2007) randomized a total of 105 patients to nefazodone (range dose = 300–600 mg/day; mean dose = 493.9 ± 128.1 mg/day) or placebo for 14 weeks. Comorbid secondary MDD was permitted if baseline scores on the MADRS were ≤19 and no risk of suicide was present. No differential improvement between the nefazodone and the placebo group was observed. Difference of remission and response rates between the nefazodone-treated group and the placebo group was not significant (31.4% vs. 23.5%).

Reboxetine

Reboxetine is an antidepressant with selective norepinephrine reuptake properties not currently marketed in the United States. The only open-label study (Atmaca, Tezcan, & Kuloglu, 2003) examining the efficacy of reboxetine (dose range = 4–8 mg/day) in SAD found statistically significant reductions in the mean Hamilton Anxiety Rating Scale (HAM-A) and total LSAS scores from baseline to the endpoint assessment at week 8. Additionally, at week 8, 63.6% were considered responders. Reboxetine was well tolerated in general.

Tricyclic Antidepressants

Based on its efficacy in the treatment of PD, imipramine was studied in SAD. However, the results of these trials failed to demonstrate its efficacy (Simpson, Schneier, Campeas, Marshall, Fallon, et al., 1998; Zitrin, Klein, Woerner, & Ross, 1983). Tricyclic antidepressants do not appear particularly useful in the treatment of SAD.

Benzodiazepines

The anxiolytic properties of benzodiazepines are useful in the treatment of GAD and PD. Therefore, a logical extrapolation was to assess their efficacy in SAD. Clinical trials have been conducted only for standing-dose treatment, although clinical experience suggests that benzodiazepines may also be used on an as-needed basis for performance fears.

Alprazolam and clonazepam are the most studied benzodiazepines. There have been two open trials and one double-blind study of alprazolam in SAD. In the first open trial, Lydiard, Laraia, Howell, and Ballenger (1988) administered alprazolam to four patients in dosages ranging from 3 to 8 mg/day. All patients had moderate to marked reduction of their symptoms. One of the patients, who had an initial partial response to alprazolam, had a full response when phenelzine was added. Reich and Yates (1988) treated 14 patients over eight weeks with alprazolam (dose range = 1–7 mg/day; mean dose = 2.9 mg/day). At the study endpoint, 14 patients were considered respondents according to the CGI-I Scale. One week after drug discontinuation, however, symptoms returned to baseline. It was unclear whether that was due, at least in part, to withdrawal symptoms from alprazolam. In the only double-blind study of alprazolam (described in the MOAI section), Gelernter et al. (1991) compared phenelzine, alprazolam (mean dose = 4.2 mg/day; *SD* = 1.3), placebo, and CBT. Only 38% of the patients taking alprazolam were considered responders after 12 weeks. When patients were reassessed two months after discontinuation of alprazolam, symptoms had returned in most cases, suggesting the low durability of already limited gains. Given the time lapsed since the discontinuation of the drug, it is unlikely that those symptoms represented benzodiazepine withdrawal.

In contrast to alprazolam, several open trials with clonazepam have obtained positive results. Versiani et al. (1989) treated 40 patients with SAD over eight weeks. Statistically significant decreases in the CGI severity and LSAS scores were noted between baseline and post-treatment assessment. Munjack, Baltazar, Bohn, Cabe, and Appleton (1990) compared the effects of clonazepam versus placebo in 10 patients with SAD, matching them for baseline severity. Of the clonazepam patients, three were very much improved and three were much improved. Although the clonazepam group also was superior to the no-treatment group on the LSAS and self-ratings of social anxiety, scores of social disability did not change.

In other open trials, Reiter, Pollack, Rosenbaum, and Cohen (1990) treated 11 patients with clonazepam. Six were very much improved and one was much improved. Ontiveros and Fontaine (1990) reported improvement in all the five patients treated with clonazepam (mean dose = 3 mg/day).

Davidson, Ford, Smith, and Potts (1991) conducted an open trial with 26 patients treated for an average of 11.3 months (range = 1–20 months). At the end of the trial, 42% of the patients were very much improved, 42% were much improved, and 15% were minimally or not improved. Subsequently, the same group showed efficacy of clonazepam in a 10-week placebo-controlled study of 75 patients (Davidson, Potts, Richichi, Krishnan, Ford, et al., 1993). At the end of the treatment, 78% of the patients taking clonazepam (range = 0.5–3 mg/day; mean = 2.4 mg/day) were classified as responders according to the CGI Scale, compared with 20% of those taking placebo.

Use of bromazepam, a benzodiazepine marketed outside the United States, has been also reported in the treatment of SAD. In the first study, Versiani et al. (1989) treated 10 patients in an eight-week open trial with bromazepam (mean dose = 26.4 mg/day; *SD* = 4.9). CGI Scale severity scores decreased from 5.0 (*SD* = 0.8) at baseline to 1.3 (*SD* = 0.5) and LSAS score improved from a baseline 69.3 (*SD* = 20.5) to 15.8 (*SD* = 9.1) at the end of treatment. In a subsequent study (Versiani, Nardia, & Figueira, 1997), bromazepam (dose up to 36 mg/day) was superior to placebo in a 12-week randomized study.

Clonazepam has also been studied as treatment augmentation of paroxetine. Seedat and Stein (2004) randomized 28 patients to paroxetine plus clonazepam or paroxetine plus placebo. More clonazepam patients (79%) than placebo patients (43%) were classified as CGI responders, but the effect was only borderline statistically significant ($p = 0.06$) in this small sample. The maximum dose of clonazepam in this study was 2.0 mg/day, rather than 3.0 mg as in the Davidson et al. (1993) trial. Clonazepam deserves further study as an augmentation or alternative treatment for patients who do not respond completely to an initial SSRI trial.

In summary, all open trials suggest that benzodiazepines are useful in the treatment of SAD. In double-blind studies, clonazepam and bromazepam, but not alprazolam, have been superior to placebo. Whether those differences are due to true differential efficacy or are related to study design and sampling requires further examination. Benzodiazepines also may be helpful on an as-needed basis for performance anxiety. The benefit of decreased anxiety must be balanced with the risk of sedation interfering with the quality of performance. It is not uncommon for patients with SAD to present with comorbid psychiatric disorders such as depression. Benzodiazepines are not recommended as monotherapy for patients with concomitant major depression, and must be used with caution in patients with a history of substance use disorders.

Beta-Adrenergic Blockers

Studies showing a connection between anxiety, signs and symptoms of peripheral arousal (i.e., tremor, palpitation, and sweating), and increased plasma levels of norepinephrine led to early trials of beta blockers in nonclinical samples of performers with high levels of anxiety, many of whom would probably be currently diagnosed as having nongeneralized social anxiety disorder. The results of those trials seemed to indicate that beta blockers were successful in decreasing the autonomic manifestations of anxiety.

Gorman, Liebowitz, Fyer, Campeas, and Klein (1985) conducted an open trial of atenolol in 10 patients with SAD. The number of patients with nongeneralized or GSAD was not reported. Five patients had a marked reduction in SAD symptoms, and four reported moderate reduction, as assessed by clinicians and patients.

Similarly, Turner, Beidel, and Jacob (1994) treated 25 patients with atenolol (25–100 mg/day), assigned 26 to flooding, and gave placebo to 21 during 12 weeks. Patients who received behavior therapy received a total of twenty 90-minute sessions of each, distributed as follows: twice a week for the first eight weeks and once a week for the last four weeks. Improvement rates were higher among patients who received flooding (89%) than in the group that received atenolol (47%) or placebo (44%). All of those who were assessed six months post-treatment had maintained most of the gains.

Beta blockers have not been proven superior to placebo in any controlled clinical trial. However, anecdotal experience and studies of analogue samples of anxious performers suggest that they are effective for specific and circumscribed performance anxiety. Beta blockers have the advantage over benzodiazepines of rarely impairing concentration or coordination. Nonselective beta blockers (affecting both $beta_1$-receptors in the heart and $beta_2$-receptors that mediate tremor), such as propranolol or nadolol, may in theory be more effective than those selective for the $beta_1$-receptor, such as atenolol or metoprolol, although this remains to be empirically tested (Schneier, 1995).

Before using a beta-blocker in a performance situation, patients should try a test dose at home, to ensure that the degree of beta-blockade is sufficient and that untoward side effects will not develop during the performance. Most individuals tolerate propranolol well, especially because the hypotensive effects will be partially balanced with the sympathetic arousal of anxiety. Propranolol (dose range = 10–40 mg) taken 45–60 minutes before the performance is sufficient for most patients.

Other Medications

Buspirone

Buspirone is an azaspirone that acts as a full agonist on the serotonin 1A ($5HT_{1A}$) autoreceptor and as a partial agonist on the postsynaptic 5-HT_{1A} receptor. Positive results of the trials with SSRIs for SAD stimulated further research with drugs that have a serotonergic effect.

Clark and Agras (1991) randomized 34 musicians with SAD to receive either six weeks of buspirone, six weeks of placebo, five sessions of group CBT plus buspirone, or CBT with placebo. The average dose of buspirone was 32 mg. There was no difference between buspirone and placebo, whereas CBT was superior to both buspirone and placebo without psychotherapy. Munjack, Bruns, Baltazar, Brown, Leonard et al. (1991) conducted a 12-week open trial of buspirone (mean dose = 48 mg/day) in 17 patients with GSAD. The overall response rate was 53% of the intent-to-treat sample.

Schneier, Saoud, Campeas, Fallon, Hollander et al. (1993) conducted another 12-week open trial with 21 patients with similar response rates (47%) to those obtained in Munjack and colleagues' study. Seventeen patients completed at least two weeks of treatment and were included in the analysis. Interestingly, responders received a higher average dose of buspirone than did nonresponders (56.9 vs. 38.3 mg/day). Van Vliet, den Boer, Westenberg, and Pian (1997) investigated further the efficacy of fixed-dose buspirone (30 mg/day) versus placebo in a 12-week placebo-controlled study of 30 patients with SAD. Only one patient receiving buspirone and another taking placebo were classified as responders. There were no statistically significant differences between the two treatment groups on any of the outcome measures.

In contrast with the promising results of the open trials, neither of the two controlled trials of buspirone was able to show its efficacy as monotherapy for SAD. Additionally, the dosage of buspirone needed seems to be in the upper range (60 mg/day), which may limit its usefulness on the basis of side effects, such as nausea or headache. Although buspirone has not proven to be superior to placebo as monotherapy, a small trial conducted by van Ameringen, Mancini, and Wilson (1996) studied buspirone (doses range = 30–60 mg/day; mean dose = 45 mg/day) as an augmenting agent on 10 patients with GSAD with a partial response to an adequate trial of an SSRI during eight weeks. Although seven patients (70%) were considered responders according to CGI criteria, this approach has not been further studied.

Pergolide

Only one small open trial of pergolide has been conducted to date. Villarreal, Johnson, and Rubey (2000) treated four subjects openly with pergolide (25–600 μg/day) but only two completed the 12 weeks of the study. Conclusions could not be drawn from such a small sample.

Anticonvulsants

Gabapentin

Gabapentin, approved since 1993 for use as adjunctive in the treatment of refractory partial epilepsy, is thought to work through voltage-gated calcium channels and to have GABAergic effects. In the only published placebo-controlled trial of gabapentin for SAD, Pande, Davidson, Jefferson, Janney, Katzelnick et al. (1999) randomized 69 patients with low levels of comorbidity to gabapentin (dose range 900–3600 mg/day) or placebo for 14 weeks. Significantly higher rates of response were observed among patients on gabapentin than for those on placebo (32% vs. 14%) in the intent-to-treat sample. Patients over 35 years old exhibited a greater degree of effect than younger patients. Dizziness and dry mouth were among the most common side effects.

Pregabalin

The anticonvulsant pregabalin has been shown to have analgesic, anxiolytic, and anticonvulsant properties. Pande, Feltner, Jefferson, Davidson, Pollack et al. (2004) randomly assigned 135 patients to pregabalin 600 mg/d, pregabalin 150 mg/d, or placebo in a 10-week double-blind trial. Pregabalin 600 mg/day, but not pregabalin 150 mg/day, was superior to placebo at endpoint. Although a total of 19 patients withdrew from the study due to adverse events, these were of mild or moderate intensity and no serious adverse event was considered related to study medication. Further studies will be needed to define the optimal dose, magnitude of the effect, and long-term effect.

Topiramate

This glutamatergic and GABAergic anticonvulsant has been used for a variety of psychiatric disorders (Dursun & Devarajan, 2001; Johnson, 2005; Tata & Kockler, 2006; Vasudev, Macritchie, Geddes, Watson, & Young, 2006). Van Ameringen, Mancini, Pipe, Oakman, and Bennett (2004) conducted a 16-week open trial to examine the efficacy of topiramate (dose range = 25–400 mg/day; mean dose = 222.8 ± 141.8 mg/day) in GSAD. The trial included 23 outpatients who could have had comorbid anxiety disorders, MDD, or attention deficit hyperactivity disorder. Of the 12 subjects who completed the trial, 9 (75%) were considered responders according to CGI-I criteria at study endpoint. However, in the intent-to-treat analysis, only 48% were considered responders and 35% remitters, as indicated by CGI-I scores. All patients experienced adverse effects, which included weight loss, paresthesias, headache, cognitive impairment, anorexia, gastrointestinal upset, tiredness, lightheadedness, agitation, and metallic taste.

Levetiracetam

Levetiracetam is a novel anticonvulsant that modulates voltage-gated calcium channels in the CNS. In the first open-label flexible dose study, Simon, Worthington, Doyle, Hoge, and Kinrys (2004) treated 20 patients with GSAD with levetiracetam (dose range = 500–3000 mg/day; mean dose = 2013 ± 948 mg/day) for eight weeks. Comorbid depressive and other anxiety disorders were permitted as long as they were considered secondary disorders for that patient. At week 8, the study found a 20-point decrease in LSAS scores. There were also decreases in CGI-S and Hamilton Rating Scale for Anxiety scores. Levetiracetam was generally well tolerated with mild and transient side effects in this study. Later on, Zhang, Connor, and Davidson (2005) randomized 18 subjects to receive either placebo or levetiracetam at flexible doses (dose range = 500–3000 mg/day; mean dose = 2279 mg/day) in a small seven-week placebo-controlled pilot study. Two subjects from the levetiracetam group dropped out because of early side effects and an additional two subjects in this group had a relatively poor tolerance to the drug. The study found no differences on a number of outcome measures.

Valproic acid

The anticonvulsant valproic acid (VPA) may have anxiolytic properties mediated by its enhancement of GABA activity in the CNS. Kinrys, Pollack, Simon, Worthington, Nardi et al. (2003) conducted a 12-week flexible-dose, open trial of VPA (range dose = 500–2500 mg/day; mean dose = 1985 ± 454 mg/day) in 17 patients with SAD. Mean reduction in the LSAS was 19.1 points for all participants. Results of the study showed 41% response rate. Side effects of VPA were mild and no severe adverse events were reported during the study.

Tiagabine

There is only one open trial of the selective GABA reuptake inhibitor tiagabine for patients with SAD. Dunlop, Papp, Garlow, Weiss, and Knight (2007) treated 54 patients in a 12-week open-label tiagabine study (dose range = 4–16 mg/day; mean dose = 12.2 ± 4.0 mg/day). At study endpoint, 63% of the completer sample and 40.7% of the intent-to-treat sample were considered responders

Atypical antipsychotics

Few antipsychotics have been tested for the treatment of SAD and none of them has been tested in large trials. These include olanzapine (Barnett, Kramer, Casat, Connor, & Davidson, 2002), quetiapine (Schutters, van Megen, & Westenberg, 2005), and risperidone (Simon, Hoge, Fischmann, Worthington, Christian, et al. 2006). Some of these studies have shown promise, but larger studies will be needed in order to clarify their effects.

PHARMACOTHERAPY IN CHILDREN AND ADOLESCENTS

Although children and adolescents with SAD often have great impairment in their social and family relationships and academic life, this often goes underdiagnosed and undertreated. Few studies of pediatric SAD have examined the efficacy of treatment modalities, making the role of pharmacotherapy for treatment of this disorder less established than for adults. The first group of studies conducted in children included a wide range of anxiety disorders and some of them concentrated on selective mutism, a condition shown to greatly overlap with SAD.

Only two studies have investigated the efficacy of benzodiazepines in this population. In a six-week open-label study, Simeon and Ferguson (1987) treated 12 children with avoidant and overanxious disorders with alprazolam (mean dose = 1.5 mg/day). Both child- and parent-rated anxiety symptoms as well as cognitive functioning decreased for both diagnostic groups. In a subsequent study, Simeon, Ferguson, and Knott (1992) randomized 30 children with avoidant and overanxious disorders to alprazolam or placebo. The maximum dosage permitted was 0.04 mg/kg/day. Differences between the groups did not reach significance, possibly due to the relatively small size of the groups.

In contrast to the scarcity of studies conducted on benzodiazepines, more data are available on the efficacy of SSRIs. Several placebo-controlled trials have been conducted that provide substantial evidence of the efficacy of SSRIs and SNRIs in children 6 to 17 years of age. However, the increasing concern about studies, most of them in depression, reporting an increased risk of suicidal ideation among adolescents treated with SSRIs or SNRIs led the FDA to add a warning in regard to the use of antidepressants in this population.

Fairbanks, Pine, Tancer, Dummit, and Kentgen (1997) treated with fluoxetine a group of children with mixed anxiety disorders who had not responded to psychotherapy. Treatment was started at 5 mg/day and increased weekly by 5–10 mg/day for six–nine weeks until improvement occurred or to a maximum of 40 mg in children younger than 12 years or 80 mg in adolescents. Eight of the 10 children with SAD were considered respondents as assessed by CGI criteria.

Some reports exist on SSRIs trials for the treatment of selective mutism, often considered a variant of SAD. Black et al. (1992) successfully treated with fluoxetine (20 mg) a 12-year-old girl with selective mutism who had failed two trials of psychotherapy. In a 12-week double-blind, placebo-controlled study of fluoxetine, Black and Uhde (1994) reported greater improvement in the fluoxetine than in the placebo group on parents' ratings of mutism change and global change but not in clinician and teacher ratings. Medication was well tolerated and no suicidal ideation was reported.

Dummit, Klein, & Tancer (1996) treated selective mutism in 21 children with diagnosis of separation anxiety, GAD, avoidant disorder, or SAD in a nine-week open trial of fluoxetine (dose range = 10–60 mg; mean dose = 28.1 mg). At study endpoint, 76% of those treated with fluoxetine were improved. Side effects were similar to those generally experienced by adults taking SSRIs and no suicidal ideation was reported in this trial.

In the first large study on the treatment of anxiety disorders in children and adolescents (Research Unit on Pediatric Psychopharmacology Anxiety Study Group, 2001), 128 individuals aged 6–17 who met criteria for SAD, separation anxiety disorder, or generalized anxiety and showed no improvement after receiving psychological treatment for three weeks were randomized to either placebo or fluvoxamine (dose range = 50–300 mg/day). After eight weeks of treatment, patients in the fluvoxamine group showed significantly greater improvement than those in the placebo group. Fluvoxamine was well tolerated with mild adverse events and no reports of suicidal ideation.

In another trial, Birmaher, Axelson, Monk, Kalas, and Clark (2003) randomized subjects 7–17 years old who met criteria for GAD, separation anxiety disorder, and/or SAD with significant impairment. Seventy-four patients were randomized to fluoxetine or placebo. Fifty-four percent of the sample had SAD. Subjects with current SAD on fluoxetine had a 76% versus 21% response rate when compared to placebo and 45.5% of children on the fluvoxamine group whereas only 10.5% in the placebo group showed significant increase in functional improvement measures.

More recently, Beidel, Turner, Sallee, Ammerman, and Crosby (2007) randomized 139 patients with SAD aged 7–17 to fluoxetine, placebo, or social effectiveness therapy for children (SET-C). More patients in the SET-C group (79%) than either those in the fluoxetine group (36%) or the placebo group (6.3%) were considered responders as assessed by the CGI score. Furthermore, fluoxetine was also showed to be significantly superior to placebo. At one-year follow-up, all treatment gains were maintained and fluoxetine and SET-C-treated patients showed continued improvement.

An eight-week open-label trial of sertraline was conducted in 14 adolescents aged 11–17 with SAD specifically (Compton, Grant, Chrisman, Gammon,

Brown, et al., 2001). At the study endpoint, 36% were considered responders, whereas an additional 29% were considered partial responders.

Wagner et al. (2004) conducted a randomized double-blind controlled multicenter trial of paroxetine (10–50 mg/day), including 322 youths with SAD. Significantly more patients taking paroxetine were considered responders (77% vs. 38%) and achieved remission (47.2% vs. 13.3%). Although no suicidal attempts were reported, four of the children treated with paroxetine expressed suicidal ideation or threatened suicide. None of these cases was serious, none involved evidence of a suicide attempt, and none of the events could be attributed to the study medication.

Isolan, Pheula, Salum, Oswald, and Rohde (2007) conducted a 12-week open trial of escitalopram (mean dose = 13 mg ± 4.1) in 20 children and adolescents (aged between 10 and 17 years old) with SAD. In the intent-to-treat analysis at week 12, 65% of the sample achieved response criteria. In addition, scores of self-report and parent report measures decreased significantly as early as week 8, with further improvement by week 12. Nevertheless, a substantial number of patients remained symptomatic at the end of the trial. Adverse effects of escitalopram were transitory and well tolerated. The most common side effects were somnolence and insomnia. No patient developed emotional liability or suicidal ideation.

In another large trial, March, Entusah, Ryan, Albano, and Tourian (2007) randomized 293 patients aged 8–17 with GSAD to venlafaxine ER (dose range = 37.5–225 mg/day) or placebo for 16 weeks. Using a CGI-I of 1 or 2 as the criterion for response, 56% of subjects treated with venlafaxine ER responded compared to 37% on placebo, a statistically significant difference. Adverse effects included nausea, anorexia, asthenia, and mydriasis. Three subjects (two during the course of treatment and one during the taper phase) in the venlafaxine ER group versus none in the placebo group developed suicidal ideation, but there were no suicide attempts.

In an eight-week open-label pilot study, Mrakotsky, Masek, Biederman, Raches, Hsin et al. (2008) administered mirtazapine (mean dose = 28.8 mg/day; *SD* = 12.4) in children with SAD aged 8–17 years. Fifty-six percent (10/18) responded to treatment and 17% (3/18) of the patients treated with mirtazapine achieved full remission. SAD symptoms improved significantly during the first two weeks of treatment, as did comorbid symptoms of depression and anxiety. Eleven patients (61%) did not complete all eight weeks of treatment. Four patients (22%) discontinued due to adverse effects, including fatigue and irritability, whereas the others discontinued due to study burden (28%), insufficient response (6%), or to pursue herbal treatment (6%). Mirtazapine treatment resulted in a significant increase in weight (mean of 3.3 kg; *SD* = 2.6).

In summary, although replication is still needed and long-term effects are still unknown, a growing body of literature supports the efficacy of pharmacological treatments in children and adolescents. SSRIs and SNRIs are the pharmacological treatment of choice in this population, with response rates ranging from 36% to 77%, but concerns regarding the emergence of suicidal ideation suggest the need for close monitoring of these treatments in this population.

RECOMMENDATIONS

Before initiating pharmacotherapy, it is essential to conduct a thorough assessment of the scope of SAD symptoms, and to help set reasonable expectations for response. In the short term, we expect to see symptomatic relief and improved social relatedness and performance. Over the long term, we hope to see decreased avoidance, increased vocational or educational functioning, and improved capacity for more satisfying relationships. Although some patients ultimately achieve a complete remission of symptoms, more commonly there is a substantial reduction that improves quality of life without altering the typical patient's self-perception as someone who tends to be shy.

Predictors of response to a particular treatment are lacking. To date, only later age of onset (in adulthood) of SAD (van Ameringen, Oakman, Mancini, Pipe, & Chung, 2004) and duration of treatment (Stein, Stein et al., 2002) seem to predict treatment response. The choice of a pharmacological agent for a specific patient depends on the diagnostic subtype of SAD, presence of comorbidity, and patient preference.

Anxiety-provoking situations in the generalized type of SAD are frequent and largely unpredictable. Since as-needed use becomes impractical for patients with generalized type, standing daily doses of medication are warranted. At present, SSRIs constitute the first-line medication treatment for GSAD. They have been most extensively tested, are generally well tolerated, and treat comorbid depression. Double-blind studies support the efficacy of drugs such as paroxetine, sertraline, fluvoxamine, and escitalopram with efficacy rates ranging from 50% to 80% after 8–12 weeks of treatment. Studies on fluoxetine have had inconsistent results, making it a less preferred treatment. The SNRI venlafaxine has also emerged as first-line therapy due to response characteristics similar to SSRIs.

Benzodiazepines remain a reasonable alternative for the treatment of the generalized type of SAD. These are commonly used in patients who cannot tolerate SSRIs or venlafaxine side effects or are unresponsive to these medications. The relatively long-acting clonazepam has shown efficacy in several studies. The role of alprazolam remains inconclusive. Benzodiazepines are not efficacious in the treatment of some of the comorbidities commonly associated with this disorder (e.g., MDD) and they should generally be avoided in most patients with a history of substance use disorders, which are moderately comorbid with SAD. In most patients, tolerance to the sedative effects of benzodiazepines develops rapidly, in most cases without loss of antianxiety efficacy.

Phenelzine has been the most studied MAOI in the treatment of SAD. It has proven to be efficacious, but the risk of hypertensive reaction and related need to follow dietary restrictions is an important limitation for its use. It is generally well tolerated, as demonstrated by several studies, and it can be reserved for patients with refractory disease. Gabapentin and pregabalin have each been studied in only a single controlled trial. Preliminary results have suggested moderate efficacy, but empirical support for their use is more limited than for SSRIs, benzodiazepines, or MAOIs. The antidepressant mirtazapine has also shown efficacy in a single controlled trial.

Cases of nongeneralized social anxiety disorder, in which feared performance situations arise only occasionally and predictably (e.g., recitals and professional presentations), can be treated initially with beta blockers such as propranolol, used on an as-needed basis about an hour before a performance. If beta blockers are ineffective or are contraindicated, an alternative is the use of a benzodiazepine. The doses needed to control anxiety may interfere with functioning when the demands of the performance are high, and may sometimes cause sedation. When performance situations arise more frequently, treatments used for GSAD might be preferable for most patients.

Few empirical data are available to guide subsequent treatment of patients who show minimal or no improvement, or of patients who show much improvement but still exhibit meaningful symptoms and impairment. The first step in managing treatment-resistant patients is to identify possible causes. Several reasons for resistance exist. For example, therapeutic failure may be caused by nonadherence to treatment resulting in suboptimal medication levels or treatment duration. The presence of a comorbid psychiatric disorder may be another reason for resistance. These are very common in patients with SAD, and are often exclusion criteria in clinical trials. The lack of information of the influence of comorbidity on treatment response can also be due to the fact that trials that allow comorbid disorders do not usually report treatment response stratified by their presence or absence of these conditions. Comorbid medical conditions and individual pharmacokinetic characteristics (drug interactions, rapid metabolizers) may be other sources contributing to resistance. Partial responses to a SSRI or a SNRI may be augmented with a benzodiazepine, gabapentin, or pregabalin (although the combination of an SSRI or a SNRI with an MAOI is absolutely contraindicated due to the risk of development of a serotonergic syndrome). The recent study by Blanco et al. (2010) as well as data from Blomhoff et al. (2001) indicate that combined CBT and medication treatment is superior to medication alone, suggesting that it may be a reasonable strategy for patients who do not respond for medication alone. However, data on sequential treatment, particularly randomized trials that compare different sequential strategies, are needed to further improve the treatment of SAD.

Another important question often raised by patients is related to the length of treatment. The available data suggest that discontinuation of medication, even after several months of treatment, can result in relatively high rates of relapse. It appears reasonable to recommend treatment for at least 6–12 months, and then to re-evaluate with the patient the advantages and disadvantages of a longer treatment versus medication discontinuation. In many cases patients prefer to continue on medication, whereas others choose a slow taper period to evaluate whether a lower dose or full discontinuation are viable alternatives. Preliminary findings suggest that the use of concomitant CBT may help maintain the gains following medication cessation, but replication of these findings is needed. Important progress over the past two decades has yielded pharmacological treatments that clearly improve the prognosis of the patient with SAD, yet remaining questions demonstrate substantial needs for further research.

REFERENCES

Allgulander, C. (1999). Paroxetine in social anxiety disorder: A randomized placebo-controlled study. *Acta Psychiatrica Scandinavica, 100*, 193–198.

Allgulander, C., Mangano, R., Zhang, J., Dahl, A. A., Lepola, U., Sjödin, I., et al. (2004). Efficacy of Venlafaxine ER in patients with social anxiety disorder: A double-blind, placebo-controlled, parallel-group comparison with paroxetine. *Human Psychopharmacology: Clinical and Experimental, 19*, 387–396.

Atmaca, M., Tezcan, E., & Kuloglu, M. (2003). An open clinical trial of reboxetine in the treatment of social phobia. *Journal of Clinical Psychopharmacology, 23*, 417–419.

Baldwin, D., Bobes, J., Stein, D. J., Scharwächter, I., & Faure, M. (1999). Paroxetine in social phobia/social anxiety disorder. Randomized double-blind, placebo-controlled study. Paroxetine Study Group. *British Journal of Psychiatry, 175*, 120–126.

Barnett, S. D., Kramer, M. L., Casat, C. D., Connor, K. M., & Davidson, J. R. (2002). Efficacy of olanzapine in social anxiety disorder: A pilot study. *Journal of Psychopharmacology, 16*, 365–368.

Beidel, D. C., Turner, S. M., Sallee, F., Ammerman, R. T., Crosby, L. A., & Pathak, S. (2007). SET-C versus Fluoxetine in the treatment of childhood social phobia. *Journal of American Academy of Child and Adolescent Psychiatry, 46*, 1622–1632.

Birmaher, B., Axelson, D. A., Monk, K., Kalas, C., Clark, D. B., Ehmann, M., et al. (2003). Fluoxetine for the treatment of childhood anxiety disorders. *Journal of American Academy of Child and Adolescent Psychiatry, 42*, 415–423.

Black, B., & Uhde, T. W. (1994). Treatment of elective mutism with fluoxetine: A double-blind, placebo-controlled study. *Journal of American Academy of Child and Adolescent Psychiatry, 33*, 1000–1006.

Black, B., Uhde, T. W., & Tancer, M. E. (1992). Fluoxetine for the treatment of social phobia. *Journal of Clinical Psychopharmacology, 12*, 293–295.

Blanco, C., Heimberg, R., Schneier, F., Fresco, D. M., Chen, H., Turk, C. L., et al. (2010). A placebo-controlled trial of phenelzine, cognitive behavioral group therapy, and their combination for social anxiety disorder. *Archives of General Psychiatry, 67*(3), 286–295.

Blanco, C., Schneier, F. R., Schmidt, A., Blanco-Jerez, C. R., Marshall, R. D., Sánchez-Lacay, A., et al. (2003). Pharmacological treatment of social anxiety disorder: A meta-analysis. *Depression and Anxiety, 18*, 29–40.

Blomhoff, S., Haug, T. T., Hellstrom, K., Holme, I., Humble, M., Madsbu, H. P., et al. (2001). Randomised controlled general practice trial of sertraline, exposure therapy and combined treatment in generalised social phobia. *British Journal of Psychiatry, 179*, 23–30.

Clark, D. B., & Agras, W. S. (1991). The assessment and treatment of performance anxiety in musicians. *American Journal of Psychiatry, 148*, 598–605.

Clark, D. M., Ehlers, A., McManus, F., Hackmann, A., Fennell, M. J., Campbell, H., (2003). Cognitive therapy versus fluoxetine in generalized social phobia: A randomized placebo-controlled trial. *Journal of Consulting and Clinical Psychology*, *71*, 1058–1067.

Compton, S. N., Grant, P. J., Chrisman, A. K., Gammon, P. J., Brown, V. L., & March, J. S. (2001). Sertraline in children with social anxiety disorder: An open trial. *Journal of American Academy of Adolescent Psychiatry*, *409*(Suppl 5), 564–571.

Crippa, J. A., Filho, A. S., Freitas, M. C., & Zuardi, A. W. (2007). Duloxetine in the treatment of social anxiety disorder. *Journal of Clinical Psychopharmacology*, *27*, 310.

Davidson, J., Yaryura-Tobias, J., DuPont, R., Stallings, L., Barbato, L. M., van der Hoop, R. G., et al. (2004). Fluvoxamine-controlled release formulation for the treatment of generalized social anxiety disorder. *Journal of Clinical Psychopharmacology*, *24*, 118–125.

Davidson, J. R., Foa, E. B., Huppert, J. D., Keefe, F. J., Franklin, M. E., Compton, J. S., et al. (2004). Fluoxetine, comprehensive cognitive behavioral therapy, and placebo in generalized social phobia. *Archives of General Psychiatry*, *61*, 1005–1013.

Davidson, J. R., Ford, S. M., Smith, R. D., & Potts, N. L. (1991). *Long-term treatment of social phobia with clonazepam. Journal of Clinical Psychiatry*, *52*(Suppl), 16–20.

Davidson, J. R. T., Potts, N. L. S., Richichi, E., Krishnan, R., Ford, S. M., Smith, R., (1993). Treatment of social phobia with clonazepam and placebo. *Journal of Clinical Psychopharmacology*, *13*, 423–428.

Dummit, E. S., III, Klein, R. G., & Tancer, N. K. (1996). Fluoxetine treatment of children with selective mutism: An open trial. *Journal of American Academy of Child and Adolescent Psychiatry*, *35*, 615–621.

Dunlop, B. W., Papp, L., Garlow, S. J., Weiss, P. S., Knight, B. T., & Ninan, P. T. (2007). Tiagabine for social anxiety disorder. *Human Psychopharmacology: Clinical and Experimental*, *22*, 241–244.

Dursun, S. M., & Devarajan, S. (2001). Accelerated weight loss after treating refractory depression with fluoxetine plus topiramate: Possible mechanisms of action?. *Canadian Journal of Psychiatry*, *46*, 287–288.

Emmanuel, N. P., Brawman-Mintzer, O., Morton, W. A., Book, S. W., Johnson, M. R., Orberbaum, J. P., (2000). Bupropion-SR in treatment of social phobia. *Depression and Anxiety*, *12*, 111–113.

Fahlen, T., Nilsson, H. L., Borg, K., Humble, M., & Pauli, U. (1995). Social phobia: The clinical efficacy and tolerability of the monoamine oxidase-A and serotonin uptake reuptake inhibitor brofaromine: A double-blind placebo-controlled study. *Acta Psychiatrica Scandinavica*, *92*, 351–358.

Fairbanks, J., Pine, D. S., Tancer, N. K., Dummit, E. S., 3rd, Kentgen, L. M., Martin, J., et al. (1997). Open fluoxetine treatment of mixed anxiety disorders in children and adolescents. *Journal of Child and Adolescent Psychopharmacology*, *7*, 17–29.

Fedoroff, I. C., & Taylor, S. (2001). Psychological and pharmacological treatments of social phobia: A meta-analysis. *Journal of Clinical Psychopharmacology*, *21*, 311–324.

Gelernter, C. S., Uhde, T. W., Cimbolic, P., Arnkoff, D. B., Vittone, B. J., Tancer, M. E., et al. (1991). Cognitive-behavioral and pharmacological treatments of social phobia: A controlled study. *Archives of General Psychiatry*, *48*, 938–945.

Gorman, J. M., Liebowitz, M. R., Fyer, A. J., Campeas, R., & Klein, D. F. (1985). Treatment of social phobia with atenolol. *Journal of Clinical Psychopharmacology*, *5*, 298–301.

Gould, R. A., Buckminster, S., Pollack, M. H., Otto, M. W., & Yap, L. (1997). Cognitive-behavioral and pharmacological treatment for social phobia: A meta-analysis. *Clinical Psychology: Science and Practice*, *4*, 291–306.

Hedges, D. W., Brown, B. L., Shwalb, D. A., Godfrey, K., & Larcher, A. M. (2007). The efficacy of selective serotonin reuptake inhibitors in adult social anxiety disorder: A meta-analysis of double-blind, placebo-controlled trials. *Journal of Psychopharmacology*, *21*, 102–111.

Heimberg, R. G., Liebowitz, M. R., Schneier, F. R., Hope, D. A., Holt, C. S., Welkowitz, L. A., et al. (1998). Cognitive-behavioral group therapy versus phenelzine in social phobia: 12-week outcome. *Archives of General Psychiatry*, *55*, 1133–1141.

Isolan, L., Pheula, G., Salum, G. A., Oswald, S., Rohde, L. A., & Manfro, G. G. (2007). An open-label trial of escitalopram in children and adolescents with social anxiety disorder. *Journal of Child and Adolescent Psychopharmacology*, *17*, 751–759.

Johnson, B. A. (2005). Recent advances in the development of treatments for alcohol and cocaine dependence: Focus on topiramate and other modulators of GABA or glutamate function. *CNS Drugs*, *19*, 873–896.

Kasper, S., Stein, D. J., Loft, H., & Nil, R. (2005). Escitalopram in the treatment of social anxiety disorder: Randomised, placebo-controlled, flexible-dosage study. *British Journal of Psychiatry*, *186*, 222–226.

Katschnig, H., Stein, M. B., & Buller, R.On behalf of the International Multicenter Clinical Trial Group on Moclobemide in Social Phobia. (1997). Moclobemide in social phobia: A double-blind, placebo-controlled clinical study. *European Archives of Psychiatry and Clinical Neuroscience*, *247*, 71–80.

Katzelnick, D. J., Kobak, K. A., Greist, J. H., Jefferson, J. W., Mantle, J. M., & Serlin, R. C. (1995). Sertraline for social phobia: A double-blind, placebo-controlled crossover study. *American Journal of Psychiatry*, *152*, 1368–1371.

Kinrys, G., Pollack, M. H., Simon, N. M., Worthington, J. J., Nardi, A. E., & Versiani, M. (2003). Valproic acid for the treatment of social anxiety disorder. *International Clinical Psychopharmacology*, *18*, 169–172.

Kobak, K. A., Greist, J. H., Jefferson, J. W., & Katzelnick, D. J. (2002). Fluoxetine in social phobia: A double-blind, placebo-controlled pilot study. *Journal of Clinical Psychopharmacology*, *22*(3), 257–262.

Lader, M., Stender, K., Burger, V., & Nil, R. (2004). Efficacy and tolerability of escitalopram in 12- and 24-week treatment of social anxiety disorder: Randomised, double-blind, placebo-controlled, fixed-dose study. *Depression and Anxiety*, *19*, 241–248.

Lepola, U., Bergtholdt, B., St, Lambert, J., Davy, K. L., & Ruggiero, L. (2004). Controlled-release paroxetine in the treatment of patients with social anxiety disorder. *Journal of Clinical Psychiatry*, *65*, 222–229.

Liebowitz, M. R., DeMartinis, N. A., Weihs, K., Londborg, P. D., Smith, W. T., Chung, H., et al. (2003). Efficacy of sertraline in severe generalized social anxiety disorder: Results of a double-blind, placebo-controlled study. *Journal of Clinical Psychiatry*, *64*, 785–792.

Liebowitz, M. R., Gelenberg, A. J., & Munjack, D. (2005). Venlafaxine extended release vs placebo and paroxetine in social anxiety disorder. *Archives of General Psychiatry*, *62*, 190–198.

Liebowitz, M. R., Mangano, R. M., Bradwejn, J., & Asnis, G. (2005). A randomized controlled trial of venlafaxine extended release in generalized social anxiety disorder. *Journal of Clinical Psychiatry*, *66*, 238–247.

Liebowitz, M. R., Schneier, F. R., Campeas, R., Hollander, E., Hatterer, J., Fyer, A., et al. (1992). Phenelzine versus atenolol in social phobia: A placebo controlled comparison. *Archives of General Psychiatry*, *49*, 290–300.

Liebowitz, M. R., Stein, M. B., Tancer, M., Carpenter, D., Oakes, R., & Pitts, C. D. (2002). A randomized, double-blind, fixed-dose comparison of paroxetine and placebo in the treatment of generalized social anxiety disorder. *Journal of Clinical Psychiatry*, *63*, 66–74.

Lott, M., Greist, J. H., Jefferson, J. W., Kobak, K. A., Katzelnick, D. J., Katz, R. J., et al. (1997). Brofaromine for social phobia: A multicenter, placebo-controlled, double-blind study. *Journal of Clinical Psychopharmacology*, *17*, 255–260.

Lydiard, R. B., Laraia, M. T., Howell, E. F., & Ballenger, J. C. (1988). Alprazolam in the treatment of social phobia. *Journal of Clinical Psychiatry*, *49*, 17–19.

March, J. S., Entusah, A. R., Rynn, M., Albano, A. M., & Tourian, K. M. (2007). A randomized controlled trial of venlafaxine ER versus placebo in pediatric social anxiety disorder. *Biological Psychiatry*, *62*(10), 1149–1154.

Marks, I. M., & Matthews, A. M. (1979). Brief standard self-rating for phobic patients. *Behaviour Research and Therapy*, *17*, 263–267.

Montgomery, S. A., Nil, R., Durr-Pal, N., Loft, H., & Boulenger, J. P. (2005). A 24-week randomized, double-blind, placebo-controlled study of escitalopram for the prevention of generalized social anxiety disorder. *Journal of Clinical Psychiatry*, *66*, 1270–1278.

Mrakotsky, C., Masek, B., Biederman, J., Raches, D., Hsin, O., Forbes, P., et al. (2008). Prospective open-label pilot trial of mirtazapine in children and adolescents with social phobia. *Journal of Anxiety Disorders*, *22*(1), 88–97.

Muehlbacher, M., Nickel, M. K., Nickel, C., Kettler, C., Lahmann, C., Pedrosa Gil, F., et al. (2005). Mirtazapine treatment of social phobia in women: A randomized, double-blind, placebo-controlled study. *Journal of Clinical Psychopharmacology*, *25*, 580–583.

Munjack, D. J., Baltazar, P. L., Bohn, P. B., Cabe, D. D., & Appleton, A. A. (1990). Clonazepam in the treatment of social phobia: A pilot study. *Journal of Clinical Psychiatry*, *51*(Suppl 5), 35–40.

Munjack, D. J., Bruns, J., Baltazar, P., Brown, R., Leonard, M., Nagy, R., (1991). A pilot study of buspirone in the treatment of social phobia. *Journal of Anxiety Disorders*, *5*, 87–98.

Noyes, R., Moroz, G., Davidson, J. T. R., Liebowitz, M. R., Davidson, A., Siegel, J., (1997). Moclobemide in social phobia: A controlled dose-response trial. *Journal of Clinical Psychopharmacology*, *17*, 247–254.

Ontiveros, A., & Fontaine, R. (1990). Social phobia and clonazepam. *Canadian Journal of Psychiatry*, *35*, 439–441.

Pallanti, S., & Quercioli, L. (2006). Resistant social anxiety disorder response to Escitalopram. *Clinical Practice and Epidemiology in Mental Health*, *13*, 35.

Pande, A. C., Davidson, J. R. T., Jefferson, J. W., Janney, C. A., Katzelnick, D. J., Weisler, R. H., et al. (1999). Treatment of social phobia with gabapentin: A placebo-controlled study. *Journal of Clinical Psychopharmacology*, *19*, 341–348.

Pande, A. C., Feltner, D. E., Jefferson, J. W., Davidson, J. R., Pollack, M., Stein, M. B., et al. (2004). Efficacy of the novel anxiolytic pregabalin in social anxiety disorder: A placebo-controlled, multicenter study. *Journal of Clinical Psychopharmacology*, *24*, 141–149.

Potts, N. L. S., & Davidson, J. R. T., (1995). Pharmacological treatments: Literature review. In R. G. Heimberg, M. R. Liebowitz, D. A. Hope (Eds.), *Social phobia: Diagnosis, assessment, and treatment* (pp. 334–366). New York: Guilford Press.

Reich, J. R., & Yates, W. (1988). A pilot study of treatment of social phobia with alprazolam. *American Journal of Psychiatry*, *145*, 590–594.

Reiter, S. R., Pollack, M. H., Rosenbaum, J. F., & Cohen, L. S. (1990). Clonazepam for the treatment of social phobia. *Journal of Clinical Psychiatry*, *51*, 470–472.

Rickels, K., Mangano, R., & Khan, A. (2004). A double-blind, placebo-controlled study of a flexible dose of venlafaxine ER in adult outpatients with generalized social anxiety disorder. *Journal of Clinical Psychopharmacology*, *24*, 488–496.

Schneier, F. R. (1995). Clinical assessment strategies for social phobia. *Psychiatric Annals*, *25*, 550–553.

Schneier, F. R., Chin, S. J., Hollander, E., & Liebowitz, M. R. (1992). Fluoxetine in social phobia (letter). *Journal of Clinical Psychopharmacology*, *12*, 62–63.

Schneier, F. R., Goetz, D., Campeas, R., Fallon, B., Marshall, R., & Liebowitz, M. R. et al. (1998). Placebo-controlled trial of moclobemide in social phobia. *British Journal of Psychiatry*, *172*, 70–77.

Schneier, F. R., Saoud, J. B., Campeas, R., Fallon, E., Hollander, E., Coplan, J., (1993). Buspirone in social phobia. *Journal of Clinical Psychopharmacology*, *13*, 251–256.

Schutters, S. I., van Megen, H. J., & Westenberg, H. G. (2005). Efficacy of quetiapine in generalized social anxiety disorder: Results from an open-label study. *Journal of Clinical Psychiatry*, *66*, 540–542.

Seedat, S., & Stein, M. B. (2004). Double-blind, placebo-controlled assessment of combined clonazepam with paroxetine compared with paroxetine monotherapy for generalized social anxiety disorder. *Journal of Clinical Psychiatry*, *65*, 244–248.

Simeon, J. G., & Ferguson, H. B. (1987). Alprazolam effects in children with anxiety disorders. *Canadian Journal of Psychiatry*, *32*, 570–574.

Simeon, J. G., Ferguson, H. B., & Knott, V. (1992). Clinical, cognitive, and neurophysiological effects of alprazolam effects in children and adolescents with overanxious disorder and avoidant disorders. *Journal of the American Academy of Child and Adolescent Psychiatry*, *31*, 29–33.

Simon, N. M., Worthington, J. J., Doyle, A. C., Hoge, E. A., Kinrys, G., Fischmann, D., et al. (2004). An open-label study of levetiracetam for the treatment of social anxiety disorder. *Journal of Clinical Psychiatry*, *65*, 1219–1222.

Simon, N. M., Hoge, E. A., Fischmann, D., Worthington, J. J., Christian, K. M., Kinrys, G., et al. (2006). An open-label trial of risperidone augmentation for refractory anxiety disorders. *Journal of Clinical Psychiatry*, *67*, 381–385.

Simon, N. M., Korbly, N. B., Worthington, J. J., Kinrys, G., & Pollack, M. H. (2002). Citalopram for social anxiety disorder: An open-label pilot in refractory and nonrefractory patients. *CNS Spectrums*, *7*, 655–657.

Simpson, H. B., Schneier, F. R., Campeas, R. B., Marshall, R. D., Fallon, B. A., Davies, S., et al. (1998). Imipramine in the treatment of social phobia. *Journal of Clinical Psychopharmacology*, *18*, 132–135.

Simpson, H. B., Schneier, F. R., Marshall, R. D., Campeas, R. B., Vermes, D., Silvestre, J., et al. (1998). Low dose selegiline (l-deprenyl) in social phobia. *Depression and Anxiety*, *7*, 126–129.

Stein, D. J., Cameron, A., Amrein, R., & Montgomery, S. A. Moclobemide Social Phobia Clinical Study Group. (2002). Moclobemide is effective and well tolerated in the long-term pharmacotherapy of social anxiety disorder with or without comorbid anxiety disorder. *International Journal of Clinical Psychopharmacology*, *17*, 161–170.

Stein, M. B., Fyer, A. J., Davidson, J. R. T., Pollack, M. H., & Wiita, B. (1999). Fluvoxamine treatment of social phobia (social anxiety disorder): A double-blind, placebo-controlled study. *American Journal of Psychiatry*, *156*, 756–760.

Stein, D. J., Kasper, S., Andersen, E. W., Nil, R., & Lader, M. (2004). Escitalopram in the treatment of social anxiety disorder: Analysis of efficacy for different clinical subgroups and symptom dimensions. *Depression and Anxiety*, *20*, 175–181.

Stein, M. B., Liebowitz, M. R., Lydiard, B., Pitts, C. D., Bushnell, W., & Gergel, I. (1998). Paroxetine treatment of generalized social phobia (social anxiety disorder): A randomized controlled trial. *JAMA*, *280*, 708–713.

Stein, D. J., Ipser, J. C., & Balkom, A. J. (2004). Pharmacotherapy for social phobia. *Cochrane Database of Systematic Reviews*, 4. CD001206.

Stein, M. B., Pollack, M. H., Bystritsky, A., Kelsey, J. E., & Mangano, R. M. (2005). Efficacy of low and higher dose extended-release venlafaxine in generalized social anxiety disorder: A 6-month randomized controlled trial. *Psychopharmacology*, *177*, 280–288.

Stein, D. J., Stein, M. B., Pitts, C. D., Kumar, R., & Hunter, B. (2002). Predictors of response to pharmacotherapy in social anxiety disorder: An analysis of 3 placebo-controlled paroxetine trials. *Journal of Clinical Psychiatry*, *63*, 152–155.

Stein, D. J., Versiani, M., Hair, T., & Kumar, R. (2002). Efficacy of paroxetine for relapse prevention in social anxiety disorder: A 24-week study. *Archives of General Psychiatry*, *59*, 1111–1118.

Sternbach, H. (1990). Fluoxetine treatment of social phobia. *Journal of Clinical Psychopharmacology*, *10*, 230–231.

Tata, A. L., & Kockler, D. R. (2006). Topiramate for binge-eating disorder associated with obesity. *Annals of Pharmacotherapy*, *40*, 1993–1997.

The Research Unit on Pediatric Psychopharmacology Anxiety Study Group. (2001). Fluvoxamine for the treatment of anxiety disorders in children and adolescents. *New England Journal of Medicine*, *344*(17), 1279–1285.

Turner, S. M., Beidel, D. C., & Jacob, R. G. (1994). Social phobia: A comparison of behavior therapy and atenolol. *Journal of Consulting and Clinical Psychology*, *62*, 350–358.

Van Ameringen, M. A., Lane, R. M., Walker, J. R., Bowen, R. C., Chokka, P. R., Goldner, E. M., et al. (2001). Sertraline treatment of generalized social phobia: A 20-week, double-blind, placebo-controlled study. *American Journal of Psychiatry*, *158*, 275–281.

Van Ameringen, M., Mancini, C., & Streitner, D. L. (1993). Fluoxetine efficacy in social phobia. *Journal of Clinical Psychiatry*, *54*, 27–32.

Van Ameringen, M., Mancini, C., Oakman, J., Walker, J., Kjernisted, K., Chokka, P., (2007). Nefazodone in the treatment of generalized social phobia: A randomized, placebo-controlled trial. *Journal of Clinical Psychiatry*, *68*, 288–295.

Van Ameringen, M., Mancini, C., Pipe, B., Oakman, J., & Bennett, M. (2004). An open trial of Topiramate in the treatment of Generalized Social Phobia. *Journal of Clinical Psychiatry*, *65*, 1674–1678.

Van Ameringen, M., Mancini, C., & Wilson, C. (1996). Buspirone augmentation of selective serotonin reuptake inhibitors (SSRIs) in social phobia. *Journal of Affective Disorders*, *39*, 115–121.

Van Ameringen, M., Oakman, J., Mancini, C., Pipe, B., & Chung, H. (2004). Predictors of response in Generalized Social Phobia: Effect of age of onset. *Journal of Clinical Psychopharmacology*, *24*, 42–48.

van der Linden, G. J., Stein, D. J., & van Balkom, A. J. (2000). The efficacy of the selective serotonin reuptake inhibitors for social anxiety disorder (social phobia): A meta-analysis of randomized controlled trials. *International Clinical Psychopharmacology*, *Suppl 2*, S15–S23.

Van Veen, J. F., Van Vliet, I. M., & Westenberg, H. G. (2002). Mirtazapine in social anxiety disorder: a pilot study. *International Clinical Psychopharmacology*, *17*, 315–317.

Van Vliet, I. M., den Boer, J. A., & Westenberg, H. G. (1992). Psychopharmacological treatment of social phobia: Clinical and biochemical effects of brofaromine, a selective MAO-A inhibitor. *European Neuropsychopharmacology*, *2*, 21–29.

Van Vliet, I. M., den Boer, J. A., & Westenberg, H. G. (1994). Psychopharmacological treatment of social phobia: A double-blind placebo controlled study with fluvoxamine. *Psychopharmacology*, *115*, 128–134.

Van Vliet, I. M., den Boer, J. A., Westenberg, H. G., & Pian, K. L. (1997). Clinical effects of buspirone in social phobia: A double-blind placebo-controlled study. *Journal of Clinical Psychiatry*, *58*, 164–168.

Vasudev, K., Macritchie, K., Geddes, J., Watson, S., & Young, A. (2006). Topiramate for acute affective episodes in bipolar disorder. *Cochrane Database of Systematic Reviews*, *1*(CD003384), 2006.

Versiani, M., Mundim, F. D., Nardi, A. E., & Liebowitz, M. R. (1988). Tranylcypromine in social phobia. *Journal of Clinical Psychopharmacology*, *8*, 279–283.

Versiani, M., Nardia, A. E., & Figueira, I. (1997). Double-blind placebo controlled trials with bromazepam. *Jornal Brasileiro de Psiquiatria*, *46*, 167–171.

Versiani, M., Nardi, A. E., & Mundim, F. D. (1989). Fobia social. *Journal Brasileiro de Psiquiatria*, *38*, 251–263.

Versiani, M., Nardi, A. E., Mundim, F. D., Alves, A. B., Liebowitz, M. R., & Amrein, R. (1992). Pharmacotherapy of social phobia: A controlled study with moclobemide and phenelzine. *British Journal of Psychiatry*, *161*, 353–360.

Villarreal, G., Johnson, M. R., & Rubey, R. (2000). Treatment of social phobia with the dopamine agonist pergolide. *Depression and Anxiety*, *11*, 45–47.

Wagner, K. D., Berard, R., Stein, M. B., Wetherhold, E., Carpenter, D. J., Perera, P., et al. (2004). A multicenter, randomized, double-blind, placebo-controlled trial of paroxetine in children and adolescents with social anxiety disorder. *Archives of General Psychiatry*, *61*, 1153–1162.

Walker, J. R., Van Ameringen, M. A., & Swinson, R. (2000). Prevention of relapse in generalized social phobia: Results of a 24-week study in responders to 20 weeks of sertraline treatment. *Journal of Clinical Psychopharmacology*, *6*, 636–644.

Westenberg, H. G., Stein, D. J., Yang, H., Li, D., & Barbato, L. M. (2004). A double-blind placebo-controlled study of controlled release fluvoxamine for the treatment of generalized social anxiety disorder. *Journal of Clinical Psychopharmacology*, *24*, 49–55.

Zhang, W., Connor, K. M., & Davidson, J. R. (2005). Levetiracetam in social phobia: A placebo controlled pilot study. *Psychopharmacology*, *19*, 551–553.

Zitrin, C. M., Klein, D. F., Woerner, M. G., & Ross, D. C. (1983). Treatment of phobias, I: a comparison of imipramine hydrochloride and placebo. *Archives of General Psychiatry*, *40*, 125–138.

Chapter 20

Treatment of Social Anxiety Disorder: A Treatments-by-Dimensions Review

Brandon J. Weiss[1]**, Debra A. Hope**[2] **and Leslie G. Cohn**[3]
[1]Department of Psychology, University of Nebraska–Lincoln, NE 68588, [2]Department of Psychology, University of Nebraska–Lincoln, NE 68588, [3]Private Practice, Seattle, WA, USA

In the past 25 years, there has been considerable research on the treatment of SAD (SP). At this writing, there are more than 35 studies evaluating psychosocial interventions with individuals who meet standard criteria in the DSM (American Psychiatric Association, 1980, 1987, 1994, 2000) for SAD. Over the years, numerous conceptual reviews of this literature have been published (Chambless & Hope, 1996; Heimberg, Dodge, & Becker, 1987; Hope, Holt, & Heimberg, 1995; Rodebaugh, Holaway, & Heimberg, 2004). Several meta-analyses have appeared as well (e.g., Feske & Chambless, 1995; Powers, Sigmarsson, & Emmelkamp, 2008). These previous conceptual and meta-analytic reviews have addressed which treatments are effective for SAD and whether there is any evidence that one treatment may be more helpful than another treatment. Occasionally, the reviews have asked more-specific questions, such as whether a cognitive intervention is essential for change (e.g., Feske & Chambless, 1995). When considering such reviews, one always struggles with which of the myriad of outcome measures should be considered the key measure(s) that accurately indexes the efficacy of the treatment.

Researchers include multiple measures of outcome because they recognize that SAD is a complex phenomenon. An individual presenting with this disorder may show a number of symptoms, including heightened physiological arousal in feared situations, high subjective anxiety/distress and behavioral avoidance, deficits in social performance or skill, cognitive bias, and excessive negative self-statements. One or more of these may be prominent in a given case. Recognition of this complexity led us to take a new approach to reviewing the treatment literature in the first edition of this volume, now updated and expanded for the second edition. This review will be organized around the

Social Anxiety: Clinical, Developmental, and Social Perspectives. DOI: 10.1016/B978-0-12-375096-9.00020-1

specific aspects of SAD, evaluating which treatments may address which symptoms most effectively. We hope this will meet two goals. First, a practitioner may use this review as a guide in treatment selection if a client presents with a particular dominant symptom cluster. Second, it is hoped that such a review will help elucidate the mechanisms underlying the best treatments, as well as identify which are broadly effective across many types of symptoms. It should be noted that not all studies that evaluated a psychosocial treatment for SAD will be reviewed because a few studies did not utilize any of the measures we examined.

TREATMENT IMPACT ON PHYSIOLOGICAL SYMPTOMS

A number of studies have included assessment of a physiological component of social anxiety in the design. Most often, researchers assess heart rate and, less frequently, blood pressure. These measures are usually taken during a behavioral test such as a brief speech or interaction task. Although many studies have found little change on physiological measures (e.g., Clark & Agras, 1991; Falloon, Lloyd, & Harpin, 1981), a few studies have found within-group changes on physiological measures, but often without any difference between various treatments.

In the pilot study of CBGT for SAD (Heimberg, Becker, Goldfinger, & Vermilyea, 1985), seven individuals were treated in a multiple baseline design and had significant reductions in heart rate during a role-played individualized behavioral test. The reductions were evident both during an anticipatory period and during the role-play, and they tended to be maintained at six-month follow-up. In their comparison of CBGT and educational-supportive therapy (ES – a credible placebo control), Heimberg et al. (1990) again measured heart rate in anticipation of and during an individualized behavioral test conducted in the laboratory at pretreatment, post-treatment, and at the six-month follow-up. Although there was no between-group difference, both treatment groups had significant reductions in heart rate at post-treatment in the range of 8–11 beats per minute (bpm). In contrast to other measures that favored CBGT at six-month follow-up, the reduction in heart rate for the ES participants only continued to be significant when compared with pretreatment measures. Unfortunately, heart rate data were not collected in the five-year follow-up study of these participants (Heimberg, Salzman, Holt, & Blendell, 1993), so it is unknown whether this pattern of results was maintained.

When CBGT was compared with exposure alone in a treatment dismantling study, heart rate in anticipation of and during the individualized behavioral test improved significantly from pre- to post-treatment, with no differences between treatments (Hope, Heimberg, & Bruch, 1995). These results were generally maintained at six-month follow-up.

A somewhat similar pattern of physiological change was also found in one of the earliest treatment studies for social anxiety. Kanter and Goldfried (1979) compared rational restructuring, self-control systematic desensitization, a combination of the two interventions, and a wait-list control group. Heart rate was measured during two separate interactions with a male or a female confederate, and the average heart rate immediately after the interaction appears to have been used in the analyses. As with Heimberg et al. (1990) and Hope, Heimberg et al. (1995), there were no differences among the groups at post-treatment. There was a significant within-group decrease in heart rate of about 10 bmp for the rational restructuring (alone) treatment from pre- to post-treatment. Heart rate did not decrease for participants who received systematic desensitization, the combined treatment, or no treatment. Physiological data do not appear to have been collected at the nine-week follow-up assessment.

Both blood pressure and heart rate were measured before and after treatment in the pilot study for social effectiveness therapy (SET), a multicomponent treatment that includes education, social skills training, individualized flooding, and homework (Turner, Beidel, Cooley, Woody, & Messer, 1994). The physiological measures were taken at two-minute intervals during a baseline period and during a speech challenge test. Despite evidence of improvement on other measures, the only significant physiological change was a decrease in diastolic blood pressure during the baseline period. Although physiological reactivity apparently was monitored within treatment sessions also, these data were not reported. However, Fink, Turner, and Beidel (1996) included a graph of in-session heart rate during imaginal exposure as part of SET for a single-subject study that included incorporation of culturally relevant factors in the treatment of an African American woman. The graph showed an across-session habituation curve, suggesting improvement in heart rate reactivity with SET. Although Turner, Beidel, and Jacob (1994) indicated the use of blood pressure and heart rate monitoring in their examination of behavior therapy versus atenolol versus placebo, they do not report any results on these measures.

Overall, very few researchers have reported that different treatments yield *differential* change on physiological measures. However, Emmelkamp, Mersch, Vissia, and van der Helm (1985) found such a difference in their comparison of *in vivo* exposure, rational emotive therapy, and self-instructional training (self-instructions and imaginal rehearsal of social situations). Using the same procedure as Kanter and Goldfried (1979), heart rate was measured during two separate interactions with a male or a female confederate at a one-minute baseline, in anticipation of the interaction, and immediately after the interaction. Surprisingly, there were no significant decreases in heart rate within the treatment groups at the completion of treatment. However, between-group comparisons at post-treatment, controlling for pretreatment heart rate, revealed that heart rate in anticipation of interactions and immediately after the interactions was more reduced for those participants in the exposure condition compared with the cognitive treatments combined. It does not appear that heart rate was assessed at the one-month follow-up assessment, and thus it is unknown whether these differences were maintained.

Recognizing the heterogeneity of the presentation of SAD, Öst and colleagues (Jerremalm, Jansson, & Öst, 1986; Öst, Jerremalm, & Johansson, 1981) investigated whether matching the type of treatment to socially anxious participants' reaction patterns may yield a better outcome. Participants were classified as physiological reactors, behavioral reactors, or cognitive reactors on the basis of their pattern of response to a role-played social interaction. Physiological reactors were expected to have a greater reduction in physiological symptoms with applied reaction compared with social skills training or self-instructional training. In contrast, socially anxious participants who were determined to be more reactive in a behavioral or cognitive sense should benefit more from social skills training or self-instructional training, respectively. Compared with pretreatment, physiological reactors, regardless of whether they received applied relaxation, social skills training, or self-instructional training, had lower heart rates (or less heart rate reactivity from baseline) at post-treatment. Neither behavioral nor cognitive reactors demonstrated change in heart rate regardless of treatment condition. The lack of change for those participants who met criteria for SAD may be attributable to floor effects, because they were initially selected as having minimal elevations in heart rate during the behavioral test. Physiological reactors assigned to a wait-list condition did not improve on heart rate, suggesting the change was not attributable to spontaneous recovery or repeated assessment.

It should be noted that the classification of physiological, behavioral, and cognitive reactors was somewhat unstable in these examinations. Also, individuals who fell between the categories, for example being moderately elevated on both physiological and cognitive indices, were excluded from these studies. However, it does appear that socially anxious participants with strong cardiac reactions to socially threatening situations will likely experience a decrease in their heart rate reactivity with either applied relaxation that targets autonomic arousal directly or social skill or cognitive intervention.

No changes in physiological reactions were noted after treatment for SAD in some studies. Falloon et al. (1981) found no habituation of heart rate from the first to the last exposure session with either role-played or *in vivo* exposure for SAIs also taking propranolol or pill placebo. Clark and Agras (1991) measured heart rate during a speech and musical performance among musicians seeking treatment for performance anxiety who also met criteria for SAD. Overall, heart rate did not change significantly from pre- to post-treatment, nor were there differences among the cognitive-behavioral, buspirone, or placebo treatments. The cognitive-behavioral treatment consisted of self-statement modification, applied relaxation, and exposure. Clark and Agras did note that heart rates during the speech, but not the musical performance, were correlated with subjective anxiety ratings.

In summary, reductions in physiological response, particularly heart rate, were noted with CBGT, exposure alone, and ES. For socially anxious participants who can be classified as physiological reactors, applied relaxation, social skills training, and self-instructional training also yielded reductions in heart rate. There is less evidence for SET resulting in changes in physiological responding, but, given that the package includes exposure and social skills training, future research may support efficacy in this area. Purely cognitive interventions may be less likely to reduce heart rates in socially threatening situations, because Emmelkamp et al. (1985) found exposure to be more effective than rational emotive therapy and self-instructional training. Only Kanter and Goldfried (1979) found rational restructuring to yield pre- to post-treatment changes in heart rate, but their study was published prior to DSM-III (American Psychiatric Association, 1980). Although their participants would likely met criteria for SAD, it is possible their sample was more heterogeneous than more recent treatment samples. However, for physiological reactors, even a purely cognitive treatment appears to be effective in reducing heart rate. Also, it is worth noting that most recent treatment studies have not used physiological assessments to measure outcome. Thus, it is unknown how more recent iterations of treatments (e.g., Hope, Heimberg, Juster, & Turk, 2000) effect physiological responses.

Some methodological issues are worth noting. Most of the studies utilized only heart rate as a physiological index. Turner and colleagues also included blood pressure, with limited results (Turner, Beidel, Cooley et al., 1994; Turner, Beidel, & Jacob, 1994). Other measures, such as skin conductance, blood flow activity/skin temperature changes (blushing), or muscle tension, may yield different results. Although all the studies assessed physiological response during a behavioral challenge, there were a variety of procedural variations (e.g., length of baseline, speech versus interaction) that make comparison among studies more difficult. Interestingly, there may be some utility to determining an individual's tendency to react physiologically. Although the treatment-matching hypotheses of Öst and colleagues (1981) were not consistently confirmed, the physiological reactors demonstrated consistently reduced heart rate after treatment.

TREATMENT IMPACT ON COGNITIVE SYMPTOMS

The interest in cognitive-behavioral treatment for SAD has been accompanied by an effort to measure cognitive change in many studies. However, cognition can be examined in various ways that actually assess several different levels of cognition. Adapting the model of Ingram and colleagues (Ingram & Kendall, 1987; Ingram & Wisnicki, 1991), this discussion will be divided into four sections: (1) cognitive propositions, or traits such as beliefs, expectancies, judgments, and attributions; (2) cognitive content accessed via an endorsement method such as self-statements; (3) cognitive products accessed via production method such as a listed thoughts; and (4) cognitive processes, such as attention.

Cognitive Propositions

Irrational Beliefs

Several studies investigating treatment of SAD have utilized a measure of Ellis's (1962) irrational beliefs. Neither the Irrational Beliefs Test (IBT) (Jones, 1969) nor the Rational Behavior Inventory (RBI) (Shorkey & Whiteman, 1977) is specific to social anxiety; instead they assess more general features of psychopathology. Six studies have used the IBT, one study has used the RBI, and one study used an apparent hybrid of the two – the Irrational Beliefs Inventory (IBI) (Koopmans, Sanderman, Timmerman, & Emmelkamp, 1994). These studies will be reviewed next.

One might expect that cognitive interventions would yield greater change in irrational beliefs than noncognitive interventions. In their comparison of rational restructuring, self-control desensitization combined rational restructuring, and self-control desensitization and a wait-list control, Kanter and Goldfried (1979) found that all active treatment groups had significantly better scores on IBT at post-treatment assessment compared with pre-treatment. However, only the rational restructuring group and the combined treatment group improved more on the IBT than the wait-list. Individuals who received rational restructuring improved more than individuals who received self-control desensitization. At nine-week follow-up, the rational restructuring group continued to have lower scores on the IBT than the self-control desensitization group. Similarly, a comparison of exposure alone, rational-emotive therapy, and self-instructional training revealed that only the two cognitive treatments resulted in change on the IBT, with continued improvement during the one-month follow-up for rational-emotive therapy only (Emmelkamp et al., 1985). Between-treatment comparisons were not significant at post-test for any of the treatments for the IBT. However, at follow-up the two cognitive treatments combined yielded lower scores on the IBT than exposure alone. Thus, it appears the interventions with a cognitive component (rational restructuring, rational-emotive therapy, or self-instructional training alone or when combined with self-control desensitization) had more impact on the IBT than the noncognitive intervention (self-control desensitization or exposure) alone in two studies.

In contrast, three studies have found that cognitive and noncognitive interventions yield similar changes in irrational beliefs, at least for individuals with many irrational beliefs. Mattick and Peters (1988) reported that individuals with social anxiety disorder who received either exposure alone or exposure combined with cognitive restructuring improved pre- to post-treatment on the modified IBT for social anxiety. Although a wait-list control group was not included in this design, a comparison to the means on the modified IBT for the wait-list group in the second Mattick study (Mattick, Peters, & Clarke, 1989) suggests this improvement was larger than would be expected by repeated assessment alone. Some continued improvement was evident for both groups between post-treatment and the three-month follow-up as well.

Stravynski, Marks, and Yule (1982), in their study of individuals with SAD assigned to social skills training with or without cognitive modification, noted that improvement on the IBT was similar between the groups, and significant within each group at both post-treatment and follow-up assessments points. Mersch, Emmelkamp, Bögels, and van der Sleen (1989) examined individuals with SAD whom they classified as cognitive (based on RBI scores) or behavioral (based on role-play performance) reactors. Half of each group received a behavioral treatment (social skills training) and the other half received a cognitive treatment (rational-emotive therapy), creating two matches and two mismatches between cognitive/behavioral reactor status and treatment condition. Between pretreatment and post-treatment, RBI scores were significantly improved for the cognitive reactors in both treatments but not for the behavioral reactors in either treatment. At the 14-month follow-up (Mersch, Emmelkamp, & Lips, 1991), all participants classified as improvers continued to improve on the RBI, whereas those classified as relapsed showed some deterioration on the RBI. These data are difficult to interpret because cognitive reactors were initially categorized on the basis of extreme score on the RBI. Regression to the mean may help explain apparent improvement on the RBI for cognitive reactors in both cognitive and noncognitive treatment.

Finally, other studies have found only modest improvements in irrational beliefs or have failed to find differences between the active treatments and wait-list controls. Using a subset of items from IBT thought to be particularly relevant for SAD, Mattick et al. (1989) failed to find differences between the wait-list individuals and participants who received exposure alone, cognitive restructuring alone, or the combination of the two treatments. The cognitive restructuring-alone group improved more on the modified IBT than the exposure-alone and combined treatment groups during the follow-up period. Mersch (1995) found a modest reduction in IBI scores (Koopmans et al., 1994) that failed to differ from the wait-list for both an exposure-alone group and an integrated-treatment group consisting of rational-emotive therapy, social skills training, and exposure. A reanalysis of these data (Mersch, Jansen, & Arntz, 1995) found no differential response to treatment for SAIs with and without DSM-III-R (American Psychiatric Association, 1987) Axis II personality disorders. Finally, seven SAIs who received Heimberg's CBGT failed to improve on the IBT from pre- to post-treatment (Heimberg et al., 1985). The IBT was dropped from the six-month follow-up assessment.

Subjective Probabilities

Some researchers have speculated that normalization of biased subjective judgments about the probabilities and costs of various social outcomes is a key mechanism of change in successful treatment of SAD (e.g., Foa, Franklin, Perry, & Herbert, 1996). "Cost bias" refers to elevated estimates about the cost if a mild negative outcome occurs. "Probability bias" refers to overestimations of the likelihood of feared outcomes. Six studies have examined the effects of treatment on the subjective judgments of individuals with SAD for positive or negative social events.

The subjective probability for aversive events was lower for SAIs who received cognitive restructuring versus associative therapy, the control condition in Taylor and colleagues' study (1997). The two groups did not differ on the subjective probability for pleasant events. Although these two groups did not differ on subjective probabilities after both received group exposure, the within-group effect sizes indicated all participants improved at the end of treatment and during the follow-up period. Lucock and Salkovskis (1988) reported that subjective probability for negative events decreased after social skills training in a small pilot study of eight participants with SAD. Foa and colleagues (1996) developed the Probability/Cost Questionnaire (PCQ), a 40-item self-report measure consisting of 20 negative nonsocial events and 20 negative social events, to investigate changes in probability and cost biases following treatment. They found that treatment (Heimberg's CBGT with an added social skills training component) reduced subjective judgments of the probability for negative social events, but their ratings were still higher than those of nonanxious controls. This reduction occurred only for social, not nonsocial, negative events. Nonanxious controls did not change their ratings across assessment points. The personal cost of negative social and nonsocial events (how bad it would be) decreased with treatment, but both were still more costly than the judgments of nonanxious controls whose ratings did not change across the two assessments. In an attempt to understand how probability and cost judgments may mediate treatment outcome, Foa et al. (1996) conducted a series of hierarchical regression analyses that revealed that change in the cost estimates for social events accounted for 58% of the variance in post-treatment SAD symptoms. Also, participants' appraisals of social evaluative danger (probability X cost estimates) decreased as a result of three weeks of intensive cognitive-behavioral treatment, but they were still higher than the appraisals of stutterers (Poulton & Andrews, 1996). McManus, Clark, and Hackmann (2000) examined subjective probability and social cost following individual cognitive therapy, drug treatment (fluoxetine plus self-exposure instructions), or pill placebo. A modified PCQ (Foa et al., 1996) was administered before and after treatment that did not include the nonsocial questions and to which McManus et al. (2000) added items of "more strongly negative social events" (p. 204). They found that participants in both treatment groups reported reduced probability and cost following treatment. Participants' post-treatment scores were also found to not significantly differ from a nonanxious control group; those who received individual cognitive therapy reported scores below the mean reported by the control group, while those who received drug treatment reported scores above, but not significantly different from, those reported by the control group. Additionally, they found that changes in both probability and cost were significantly correlated with responder/nonresponder status, as determined by mean change in social anxiety symptoms. Also, similarly to Foa et al., they conducted separate hierarchical regression analyses to determine the comparative value of change in probability versus change in cost in symptom reduction, defined by several standard self-report measures of social anxiety and fear of negative evaluation. In contrast to the findings reported by Foa et al. (1996), these analyses indicated that changes in probability played a more prominent role than changes in cost in social anxiety symptom change.

More recently, Hofmann (2004) investigated the impact of treatment on estimated social cost. Participants were randomly assigned to receive either CBGT or exposure-only group therapy (which included video feedback) or to a wait-list control group. Estimated social cost was measured using the social events subscale of the PCQ (Foa et al., 1996), which consists of 10 performance situations and 10 nonperformance social situations of which respondents rate the perceived social cost. Hofmann found that both CBGT and exposure-only group therapy led to significant reductions in estimated social cost and that pre–post changes in estimated social cost were significantly correlated with pre- to six-month follow-up changes for those who received CBGT but not for those who received the exposure-only treatment. Finally, Smits, Rosenfield, McDonald, and Telch (2006) examined the effects of exposure-based treatment on probability and cost biases. Participants were randomly assigned to receive exposure treatment plus videotape feedback of performance, exposure treatment plus videotape feedback of audience reactions, exposure treatment without feedback, or credible placebo. All exposure trials consisted of repeated public speaking exercises, and participants receiving exposure-based treatments were aggregated for analyses examining probability and cost biases. Probability and cost biases were measured using a modified version of the Appraisal of Social Concerns Scale (ASC; Telch et al., 2004), which asks participants to rate the probability and cost of the following outcomes during the public speaking exposures: sweating, blushing, trembling, poor voice quality, mind going blank, losing control, appearing stupid, appearing incompetent, being incoherent, and people ridiculing you. Smits et al. found that exposure treatment led to significant reductions in both probability and cost biases; further, reductions in probability bias predicted fear reduction, which predicted additional reduction in probability bias, while reductions in cost bias did not predict but were predicted by fear reduction.

Attributions and Locus of Control

Four studies have examined attributions and locus of control. Two studies used a modification of the well-known Attributional Style Questionnaire (ASQ) (Peterson et al., 1982). Heimberg et al. (1985) reported that seven SAIs treated with an early version of CBGT changed their attribution of negative outcomes by making fewer internal and stable attributions and by placing less blame on themselves for negative outcomes at post-treatment. Using ASQ items related to self-blame (internal attributions for aversive social events), Taylor and colleagues (1997) reported improvement for individuals who received either cognitive restructuring or the control therapy (which was associative therapy), with no difference between the two groups. Review of the effect sizes indicates additional improvement during group exposure treatment, which followed cognitive restructuring or associative therapy, with no differential effects for initial treatment condition of cognitive restructuring or associative therapy.

Wlazlo, Schroeder-Hartwig, Hand, Kaiser, and Munchau (1990) used a German attributional measure identified as the IE-SV-F, which examines "internal versus external and stable versus variable attributions in successful and nonsuccessful situations" (p. 184). The study design included personal effectiveness training, a social skills intervention developed by Liberman, King, De Risi, and McCann (1975), and individual and group exposure. The attributional measure is available at several assessment points for the group participants but only at 2.5-year follow-up assessment for all participants. The three treatment groups did not differ in attributions at follow-up. However, an examination of various assessment points for the individuals receiving group exposure revealed significant improvement. Group exposure participants' self-attributions for successful outcomes due to internal factors were increased, and successful outcomes that were attributed to external factors were decreased. Attributions related to situational difficulty did not change. In those situations considered unsuccessful, causation related to internal factors and situational difficulty was decreased, whereas attributions based on lack of effort and external factors did not change. Two concerns about the design of this study should be noted. First, the exposure and social skills interventions purposefully contained overlapping procedures. Second, participants were not randomly assigned; instead, they were assigned based on the year they arrived for treatment.

The Levenson Locus of Control Scale (Levenson, 1973) assesses perceptions of internality as well as attributions regarding powerful others or chance as causes for events. Individuals with GSAD with and without DSM-III-R APD and participants with nongeneralized social anxiety disorder who were treated with Heimberg's CBGT apparently improved on all three subscales (detailed results not given) despite initial differences on the subscales (Brown, Heimberg, & Juster, 1995). No follow-up data were reported.

Conclusions about Cognitive Propositions

In summary, this review demonstrates that cognitive propositions, including beliefs, attributions, and judgments of probability and cost, may change with treatment for SAD. The results for modification of irrational beliefs are mixed, perhaps because many of the scales are broader measures of psychopathology. Not all of the beliefs would be addressed in treatments that focus on social anxiety. It is worth noting that the findings are more consistent for irrational beliefs related to SAD as found in the studies by Mattick and colleagues. Purely cognitive treatments do appear to have a positive impact on irrational beliefs, especially in the earlier studies. Inclusion of a nonanxious control group (Foa et al., 1996; Poulton & Andrews, 1996) reveals that significant improvement in judgments of probability and cost may not mean that the participants treated for SAD are in the normative range, though participants in McManus et al. (2000) reported scores in the normative range following individual cognitive therapy. However, the studies by Hofmann (2004) and Smits and colleagues (2006) suggest that changes in cost and probability biases may be important mediators of clinical improvement following exposure-based treatment. Changes in these biases may be a key mechanism and suggest that such faulty appraisals must be altered in order for treatment to be effective and for gains to be maintained.

Cognitive Content

Cognitive content refers to the self-statements that an individual is able to report about a particular experience or within a particular time frame. With cognitive therapy models, the self-statements are usually classified as positive (facilitating functioning) or negative (inhibiting functioning). Over thirty years ago, Cacioppo, Glass, and Merluzzi (1979) demonstrated that socially anxious and nonanxious individuals could list the thoughts they experienced in anticipation of a stressful social interaction. Anxious individuals listed more negative and fewer positive thoughts when compared with nonanxious individuals. However, scoring the protocols from unstructured thought-listing exercises is quite time-consuming and requires training. Consequently, inventories of common positive and negative thoughts for a particular problem were developed. The response format on these inventories requires the respondent to indicate the frequency with which they have experienced each thought. The most commonly used self-statement inventory in research on SAD is the SISST (Glass, Merluzzi, Biever, & Larsen, 1982). Both thought-listing procedures and self-statement inventories have been used as measures of the efficacy of treatment for SAD.

Endorsement – SISST

Only two treatment studies have utilized the SISST without modification of items or instructions. Gelernter et al. (1991) had participants complete the SISST after an individualized behavioral test based on a primary feared situation. Individuals across all treatment conditions improved in the expected direction from pretreatment through post-treatment and two-month follow-up on the SISST. As with most measures in this study, there were no differences on the SISST among the treatment conditions – CBGT, alprazolam, phenelzine, and pill placebo. All treatment conditions included homework exposure instructions. As will be shown later, when the SISST is used for situations other than heterosocial conversations, for which it was developed, researchers typically adjust the items to reflect the content of the behavioral challenge. That does not appear to have been done in this study, so it is unclear how applicable the SISST items were for participants whose individualized behavioral test involved a different type of interaction, such as a speech or writing while being observed.

The SISST was used to assess self-statements after three behavioral tests – two interactions and one speech – in a study examining the role of self-focused attentional shifts in the treatment of SAD (Woody, Chambless, & Glass, 1997). Items on the SISST were modified for the speech. Unfortunately, the various outcome measures for this study were subjected to factor analysis, and results were reported in terms of the factor scores, not individual measures. Only the negative subscale of the SISST was used, and it loaded on a factor labeled "self-judgment." The authors reported a significant pre- to post-treatment change in this factor for Heimberg's CBGT with added components of breathing retraining and attentional training. Therefore, it seems likely that this treatment resulted in a reduction of negative self-statements on the SISST.

In addition to the speech behavioral test in Woody et al. (1997), five other studies have adapted the SISST for use with a speech. Turner and colleagues (Turner, Beidel, Cooley et al., 1994; Turner, Beidel, & Jacob, 1994) modified the SISST items to reflect thoughts during a speech as part of their standard behavioral test. In the first study, socially anxious participants treated with flooding reported fewer negative and more positive self-statements at post-treatment than socially phobic participants treated with atenolol or pill placebo. At the six-month follow-up, individuals in the flooding condition reported more positive self-statements than individuals in the atenolol condition, with no between-group difference on negative self-statements. Both positive and negative self-statements improved from pre- to post-treatment in Turner and colleagues' SET (Turner, Beidel, Cooley et al., 1994); however, the SISST was not included in their two-year follow-up (Turner, Beidel, & Cooley-Quille, 1995).

Using a similar modification of the SISST for a speech task, Taylor et al. (1997) compared positive and negative cognitions among GSAD participants who received cognitive therapy with participants who received an attentional-control treatment called associative therapy, which involved thinking about social anxiety but not attempting to modify cognitions. Both treatments were followed by exposure therapy, but systematic exposure was explicitly omitted during the first phase of treatment. At the end of the first phase, participants who had completed cognitive therapy reported fewer negative self-statements and more positive self-statements on the modified SISST than participants who had completed associative therapy. Despite the authors' hypothesis that cognitive therapy would facilitate later exposure, there were no differences between the two treatment groups on the SISST subscales after both had received exposure.

An examination of the effect sizes after the first phase of treatment suggests that associative therapy yielded a modest decrease in negative self-statements, but only cognitive therapy yielded an increase in positive self-statements.

Hofmann and DiBartolo (2000) fully adapted the SISST for public speaking situations. The SSPS includes five negative and five positive cognitions. Socially phobic participants whose worst fear involved public speaking were treated for this fear in a purely behavioral treatment involving speaking skills training and exposure or they were assigned to a wait-list control (Newman, Hofmann, Trabert, Roth, & Taylor, 1994). Treated participants, but not wait-list controls, demonstrated a reduction in anxiety-related cognitions on an earlier version of the SSPS. A subset of these participants was included in a later study comparing SAIs with and without APD (Hofmann, Newman, Becker, Taylor, & Roth, 1995). Participants reported fewer anxiety-related cognitions at the end of treatment, irrespective of APD diagnosis. Another study further showed that negative cognitions were particularly sensitive to treatment change (Hofmann & DiBartolo, 2000).

Finally, Heimberg et al. (1990) used the SISST with instructions to study participants to rate the items in general, rather than reference to a specific interaction, in a comparison of CBGT and an educational-supportive group intervention. The results showed no between-group differences. Overall, positive self-statements increased from pre- to post-treatment with little change in the negative subscale.

Endorsement Other than SISST

A variety of endorsement-style measures other than the SISST have been used in treatment-outcome studies. Unlike the original SISST, these measures assess cognitions in a variety of situations, not just heterosocial interaction.

In their study of musicians who met DSM-III-R criteria for SAD, Clark and Agras (1991) utilized the Self-Statement Questionnaire (Steptoe & Fidler, 1987) to compare various combinations of cognitive-behavioral treatment, buspirone, and placebo. Overall, the results suggested that the placebo with and without CBT resulted in fewer negative and more positive thoughts than buspirone alone at post-treatment assessment.

Mersch and colleagues (1989) also examined self-statements based on a measure designed by Jerremalm et al. (1986) to assess cognitions during a behavioral test for individuals classified as cognitive or behavioral reactors who received social skills training or rational-emotive therapy. There were no between-group differences at post-test. Only three of the four treatment groups demonstrated significant pre- to post-treatment change in self-statements. Cognitive reactors who received both treatments, and behavioral reactors who received social skills training, had more positive self-statements at post-test. Behavioral reactors who received rational-emotive therapy did not demonstrate improvement in self-statements. There was no further change at the six-week follow-up assessment.

Six studies have utilized a Dutch self-statement questionnaire, the Social Anxiety Self-Statement Inventory (SASSI), derived from positive and negative thoughts reported during social interactions in a behavioral test (Mersch et al., 1996). Similarly to the SISST, the SASSI has positive and negative subscales, and respondents indicate the frequency of the various thoughts.

In Mersch's (1995) study, socially anxious participants were assigned to one of three conditions: *in vivo* exposure alone; an integrated treatment of *in vivo* exposure, rational-emotive therapy, and social skills training; or wait-list control. There was a reduction in negative self-statements (the positive subscale was not reported) for both active treatment groups but not for the wait-list group. There was no difference between *in vivo* exposure and the integrated treatment at post-test or 1.5-year follow-up, but gains were maintained.

Scholing and Emmelkamp (1993a, 1993b, 1996a, 1996b) combined the negative subscale of the SASSI with the Social Cognition Inventory (SCI) as a composite measure of cognitive change. The SCI appears to be more of an attitudinal or belief measure than a self-statement measure, so these results do not strictly fall in the category of endorsement methods of analyzing self-statements. In the first series of studies (1993a, 1996a), Scholing and Emmelkamp examined participants diagnosed with SAD who also had particular fears of blushing, sweating, or trembling. Participants were treated in an individual format with *in vivo* exposure and cognitive therapy presented either sequentially in four-week blocks (exposure, then cognitive therapy, and vice versa) or in an integrated fashion. All three treatment groups demonstrated improvement at four weeks and at post-test, with change generally maintained at the 3- and 18-month follow-ups. There were no differences among the treatment conditions; the two sequential treatments and the integrated treatment package were equally effective in producing cognitive change.

Using a similar design, Scholing and Emmelkamp (1993b, 1996b) again used the composite SCI and SASSI. Participants with GSAD were randomly assigned to group or individual treatment and to (1) *in vivo* exposure alone; (2) sequential cognitive therapy, then *in vivo* exposure; or (3) an integrated cognitive and exposure package. Cognitions were less negative for all treatment groups after 8 and 16 sessions of treatment and at the three-month follow-up. Data were not presented separately for the composite cognitive measure at the 18-month follow-up, but gains were generally maintained across measures. There were few differences among the six treatment conditions across measures. However, when rank-ordering the effectiveness of the six treatment conditions at the three-month follow-up, the group sequential treatment (cognitive therapy then *in vivo* exposure) yielded the largest improvement on the cognitive measure, and the integrated group treatment yielded the smallest improvement. It appears these differences may have been maintained, because a somewhat similar pattern appeared at the 18-month follow-up, but, again, results for the cognitive measure were not presented separately.

Finally, Jerremalm and colleagues (1986) used an apparently unvalidated list of 10 positive and 10 negative thoughts that were rated for frequency of occurrence during a social interaction test. The items were combined to yield one measure of cognition. In this study, the socially anxious participants were classified as cognitive reactors (on the basis of this scale) or physiological reactors (on the basis of their heart rates) to the behavioral test. The treatment conditions in this study were applied relaxation, self-instructional training, and a wait-list control. Physiological reactors who received self-instructional training, but not applied relaxation, improved significantly from pre- to post-treatment and differed from the wait-list control. Cognitive reactors improved whether they received applied relaxation or self-instructional training, but only those in the latter treatment differed from the wait-list control. Changes for the cognitive reactors must be treated with some caution because their initial classification was determined by extreme scores on the thought measure. Thus, regression toward the mean could have accounted for some of the positive effects.

Conclusions about Endorsement Methods

Although a variety of inventories have been used to tap self-statements among SAIs, changes in self-statements using endorsement methodology are surprisingly consistent. Across active treatment modalities, reductions in negative self-statements and sometimes increases in positive self-statements are achieved by post-treatment assessment. Gains are typically maintained into the follow-up period. Active treatments consistently differ from attentional control or wait-list control conditions. Two exceptions to this pattern involve studies in which a subgroup of participants was identified as behavioral (Mersch et al., 1989) or physiological (Jerremalm et al., 1986) reactors. Behavioral reactors who received a matched behavioral intervention (social skills training), but not a mismatched cognitive intervention (rational-emotive therapy), improved on the self-statement inventory. In contrast, physiological reactors in the mismatched self-instructional training, but not the matched applied relaxation intervention, improved on the self-statement inventory.

Production Methods of Assessing Cognitive Content

Heimberg and colleagues have often used a thought-listing procedure to assess self-statements in their treatment studies. The thought-listing procedure, developed for social anxiety assessment by Cacioppo et al. (1979), requires participants to record their thoughts in boxes after a behavioral test. The thoughts are then classified by research assistants as positive, negative, or neutral. Typically, the thoughts are reported as a percentage of the total thoughts listed or as a positive/negative ratio.

In Heimberg and colleagues' (1990) comparison of CBGT and ES group therapy, all participants demonstrated an increase in percentage of positive thoughts and a decrease in negative thoughts at post-treatment. However, at the six-month follow-up, decreases in negative thoughts were still significant only for participants who had received CBGT. Additionally, at the six-month follow-up, CBGT participants reported more positive and fewer negative thoughts than ES group participants. Bruch, Heimberg, and Hope's (1991) reanalysis of these data using a thought ratio yielded similar results, with both groups showing improvement at post-treatment, but ES group participants relapsed on this measure during the six-month follow-up. At the five-year follow-up, the two groups did not differ on percentage of positive or negative thoughts listed (Heimberg et al., 1993). In a comparison of CBGT to exposure alone and a wait-list control, Hope, Heimberg, et al. (1995) found a small, but significant, pre- to post-treatment change on percentage of negative thoughts for CBGT only. Percentage of positive thoughts and follow-up data were not reported.

Rather than examining the valence of thoughts, Hofmann, Moscovitch, Kim, and Taylor (2004) utilized the thought-listing procedure to examine the focus of the thoughts (i.e., self-focused versus other-focused). In their study, participants were randomly assigned to receive CBGT or exposure-only group therapy or to a wait-list control group. Participants completed three social tasks pre- and post-treatment (giving a speech, initiating and maintaining a conversation with an unfamiliar person, and solving simple mathematical problems on a chalkboard while being observed) and were asked to write down any thoughts that entered their mind during a three-minute anticipation period preceding each task. Thoughts were coded by trained raters and classified as either self-focused or other-focused. They found that both CBGT and exposure-only group therapy resulted in a significant reduction in negative self-focused thoughts, with no differences between the two groups at post-treatment.

In contrast with endorsement methods of self-statement assessment, thought-listing may be more sensitive to differences between active treatments. In the Heimberg and Hope studies described above, the intervention with a cognitive component showed more evidence of improvement in thoughts than a nonbehavioral or strictly behavioral intervention, though these differences may fade at long-term follow-up. However, the study by Hofmann et al. (2004) suggests that both cognitive-behavioral and exposure-based treatments resulted in significant reductions in negative self-focused thoughts. Thus, it appears that the focus of the thoughts may be just as important as their valence.

Cognitive Process

Relatively few studies have assessed treatment effects on cognitive processes such as attention or memory. Mattia, Heimberg, and Hope (1993) reported that interference for social threat cues on the emotional Stroop color-naming task (which is thought to be a measure of attentional bias) was reduced after successful treatment, but not unsuccessful treatment, for SAD. The study did not distinguish color-naming performance among the possible treatments – CBGT, phenelzine, or pill placebo. Woody et al. (1997) found that self-reported, self-focused attention decreased during CBGT that was modified to include diaphragmatic breathing and instruction in external focus of attention. Improvement in self-focus was associated with positive change on some other outcome measures, particularly for individuals with public speaking anxiety. Similarly, Hofmann (2000) reported that changes in negative self-perception covary significantly with changes in social anxiety.

A recent study by Amir et al. (2009) focused on treating SAD by directly altering attention mechanisms. Amir and colleagues developed a computer-delivered attention modification protocol that utilizes a modified dot probe paradigm (MacLeod, Mathews, & Tata, 1986), where a fixation point was followed by images of two faces (either neutral or displaying disgust or both neutral). These images were followed by presentation of a probe (either "E" or "F") in the location of one of the two faces, and participants identified which probe they were presented with. Participants in the study were randomly assigned to a condition where the probe appeared with 80% frequency in the location of the disgust face (AMP) or a condition where the probe appeared with equal frequency in the location of the disgust face or neutral face (attention control condition; ACC). Attentional bias was assessed by a modified Posner paradigm (Posner, 1980), where social threat or neutral cue words are presented on opposite sides of a computer screen, following a fixation point in the center of the screen, and are then replaced by a probe ("*") in the location of one of the two words. Participants identified the location of the probe, and response latency was recorded. Longer response latencies when the probe was located opposite the location of a social threat word suggested that the participant had difficulty shifting attention from the threat word. Amir et al. found that participants in the AMP group displayed significantly reduced response latencies following treatment, whereas response latency did not significantly differ among participants in the ACC group pre- to post-treatment. Thus, preliminary evidence suggests that computerized attentional training can result in reduced attention bias for threat cues.

Conclusions about Cognitive Change

Overall, this review reveals that the cognitions of SAIs with a variety of targeted fears are responsive to interventions. It appears that beliefs and self-statements related to social anxiety may be easier to change than broader dysfunctional beliefs. Surprisingly, both cognitive and non-cognitive interventions are about equally effective in changing cognition. There were some hints in Scholing and Emmelkamp's studies (1993b, 1996b) with participants with GSAD in group therapy that it may be more helpful to do cognitive interventions followed by exposure, rather than fully integrating the two components. In contrast, Taylor and colleagues (1997) did not find that early cognitive therapy followed by exposure facilitated self-statement change, but the designs of the two studies are not strictly comparable. Also, change in self-statements among SAIs who are characterized by strong physiological reactions to feared situations may be facilitated with a cognitive intervention, compared with applied relaxation alone. Additionally, several recent studies provide evidence that changes in probability and cost biases may be important mediators of clinical improvement. Finally, preliminary evidence suggests that directly altering attention patterns can result in reduced social anxiety symptoms.

Fear of Negative Evaluation

The core feature of SAD is concern with being negatively evaluated by other people (American Psychiatric Association, 1994; Rapee, 1995). Butler (1989) argued that fear of negative evaluation is essentially a cognitive construct and thus may be particularly amenable to cognitive interventions. As will be discussed later, this has not proven to be true. However, Mattick and colleagues (Mattick & Peters, 1988; Mattick et al., 1989) found that change in fear of negative evaluation predicted long-term success in treatment. A review of treatment-outcome studies that included a wait-list control condition revealed that fear of negative evaluation generally does not improve spontaneously over a few weeks or months (e.g., Kanter & Goldfried, 1979; Mattick et al., 1989; Newman et al., 1994). Any spontaneous changes that have appeared in the literature are very small and of little clinical significance (e.g., Hope, Heimberg, et al., 1995).

Typically, the fear of negative evaluation has been assessed with the Watson and Friend (1969) self-report questionnaire, entitled the Fear of Negative Evaluation Scale (FNE), or the brief version of the scale, the Brief Fear of Negative Evaluation Scale (BFNE) (Leary, 1983). Only occasionally are other measures, such as fear of negative evaluation ratings for the situations on an individualized Fear and Avoidance Hierarchy (Hope, Heimberg, et al., 1995) or a subscale of the Fear Survey Schedule (Wolpe & Lang, 1964), used to assess social-evaluative concerns.

Cognitive interventions target dysfunctional assumptions about other people's negative evaluations of the individual with SAD. Thus, one would expect that cognitive interventions on their own would lead to reductions in fear of negative evaluation. Socially anxious participants in Kanter and Goldfried's (1979) study who received systematic rational restructuring demonstrated significant pre- to post-treatment change on the FNE. These scores were lower than for individuals who had been on the wait-list. Similarly, Mattick et al. (1989) found that individuals diagnosed with SAD who received cognitive restructuring without exposure for severe fears of scrutiny by others improved on the FNE at post-treatment. Taylor and colleagues (1997) compared cognitive restructuring to a control intervention – associative therapy. Individuals receiving cognitive therapy made more improvement on the BFNE (Leary, 1983) than individuals receiving associative therapy. The changes were small but significant from pre- to post-treatment for the cognitive restructuring group.

Clark's cognitive therapy (CT; Clark, 1997) emphasizes the Clark and Wells (1995) model of maintenance of SAD and focuses on a number of components: (1) developing a personal model of SAD for each client, (2) safety behaviors and self-focused attention experiments, (3) shifting of attention focus, (4) video feedback, (5) behavioral experiments, (6) problematic anticipatory and PEP, and (7) challenging dysfunctional assumptions. In the first study evaluating this treatment, Clark et al. (2003) compared CT to fluoxetine plus self-exposure and placebo plus self-exposure. They found that CT led to a greater reduction in fear of negative evaluation compared to the other treatments, which did not differ from each other, at post-treatment and 12-month follow-up. Clark and colleagues (2006) compared CT to exposure plus applied relaxation (Butler, 1985; Öst, 1987) and a wait-list control group. Participants in both the CT and exposure plus applied relaxation groups reported significant reductions in FNE scores at post-treatment and compared to the wait-list control group. This reduction was significantly greater for participants who received CT compared to exposure plus applied relaxation at post-treatment and three-month follow-up; however, there was no significant difference in FNE scores at one-year follow-up.

Despite its utility, a cognitive intervention may not be essential to reduce fear of negative evaluation. A number of studies employed exposure-alone conditions that were carefully constructed to avoid the inclusion of cognitive interventions. Taylor et al. (1997) followed cognitive restructuring or associative therapy with an exposure-alone group treatment. Two studies by Mattick and colleagues (Mattick & Peters, 1988; Mattick et al., 1989) included an exposure-alone treatment condition for socially anxious participants who had severe fears of scrutiny. Hope, Heimberg, et al. (1995) used exposure-alone with a heterogeneous group of socially phobic participants on two measures of fear of negative evaluation – the FNE and fear of negative evaluation ratings for situations on an individualized Fear and Avoidance Hierarchy. Mersch used the BFNE and exposure with a heterogeneous group of individuals with SAD (Mersch, 1995) or who had comorbid personality disorders (Mersch et al., 1995). Salaberria and Echeburua (1998) used a translation of the FNE with SAD participants in the Basque region of Spain who received exposure with or without a self-help manual (which had no effect). Butler, Cullington, Munby, Amies, and Gelder (1984) utilized an exposure-alone treatment condition that included some filler material to equalize time spent in a combined exposure-plus-anxiety-management treatment condition also included in the study. Haug and colleagues (2003) used the FNE to compare sertraline,

sertraline plus exposure, exposure therapy plus placebo, and a pill placebo. Finally, Nortje, Posthumus, and Moller (2008) used the FNE with social phobic participants (generalized type) following an exposure-alone treatment and at three-months post-treatment. The results of these studies are mixed. Participants in both Mattick studies, in Hope, Heimberg, et al., in Mersch, and in Mersch et al. demonstrated improvement in fear of negative evaluation from pre- to post-treatment. Mersch, and Salaberria and Echeburua also reported additional improvement over the extended follow-up period (1 to 1.5 years). Haug et al. reported significant reductions in FNE scores up to one year following exposure treatment, with participants in the exposure therapy plus placebo group showing the greatest long-term reduction. In Taylor et al., exposure resulted in substantial additional improvement in fear of negative evaluation, regardless of whether participants had originally received cognitive therapy or the associative therapy. However, Butler and colleagues reported little change on the FNE for the exposure-plus-filler-material treatment. Also, Nortje and colleagues found no significant reductions in FNE scores at post-treatment or follow-up.

Other noncognitive treatments may also result in improvements in fear of negative evaluation. Systematic desensitization in Marzillier, Lambert, and Kellet (1976) resulted in more improvement in fear of negative evaluation than a wait-list control condition. In Turner, Beidel, and Jacob (1994), flooding produced modest change on the FNE at post-treatment, but additional change was evidenced at six-month follow-up. Although self-control desensitization in Kanter and Goldfried (1979) yielded pre- to post-treatment change in fear of negative evaluation, this condition did not differ from the wait-list control at posttest. Social skills training for SAD also led to changes in fear of negative evaluation in Marzillier et al. and Stravynski et al. (1982). However, these data are somewhat difficult to interpret given changes in the diagnostic criteria for SAD. The Kanter and Goldfried and Marzillier et al. studies were conducted before the advent of modern DSM diagnostic criteria. The Kanter and Goldfried participants were described as a community sample with social anxiety. The participants in Marzillier et al. were described as "socially inadequate psychiatric patients" who appear to have been social phobic. Stravynski et al.'s participants were described as "socially dysfunctional neurotic outpatients" who met DSM-III (American Psychiatric Association, 1980) criteria for SAD and APD.

As has been noted elsewhere, many of the treatment outcome studies for SAD included a combination treatment condition. Overall, the various combinations of treatment appear to be effective in reducing fear of negative evaluation. Heimberg's CBGT, which combines cognitive restructuring and exposure, leads to significant improvement in fear of negative evaluation across several studies (Cox, Ross, Swinson, & Direnfeld, 1998; Gelernter et al., 1991; Heimberg et al., 1985; Heimberg et al., 1990; Heimberg et al., 1998; Hope,

Heimberg, et al., 1995; Hope, Herbert, & White, 1995). These changes were maintained at follow-up with the exception of the five-year follow-up, in which improvement in fear of negative evaluation had diminished somewhat (Heimberg et al., 1993). Participant characteristics such as subtype of SAD or comorbid APD do not appear to affect the outcome of CBGT on fear of negative evaluation (Brown et al., 1995; Hope, Herbert et al., 1995). Similarly, Ledley et al. (2009) found that an individualized version of CBGT (Hope et al., 2000; Hope, Heimberg, & Turk, 2006) was effective in significantly reducing fear of negative evaluation at post-treatment and three-month follow-up. Other treatment packages that combined exposure and a cognitive intervention yielded similar changes in fear of negative evaluation (Mattick & Peters, 1988; Mattick et al., 1989; Mersch, 1995). Rapee, Abbott, Baillie, and Gaston (2007) compared CBGT (consisting of a combination of cognitive restructuring, exposure, attention training, and "realistic feedback of social performance" (p. 247)), pure self-help (Rapee, 1998), therapist-augmented self-help (self-help plus five group treatment sessions focusing on discussion of treatment principles), and a wait-list control group. They found that each treatment group resulted in significant reduction in BFNE scores at post-treatment, and these gains were maintained at three-month follow-up for the CBGT and therapist-augmented self-help groups. In contrast to these positive findings, in a multiple baseline study of scriptophobia, change on FNE was only noted in one of three participants at nine-month follow-up (Biran, Agusto, & Wilson, 1981). Also, Mortberg, Karlsson, Fyring, and Sundin (2006) found no significant changes in FNE scores at post-treatment or 3-, 6-, and 12-month follow-ups following intensive (three weeks) CBGT that included cognitive restructuring, applied relaxation (Öst, 1987), and public speaking exposures. Additionally, Nortje and colleagues (2008) found no improvement in fear of negative evaluation following a combined cognitive restructuring and exposure treatment at post-treatment or three-month follow-up.

Newman et al. (1994) reported that a combination of exposure and skills training for individuals with public speaking fears produced reductions on the FNE. No follow-up data were reported. Basque participants with SAD who received a combined exposure and cognitive-restructuring intervention improved on the FNE at post-test and continued to improve through the one-year follow-up (Salaberria & Echeburua, 1998). Combining rational restructuring with self-control desensitization (Kanter & Goldfried, 1979) or social skills training (Stravynski et al., 1982) was effective in reducing fear of negative evaluation. Socially phobic participants who received Turner and colleagues' SET (Turner, Beidel, Cooley et al., 1994), which combines exposure, social skills training, education, and programmed practice, reported significant reductions in fear of negative evaluation at post-treatment. The FNE was not included in the two-year follow-up, so durability of this result is not known (Turner et al., 1995). Butler et al.'s (1984) combination of exposure and anxiety management (relaxation, rational self-talk, and distraction) yielded larger reductions in fear of negative evaluation than the wait-list control. These gains were maintained at six-month follow-up. Finally, Herbert, Rheingold, Guadiano, and Myers (2004) found that a combination of CBGT and social skills training resulted in significantly lower BFNE scores at post-treatment and three-month follow-up.

Across studies it is rare to find that two active treatments differed in their impact on fear of negative evaluation. When present, such differences tend to be small and fail to maintain at later assessment points. Although changes in fear of negative evaluation for CBGT were sometimes not as strong as exposure-alone (Hope, Heimberg, et al., 1995) or phenelzine (Heimberg et al., 1998) at post-test, these differences dissipated during the follow-up periods (Liebowitz et al., 1998). Also, Herbert and colleagues (2005) found that a combination of CBGT and social skills training was superior to CBGT without social skills training in reduction of BFNE scores at post-treatment and three-month follow-up. In contrast, the ES treatment used as an attentional control in Heimberg's work resulted in similar or smaller changes in fear of negative evaluation compared with CBGT. In the study by Kanter and Goldfried (1979), rational restructuring both with and without self-control desensitization alone did not differ from the wait-list control. Similarly, in Butler et al. (1984), the combined exposure-plus-anxiety-management treatment, but not exposure-alone, differed from the wait-list control.

To conclude, it appears that nearly all of the treatments employed across studies yielded some change in fear of negative evaluation. If social-evaluative concern is the core feature of SAD, then it appears that there may be several paths to modify that concern. Any of these treatments are likely to yield positive results on the standard measures of fear of negative evaluation, although the data are weakest for social skills training alone. To date there is no evidence that individuals with certain characteristics would benefit from one treatment or another in changing fear of negative evaluation. However, little research addressing this question has been conducted.

TREATMENT IMPACT ON OVERT BEHAVIORAL PERFORMANCE

Individuals presenting with SAD often report longstanding patterns of avoidance or escape from feared situations. When they do enter feared situations, SAIs often report that they lack social skills and perform poorly (e.g., Hope, Burns, Hayes, Herbert, & Warner, 2010; Norton & Hope, 2001b; Stopa & Clark, 1993). However, there is some evidence that they may underestimate the quality of their performance (Hope, Heimberg, et al., 1995). Over the years a number of treatment studies have tested whether treatment impacts overt behavior, including avoidance/escape and performance quality, or social skills. This review will address only those studies that included a behavioral challenge of some type, including *in vivo* or role-played social interactions or speeches and behavioral-approach tests. Additional studies included self-report measures of behavior, but these will not be included here in order to emphasize objective ratings, uninfluenced by self-report biases.

Escape and Avoidance

Two primary paradigms have been used to assess escape and avoidance in SAD. Beidel and Turner developed a standardized public speaking task during which they allow escape after the first three minutes. The primary behavioral index is the time before escape, and this appears to be a valid measure of behavioral performance, even for SAIs for whom public speaking is not the primary complaint (Beidel, Turner, Jacob, & Cooley, 1989). The second approach to assessing avoidance in SAD is the behavioral avoidance test, or BAT (e.g., Mattick & Peters, 1988). Following the construction of a hierarchy of feared situations, the individual indicates the highest-ranked situation that could be completed without excessive anxiety. That situation is then enacted, usually *in vivo*. Working on the assumption that lower situations could also be completed, the primary measure is the percentage of hierarchy items that can be completed.

Cognitive restructuring alone does not appear to lead to strong changes on the BAT. In their study of scriptophobia, Biran and colleagues (1981) found little improvement on the BAT for the cognitive-restructuring portion of the treatment. Mattick et al. (1989) reported that cognitive restructuring alone was better than the wait-list on the BAT, but change was slower and never equaled improvement with the combined cognitive and exposure intervention at follow-up.

Pure exposure treatments, either graduated or flooding, yield positive changes in escape/avoidance behavior. Exposure-alone was better than the wait-list on the BAT; however, it was less effective than combined exposure and cognitive restructuring at three-month follow-up (Mattick & Peters, 1988; Mattick et al., 1989). Biran et al. (1981) found exposure-alone resulted in less avoidance on the BAT than cognitive restructuring for scriptophobia, but Mattick and colleagues (1989) found the two treatments equally effective on the BAT. Flooding resulted in more improvement (greater delay to escape) when compared with atenolol and placebo at post-test (Turner, Beidel, & Jacob, 1994). Follow-up data were not reported. Shaw (1979) found flooding, systematic desensitization, and social skills training yielded similar gains on the BAT, and gains were maintained through the six-month follow-up.

Several studies have examined the impact of combination treatments on avoidance and escape. As noted previously, Mattick and colleagues (Mattick & Peters, 1988; Mattick et al., 1989) twice found that the combination of exposure and cognitive restructuring yielded the best results on the BAT, compared with exposure or cognitive-restructuring alone, especially at six-month follow-up. Turner and colleagues' SET yielded a substantial increase in speaking time (delayed escape) in a single subject study (Fink et al., 1996), but there was no change in speaking time in a larger study of SET (Turner, Beidel, Cooley et al., 1994). Speaking time did not improve pre- to post-treatment or differ from wait-list controls with a combined treatment of exposure and speaking skills training (Newman et al., 1994). This null result was unaffected by comorbid APD (Hofmann et al., 1995). Hofmann (2004) found that premature termination during a speech BAT was significantly reduced following either CBGT or exposure-alone group therapy compared with a waitlist control group. Slightly more participants in the exposure-alone group prematurely terminated the BAT compared to the CBGT group, though the difference between the two groups was not significant. A similar pattern of results was found for speech duration (Hofmann et al., 2004).

Conclusions about Escape/Avoidance

Only a few studies have included a behavioral measure of escape or avoidance of feared situations. Cognitive restructuring alone does not appear to be the treatment of choice to reduce avoidance behavior. Combined cognitive and exposure treatments have shown the most positive results for avoidance. Exposure alone may be as effective, but there is no evidence that it is more effective than combination treatments. One older study examined systematic desensitization and social skills training and found reductions in avoidance, but, given the sample characteristics, these would probably not be the first treatments of choice for most DSM-IV-diagnosed individuals with SAD.

Surprisingly, time to escape from a public speaking task has not shown improvement in any of the studies, with the exception of the one case using SET. This lack of change is difficult to interpret because participants in those studies changed on other measures, including some behavioral measures such as performance quality.

Behavioral Ratings of Performance Quality

Ratings of the quality of performance in social interactions have typically been the sum of micro ratings of social behaviors (e.g., voice loudness, eye contact) or macro ratings of overall skill or quality. In the literature on social skills assessment, there has been a surprising lack of concordance between micro and macro ratings, suggesting that the overall ratings are more than the sum of the individual components (see Meier & Hope, 1998; Norton & Hope, 2001a). Furthermore, measures of apparently similar constructs appear by different names in the literature on SAD treatment, including "social skill" and "performance quality." Because social skill infers that deficits are attributable to a lack of skill, as opposed to an anxiety-based performance decrement, the more general term "performance quality" will be used here. Given the inherent biases in self ratings, only ratings by independent observers will be included.

Social skills training is designed specifically to address observable social behavior, so it is not surprising that studies of social skills treatments have tended to include behavioral ratings of performance quality. In their comparison of social skills training and systematic desensitization, Marzillier and colleagues (1976) found no difference between treatments on pre- to post-treatment change scores for videotape ratings of overall conversation skills during a role-played behavioral test. The active treatments did not differ from the wait-list control apparently because all participants showed some improvement on this measure. In contrast, Mersch et al. (1989) found improvements in social skill[1] in videotaped reactions to brief social scenarios for both behavioral and cognitive reactors who received social skills training. Individuals who received rational-emotive therapy, regardless of classification as behavioral or cognitive reactors, did not improve in social skill. Despite the within-group change for social skills training, there were no significant differences among the treatment groups at post-test. Follow-up data are not reported on this measure. In summary, it appears that improvement in performance quality as a result of social skills training has been seen only in limited social exchanges but not in more extended social interactions. It should be noted, however, that Marzillier et al. was completed prior to DSM-III, so the samples may not be comparable on diagnostic status.

Marzillier et al. (1976) is the only study to examine performance quality ratings for systematic desensitization. As noted, the treatment was not particularly effective in improving performance.

Only three studies have examined performance quality following either cognitive therapy alone or exposure-alone as the primary treatment. As noted previously, Mersch et al. (1989) found no improvement in social skills for cognitive or behavioral reactors who received rational-emotive therapy. Individuals who received exposure without a cognitive intervention demonstrated pre- to post-treatment improvement on a consensus rating of performance quality based on videotapes of individualized behavioral tests (Hope, Heimberg, et al., 1995). Exposure-alone and combined cognitive and exposure treatment did not differ, but both active treatments showed more improvement on performance quality than the wait-list control. In the Newman et al. (1994) study, SAIs receiving treatment for public speaking anxiety with an intervention consisting of exposure and some speech skills training improved on overall speaking skills as rated by briefly trained audience members. However, these participants did not differ from the wait-list control group, who also improved somewhat. Participants with and without APD did not differ on improvement in speaking skills in the Hofmann et al. (1995) study.

---

[1]These ratings were made by confederates, not independent observers, due to equipment malfunction. However, the authors demonstrated that confederate and independent ratings were highly correlated, so the study is included.

Several studies of multicomponent treatment have included a performance quality measure as an outcome variable. Overall effectiveness of social skill was rated by independent raters for two social interactions in Turner, Beidel, Cooley et al.'s (1994) evaluation of SET. Participants demonstrated significant improvement in social skills at midtreatment, following the social skills intervention. Gains were maintained but not increased at post-test after the exposure portion of the intervention. Follow-up data were not reported. Similar improvement in social skill was seen in the single-subject study using this intervention (Fink et al., 1996). Herbert and colleagues (2005) found that CBGT plus social skills training resulted in significantly greater improvement in a composite of independently rated verbal, nonverbal, paralinguistic, and overall social performance than CBGT without social skills training during a role-played interaction with a confederate, while there was a trend toward a significant difference for a role-played interaction with two confederates and an impromptu speech task.

Heimberg's CBGT has been examined in three studies that included a performance quality measure. As noted, Hope, Heimberg, et al. (1995) reported significant improvement in consensus ratings of performance quality for CBGT compared with the wait-list control. However, CBGT did not differ from exposure-alone. Although a performance quality rating was not included in the original study comparing CBGT and the attention-control intervention consisting of education and support (Heimberg et al., 1990), at five-year follow-up (Heimberg et al., 1993), individuals who had received CBGT received higher consensus ratings of performance quality than individuals who had received the control treatment. CBGT also yielded improvement on an overall social skills rating using trained observers of videotaped interactions (Hope, Herbert, et al., 1995). No differential improvement was seen based on SAD subtype or the presence of APD. No follow-up data were reported for this measure. When CBGT was expanded to include diaphragmatic breathing and attentional instruction, pre- to post-treatment change was observed on a composite variable of independent ratings of skill and anxiety for three behavioral tests (Woody et al., 1997). Finally, Clark and Agras (1991) reported that cognitive therapy combined with exposure was more effective in improving the performance of anxious musicians then buspirone or placebo.

Conclusion about Performance Quality

Despite the obvious conceptual link between social skills interventions and clinical changes on the quality of observable performance in social interactions, the evidence supporting social skills training is not strong. Perhaps the best support for social skills training is as part of SET, given that Turner and colleagues (1994) found improved performance following the initial treatment phase. There is little support for systematic desensitization or cognitive interventions alone in improving overt performance. Exposure-alone may be more effective than cognitive therapy alone, but the most consistent results are for combined interventions. CBGT, in particular, has consistently led to more improvement in performance quality than wait-list or attention controls, regardless of diagnostic subtype or the presence of comorbid APD.

OVERALL CONCLUSIONS

Previous reviews (e.g., Chambless & Hope, 1996; Heimberg & Juster, 1995) and meta-analyses (e.g., Feske & Chambless, 1995; Powers, Sigmarsson, & Emmelkamp, 2008) have concluded that there are effective treatments for SAD. In this chapter we hoped to examine whether there were differential effects for various treatments on certain aspects of SAD. A summary of the review appears in Table 20.1. Although overall most treatments were helpful for most of the constructs we examined, some differences did emerge. Furthermore, some aspects of SAD have not been regularly assessed in outcome studies, so final conclusions remain elusive. We will summarize what we can conclude with some confidence.

CBGT, exposure-alone, and a nonbehavioral treatment of education and supportive group therapy appear to be helpful in decreasing physiological arousal, particularly heart rate. The limited current evidence is not particularly supportive of SET in the reduction of physiological arousal, but, because SET contains therapeutic elements that have been effective in other studies, future research may support it as well.

Cognitive propositions such as irrational beliefs, dysfunctional attributions, locus of control, and cost and probability judgments appear to respond to most active treatments. Even cognitive restructuring without any exposure to feared situations seems to yield some benefit. Improvement appears to be more pronounced for beliefs that are closely related to social anxiety rather than more general irrational beliefs, presumably because the former are more likely to be targeted by treatment. Improvement in cognitive propositions may not mean achievement of scores in the normal range, however.

Self-statements – cognitive content in Ingram and colleagues' terminology (Ingram & Kendall, 1987; Ingram & Wisnicki, 1991) – appear to be quite responsive to any of the interventions, except those identified as attention controls. Typically negative self-statements decrease, sometimes accompanied by an increase in positive self-statements. Thought-listing may be more sensitive to differences among treatments, with some evidence that cognitive interventions add to the efficacy of exposure-alone. When examining such thoughts, it is useful to consider its focus (i.e., self- vs. other-focused) in addition to valence.

Fear of negative evaluation, which is thought to be the core feature of SAD, appears to respond to all of the interventions examined. The evidence is weakest for social skills training. Furthermore, there is little evidence that individuals with certain characteristics respond more or less positively on fear of negative evaluation measures with a given intervention.

TABLE 20.1 Overall Summary of Treatments by Interventions[a]

Dimension	Cognitive Intervention	Exposure Alone	Systematic Desensitization	Social Skills Training	Combined Exposure and Cognitive Intervention	Combined Exposure and Social Skills Training
Physiology	+/−	+	−		+/−	−
Cognitive propositions	+	+/−		+	+	
Cognitive content	+	+/−		+	+	
Cognitive processes				+		
Fear of negative evaluation	+	+	+/−	+	+	−
Escape/avoidance behavior	+/−	+	+/−	+	+	−
Performance quality		+/−	−	+/−	+	+/−

Note: + = *Studies generally were supportive that this intervention yielded positive change on this dimension, which differs from a wait-list or attention control group (if available).* +/ − = *Some studies indicate that this intervention yielded positive change on this dimension, but other studies found no change or a failure to differ from the wait-list or attention control group (if available).* − = *Studies generally failed to find that this intervention yielded positive change on this dimension. A blank cell in the table indicates no studies are available.*

[a]*See text of chapter for nuances such as important subgroups, number and quality of studies supporting a rating, and extent of change.*

Cognitive restructuring alone does not appear to be the treatment of choice to reduce behavioral avoidance or to improve performance. Both combined cognitive restructuring and exposure and exposure-alone appear to be effective for avoidance behavior, but the combined treatment may be best for improving overt behavioral performance. The evidence does not support using social skills training alone as a first choice of treatment for improvement of performance in social interactions. Because few studies have included behavioral measures, the strongest case can be made for CBGT having a positive impact on performance quality. Escape behavior has rarely been assessed, but so far no treatment has demonstrated change on this variable, except for a single case study.

Subgroups

Examination of subgroups of individuals diagnosed with SAD yielded some differential treatment recommendations. Behavioral reactors improved more on self-statements and performance quality when they received social skills training than when they received rational-emotive therapy. Socially anxious participants with high physiological reactivity may also benefit from applied relaxation, social skills training, or self-instructional training to reduce their arousal. Physiological reactors improved more on self-statements with self-instructional training than with applied relaxation alone. Individuals for whom irrational beliefs are particularly problematic (cognitive reactors) made progress on irrational beliefs with both cognitive intervention and social skills training, a noncognitive intervention. However, social skills training, but not rational-emotive therapy, was effective in changing performance quality for cognitive reactors. There is little evidence that diagnostic subtype or a status of APD impacted the effectiveness of treatment.

Changes in Measures and Research Questions Over Time

In updating this review, it has become apparent that the types of measures used to assess treatment outcome have changed somewhat over time. Early studies often emphasized a measure of cognitive content including self-statement questionnaires and thought-listing. Such measures tend to be absent from current studies that are more likely to assess cognitive propositions such as cost and probability judgments, including the PCQ (Foa et al., 1996) and its variations (e.g., McManus et al., 2000). Few of the most recent studies assessed physiological processes such as heart rate. Assessing fear of negative evaluation has been consistent over time, though most recent studies use the abbreviated BFNE. Many early studies compared different treatments with different hypothesized mechanisms of actions such as social skills training versus exposure therapy. The abundant evidence for the efficacy of exposure-based treatments has resulted in research questions that test whether adding certain components to exposure (such as social skills training) or conducting exposure in a different way within a different theoretical model (Clark's cognitive therapy) adds to the efficacy of treatment. Finally, several recent studies (e.g., Hofmann, 2004; Smits et al., 2006) have focused on hypothesized mechanisms of change (see Rodebaugh, Holaway, & Heimberg, 2004, for a review).

SUMMARY

This review has focused on how various treatments impact specific dimensions of SAD. As noted earlier, many reviews have compared which interventions are most effective in producing overall clinical improvement. It is hoped that practitioners may find this chapter useful in selecting a treatment when a particular dimension of SAD is prominent in the clinical presentation. At the same time, one might question whether certain dimensions must change before overall clinical improvement occurs. A full discussion of this issue is beyond the bounds of the chapter. However, it is worth noting that Mattick and colleagues (Mattick & Peters, 1988; Mattick et al., 1989) found that greater change in fear of negative evaluation was associated with a more positive treatment outcome. Foa et al. (1996) reported that improvement in cost estimates for social events accounted for a substantial portion of the variance in post-treatment symptoms of SAD. However, Smits et al. (2006) found more evidence for the importance of change in probability biases than cost biases. The role of change in probability and cost biases as important mechanisms of effective treatment should be explored further. On the other hand, change on some dimensions, such as behavioral avoidance, is typically defined as a key part of clinically significant change.

It is hoped that future studies will include more comprehensive assessment of the full range of symptoms of SAD with less reliance on self-report measures. A surprisingly small proportion of the studies of treatment of SAD have included a measure of overt behavior such as performance quality or behavioral avoidance. Although these measures are more time-consuming to administer than self-report questionnaires, it is essential that an intervention not be judged successful unless it remediates any performance deficits or avoidance of feared situations. Despite a growing body of literature on cognitive processes, little is known about how attentional biases toward social-threat cues change over the course of treatment, though preliminary data are available. Given the theoretical importance of cognitive processes, it is hoped that future treatment studies will include these measures. Finally, physiological arousal provides an objective index of fear that does not rely on self-report and is a key part of SAD. However, few studies have included measures of physiological arousal despite improvements that make ambulatory monitoring more feasible.

REFERENCES

American Psychiatric Association. (1980). *Diagnostic and statistical manual of mental disorders* (3rd ed.) (DSM-III). Washington, DC: Author.

American Psychiatric Association. (1987). *Diagnostic and statistical manual of mental disorders* (3rd ed., rev.) (DSM-III-R). Washington, DC: Author.

American Psychiatric Association. (1994). *Diagnostic and statistical manual of mental disorders* (4th ed.) (DSM-IV). Washington, DC: Author.

American Psychiatric Association. (2000). *Diagnostic and statistical manual of mental disorders* (4th ed., text rev.) (DSM-IV-R). Washington, DC: Author.

Amir, N., Beard, C., Taylor, C. T., Klumpp, H., Elias, J., Burns, M., et al. (2009). Attention training in individuals with generalized social phobia: A randomized controlled trial. *Journal of Consulting and Clinical Psychology*, *77*, 961–973.

Beidel, D. C., Turner, S. M., Jacob, R. G., & Cooley, M. R. (1989). Assessment of social phobia: Reliability of an impromptu speech task. *Journal of Anxiety Disorders*, *3*, 149–158.

Biran, M., Agusto, F., & Wilson, G. T. (1981). *In vivo* exposure vs. cognitive restructuring in the treatment of scriptophobia. *Behaviour Research and Therapy*, *19*, 525–532.

Brown, E. J., Heimberg, R. G., & Juster, H. R. (1995). Social phobia subtype and avoidant personality disorder: Effect on severity of social phobia, impairment, and outcome of cognitive behavioral treatment. *Behavior Therapy*, *26*, 467–486.

Bruch, M. A., Heimberg, R. G., & Hope, D. A. (1991). States of mind model and cognitive change in treated social phobics. *Cognitive Therapy and Research*, *15*, 429–441.

Butler, G. (1985). Exposure as a treatment for social phobia: Some instructive difficulties. *Behaviour Research and Therapy*, *23*, 651–657.

Butler, G. (1989). Issues in the application of cognitive and behavioral strategies to the treatment of social phobia. *Clinical Psychology Review*, *9*, 91–106.

Butler, G., Cullington, A., Munby, M., Amies, M., & Gelder, M. (1984). Exposure and anxiety management in the treatment of social phobia. *Journal of Consulting and Clinical Psychology*, *52*, 642–650.

Cacioppo, J. T., Glass, C. R., & Merluzzi, T. V. (1979). Self-statements and self-evaluations: A cognitive-response analysis of heterosocial anxiety. *Cognitive Therapy and Research*, *3*, 249–262.

Chambless, D. L., & Hope, D. A. (1996). Cognitive approaches to the psychopathology and treatment of social phobia. In P. Salkovskis (Ed.), *Frontiers in cognitive therapy* (pp. 345–382). New York: Guilford Press.

Clark, D. B., & Agras, W. S. (1991). The assessment and treatment of performance anxiety in musicians. *American Journal of Psychiatry*, *148*, 598–605.

Clark, D. M. (1997). Cognitive therapy for social phobia: Some notes for therapists. Unpublished manuscript.

Clark, D. M., Ehlers, A., Hackmann, A., McManus, F., Fennell, M., Grey, N., et al. (2006). Cognitive therapy versus exposure and applied relaxation in social phobia: A randomized controlled trial. *Journal of Consulting and Clinical Psychology*, *74*, 568–578.

Clark, D. M., Ehlers, A., McManus, F., Hackmann, A., Fennell, M., Campbell, H., et al. (2003). Cognitive therapy versus fluoxetine in generalized social phobia: A randomized placebo-controlled trial. *Journal of Consulting and Clinical Psychology*, *71*, 1058–1067.

Clark, D. M., & Wells, A. (1995). A cognitive model of social phobia. In R. Heimberg, M. Liebowitz, D. A. Hope, & F. R. Schneier (Eds.), *Social phobia: Diagnosis, assessment, and treatment* (pp. 69–93). New York: Guilford Press.

Cox, B. J., Ross, L., Swinson, R. P., & Direnfeld, D. M. (1998). A comparison of social phobia outcome measures in cognitive behavioral group therapy. *Behavioral Modification*, *22*, 285–297.

Ellis, A. (1962). *Reason and emotion in psychotherapy*. New York: Lyle Stuart.

Emmelkamp, P. M. G., Mersch, P. P., Wissia, E., & van der Helm, M. (1985). Social phobia: A comparative evaluation of cognitive and behavioral interventions. *Behaviour Research and Therapy*, *23*, 365–369.

Falloon, I. R. H., Lloyd, G. G., & Harpin, R. E. (1981). The treatment of social phobia: Real-life rehearsal with nonprofessional therapists. *Journal of Nervous and Mental Disease*, *169*, 180–184.

Feske, U., & Chambless, D. L. (1995). Cognitive behavioral versus exposure only treatment for social phobia: A meta-analysis. *Behavior Therapy*, *26*, 695–720.

Fink, C. M., Turner, S. M., & Beidel, D. C. (1996). Culturally relevant factors in the behavioral treatment of social phobia: A case study. *Journal of Anxiety Disorders*, *10*, 201–209.

Foa, E. B., Franklin, M. E., Perry, K. J., & Herbert, J. D. (1996). Cognitive biases in generalized social phobia. *Journal of Abnormal Psychology*, *105*, 433–439.

Gelernter, C. S., Uhde, T. W., Cimbolic, P., Arnkoff, D. B., Vittone, B. J., Tancer, M. E., et al. (1991). Cognitive-behavioral and pharmacological treatment of social phobia: A controlled study. *Archives of General Psychiatry*, *48*, 938–945.

Glass, C. R., Merluzzi, T. V., Biever, J. L., & Larsen, K. H. (1982). Cognitive assessment of social anxiety: Development and validation of a self-statement questionnaire. *Cognitive Therapy and Research*, *6*, 37–55.

Haug, T. T., Blomhoff, S., Hellstrom, K., Holme, I., Humble, M., Madsbu, H. P., et al. (2003). Exposure therapy and sertraline in social phobia: 1-year follow-up of a randomised controlled trial. *British Journal of Psychiatry*, *182*, 312–318.

Heimberg, R. G., Becker, R. E., Goldfinger, K., & Vermilyea, J. A. (1985). Treatment of social phobia by exposure, cognitive restructuring, and homework assignments. *Journal of Nervous and Mental Disease*, *173*, 236–245.

Heimberg, R. G., Dodge, C. S., & Becker, R. E. (1987). Social phobia. In L. Michelson & L. M. Ascher (Eds.), *Anxiety and stress disorders: Cognitive-behavioral assessment and treatment* (pp. 220–309). New York: Guilford Press.

Heimberg, R. G., Dodge, C. S., Hope., D. A., Kennedy, C. R., Zollo, L. J., & Becker, R. E. (1990). Cognitive behavioral group treatment for social phobia: Comparison with a credible placebo control. *Cognitive Therapy and Research*, *14*, 1–23.

Heimberg, R. G., & Juster, H. R. (1995). Cognitive-behavioral treatments: Literature review. In R. G. Heimberg, L. R. Liebowitz, D. A. Hope, & F. R. Schneier (Eds.), *Social phobia: Diagnosis, assessment, and treatment* (pp. 261–309). New York: Guilford Press.

Heimberg, R. G., Liebowitz, M. R., Hope, D. A., Schneier, F. R., Holt, C. S., Welkowitz, L. A., et al. (1998). Cognitive behavioral group therapy vs. phenelzine therapy for social phobia. *Archives of General Psychiatry*, *55*, 1133–1141.

Heimberg, R. G., Salzman, D., Holt, C. S., & Blendell, K. (1993). Cognitive behavioral group treatment of social phobia: Effectiveness at 5-year follow-up. *Cognitive Therapy and Research*, *17*, 325–329.

Herbert, J. D., Guadiano, B. A., Rheingold, A. A., Myers, V. H., Dalrymple, K., & Nolan, E. (2005). Social skills training augments the effectiveness of cognitive behavioral group therapy for social anxiety disorder. *Behavior Therapy*, *36*, 125–138.

Herbert, J. D., Rheingold, A. A., Guadiano, B. A., & Myers, V. H. (2004). Standard versus extended cognitive behavior therapy for social anxiety disorder: A randomized-controlled trial. *Behavioural and Cognitive Psychotherapy*, *32*, 131–147.

Hofmann, S. G. (2000). Self-focused attention before and after exposure treatment of social phobia. *Behaviour Research and Therapy, 38*, 717–725.

Hofmann, S. G. (2004). Cognitive mediation of treatment change in social phobia. *Journal of Consulting and Clinical Psychology, 72*, 392–399.

Hofmann, S. G., & DiBartolo, P. M. (2000). An instrument to assess self-statements during public speaking: Scale development and preliminary psychometric properties. *Behavior Therapy, 31*, 499–515.

Hofmann, S. G., Moscovitch, D. A., Kim, Y., & Taylor, A. N. (2004). Changes in self-perception during treatment of social phobia. *Journal of Consulting and Clinical Psychology, 72*, 588–596.

Hofmann, S. G., Newman, M. G., Becker, E., Taylor, C. B., & Roth, W. T. (1995). Social phobia with and without avoidant personality disorder: Preliminary behavior therapy outcome findings. *Journal of Anxiety Disorders, 9*, 427–438.

Hope, D. A., Burns, J., Hayes, S. A., Herbert, J., & Warner, M. D. (2010). Automatic thoughts and cognitive restructuring in cognitive-behavioral group therapy for social anxiety disorder. *Cognitive Therapy and Research, 34*, 1–12.

Hope, D. A., Heimberg, R. G., & Bruch, M. A. (1995). Dismantling cognitive-behavioral group therapy for social phobia. *Behaviour Research and Therapy, 33*, 637–650.

Hope, D. A., Heimberg, R. G., Juster, H. R., & Turk, C. (2000). *Managing social anxiety: A cognitive-behavioral therapy approach (Client Workbook)*. The Psychological Corporation.

Hope, D. A., Heimberg, R. G., & Turk, C. (2006). *Managing social anxiety: A cognitive-behavioral therapy approach (Therapist Guide)*. New York: Oxford University Press.

Hope, D. A., Herbert, J. D., & White, C. (1995). Diagnostic subtype, avoidant personality disorder, and efficacy of cognitive-behavioral group therapy for social phobia. *Cognitive Therapy and Research, 19*, 399–417.

Hope, D. A., Holt, C. S., & Heimberg, R. G. (1995). Social phobia. In T. R. Giles (Ed.), *Handbook of effective psychotherapy* (pp. 227–251). New York: Plenum.

Ingram, R. E., & Kendall, P. C. (1987). The cognitive side of anxiety. *Cognitive Therapy and Research, 11*, 523–536.

Ingram, R. E., & Wisnicki, K. (1991). Cognition and depression. In P. A. Magaro (Ed.), *Cognitive bases of mental disorders* (Vol. 1, pp. 187–239). Newburn Park, CA: Sage.

Jerremalm, A., Jansson, L., & Öst, L. G. (1986). Cognitive and physiological reactivity and the effects of different behavioral methods in the treatment of social phobia. *Behaviour Research and Therapy, 24*, 171–180.

Jones, R. G. (1969). A factored measure of Ellis' rational beliefs system with personality and maladjustment correlates (University Microfilms No. 69-64443). *Dissertation Abstracts International, 29*, 4379B–4380B.

Kanter, N. J., & Goldfried, M. R. (1979). Relative effectiveness of rational restructuring and self-control desensitization in the reduction of interpersonal anxiety. *Behavior Therapy, 10*, 472–490.

Koopmans, P. C., Sanderman, R., Timmerman, G. H., & Emmelkamp, P. M. G. (1994). The irrational beliefs inventory: Development and psychometric evaluation. *European Journal of Psychological Assessment, 10*, 15–27.

Leary, M. R. (1983). A brief version of the fear of negative evaluation scale. *Personality and Social Psychology Bulletin, 9*, 371–375.

Ledley, D. R., Heimberg, R. G., Hope, D. A., Hayes, S. A., Zaider, T. I., Dyke, M. V., et al. (2009). Efficacy of a manualized and workbook-driven individual treatment for social anxiety disorder. *Behavior Therapy, 40*, 414–424.

Levenson, H. (1973). Multidimensional locus of control in psychiatric patients. *Journal of Consulting and Clinical Psychology*, *41*, 397–404.

Liberman, R. P., King, L. W., De Risi, W. J., & McCann, M. (1975). *Personal effectiveness: Guiding people to assert themselves and improve their social skills.* Champaign, IL: Research Press.

Liebowitz, M. R., Heimberg, R. G., Schneier, F. R., Hope, D. A., Davies, S., Holt, C. S., et al. (1998). Cognitive-behavioral group therapy versus phenelzine in social phobia: Long-term outcome. *Depression and Anxiety*, *10*, 89–98.

Lucock, M. P., & Salkovskis, P. M. (1988). Cognitive factors in social anxiety and its treatment. *Behaviour Research and Therapy*, *14*, 225–238.

MacLeod, C., Mathews, A., & Tata, P. (1986). Attentional bias in emotional disorders. *Journal of Abormbal Psychology*, *95*, 15–20.

Marzillier, J. S., Lambert, C., & Kellet, J. (1976). A controlled evaluation of systematic desensitization and social skills training for socially inadequate psychiatric patients. *Behaviour Research and Therapy*, *14*, 225–238.

Mattia, J. I., Heimberg, R. G., & Hope, D. A. (1993). The revised Stroop color-naming task in social phobics. *Behaviour Research and Therapy*, *31*, 305–313.

Mattick, R. P., & Peters, L. (1988). Treatment of severe social phobia: Effects of guided exposure with and without cognitive restructuring. *Journal of Consulting and Clinical Psychology*, *56*, 251–260.

Mattick, R. P., Peters, L., & Clarke, J. C. (1989). Exposure and cognitive restructuring for social phobia: A controlled study. *Behavior Therapy*, *20*, 3–23.

McManus, F., Clark, D. M., & Hackmann, A. (2000). Specificity of cognitive biases in social phobia and their role in recovery. *Behavioral and Cognitive Psychotherapy*, *28*, 201–209.

Meier, V. J., & Hope, D. A. (1998). Assessment of social skills. In A. S. Bellack & M. Hersen (Eds.), *Behavioral assessment: A practical handbook* (pp. 232–255). Needham Heights, MA: Allyn & Bacon.

Mersch, P. P. A. (1995). The treatment of social phobia: The differential effectiveness of exposure *in vivo* and an integration of exposure *in vivo*, rational emotive therapy, and social skills training. *Behaviour Research and Therapy*, *33*, 259–269.

Mersch, P.P.A., Bögels, S.M., Hofmann, A., van Hout, W.J.P.J., Scholing, A., & Arntz, A.R. (1996). *Construction and validation of the social anxiety self-statements inventory (SASSI).* Unpublished manuscipt.

Mersch, P. P. A., Emmelkamp, P. M. G., Bögels, S. M., & van der Sleen, J. (1989). Social phobia: Individual response patterns and the effects of behavioral and cognitive interventions. *Behaviour Research and Therapy*, *27*, 421–434.

Mersch, P. P. A., Emmelkamp, P. M. G., & Lips, C. (1991). Social phobia: Individual response patterns and the long term effects of behavior and cognitive interventions. A follow-up study. *Behaviour Research and Therapy*, *29*, 357–362.

Mersch, P. P. A., Jansen, M. A., & Arntz, A. (1995). Social phobia and personality disorder: Severity of complaint and treatment effectiveness. *Journal of Personality Disorders*, *9*, 143–159.

Mortberg, E., Karlsson, A., Fyring, C., & Sundin, O. (2006). Intensive cognitive-behavioral group treatment (CBGT) of social phobia: A randomized controlled study. *Journal of Anxiety Disorders*, *20*, 646–660.

Newman, M. G., Hofmann, S. G., Trabert, W., Roth, W. T., & Taylor, C. B. (1994). Does behavioral treatment of social phobia lead to cognitive changes? *Behavior Therapy*, *25*, 503–517.

Nortje, C., Posthumus, T., & Moller, A. T. (2008). Comparison of integrated cognitive restructuring plus exposure with exposure alone in group treatment of generalized social anxiety disorder. *South African Journal of Psychology*, *38*, 647–658.

Norton, P. J., & Hope, D. A. (2001a). Analogue observational methods in the assessment of social functioning in adults. *Psychological Assessment*, *13*, 59–72.

Norton, P. J., & Hope, D. A. (2001b). Kernels of truth or distorted perceptions: Self and observer ratings of social anxiety and performance. *Behavior Therapy*, *32*, 765–786.

Öst, L. G. (1987). Applied relaxation: Description of a coping technique and review. *Behaviour Research and Therapy*, *23*, 397–409.

Öst, L. G., Jerremalm, A., & Johansson, J. (1981). Individual response patterns and the effects of different behavioral methods in the treatment of social phobia. *Behaviour Research and Therapy*, *19*, 1–16.

Peterson, C., Semmel, A., von Baeyer, C., Abramson, L. Y., Metalsky, G. I., & Seligman, M. E. P. (1982). The attributional style questionnaire. *Cognitive Therapy and Research*, *6*, 287–300.

Posner, M. I. (1980). Orienting of attention. *Quarterly Journal of Experimental Psychology*, *32A*, 3–25.

Poulton, R. G., & Andrews, G. (1996). Change in danger cognitions in agoraphobia and social phobia during treatment. *Behaviour Research and Therapy*, *34*, 413–421.

Powers, M. B., Sigmarsson, S. R., & Emmelkamp, P. M. G. (2008). A meta-analytic review of psychological treatments for social anxiety disorder. *International Journal of Cognitive Therapy*, *1*, 94–113.

Rapee, R. M. (1995). Descriptive psychopathology of social phobia. In R. G. Heimberg, L. R. Liebowitz, D. A. Hope, & F. R. Schneier (Eds.), *Social phobia: Diagnosis, assessment, and treatment* (pp. 41–68). New York: Guilford Press.

Rapee, R. M. (1998). *Overcoming shyness and social phobia: A step by step guide*. Bristol, UK: Lifestyle Press.

Rapee, R. M., Abbott, M. J., Baillie, A. J., & Gaston, J. E. (2007). Treatment of social phobia through pure self-help and therapist-augmented self-help. *British Journal of Psychiatry*, *191*, 246–252.

Rodebaugh, T. L., Holaway, R. M., & Heimberg, R. G. (2004). The treatment of social anxiety disorder. *Clinical Psychology Review*, *24*, 883–908.

Salaberria, K., & Echeburua, E. (1998). Long-term outcome of cognitive therapy's contribution to self-exposure *in vivo* to the treatment of generalized social phobia. *Behavior Modification*, *22*, 262–284.

Scholing, A., & Emmelkamp, P. M. G. (1993a). Cognitive and behavioural treatments of fear of blushing, sweating, or trembling. *Behaviour Research and Therapy*, *31*, 155–170.

Scholing, A., & Emmelkamp, P. M. G. (1993b). Exposure with and without cognitive therapy for generalized social phobia: Effects of individual and group treatment. *Behaviour Research and Therapy*, *31*, 667–681.

Scholing, A., & Emmelkamp, P. M. G. (1996a). Treatment of fear of blushing, sweating, or trembling: Results at long-term follow-up. *Behavior Modification*, *20*, 338–356.

Scholing, A., & Emmelkamp, P. M. G. (1996b). Treatment of generalized social phobia: Results at long-term follow-up. *Behaviour Research and Therapy*, *34*, 447–452.

Shaw, P. (1979). A comparison of three behavior therapies in the treatment of social phobia. *British Journal of Psychiatry*, *134*, 620–623.

Shorkey, C. T., & Whiteman, V. L. (1977). Development of the rational behavior inventory: Initial validity and reliability. *Educational and Psychological Measurement*, *37*, 527–534.

Smits, J. A. J., Rosenfield, D., McDonald, R., & Telch, M. J. (2006). Cognitive mechanisms of social anxiety reduction: An examination of specificity and temporality. *Journal of Consulting and Clinical Psychology*, *74*, 1203–1212.

Steptoe, A., & Fidler, H. (1987). Stage fright in orchestral musicians: A study of cognitive and behavioral strategies in performance anxiety. *British Journal of Psychology*, *78*, 241–249.

Stopa, L., & Clark, D. M. (1993). Cognitive processes in social phobia. *Behaviour Research and Therapy*, *31*, 255–267.

Stravynski, A., Marks, I., & Yule, W. (1982). Social skills problems in neurotic outpatients: Social skills training with and without cognitive modification. *Archives of General Psychiatry*, *39*, 1378–1385.

Taylor, S., Woody, S., Koch, W. J., McLean, P., Paterson, R. J., & Anderson, K. W. (1997). Cognitive restructuring in the treatment of social phobia. *Behavior Modification*, *21*, 487–511.

Telch, M. J., Lucas, R. A., Smits, J. A. J., Powers, M. B., Heimberg, R. G., & Hart, T. A. (2004). The Appraisal of Social Concerns (ASC): A cognitive assessment instrument for social phobia. *Depression and Anxiety*, *19*, 217–224.

Turner, S. M., Beidel, D. C., Cooley, M. R., Woody, S. R., & Messer, S. C. (1994). A multicomponent behavioral treatment for social phobia: Social effectiveness therapy. *Behaviour Research and Therapy*, *32*, 381–390.

Turner, S. M., Beidel, D. C., & Cooley-Quille, M. R. (1995). Follow-up of social phobics treated with social effectiveness therapy. *Behaviour Research and Therapy*, *33*, 553–555.

Turner, S. M., Beidel, D. C., & Jacob, R. G. (1994). Social phobia: A comparison of behavior therapy and atenolol. *Journal of Consulting and Clinical Psychology*, *62*, 350–358.

Watson, D., & Friend, R. (1969). Measurement of social-evaluative anxiety. *Journal of Consulting and Clinical Psychology*, *33*, 448–457.

Wlazlo, Z., Schroeder-Hartwig, K., Hand, I., Kaiser, G., & Munchau, N. (1990). Exposure *in vivo* vs. social skills training for social phobia: Long term outcome and differential effects. *Behaviour Research and Therapy*, *28*, 181–193.

Wolpe, J., & Lang, P. J. (1964). A fear schedule for use in behavior therapy. *Behaviour Research and Therapy*, *2*, 27–30.

Woody, S. R., Chambless, D. L., & Glass, C. R. (1997). Self-focused attention in the treatment of social phobia. *Behaviour Research and Therapy*, *35*, 117–129.

Chapter 21

Comparison between Psychosocial and Pharmacological Treatments

Mark B. Powers[1], Michelle C. Capozzoli[1], Pamela Handelsman[2], and Jasper A.J. Smits[2]
[1]*Center for the Treatment and Study of Anxiety, University of Pennsylvania, Philadelphia, PA 19104,*
[2]*Anxiety Research and Treatment Program, Southern Methodist University, Dallas, TX 75205*

In this chapter we summarize the data to date comparing pharmacological and psychosocial treatments for SAD. First we briefly describe the pharmacological and psychosocial treatments of choice and support for their efficacy. We limit our discussion primarily to those treatments with significant empirical support. Next, we present data from meta-analyses and individual trials comparing both treatment modalities (alone and in combination). We then present data on novel pharmacological and psychosocial treatment combinations that are born from learning theory and translational research. Finally, we describe how these findings may affect clinical practice. In short, pharmacotherapy, psychosocial treatment, and their combination offer roughly equivalent outcomes overall. Thus, decisions to employ one strategy over the other must rely on other factors (cost, side-effects, long-term outcome, etc.).

PSYCHOSOCIAL TREATMENTS

The current psychosocial treatment of choice is CBT. CBT is a family of learning-based approaches targeted to helping patients eliminate the core fears and associated avoidance and anticipatory anxiety that help maintain anxiety disorders. These treatments can be delivered in both individual and group formats. Although anxiety management skills such as muscle relaxation and breathing retraining can provide benefit, CBT currently emphasizes helping patients relearn a sense of safety with, rather than simply coping with, feared situations and events (Otto, Smits, & Reese, 2004). This systematic relearning utilizes informational, cognitive, and exposure strategies. In exposure-based procedures, patients are repeatedly exposed to feared stimuli under controlled conditions, allowing fears to dissipate (extinguish) as patients acquire a sense

Social Anxiety: Clinical, Developmental, and Social Perspectives. DOI: 10.1016/B978-0-12-375096-9.00021-3

of safety in the presence of these stimuli. To achieve this type of learning, CBT protocols, usually 12–15 weeks in length, emphasize education about anxiety psychopathology as well as repeated exposure to fear-eliciting cues, often in combination with restructuring of false threat appraisals. For example, exposure therapy for patients with SAD might include giving a speech, attending social engagements, or creating embarrassing situations in which they must engage until anxiety dissipates. From a neurobiological perspective, Gorman, Kent, Sullivan, and Coplan (2000) proposed that CBT deconditions contextual fear at the level of the hippocampus and enhances the ability of the prefrontal cortex to inhibit the amygdala.

A recent meta-analysis of randomized placebo-controlled trials indicated that CBT protocols of this nature are associated with clinically meaningful improvements at the conclusion of acute-phase treatment in SAD and other anxiety disorders (Hofmann & Smits, 2008). Although long-term follow-up studies are sparse in SAD (as in other disorders), the available data suggest that the gains achieved with CBT can be durable over time (Gould, Buckminster, Pollack, Otto, & Yap, 1997). Similar results were found in a meta-analysis by Powers, Sigmarsson, and Emmelkamp (2008). Their literature search produced 32 randomized controlled trials ($n = 1479$) that were included in the final analyses. There was a clear overall advantage of treatment compared to wait-list ($d = 0.86$), psychological placebo ($d = 0.34$), and pill placebo ($d = 0.36$) conditions at post-treatment on the primary outcome measures. The average treated participant scored better than 80% of the wait-list and 66% of the placebo participants. Treatment also fared better than control conditions across secondary outcomes including cognitive measures ($d = 0.55$), behavioral measures ($d = 0.62$), and general subjective distress measures ($d = 0.47$). Treatment gains were maintained at follow-up ($d = 0.76$). Combined exposure and cognitive therapy (vs. control: $d = 0.61$) was not significantly different from exposure (vs. control: $d = 0.89$; $p = 0.33$) or cognitive treatments (vs. control: $d = 0.80$; $p = 0.70$). Likewise, group treatments (vs. control: $d = 0.68$) were not significantly different from individual treatments (vs. control: $d = 0.69$; $p = 0.62$). Effect sizes were not associated with treatment dose ($p = 0.91$), sample size ($p = 0.53$), or publication year ($p = 0.77$). The results add confidence to previous meta-analytic findings supporting the use of psychological treatments for SAD with no significant differences in treatment type or format.

The trajectory of outcome over follow-up periods suggests that during acute treatment patients learn a method for approaching their social fears and avoidance, such that patients continue to increase the magnitude of their treatment gains over time (Heimberg, Salzman, Holt, & Blendell, 1993). Additional psychotherapies that are not discussed further due to limited data at this time include interpersonal psychotherapy (IPT) and psychodynamic therapy, among others.

PHARMACOLOGICAL TREATMENTS

In contrast to CBT, pharmacological interventions aim to directly target biochemical pathways underlying the anxiety by decreasing activity in the amygdala (Gorman et al., 2000). The hypothesized mechanism of action in pharmacotherapy for anxiety disorders is the modulation of anxiety via specific biochemical pathways when anxiety is elicited by disorder-specific cues, such as social scrutiny in SAD (e.g., Otto, Safren, Nicolaou, & Pollack, 2003). The first-line pharmacological treatments for SAD include MAOIs, SSRIs, tricyclic antidepressants, benzodiazepines, and beta-adrenergic blockers (Lydiard, Brawman-Mintzer, & Ballenger, 1996; Smoller & Pollack, 1996). However, currently, the largest evidence base supports the use of MAOIs (e.g. phenelzine sulfate) and SSRIs (i.e. fluvoxamine, sertraline, paroxetine, citalopram, escitalopram, and fluoxetine).

COMPARISON OF PSYCHOSOCIAL AND PHARMACOLOGICAL TREATMENTS: META-ANALYSES

The first major meta-analysis to compare CBT and pharmacotherapy for SAD included 24 studies with 1079 participants (Gould et al., 1997). Sixteen studies included cognitive behavioral interventions and 10 studies included pharmacotherapy. Only two studies included a combined approach (pharmacotherapy with psychosocial treatment). The mean duration of SAD in these trials was 15.92 years. Overall, they found that both treatments were effective with no significant differences between CBT (ES = 0.74) and pharmacological (ES = 0.62) treatments (see Figure 21.1).

Among CBT interventions, exposure showed the largest effect size (ES = 0.89) and SSRIs had the largest effect size (ES = 1.89) of the pharmacotherapies.

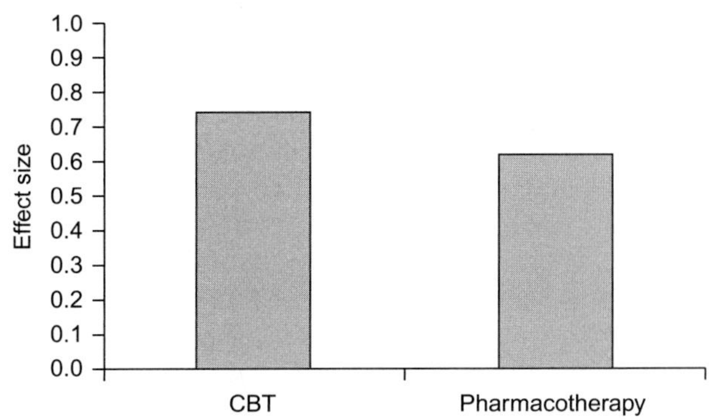

FIGURE 21.1 Mean effect sizes for CBT and pharmacotherapy in social anxiety disorder trials. *(Data from Gould et al., 1997.)*

A cost projection analysis showed that group CBT was by far the most cost-effective treatment option. In 1997 dollars, the authors estimated the total cost for CBGT to be approximately $600 compared to a yearly cost of $1000 for the cheapest pharmacological intervention (clonazapam). A larger meta-analysis of 108 trials showed that benzodiazepines and SSRIs were equipotent and more effective than applied relaxation and control conditions at post-treatment (Fedoroff & Taylor, 2001). Finally, a recent meta-analysis compared the post-acute efficacy of CBT plus pharmacotherapy with CBT plus pill placebo for the range of anxiety disorders (Hofmann, Sawyer, Korte, & Smits, 2009). The effect size for SAD was small and not significant ($ES = 0.16$). Unfortunately, there were insufficient follow-up data to determine long-term outcome. Taken together, meta-analyses suggest that medications and CBT are both effective and not significantly different from each other. Combined strategies are not significantly better than monotherapies. Thus, based on current data, treatment decisions must be based on other factors (cost, long-term commitment, history, comorbidity, etc.). Next we examine individual trials for more information on the relative efficacy of pharmacological and psychosocial treatments alone and in combination.

COMPARISON OF PSYCHOSOCIAL AND PHARMACOLOGICAL TREATMENTS: INDIVIDUAL TRIALS

Here we briefly discuss eight randomized controlled trials that included both psychosocial and pharmacological treatments for social anxiety along with their follow-up studies where available. See Table 21.1 for a summary of these trials.

First, Clark and Agras (1991) randomized 94 participants with SAD (DSM-III-R) to CBT plus buspirone, CBT plus placebo, buspirone alone, or placebo only over a six-week period. The CBT consisted of five group sessions. Overall, results favored the CBT conditions (with and without buspirone). Both CBT groups showed lower fear ratings during behavioral tasks and on other measures compared to buspirone alone and placebo alone. Buspirone was not significantly superior to placebo in this trial. Thus, this trial clearly supports the use of CBT (with or without buspirone) over buspirone alone.

Next, Gelernter et al. (1991) randomized 65 participants with SAD (DSM-III-R) to one of four conditions: alprazolam with self-exposure instructions, phenelzine with self-exposure instructions, placebo with self-exposure instructions, or CBT alone. Results showed that all four conditions resulted in significant improvement in social anxiety symptoms. However, they found no differences between any of the treatments. The one consistent component across all four treatments was the inclusion of exposure (in addition to non-specific factors). Thus, the results suggest that there was no added benefit of adding pharmacotherapy to exposure. However, the lack of a no treatment comparison group suggests caution in interpreting these results in this way.

TABLE 21.1 Randomized Controlled Trials of Psychotherapy and Pharmacotherapy

Study	Conditions	*n*	Overall Outcome
Clark & Agras, 1991	CBT + BUSCBT + PLBUSPL	94	CBT + BUS = CBT + PL > BUS = PL
Gelernter et al., 1991	SE + AlpSE + PhenSE + PLCBT	65	SE + Alp = SE + Phen = SE + PL = CBT
Turner et al., 1994	ExpAtenololPL	72	Exp > Atenolol = PL
Heimberg et al., 1998; Liebowitz et al., 1999	CBGTPhenPsych PLPL	133	CBGT = Phen > Psych PL = PL
Blomhoff et al., 2001; Haug et al., 2003	Exp + SertExp + PLSertPL	387	Exp + Sert = Exp + PL > Sert > PL
Clark et al., 2003	CTSE + FluSE + PL	60	CT > SE + Flu = SE + PL
Davidson et al., 2004	CBT + FluCBT + PLCBTFluPL	295	CBT = CBT + Flu = CBT + PL = Flu > PL
Blanco et al., 2010	CBGT + PhenCBGTPhenPL	128	CBGT+ Phen > CBGT = Phen > PL

Note: Alp = alprazolam; BUS = buspirone; CBGT = cognitive behavioral group therapy; Exp = exposure; Flu = fluoxetine; Phen = phenelzine; PL = pill placebo; Psych PL = psychological placebo; SE = instructions for self exposure; sert = sertraline.

Turner, Beidel, and Jacob (1994) randomized participants with SAD to exposure only, atenolol, or placebo. Treatment proceeded over a three-month period and the trial included a six-month follow-up. Overall, exposure was superior to both atenolol and placebo. In fact, atenolol did not outperform placebo in this trial. However, atenolol is not considered a first-line treatment for social anxiety. Thus, many researchers point out that the outcome of this trial is not surprising.

Heimberg et al. (1998) randomized 72 participants with SAD (n = 133) to one of four treatments: CBGT, phenelzine, psychological placebo, or pill placebo. The psychological placebo was an educational supportive group and showed equal credibility to the CBGT condition. The participants were then followed for one-year post-treatment (Liebowitz et al. 1999). This follow-up included a six-month maintenance phase followed by a six-month treatment-free phase. Overall, the CBGT and phenelzine conditions were roughly equivalent over the course of the trial and both were clearly superior to the control conditions. Phenelzine outperformed CBGT on some measures during the acute phase. However, phenelzine also showed a trend for greater relapse during the treatment-free follow-up. In addition, phenelzine is an MAOI and therefore requires dietary restrictions to prevent a hypertensive crisis (i.e., cheese, lunch meats, snow peas, beer and red wine, etc.).

In an interesting community/general practice double-masked design, Blomhoff et al. (2001) randomized 387 treatment-seeking participants with generalized SAD (DSM-IV) to exposure plus sertraline, exposure plus placebo, sertraline alone, or placebo alone. The treatments were provided by 47 trained physicians with private practices. The exposure treatment was manualized and monitored for adherence. Participants were followed for one year post-treatment (Haug et al., 2003). It should be noted that funding was provided for this trial by Pfizer. The results showed an advantage of sertraline and exposure plus sertraline during the acute phase of treatment. Response rates at the end of acute phase-treatment were 45.5% (sertraline + exposure), 40.2% (sertraline), 33% (placebo + exposure), and 24% (placebo). These findings suggest that sertraline can augment the effects of exposure treatment, particularly when exposure treatment is delivered with minimal therapist contact (i.e., eight 20-minute sessions involving instructions for homework exposures). However, relative to CBT alone, these benefits of combined treatment were no longer evident at a one-year follow-up evaluation (Haug et al., 2003). During the treatment-free phase, the exposure-alone condition showed substantial continued improvement, whereas the sertraline conditions showed considerable deterioration. This finding is consistent with similar trials in other anxiety disorders. More specifically, treatment gains obtained during CBT while in a medication context may not transfer to the nonmedication context (Barlow, Gorman, Shear, & Woods, 2000; Liebowitz et al., 1999; Marks et al., 1993). This phenomenon will be discussed in greater detail later in the chapter. The authors concluded that: (1) sertraline, exposure therapy, and their combination are all effective treatments for SAD; (2) treatment with exposure therapy appears to confer longer-lasting gains than sertraline; and (3) exposure alone is more effective in the long term than when given in combination with sertraline. Thus, exposure alone was the treatment of choice in this trial.

Clark et al. (2003) randomly assigned 60 participants with generalized SAD (DSM-IV) to one of three conditions: cognitive therapy, fluoxetine plus self-exposure instructions, or placebo plus self-exposure instructions. Acute treatment occurred over 16 weeks and participants were followed for one year post-treatment. Significant improvement was observed in all three conditions. On SAD measures there was a clear advantage for the cognitive therapy group compared to both the fluoxetine plus exposure and placebo plus exposure conditions. The fluoxetine/exposure and placebo/exposure conditions were not significantly different from each other.

In a more recent large trial, Davidson and associates (2004) randomized patients with generalized SAD ($n = 295$) to one of five conditions: CBT alone, fluoxetine alone, CBT plus fluoxetine, CBT plus placebo, or placebo alone. All active treatments were superior to placebo on primary outcomes, but investigators found less than a 3% improvement in response rates with the addition of fluoxetine to CBT. Patients treated with CBT plus fluoxetine demonstrated an intent-to-treat response rate of 54% relative to intent-to-treat response rates of 52% for CBT alone, 51% for fluoxetine alone, and 32% for the pill-placebo condition. Overall, at the end of the 14-week trial all active treatments showed significant improvement relative to placebo alone. However, there were no significant differences between active treatments.

In the most recent trial to date, Blanco et al. (2010) randomly assigned 128 participants with SAD (DSM-IV) to CBGT plus phenelzine, CBGT alone, phenelzine alone, or pill placebo alone. The study included four phases: acute phase (12 weeks), continuation phase (12 weeks), maintenance phase (28 weeks), and a 12-month naturalistic follow-up. The data presented in this article (Blanco et al., 2010) only included the acute and continuation phases. Results clearly supported the superiority of combined treatment (CBGT plus phenelzine) throughout the acute and continuation phases. The response rates at the 24 week assessment were 78% (CBGT + phenelzine), 53% (CBGT), 49% (phenelzine), and 33% (placebo) (see Figure 21.2).

However, it should be noted that these assessments took place while participants were still in continuation treatment. It will be interesting to find out how the treatments compare after the naturalistic follow-up results are published. Thus, the combined approach was more effective during the acute and continuation phases but it remains unclear how the participants will fare in the long run.

In summary, the individual randomized controlled trials support the efficacy of both psychosocial and pharmacological approaches. The decision to apply one treatment over the other must then rely on other factors such as cost, long-term outcome, side effects, etc. Next we discuss some advantages of each approach to treatment.

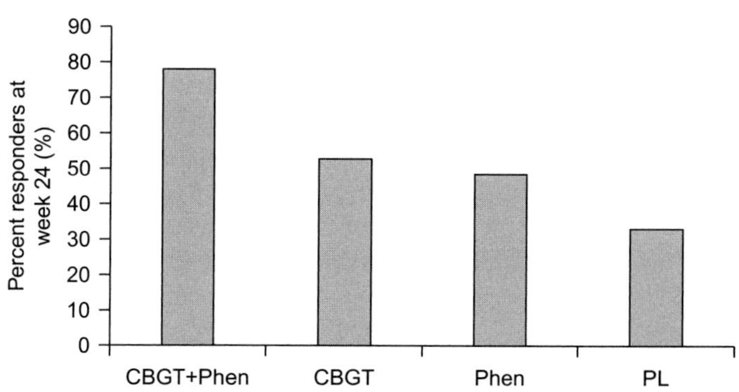

FIGURE 21.2 Percent responders by treatment condition at week 24. *(Data from Blanco et al., 2010.)*

ADVANTAGES OF PSYCHOSOCIAL TREATMENTS

One of the consistent features of the effects of CBT in anxiety disorders is that it has strong relapse-prevention effects. This is a particularly important feature when cost-effectiveness is assessed relative to medications; short-term CBT is associated with strong maintenance of treatment gains, whereas pharmacotherapy often requires ongoing treatment to prevent relapse (e.g., Antonuccio, Thomas, & Danton, 1997; Haug et al., 2003; Otto, Pollack, & Maki, 2000).

Across diagnostic domains, there is some suggestion that CBT is a more tolerable treatment relative to medications and is cost-effective, particularly when the long-term outcomes provided by CBT are considered (e.g., Antonuccio et al., 1997; Hofmann et al., 1998; Otto et al., 2000). Indeed, review of dropout rates, as evaluated in meta-analytic reviews of acute pharmacotherapy and CBT trials, indicates that CBT is equal to or more tolerable than pharmacological alternatives across the anxiety disorders.

In addition, CBT has been shown to be an effective treatment for individuals who have failed to respond to medication treatment for PTSD (Otto, Hinton et al., 2003), OCD (Kampman, Keijsers, Hoogdiun, & Verbraak, 2002), and PD (Otto, Pollack, Penava, & Zucker, 1999; Pollack, Otto, Kaspi, Hammerness, & Rosenbaum, 1994; Heldt et al., 2006). For example, Heldt et al. (2006) offered 12-weekly sessions of group CBT to individuals with PD who had remained symptomatic despite an average of three years of pharmacotherapy. At one-year follow-up, nearly two-thirds of the participants met remission criteria. Given that psychiatrists and primary care physicians greatly outnumber psychologists trained in CBT, the most readily available treatment for the anxiety disorders is often medication. Thus, the use of CBT as a treatment strategy for individuals who have not benefited from medication may be a practical solution when treatment resources are limited.

Treatment-free follow-up data suggest that pharmacotherapy is a long-term commitment; relapse is common following medication discontinuation (e.g., Mavissakalian & Perel, 1992; Noyes, Garvey, Cook, & Suelzer, 1991; Stein, Versiani, Hair, & Kumar, 2002; Walker et al., 2000). For the average patient, this attenuation of the anxiety response appears to work as long as medication treatment is continued. However, when treatment is discontinued, relapse is common (Noyes, Garvey, Cook, & Samuelson, 1989; Noyes et al., 1991; Pollack & Smoller, 1996), although studies of PD indicate that relapse rates are attenuated the longer a patient is kept on medication (Mavissikalian & Perel, 1993). Furthermore, although a long-term proposition, patients often fail to adhere to pharmacological prescriptions over the long run (Cowley, Ha, & Roy-Byrne, 1997; Sirey et al., 1999; Weilburg, O'Leary, Meigs, Hennen, & Stafford 2003).

ADVANTAGES OF PHARMACOLOGICAL TREATMENT

A striking advantage of pharmacological treatment is that it requires far less effort and time than psychosocial interventions. Patients who are too busy or not committed to a full course of CBT may be particularly well suited for this option. Once they have reached a therapeutic dose, they only need periodic appointments for assessments and refills.

In addition, there is evidence that pharmacotherapy may be effective when CBT fails. For example, Kampman, Keijsers, Hoogduin, and Hendriks (2002) randomly assigned individuals with PD who remained symptomatic after 15 sessions of CBT to continued CBT plus paroxetine, or CBT plus placebo. Those subjects who received the paroxetine experienced significant improvement on measures of avoidance and anxiety whereas those who received placebo did not.

NOVEL THERAPEUTICS: COMBINING "COGNITIVE ENHANCERS" WITH PSYCHOSOCIAL TREATMENT

The combination treatment strategies reviewed above represent the application of two independent strategies, each designed to treat disorders on its own. However, are there alternative ways to conceptualize the combination of psychosocial and pharmacological strategies? Rather than focusing on the anxiolytic, antidepressant, or mood-stabilizing effects of pharmacotherapy, can medication be used to more directly enhance the change processes specific to psychotherapy? One such strategy relies not on anxiolysis, but on the enhancement of the extinction learning that occurs in CBT.

This approach grew out of advances in animal research that have mapped some of the core pathways and neurotransmitters involved in fear extinction (e.g., Davis, Falls, & Gewirtz, 2000; Davis & Myers, 2002). Specifically, animal studies suggest that fear learning and extinction are both blocked by antagonists at the glutamatergic NMDA receptor. D-cycloserine (DCS), a partial NMDA agonist, appears to augment learning in animal trials (for review see Davis, 2002; Richardson, Ledgerwood, & Cranney, 2004). That is, the process of extinction of conditioned fear is facilitated by DCS given in individual doses prior to or soon after extinction (exposure) trials in animals, and may even aid the generalization of extinction to related cues (Ledgerwood, Richardson, & Cranney, 2005).

In a groundbreaking study, Ressler et al. (2004) randomly assigned acrophobic patients ($n = 28$) to one of three treatment conditions: (1) virtual-reality exposure (VRE) therapy plus DCS 500 mg; (2) VRE plus DCS 50 mg; or (3) VRE plus a pill placebo. Pills were administered in a double-blind fashion one hour prior to each of two weekly virtual-reality exposure sessions. Results indicated that, by the second exposure session, patients who had received DCS reported significantly greater reductions in acrophobia symptoms and skin conductance levels during virtual exposures, as well as greater improvement on general acrophobia symptoms as applied to real-world situations relative to those treated with placebo. Furthermore, this differential benefit was maintained at three months following treatment termination.

Thus far, two published studies have examined the ability of DCS to enhance the effects of exposure in the treatment of SAD (see Table 21.2).

Hofmann et al. (2006) examined the efficacy of adjunctive DCS in a placebo-controlled trial of CBT for SAD. The use of patients with SAD represents the application of adjunctive DCS to a disorder known for its marked disability and distress that has been the target of more-traditional combination treatment strategies discussed earlier in the chapter (e.g., Davidson et al., 2004). Furthermore, it examined DCS as applied to a longer course of treatment: a total of five sessions of exposure-based CBT, with DCS or placebo administration one hour before four of these sessions. A total of 27 participants were randomized in a double-blind fashion to receive treatment, and results indicated that patients in the DCS group reported significantly more gains from exposure treatment than those who had received adjunctive placebo plus exposure. These benefits were seen both at post-treatment and at the one-month follow-up assessment. Between-group effect sizes for the advantage of adjunctive DCS versus placebo were in the range from medium ($d = 0.72$) to large ($d = 1.43$) according to Cohen's standards. In a second study, Guastella et al. (2008) randomized 56 participants with SAD to exposure plus DCS or exposure plus placebo. Consistent with previous findings, the participants who received DCS prior to exposures reported greater improvement in symptoms of social anxiety, dysfunctional cognitions, and life impairment compared to those who received placebo.

The use of adjunctive DCS to enhance therapeutic learning from exposure is fully congruent with concerns against affect modulation and context effects in combination treatments. DCS is taken only prior to sessions, and hence exposure practice following each week of therapy is during a drug-free state. Moreover, even during acute administration DCS is not an anxiolytic and in the 50 mg dose range appears to be virtually free of side effects (e.g., D'Souza et al., 2000; Heresco-Levy et al., 2002; Hofmann et al., 2006; van Berckel et al., 1998). Accordingly, DCS emerges, at this early stage, as a particularly promising candidate for enhancing CBT.

Ongoing work is seeking to document the efficacy of adjunctive DCS across the anxiety disorders. One aspect of DCS treatment that is not known

TABLE 21.2 Randomized Controlled Trials of Psychotherapy Augmentation

Study	Conditions	*n*	Overall Outcome
Hofmann et al., 2006	Exp + DCSExp + PL	27	Exp + DCS > Exp + PL
Guastella et al., 2008	Exp + DCSExp + PL	56	Exp + DCS > Exp + PL
Guastella et al., 2009	Exp + oxytocinExp + PL	25	Exp + oxytocin = Exp + PL

Note: DCS = D-cycloserine; Exp = exposure; PL = pill placebo.

is the number of times it can be used successfully within a treatment episode. Investigations of isolated versus chronic dosing (i.e., 20 minutes prior to testing versus daily for 15 days prior) of DCS in animal paradigms has revealed limitations for chronic dosing (Parnas, Weber, & Richardson, 2005; Quartermain, Mower, Rafferty, Herting, & Lanthorn, 1994). As suggested by Ressler et al. (2004), DCS may need to be taken on an isolated rather than a chronic dosing schedule in order for it to have its intended effect on NMDA receptor activity. To date, the use of DCS on four weekly occasions in the Hofmann et al. (2006) protocol represents the most frequent isolated-dose use of DCS with positive results. Further research will need to be conducted to determine whether use beyond this amount provides any additional benefit.

Another interesting augmentation candidate for exposure-based treatments is the use of intranasal oxytocin. Oxytocin is known to be involved in several social processes, including bonding, communication, social threat, and encoding of positive social cues. Guastella, Howard, Dadds, Mitchell, and Carson (2009) randomized 25 participants with SAD to exposure with oxytocin or exposure with a placebo. Results showed improvements in both groups. However, the oxytocin condition did not significantly outperform the placebo condition on primary outcome measures for SAD. Thus, it is unclear whether oxytocin will be a viable augmentation agent at this time.

Translational research also provides support for administration of yohimbine hydrochloride (an alpha$_2$-receptor antagonist) as an alternative strategy for enhancing extinction learning (Cain, Blouin, & Barad, 2004). Yohimbine is a rapid-acting compound with an absorption half-time of 10 minutes and an elimination half-life of 36 minutes. Cain et al. (2004) found that fear extinction in mice was accelerated (from 30 trials to 5 trials) following injection of yohimbine hydrochloride (5 mg/kg). Additionally, the mice treated with yohimbine hydrochloride were protected from the negative effects of spacing extinction trials (20-minute intertrial intervals) in comparison to mice treated with placebo.

The theorized mechanism whereby yohimbine hydrochloride's effects emerge is stimulation of the MPFC, signaling safety both during and following extinction trials. Specifically, yohimbine hydrochloride stimulates c-Fos expression in the mPFC, making it capable of accelerating fear reduction and enhancing subsequent recall of safety learning. Yohimbine blocks inhibition of norepinephrine release thus increasing norepinephrine in the forebrain regions important for fear extinction including the hippocampus, amygdala, and prefrontal cortex. Indeed, the animal literature indicates that mPFC is implicated strongly in extinction learning (Morgan, Romanski, & LeDoux, 1993; Quirk, Russo, Barron, & Lebron, 2000). For example, mPFC activity in healthy rats increases (thereby signaling safety) during testing on the day following extinction learning (Milad & Quirk, 2002), and stimulation of the mPFC in rats enhances extinction learning (Herry & Garcia, 2002; Milad & Quirk, 2002). Likewise, removal of the mPFC in rats precludes the continuation of successful extinction from one day to the next (Morgan et al., 1993; Quirk et al., 2000). In a randomized controlled study, Powers, Smits, Otto, Sanders, and Emmelkamp (2009) examined the potential exposure-enhancing effect of yohimbine in claustrophobic humans. Participants displaying marked claustrophobic fear ($n = 24$) were randomized to take 10.8 mg yohimbine or placebo before being treated with two one-hr *in vivo* exposure sessions. Both groups improved equally at post-treatment. Consistent with predictions, the group that took yohimbine showed significantly greater improvement at the one-week follow-up. This pilot study provides support for the use of yohimbine to enhance exposure therapy. Trials are currently under way to determine whether yohimbine also enhances fear reduction in SAD.

CLINICAL IMPLICATIONS AND DISCUSSION

As discussed above, the data suggest that pharmacotherapy, CBT, and their combination are effective treatments for the symptoms of SAD. There are few differences between treatment modalities when compared directly. There is some suggestion that a combined approach may yield faster results in acute treatment and after treatment discontinuation there may be less relapse with CBT. In reality, most patients are given pharmacotherapy as a first-line treatment for social anxiety. Thus, if they do arrive at a psychotherapy clinic they are most likely taking medication. This partly reflects the fact that primary care physicians far outnumber experts in delivery of CBT for SAD. In addition, patients typically approach their primary care doctor for advice about anxiety first. If full programs of CBT are not available, should elements of CBT be added to pharmacotherapy? Research shows that instruction in stepwise exposure offers benefits similar to therapist-guided exposure for some disorders, and that the addition of *elements* of CBT, particularly instruction in stepwise exposure, has been shown to enhance pharmacological treatment in both specialty care and primary care settings (Craske et al., 2005; Marks et al., 1988; Mavissakalian & Michelson, 1986; Telch, Agras, Taylor, Roth, & Gallen, 1985). Indeed, the "prescription" of exposure assignments conjoint with medications has been recommended as standard practice in pharmacotherapy for SAD (Sutherland & Davidson, 1995). Accordingly, one strategy for combination treatment is to consider elements of CBT as "add ons" to pharmacotherapy, helping to ensure that patients have a framework for re-entering and persisting in avoided situations. This approach has the advantage of extending the benefit of pharmacotherapy without substantially increasing costs when a CBT specialist is not available for a full program of treatment. However, it has the limitation of failing to use the more comprehensive programs of CBT that have shown particular acceptability, tolerability, efficacy, and cost-efficacy on their own (Deacon & Abramowitz, 2005; Heuzenroeder et al., 2004; Otto et al., 2000).

The issue of adding pharmacotherapy to full packages of CBT requires greater consideration of whether core fears associated with anxiety disorders can be treated adequately when these fears are being attenuated by medication. A number of accounts of the fear reductions from exposure stress the importance of evoking anxiety during exposure (for review, see Powers, Smits, Leyro, & Otto, 2006). For example, in their emotional processing theory, Foa and Kozak (1986) stress the importance of adequate activation of fear-related memories so that new (safety) information can be incorporated in these memories. Adequate activation depends in part on whether the exposure procedures are a realistic representation of the feared event or situation, including the elicitation of fear itself during exposure. This theoretical account is consistent with findings showing that attenuation of the perceived threat of the exposure situation also attenuates the efficacy of exposure. For example, the availability of escape strategies (Powers, Smits, & Telch, 2004) or strategies such as distraction from the feared stimulus (e.g., Kamphuis & Telch, 2000; Rodriguez & Craske, 1993) or "playing it safe" in the presence of the stimulus (Sloan & Telch, 2002) can each reduce the efficacy of exposure.

Another possible reason for the increased risk of relapse following termination of combined exposure-based and pharmacological treatment is the role of context (for review, see Bouton, 2002; Powers, Smits, Leyro, & Otto 2006). Specifically, animal studies have shown that extinction learning, which involves procedures similar to exposure-based treatments, is context-specific (Bouton, 2002). That is, extinction of fear that occurs in one context (e.g., room A) may not generalize to a second context (e.g., room B). Accordingly, shifts in context such as medication discontinuation (i.e., the drug-state is withdrawn) may account for the loss of gains apparent during acute-phase treatment (i.e., the extinction memory is specific to the state of being on medication). Mystkowski, Mineka, Vernon, and Zinbarg (2003) tested this hypothesis using a sample of participants fearful of spiders. They randomly allocated these participants to ingest either caffeine or a pill placebo before receiving treatment involving exposure to live spiders, and outcome was assessed by means of a behavioral approach task immediately following treatment completion. To test the hypothesis that extinction learning during CBT is context-specific, and thus would be lost as a result of changing the drug state, the investigators retested participants one week following treatment under conditions of either the same or opposite drug context. Consistent with predictions, participants who were tested under the incongruent condition (e.g., treated while taking caffeine and later tested while taking placebo) displayed greater return of fear compared to those tested under the congruent condition (e.g., treated while taking caffeine and later tested while taking caffeine).

Self-efficacy theory (Bandura, 1977) offers a possible alternative or complementary mechanism underlying the negative effects of medication on long-term effects of CBT. Self-efficacy theory posits that phobic behavior is a function of one's perceived inability to execute effective coping behavior in response to potential phobic threats (Bandura, 1977). It seems plausible that medication-taking may cause patients to attribute their gains to the medication instead of their own efforts and accomplishments, thereby undermining self-efficacy enhancement. Indeed, patients with anxiety disorders tend to attribute treatment gains to external factors (Adler & Price, 1985; Anderson & Arnoult, 1985; Broadbeck & Michelson, 1987; Cloitre, Heimberg, Liebowitz, & Gitow, 1992; Emmelkamp & Cohen-Kettenis, 1975; Hoffart & Martinsen, 1990). The influence of patients' attributions of treatment gains to medication on the outcome of combined treatments has been examined in a few studies. Basoglu, Marks, Kilic, Brewin, and Swinson (1994) reported that attributions of improvement to the medication (i.e., alprazolam or placebo) significantly predicted relapse in PD patients treated with exposure in combination with medication. Interestingly, Biondi and Picardi (2003) reported that making external/medication attributions in PD treatment was associated with a 60% relapse rate, whereas making internal attributions was associated with a 0% relapse rate.

Perhaps the strongest evidence for the causal role of external attributions in relapse following the discontinuation of combined treatments comes from a recent analogue study by Powers, Smits, Whitley, Bystritsky, and Telch (2008). Using an experimental design, the investigators first randomly assigned participants displaying marked claustrophobic fear to one of four conditions: wait-list, psychological placebo, exposure-based treatment, or exposure-based treatment plus an inactive pill. Following post-treatment assessment, which revealed an advantage of exposure over control conditions and no effects of pill-taking, they manipulated attributions concerning medication-taking by randomly assigning participants in the exposure-based treatment plus pill-placebo condition to one of three instructional sets: (1) the pill was described as a sedating herb that likely made exposure treatment easier; (2) the pill was described as a stimulating herb that likely made exposure treatment more difficult; or (3) the pill was described as a placebo that had no effect on exposure treatment. Assessments at follow-up showed a relapse rate of 39% among participants who believed that the pill had a sedating effect, whereas a relapse rate of 0% was observed among participants in the other two conditions involving medication-taking. Moreover, reduced self-efficacy accounted for the elevated relapse rates associated with the sedating instructional set.

Collectively, these findings suggest that the practice of acute-phase combined treatments may warrant the utilization of specific relapse prevention strategies, including the assessment and possible modification of patient attributions regarding the improvements achieved with treatment as well the continuance of exposure practice following the termination of medication treatment. Indeed, research suggests that, for patients who would like to discontinue medication following successful CBT, a slow taper coupled with reapplication of exposures during the taper reduces relapse (e.g. Otto et al., 1993; Whittal, Otto, & Hong, 2001).

Based on the available data as well as cost–benefit considerations (see Otto et al., 2000; McHugh et al., 2007), it appears that there is no strong justification for recommending that combined treatment be adopted as a standard, first-line treatment for optimizing acute outcomes for the SAD. Whether combination treatments are indicated for certain subgroups of patients (e.g., those with comorbid depressive disorders) or in settings where CBT cannot be delivered in its most optimized form (e.g., primary care) are questions that deserve further inquiry. Although the evidence to date provides no justification for recommending combined treatments as a first-line intervention for anxiety disorders, it does not rule out that the combined approach holds great value for many patients suffering from SAD.

It appears that the utility of combined treatments may vary depending on the combination of a number of factors, including, but not limited to, patient preferences with respect to pharmacotherapeutic approaches, availability of state-of-the-art CBT, and the presence of comorbid conditions at presentation. Another consideration is attenuation. Recent large-scale studies of SAD (Davidson et al., 2004) and OCD (Foa et al., 2005) reveal trends toward a higher dropout rate in combination treatment than CBT, but this trend was not evident in a multicenter trial of PD (Barlow et al., 2000). Given these mixed data, a conservative conclusion is that combination treatment offers no reliable advantages to CBT in terms of the acute retention of patients. Considering the availability, tolerability, and efficacy of combined treatment strategies for anxiety disorders, we believe the available evidence supports the following conclusions. Elements of CBT, particularly instruction in stepwise exposure, offer fairly reliable benefit to ongoing pharmacotherapy. To the extent that these treatment elements can be provided as part of the care of the pharmacotherapy team and do not require resources from clinicians who otherwise would provide full packages of CBT, routine application of this strategy appears indicated. In contrast, when state-of-the-art CBT is available, this intervention can be offered alone and achieve results that rival combination treatment in many cases and offer the potential for greater durability of treatment and lower cost (e.g., Heuzenroeder et al., 2004; Otto, Pollack, & Sabatino, 1996). As such, clinicians should be cautious about recommending routine combination treatment when full packages of CBT can be provided.

Nonetheless, combination treatment should be considered when nonresponse is encountered in singular treatment modalities. In cases in which the patient wishes to discontinue psychopharmacological-only treatment, beginning CBT before the medication has been discontinued can be beneficial. Furthermore, therapists should take special care with patients who wish to discontinue medication during therapy.

REFERENCES

Adler, D., & Price, J. H. (1985). Relation of agoraphobics' health locus of control orientation to severity of agoraphobia. *Psychological Reports*, *56*, 619–625.

Anderson, C. A., & Arnoult, L. H. (1985). Attributional style and everyday problems in living: Depression, loneliness, and shyness. *Social Cognition*, *3*, 16–35.

Antonuccio, D. O., Thomas, M., & Danton, W. G. (1997). A cost-effectiveness analysis of cognitive behavior therapy and fluoxetine (Prozac) in the treatment of depression. *Behavior Therapy*, *28*, 187–210.

Bandura, A. (1977). Self-efficacy: toward a unifying theory of behavioral change. *Psychological Review*, *84*(2), 191–215.

Barlow, D. H., Gorman, J. M., Shear, M. K., & Woods, S. W. (2000). Cognitive-behavioral therapy, imipramine, or their combination for panic disorder: A randomized controlled trial. *Journal of the American Medical Association*, *283*, 2529–2536.

Basoglu, M., Marks, I. M., Kilic, C., Brewin, C. R., & Swinson, R. P. (1994). Alprazolam and exposure for panic disorder with agoraphobia attribution of improvement to medication predicts subsequent relapse. *British Journal of Psychiatry*, *164*, 652–659.

Biondi, M., & Picardi, A. (2003). Attribution of improvement to medication and increased risk of relapse of panic disorder with agoraphobia. *Psychotherapy and Psychosomatics*, *72*, 110–111.

Blanco, C., Heimberg, R. G., Schneier, F. R., Fresco, D. M., Chen, H., Turk, C. L., et al. (2010). A placebo-controlled trial of phenelzine, cognitive behavioral group therapy, and their combination for social anxiety disorder. *Archives of General Psychiatry*, *67*(3), 286–295.

Blomhoff, S., Haug, T. T., Hellström, K., Holme, I., Humble, M., Madsbu, H. P., et al. (2001). Randomised controlled general practice trial of sertraline, exposure therapy and combined treatment in generalized social phobia. *British Journal of Psychiatry*, *179*, 23–30.

Bouton, M. E. (2002). Context, ambiguity, and unlearning: Sources of relapse after behavioral extinction. *Biological Psychiatry*, *52*, 976–986.

Broadbeck, C., & Michelson, L. (1987). Problem-solving skills and attributional styles of agoraphobics. [10.1007/BF01183861]. *Cognitive Therapy and Research*, *V11*(5), 593–610.

Cain, C. K., Blouin, A. M., & Barad, M. (2004). Adrenergic transmission facilitates extinction of conditional fear in mice. *Learning & Memory*, *11*, 179–187.

Clark, D. B., & Agras, W. S. (1991). The assessment and treatment of performance anxiety in musicians. *American Journal of Psychiatry*, *148*(5), 598–605.

Clark, D. M., Ehlers, A., McManus, F., Hackmann, A., Fennell, M., Campbell, H., et al. (2003). Cognitive therapy versus fluoxetine in generalized social phobia: A randomized placebo-controlled trial. *Journal of Consulting and Clinical Psychology*, *71*(6), 1058–1067.

Cloitre, M., Heimberg, R. G., Liebowitz, M. R., & Gitow, A. (1992). Perceptions of control in panic disorder and social phobia. *Cognitive Therapy and Research*, *16*, 569–577.

Cowley, D. S., Ha, E. H., & Roy-Byrne, P. P. (1997). Determinants of pharmacologic treatment failure in panic disorder. *Journal of Clinical Psychiatry*, *58*(12), 555–561.

Craske, M. G., Golinelli, D., Stein, M. B., Roy-Byrne, P., Bystritsky, A., & Sherbourne, C. (2005). Does the addition of cognitive behavioral therapy improve panic disorder treatment outcome relative to medication alone in the primary-care setting? *Psychological Medicine*, *35*, 1645–1654.

D'Souza, D. C., Gil, R., Cassello, K., Morrissey, K., Abi-Saab, D., White, J., et al. (2000). IV glycine and oral D-cycloserine effects on plasma and CSF amino acids in healthy humans. *Biological Psychiatry*, *47*, 450–462.

Davidson, J. R. T., Foa, E. B., Huppert, J. D., Keefe, F. J., Franklin, M. E., Compton, J. S., et al. (2004). Fluoxetine, comprehensive cognitive behavioral therapy, and placebo in generalized social phobia. *Archives of General Psychiatry*, *61*, 1005–1013.

Davis, M. (2002). Role of NMDA receptors and MAP kinase in the amygdala in extinction of fear: Clinical implications for exposure therapy. *European Journal of Neuroscience*, *16*, 395–398.

Davis, M., Falls, W. A., & Gewirtz, J. (2000). Neural systems involved in fear inhibition: Extinction and conditioned inhibition. In M. Myslobodsky & I. Weiner (Eds.), *Contemporary issues in modeling psychopathology* (pp. 113–142). Boston: Kluwer Academic Publishers.

Davis, M., & Myers, K. M. (2002). The role of glutamate and gamma-aminobutyric acid in fear extinction: Clinical implications for exposure therapy. *Biological Psychiatry*, *52*, 998–1007.

Deacon, B. J., & Abramowitz, J. S. (2005). Patients' perceptions of pharmacological and cognitive-behavioral treatments for anxiety disorders. *Behavior Therapy*, *36*, 139–145.

Emmelkamp, P. M., & Cohen-Kettenis, P. T. (1975). Relationship of locus of control to phobic anxiety and depression. *Psychological Reports*, *36*, 390.

Fedoroff, I. C., & Taylor, S. (2001). Psychological and pharmacological treatments of social phobia: a meta-analysis. *Journal of Clinical Psychopharmacology*, *21*(3), 311–324.

Foa, E. B., & Kozak, M. J. (1986). Emotional processing of fear: Exposure to corrective information. *Psychological Bulletin*, *99*, 20–35.

Foa, E. B., Liebowitz, M. R., Kozak, M. J., Davies, S., Campeas, R., Franklin, M. E., et al. (2005). Randomized, placebo-controlled trial of exposure and ritual prevention, clomipramine, and their combination in the treatment of obsessive-compulsive disorder. *American Journal of Psychiatry*, *162*(1), 151–161.

Gelernter, C. S., Uhde, T. W., Cimbolic, P., Arnkoff, D. B., Vittone, B. J., Tancer, M. E., et al. (1991). Cognitive-behavioral and pharmacological treatments of social phobia: A controlled study. *Archives of General Psychiatry*, *48*(10), 938–945.

Gorman, J. M., Kent, J. M., Sullivan, G. M., & Coplan, J. D. (2000). Neuroanatomical hypothesis of panic disorder, revised. *American Journal of Psychiatry*, *157*(4), 493–505.

Gould, R. A., Buckminster, S., Pollack, M. H., Otto, M. W., & Yap, L. (1997). Cognitive-behavioral and pharmacological treatment for social phobia: A meta-analysis. *Clinical Psychology: Science and Practice*, *4*, 291–306.

Guastella, A. J., Howard, A. L., Dadds, M. R., Mitchell, P., & Carson, D. S. (2009). A randomized controlled trial of intranasal oxytocin as an adjunct to exposure therapy for social anxiety disorder. *Psychoneuroendocrinology*, *34*(6), 917–923.

Guastella, A. J., Richardson, R., Lovibond, P. F., Rapee, R. M., Gaston, J. E., Mitchell, P., et al. (2008). A randomized controlled trial of D-cycloserine enhancement of exposure therapy for social anxiety disorder. *Biological Psychiatry*, *63*(6), 544–549.

Haug, T. T., Blomhoff, S., Hellström, K., Holme, I., Humble, M., Madsbu, H. P., et al. (2003). Exposure therapy and sertraline in social phobia: One-year follow-up of a randomised controlled trial. *British Journal of Psychiatry*, *182*, 312–318.

Heimberg, R., Liebowitz, M. R., Hope, D. A., Schneier, F. R., Holt, C. S., Welkowitz, L. A., et al. (1998). Cognitive behavioral group therapy vs. phenelzine therapy for social phobia: 12-week outcome. *Archives of General Psychiatry*, *55*(12), 1133–1141.

Heimberg, R. G., Salzman, D. G., Holt, C. S., & Blendell, K. A. (1993). Cognitive-behavioral group treatment for social phobia: Effectiveness at five-year follow-up. *Cognitive Therapy and Research*, *17*, 325–339.

Heldt, E., Manfro, G. G., Kipper, L., Blaya, C., Isolan, L., & Otto, M. W. (2006). One-year follow-up of pharmacotherapy-resistant patients with panic disorder treated with cognitive-behavior therapy: Outcome and predictors of remission. *Behaviour Research and Therapy*, *44*, 657–665.

Heresco-Levy, U., Kremer, I., Javitt, D. C., Goichman, R., Reshef, A., Blanaru, M., et al. (2002). Pilot-controlled trial of D-cycloserine for the treatment of post-traumatic stress disorder. *International Journal of Neuropsychopharmacology*, *5*, 301–307.

Herry, C., & Garcia, R. (2002). Prefrontal cortex long-term potentiation, but not long-term depression, is associated with the maintenance of extinction of learned fear in mice. *Journal of Neuroscience*, *22*, 577–583.

Heuzenroeder, L., Donnelly, M., Haby, M. M., Mihalopoulos, C., Rossell, R., Carter, R., et al. (2004). Cost-effectiveness of psychological and pharmacological interventions for generalized anxiety disorder and panic disorder. *Australian and New Zealand Journal of Psychiatry, 38*, 602–612.

Hoffart, A., & Martinsen, E. W. (1990). Agoraphobia, depression, mental health locus of control, and attributional styles. *Cognitive Therapy and Research, 14*, 343–351.

Hofmann, S. G., Barlow, D. H., Papp, L. A., Detweiler, M. F., Ray, S. E., Shear, M. K., et al. (1998). Pretreatment attrition in a comparative treatment outcome study on panic disorder. *American Journal of Psychiatry, 155*, 43–47.

Hofmann, S. G., Meuret, A. E., Smits, J. A. J., Simon, N. M., Pollack, M. H., Eisenmenger, K., et al. (2006). Augmentation of exposure therapy with d-cycloserine for social anxiety disorder. *Archives of General Psychiatry, 63*, 298–304.

Hofmann, S. G., Sawyer, A. T., Korte, K. J., & Smits, J. A. J. (2009). Is it beneficial to add pharmacotherapy to cognitive-behavioral therapy when treating anxiety disorders? A meta-analytic review. *International Journal of Cognitive Therapy, 2*, 160–175.

Hofmann, S. G., & Smits, J. A. J. (2008). Cognitive-behavioral therapy for adult anxiety disorders: a meta-analysis of randomized placebo-controlled trials. *Journal of Clinical Psychiatry, 69*, 621–632.

Kamphuis, J. H., & Telch, M. J. (2000). Effect of distraction and guided threat reappraisal on fear reduction during exposure-based treatments for specific fears. *Behaviour Research and Therapy, 38*(12), 1163–1181.

Kampman, M., Keijsers, G. P., Hoogduin, C. A., & Hendriks, G. J. (2002). A randomized, double-blind, placebo-controlled study of the effects of adjunctive paroxetine in panic disorder patients unsuccessfully treated with cognitive-behavioral therapy alone. *Journal of Clinical Psychiatry, 63*, 772–777.

Kampman, M., Keijsers, G.. P. J., Hoogdiun, C. A. L., & Verbraak, M. J. P. M. (2002). Addition of cognitive-behaviour therapy for obsessive-compulsive disorder patients non-responding to fluoxetine. *Acta Psychiatrica Scandinavica, 106*, 314–319.

Ledgerwood, L., Richardson, R., & Cranney, J. (2005). D-cycloserine facilitates extinction of learned fear: effects of reacquisition and generalized extinction. *Biological Psychiatry, 57*, 841–847.

Liebowitz, M. R., Heimberg, R. G., Schneier, F., Hope, D. A., Davies, S., Holt, C. S., et al. (1999). Cognitive-behavioral group therapy versus phenelzine in social phobia: long term outcome. *Depression and Anxiety, 10*, 89–98.

Lydiard, R. B., Brawman-Mintzer, O., & Ballenger, J. C. (1996). Recent developments in the psychopharmacology of anxiety disorders. *Journal of Consulting and Clinical Psychology, 64*, 660–668.

Marks, I. M., Lelliott, P., Basoglu, M., Noshirvani, H., Monteiro, W., Cohen, D., et al. (1988). Clomipramine, self-exposure and therapist-aided exposure for obsessive-compulsive rituals. *British Journal of Psychiatry, 152*, 522–534.

Marks, I. M., Swinson, R. P., Basaglu, M., Kuch, K., Nasirvani, H., O'Sullivan, G., et al. (1993). Alprazolam and exposure alone and combined in panic disorder with agoraphobia: A controlled study in London and Toronto. *British Journal of Psychiatry, 162*, 776–787.

Mavissakalian, M., & Michelson, L. (1986). Agoraphobia: Relative and combined effectiveness of therapist-assisted in vivo exposure and imipramine. *Journal of Clinical Psychiatry, 47*(3), 117–122.

Mavissakalian, M., & Perel, J. M. (1992). Clinical experiments in maintenance and discontinuation of imipramine therapy in panic disorder with agoraphobia. *Archives of General Psychiatry, 49*, 318–323.

Mavissikalian, M., & Perel, J. M. (1993). Clinical experience in maintenance and discontinuation of imipramine therapy in panic disorder with agoraphobia. *Archives General Psychiatry, 49*, 318–323.

McHugh, R. K., Otto, M. W., Barlow, D. H., Gorman, J. M., Shear, M. K., & Woods, S. W. (2007). Cost-efficacy of individual and combined treatments of panic disorder. *Journal of Clinical Psychiatry, 68*, 1038–1044.

Milad, M. R., & Quirk, G. J. (2002). Neurons in medial prefrontal cortex signal memory for fear extinction. *Nature, 420*, 70–74.

Morgan, M. A., Romanski, L. M., & LeDoux, J. E. (1993). Extinction of emotional learning: Contribution of medial prefrontal cortex. *Neuroscience Letters, 163*, 109–113.

Mystkowski, J. L., Mineka, S., Vernon, L. L., & Zinbarg, R. E. (2003). Changes in caffeine states enhance return of fear in spider phobia. *Journal of Consulting and Clinical Psychology, 71*, 243–250.

Noyes, R., Garvey, M. J., Cook, B. L., & Samuelson, L. (1989). Problems with tricyclic antidepressant use in patients with panic disorder or agoraphobia: Results of a naturalistic follow-up study. *Journal of Clinical Psychiatry, 50*, 163–169.

Noyes, R., Garvey, M. J., Cook, B., & Suelzer, M. (1991). Controlled discontinuation of benzodiazepine treatment for patients with panic disorder. *American Journal of Psychiatry, 148*, 517–523.

Otto, M. W., Hinton, D., Korbly, N. B., Chea, A., Phalnarith, B., Gershuny, B. S., et al. (2003). Treatment of pharmacotherapy-refractory posttraumatic stress disorder among Cambodian refugees: A pilot study of combination treatment with cognitive-behavior therapy vs. sertraline alone. *Behaviour Research and Therapy, 41*, 1271–1276.

Otto, M. W., Pollack, M. H., & Maki, K. M. (2000). Empirically-supported treatment for panic disorder: Costs, benefits, and stepped care. *Journal of Consulting and Clinical Psychology, 68*, 556–563.

Otto, M. W., Pollack, M. H., Penava, S. J., & Zucker, B. G. (1999). Cognitive-behavior therapy for patients failing to respond to pharmacotherapy for panic disorder: A clinical case series. *Behaviour Research and Therapy, 37*, 763–770.

Otto, M. W., Pollack, M. H., & Sabatino, S. A. (1996). Maintenance of remission following cognitive-behavior therapy for panic disorder: Possible deleterious effects of concurrent medication treatment. *Behavior Therapy, 27*, 473–482.

Otto, M. W., Pollack, M. H., Sachs, G. S., Reiter, S. R., Meltzer-Brody, S., & Rosenbaum, J. F. (1993). Discontinuation of benzodiazepine treatment: Efficacy of cognitive-behavioral therapy for patients with panic disorder. *American Journal of Psychiatry, 150*(10), 1485–1490.

Otto, M. W., Safren, S. A., Nicolaou, D. C., & Pollack, M. H. (2003). Considering mechanisms of action in the treatment of social anxiety disorder. In M. H. Pollack, N. M. Simon, & M. W. Otto (Eds.), *Social Phobia: Presentation, course, and treatment*. New York: Castle Connolly Graduate Medical Publishing.

Otto, M. W., Smits, J. A. J., & Reese, H. E. (2004). Cognitive-behavioral therapy for the treatment of anxiety disorders. *Journal of Clinical Psychiatry, 65*(Suppl 5), 34–41.

Parnas, A. S., Weber, M., & Richardson, R. (2005). Effects of multiple exposures to D-cycloserine on extinction of conditioned fear in rats. *Neurobiology of Learning and Memory, 83*(3), 224–231.

Pollack, M. H., Otto, M. W., Kaspi, S. P., Hammerness, P. G., & Rosenbaum, J. F. (1994). Cognitive-behavior therapy for treatment-refractory panic disorder. *Journal of Clinical Psychiatry, 55*, 200–205.

Pollack, M. H., & Smoller, J. W. (1996). Pharmacologic approaches to treatment resistant panic disorder. In M. H. Pollack & M. W. Otto (Eds.), *Challenges in clinical practice: Pharmacological and psychosocial strategies* (pp. 89–112). New York: Guilford Press.

Powers, M. B., Sigmarsson, S. R., & Emmelkamp, P. M. G. (2008). A meta-analytic review of social phobia treatments. *International Journal of Cognitive Therapy, 1*, 94–113.

Powers, M. B., Smits, J. A. J., Leyro, T. M., & Otto, M. (2006). Translational research perspectives on maximizing the effectiveness of exposure therapy. In D. C. S. Richard & D. Lauterbach (Eds.), *Comprehensive handbook of the exposure therapies* (109–126). New York: Academic Press.

Powers, M. B., Smits, J. A. J., Otto, M. W., Sanders, C., & Emmelkamp, P. M. G. (2009). Facilitation of fear extinction in phobic participants with a novel cognitive enhancer: A randomized placebo controlled trial of yohimbine augmentation. *Journal of Anxiety Disorders, 23*(3), 350–356.

Powers, M. B., Smits, J. A., & Telch, M. J. (2004). Disentangling the effects of safety-behavior utilization and safety-behavior availability during exposure-based treatment: A placebo-controlled trial. *Journal of Consulting and Clinical Psychology*, *72*(3), 448–454.

Powers, M. B., Smits, J. A., Whitley, D., Bystritsky, A., & Telch, M. J. (2008). The effect of attributional processes concerning medication taking on return of fear. *Journal of Consulting & Clinical Psychology*, *76*, 478–490.

Quartermain, D., Mower, J., Rafferty, M. F., Herting, R. L., & Lanthorn, T. H. (1994). Acute but not chronic activation of the NMDA-coupled glycine receptor with D-cycloserine facilitates learning and retention. *European Journal of Pharmacology*, *157*, 7–12.

Quirk, G. J., Russo, G. K., Barron, J. L., & Lebron, K. (2000). The role of ventromedial prefrontal cortex in the recovery of extinguished fear. *Journal of Neuroscience*, *20*, 6225–6231.

Ressler, K. J., Rothbaum, B. O., Tannenbaum, L., Anderson, P., Graap, K., Zimand, E., et al. (2004). Cognitive enhancers as adjuncts to psychotherapy: Use of D-cycloserine in phobics to facilitate extinction of fear. *Archives of General Psychiatry*, *61*(11), 1136–1144.

Richardson, R., Ledgerwood, L., & Cranney, J. (2004). Facilitation of fear extinction by D-cycloserine: Theoretical and clinical implications. *Learning and Memory*, *11*, 510–516.

Rodriguez, B. I., & Craske, M. G. (1993). The effects of distraction during exposure to phobic stimuli. *Behaviour Research and Therapy*, *31*, 549–558.

Sirey, J. A., Meyers, B. S., Bruce, M. L., Alexopoulos, G. S., Perlick, D. A., & Raue, P. (1999). Predictors of antidepressant prescription and early use among depressed outpatients. *American Journal of Psychiatry*, *156*(5), 690–696.

Sloan, T., & Telch, M. J. (2002). The effects of safety-seeking behavior and guided threat reappraisal on fear reduction during exposure: An experimental investigation. *Behaviour Research and Therapy*, *40*, 235–251.

Smoller, J. W., & Pollack, M. H. (1996). Pharmacologic approaches to treatment resistant social phobia and generalized anxiety disorder. In M. H. Pollack & M. W. Otto (Eds.), *Challenges in Clinical Practice: Pharmacological and Psychosocial Strategies* (pp. 141–170). New York: Guilford Press.

Stein, D. J., Versiani, M., Hair, T., & Kumar, R. (2002). Efficacy of paroxetine for relapse prevention in social anxiety disorder. *Archives of General Psychiatry*, *59*, 1111–1118.

Sutherland, S. M., & Davidson, J. R. T. (1995). β-blockers and benzodiazepines in pharmacotherapy. In M. B. Stein (Ed.), *Social phobia: Clinical and research perspectives* (pp. 323–326). Washington, DC: American Psychiatric Press.

Telch, M. J., Agras, W. S., Taylor, C. B., Roth, W. T., & Gallen, C. (1985). Combined pharmacological and behavioral treatment for agoraphobia. *Behaviour Research and Therapy*, *23*, 325–335.

Turner, S. M., Beidel, D. C., & Jacob, R. G. (1994). Social phobia: A comparison of behavior therapy and atenolol. *Journal of Consulting and Clinical Psychology*, *62*(2), 350–358.

van Berckel, B. N., Lipsch, C., Gispen-de Wied, C., Wynne, H. J., Blankenstein, M. A., van Ree, J. M., et al. (1998). The partial NMDA agonist D-cycloserine stimulates LH secretion in healthy volunteers. *Psychopharmacology (Berl)*, *138*, 190–197.

Walker, J. R., van Ameringen, M. A., Swinson, R., Bowen, R. C., Chokka, P. R., Goldner, E., et al. (2000). Prevention of relapse in generalized social phobia: Results of a 24-week study in responders to 20 weeks of sertraline treatment. *Journal of Clinical Psychopharmacology*, *20*, 636–644.

Weilburg, J. B., O'Leary, K. M., Meigs, J. B., Hennen, J., & Stafford, R. S. (2003). Evaluation of the adequacy of outpatient antidepressant treatment. *Psychiatric Services*, *54*(9), 1233–1239.

Whittal, M. L., Otto, M. W., & Hong, J. J. (2001). Cognitive-behavior therapy for discontinuation of SSRI treatment of panic disorder: A case series. *Behaviour Research and Therapy*, *8*, 939–945.

Chapter 22

Mechanisms of Action in the Treatment of Social Anxiety Disorder

Michael W. Otto, Bridget A. Hearon, and Steven A. Safren
Center for Anxiety and Related Disorders, Boston University, MA 02215

Treatment outcome studies for SAD have provided consistent evidence for the efficacy of two modalities of treatment: CBT and pharmacotherapy (for reviews see Gould & Otto, 1996; Heimberg & Juster, 1995; Jorstad-Stein & Heimberg, 2009; Potts & Davidson, 1995). Comparison-treatment studies (e.g., Davidson et al., 2004; Heimberg et al., 1998; Otto et al., 2000), as well as a meta-analytic review of the treatment outcome literature (Gil, Carrillo, & Meca, 2001; Gould, Buckminster, Pollack, Otto, & Yap, 1997) suggest that, on average, these treatment modalities provide equivalent outcomes.

Among pharmacological treatments, the MAOIs, SSRIs, and benzodiazepines have the highest estimates of efficacy (Gould et al., 1997; van Ameringen, Mancini, Patterson, & Simpson, 2009; van der Linden, Stein, & van Balkom, 2000). Among cognitive behavioral treatments, there is evidence that exposure-based and combined cognitive-restructuring and exposure treatments can outperform cognitive interventions alone, and that these treatments are more powerful than relaxation-based treatment and social skills training alone (for reviews see Feske & Chambless, 1995; Gould et al., 1997; Heimberg & Juster, 1995; Jorstad-Stein & Heimberg, 2009; Taylor, 1996).

In addition to approximately equal outcome, there is evidence that cognitive behavioral and pharmacological interventions are equally tolerable to patients, at least as assessed by dropout rates, with an overall 10% dropout rate for CBT and 14% for pharmacotherapy (Fedoroff & Taylor, 2001; Gould et al., 1997). Moreover, to date there appears to be little evidence for differential predictors of response for these two modalities of treatment. For example, Otto et al. (2000) examined demographic, diagnostic, and symptom-severity predictors of outcome in patients undergoing either group CBT or treatment

Social Anxiety: Clinical, Developmental, and Social Perspectives. DOI: 10.1016/B978-0-12-375096-9.00022-5

with clonazepam. Severity of the disorder, as assessed by a range of SAD symptom measures, was a reliable predictor of poorer outcome, but there was no consistent evidence for differential prediction based on treatment modality.

The fact that two different modalities of treatment have similar rates of efficacy and similar predictors of outcome presents an interesting and difficult challenge for the identification of mechanisms of action for these treatments. Given this challenge, it is helpful to consider potential mechanisms of action within a model of the cognitive, behavioral, and physiological components of SAD that must be modified to return an individual to more normal social functioning. Interventions may differ in the way in which one or more of these components are targeted, but, for remission of the disorder, it is these patterns that must be normalized. In addition to the material presented here, discussions of the cognitive, behavioral, and affective patterns that characterize and maintain SAD are provided by Heimberg, Brozovic, and Rapee (Chapter 15 in this volume); Clark and Wells (1995); Heimberg and Barlow (1991); Hofmann (2000); Otto (1999); and Rapee and Heimberg (1997).

A MODEL OF SOCIAL ANXIETY DISORDER

Perhaps one of the most salient features of SAD is the negative and catastrophic expectations that socially phobic individuals bring to social situations. Fears and expectations of poor social performance ("I won't think of anything to say," "I will be humiliated"), negative evaluations from others ("They will think I am stupid"), and uncontrollable anxiety ("I will tremble so much I won't be able to finish the talk") predominate. Accordingly, models of SAD attend to the emotional consequences of such cognitions and other distortions in the interpretation and processing of socially relevant information (Clark & Wells, 1995; Heimberg, 2001; McNally, 1996; Rapee & Heimberg, 1997; see also Heimberg et al., Chapter 15, this volume). The natural result of these fears and negative expectations is that the socially phobic individual enters social situations with anxious apprehension: hoping that negative outcomes will not occur, but being excessively vigilant to feared negative or catastrophic outcomes. In addition to the fear of negative evaluation, recent studies also provide support for a more general fear of evaluation that would also include fears of positive evaluation, suggesting that socially phobic individuals are not necessarily preoccupied by a desire for praise but rather a desire to remain inconspicuous (Weeks, Heimberg, Rodebaugh, & Norton, 2008).

Inherent to many of these fears are the tendencies to exaggerate the perceived consequences of performing inadequately in social situations, to underestimate one's ability to cope in social situations, and to rehearse self-defeating and global attributions about oneself and future social behavior (Clark & Wells, 1995; Rapee & Heimberg, 1997). Salient negative core beliefs (see Beck, Emery, & Greenberg, 1985) such as "I am worthless," "Others will not like me," or "Because I have anxiety, I am inadequate," are at the heart of SAD, and they become activated when individuals with SAD are confronted by social situations. Moreover, these beliefs may include catastrophic interpretations of the meaning of minor mistakes or anxiety in social situations that further amplify negative emotional reactions to these events. Particularly important may be beliefs about the meaning of anxiety itself. Fears that anxiety symptoms will be perceived by others form their own factor on social anxiety scales (Safren, Heimberg, & Turk, 1998), and there is evidence that SAIs overestimate the degree to which their anxiety symptoms are noticed by others (e.g., McEwan & Devins, 1983). The belief that anxiety in social situations is a sign of personal failure is one of three "amplifying cognitions" identified by Otto (1999). Figure 22.1 presents the putative role of these amplifying cognitions in ensuring that initial signs of anxiety or errors in social situations engender more-intense feelings of anxiety, failure, and shame.

In addition to increasing anxiety, these negative and catastrophic expectations also act to direct attention to signs of negative outcomes. This vigilance to perceived danger has the additional destructive effect of distracting individuals from more-relevant information processing. Instead of attending to relevant social cues (e.g., the enjoyment of a conversation, the topic at hand, additional conversation items), negative expectations and vigilance to potential negative outcomes direct attention to a wide range of "off task" thoughts and events. These include fears such as whether one is about to flush, sweat, pause too long in a conversation, or otherwise do something embarrassing or humiliating.

These patterns – negative social expectations, vigilance to negative outcomes, rising symptoms, and negative interpretations of symptoms and

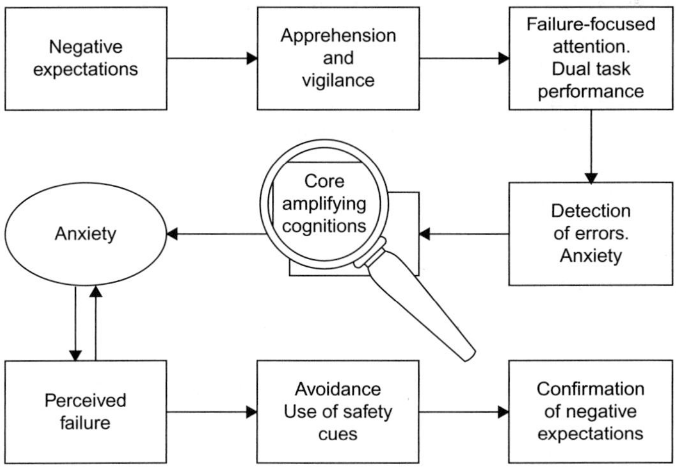

FIGURE 22.1 Amplifying cognitions in social phobia. *(From M. W. Otto, Cognitive-behavioral therapy for social anxiety disorder: Model, methods, and outcome. Journal of Clinical Psychiatry, 60(Suppl 9) (page 15), 1999. Copyright 1999, Physicians Postgraduate Press. Reprinted by permission.)*

outcomes – motivate escape from and avoidance of social situations. Avoidance itself offers the potential of rapid reduction in anxiety at the cost of severe disruptions in quality of life (Bogels & Mansell, 2004; Safren, Heimberg, Brown, & Holle, 1997) and the maintenance of anxiety by preventing the disconfirmation of negative expectations. Consequently, fears of future social situations are enhanced, distorted cognitions are strengthened, and SAD continues.

There is also evidence that even subtle avoidance behaviors, termed safety behaviors by Wells et al. (1995), can have similar deleterious effects with respect to the maintenance of SAD. Safety behaviors include such strategies as holding a drink or clenching one's hands to hide trembling, talking quickly, avoiding eye contact, or taking shallow breaths to avoid freezing up in a conversation. These safety behaviors, like other avoidance behaviors, offer anxiety reduction at the cost of maintained social fears. In an elegant study, Wells et al. found that the use of safety behaviors impaired anxiety reduction from exposure, perhaps by hampering the disconfirmation of fears. More recently, Kim (2005) found that exposures in which patients were encouraged to drop safety behaviors when a cognitive rationale was provided proved most efficacious for reducing anxiety when compared to patients who dropped safety behaviors with an extinction rationale as well as those who were not encouraged to change safety behaviors.

Accordingly, a number of targets for treatment can be translated from this model of the maintenance of SAD. These include: (1) direct modulation of the anxiety evoked in social situations; (2) correction of the dysfunctional thoughts that create apprehension and anxiety, including core amplifying cognitions that intensify anxiety experiences in social situations; (3) elimination of failure-focused attention and the perceived social cost of these failures; (4) elimination of safety behaviors; and (5) development of accurate evaluation of performance in social situations. Direct modulation of the anxiety experience is most frequently associated with pharmacological approaches to treatment, whereas modification of patterns creating or sustaining this anxiety is typically the target of cognitive behavioral interventions.

MECHANISMS OF TREATMENT: PHARMACOTHERAPY

The absence of consistent differences between individuals with SAD and healthy control subjects in studies using chemical and naturalistic provocations (see Tancer, Lewis, & Stein, 1995) makes a detailed biological model of SAD difficult to construct. This difficulty is exacerbated by the wide range of agents that successfully treat the disorder. There is an abundance of evidence that patients can improve from MAOI, SSRI, and tricyclic antidepressants, as well as benzodiazepine treatment (Gould et al., 1997; van Ameringen et al., 2009; van der Linden et al., 2000). Historically, the success of dopaminergic agents led to emphasis on dopaminergic pathways in the pathogenesis of SAD (Liebowitz, Campeas, & Hollander, 1987). Likewise, the more recent success of the SSRIs has directed attention to serotonergic contributions to the disorder (Tancer et al., 1995). However, these findings do little to account for the etiology and nature of SAD. Instead their empirical support and explanatory value appear to be limited to identification of some of the neurophysiologic pathways that may help regulate anxious affect, regardless of whether it arises in the context of SAD or other anxiety conditions.

Both pathways, serotonergic and dopaminergic, have received attention in Gray's (1982a, 1982b) neuropsychological theory of anxiety. These neurotransmitters are hypothesized to play an important role in chemically labeling information delivered to the "behavioral inhibition system" (BIS). The BIS is hypothesized to be the core component of an anxiety system that includes the septohippocampal system, the Papez circuit, the prefrontal cortex, and ascending monoaminergic pathways enervating this cortex. The BIS is hypothesized to respond to potentially anxiety-provoking stimuli – novel stimuli, stimuli associated with punishment, and stimuli associated with nonreward – by increasing arousal, increasing attention to the environment, and inhibiting ongoing behavior. Regarding anxiety conditions such as SAD, the BIS is assumed to be overactive as a product of conditioning experiences or overactive serotonergic or noradrenergic inputs to the septohippocampal system. Gray hypothesizes that serotonergic afferents may be especially important for labeling stimuli as aversive and for fostering motor inhibition but notes that differentiation of the relative contributions of serotonergic and noradrenergic functions is difficult at best. Nonetheless, the action of antidepressant treatment of anxiety conditions is assumed to be a function of reductions in the intensity of serotonergic and noradrenergic signals reaching the septohippocampal system. Benzodiazepine treatment, on the other hand, is assumed to have more general antianxiety effects by facilitating GABA, an inhibitory neurotransmitter that may modulate the effects of the BIS through any of a number of mechanisms (Gray, 1982a, 1982b). In short, pharmacological treatments have, as a core treatment effect for SAD, the ability to reduce or eliminate the pathologic anxiety signal in social situations.

Elimination of the severe anxiety in social situations would, according to the model of SAD presented previously, have a number of significant additional effects. First, with the successful blockade of severe anxiety responses, patients gain control over one aspect of their social fears: the fear of uncontrolled anxiety in social situations. This should substantially reduce the fears of negative evaluations from others ("They will see me tremble and think I am weird") as well as negative self-evaluations ("I feel so nervous; I am really failing") that depend on the socially catastrophic interpretations of anxious affect and anxiety symptoms. Second, with anxiety under at least partial control, patients have the ability to feel more comfortable entering social situations, and, potentially, to experience more-normal social interactions. With each successful social outing, patients responding to medication treatment have the potential to achieve greater confidence in their social abilities and effectiveness, as well as reductions in negative expectations and anticipatory anxiety before future social events. Failure-focused attention should therefore diminish over time, to be replaced by more-normal information processing that focuses attention on the true social demands at hand. Accordingly, it is important to note that pharmacological treatment of SAD, at least treatment that encourages patients to re-enter social situations, tends to achieve reductions in fears of negative evaluation, at least to the levels achieved by cognitive behavioral interventions (Mattia, Heimberg, & Hope, 1993; Otto et al., 2000). Similar evidence is available for changes in the processing of social threat information. Using an emotional Stroop color-naming task, Mattia et al. (1993) found that socially phobic individuals who responded to treatment achieved normalization of response latencies to social threat words, regardless of whether improvement was achieved from CBGT or from phenelzine treatment.

According to the model presented thus far, medication treatment gains are initiated by reductions in anxious affect and are followed by broader changes in dysfunctional patterns, mediated by the effects of successful reentry and performance in social situations. This model suggests that the degree of treatment gains would be associated with the degree of social exposure practiced while taking medications. Future research should test this hypothesis explicitly; nonetheless, tentative support is provided by a study of the treatment of PD with agoraphobia. Telch, Agras, Taylor, Roth, and Gallen (1985) showed that most of the beneficial effects of imipramine treatment could be greatly attenuated by instructions from clinicians that discouraged step-by-step exposure. Without exposure, patients did not have a mechanism to translate anxiety suppression into the fuller reduction of fears and impairment that is produced by learning that feared situations are again safe.

Given this model of the efficacy of pharmacotherapy, the question arises why relaxation treatments, targeted directly to the modification of anxious arousal, are not more effective (see Gould et al., 1997; Taylor, Koch, Woody, & McLean, 1996, for efficacy estimates). For example, Alstrom, Nordlund, Persson, Harding, and Ljungquist (1984) found that relaxation training was ineffective, with poorer outcome than the exposure and supportive therapy comparison conditions, and no better than a control condition. One answer to this question is that, although both relaxation training and pharmacological treatment can reduce anxiety, relaxation training requires active, in-situation effort. This effort to relax in social situations may have the untoward effects of further distracting attention from relevant social cues ("I am getting nervous, I need to relax my shoulders") and providing safety behaviors ("I will be OK, because I can relax my shoulders") that help in the moment but may maintain fears of social situations over the long term ("If not for my relaxation, it would have been a disaster"). In contrast, medication use does not require in-situation behaviors; instead, medications are taken well before the social situation, and the individual is left to focus on relevant social behaviors with an increased sense of confidence ("I will probably be OK; I took my medication").

Of course, these considerations imply that patients treated with pharmacotherapy will be entering situations under conditions of a safety cue (taking medication), and accordingly they should be at risk for relapse upon medication discontinuation. That is, patients taking medication may never learn that social situations are truly safe, but only that they are conditionally safe as long as medication is controlling anxious affect. These considerations have received particular attention in PD (see Otto, Pollack, & Sabatino, 1996; Westra & Stewart, 1998), and they are consistent with high rates of relapse after medication discontinuation in SAD (Davidson, Tupler, & Potts, 1994; Sutherland, Tupler, Colket, & Davidson, 1996) and tentative observations of poorer longer-term efficacy for medications over time (Heimberg et al., 1994). In fact, based on these relapse rates, a recent review suggests that pharmacotherapy should be continued for at least 12 months to maintain gains (Davidson, 2003).

Thus far, we have discussed the cognitive effects of medication as an indirect effect of successful exposure: When patients observe the blockade of feared anxiety responses and the success of initial social exposures, their negative expectations and self-evaluations diminish. There is also evidence that medications may have a more direct influence on cognitions, perhaps as a direct function of the modulation of affect.

There is evidence that negative affect may increase the severity of typical anxiety-related cognitions. For example, Ball, Otto, Pollack, Uccello, and Rosenbaum (1995) found that the presence of major depression was associated with increased fears of negative evaluation and lower assertiveness among patients with SAD, and depressed mood appears to increase scores on other measures of dysfunctional attitudes characteristic of SAD (Bruch, Mattia, Heimberg, & Holt, 1993; Ingram, 1989).

This evidence for mood state effects on anxiety-related cognitions is complemented by a wealth of evidence from the study of major depression. Successful pharmacological treatment of major depression is associated with significant reductions in negative thoughts and dysfunctional attitudes (Dohr, Rush, & Bernstein, 1989; Fava, Bless, Otto, Pava, & Rosenbaum, 1994; Peselow, Robins, Block, Barouche, & Fieve, 1990; Szentagotai, David, Lupu, & Cosman, 2008), suggesting that some of these negative beliefs are mood-state-dependent (see also Miranda, Persons, & Byers, 1990). Likewise, the presence of major depression is associated with elevations or greater fears of anxiety sensations (anxiety sensitivity), which decrease significantly after the pharmacological treatment of depression (Otto, Pollack, Fava, Uccello, & Rosenbaum, 1995; see also Taylor et al., 1996). Presumably, this finding may reflect the contribution – and subsequent elimination of the contribution – of negative affectivity to the negative and catastrophic evaluations of anxiety sensations. Extending these considerations to SAD, pharmacotherapy may exert more-direct effects on fears of negative evaluation and other anxiogenic cognitions by reducing negative affect. With less negative affect, catastrophic expectations

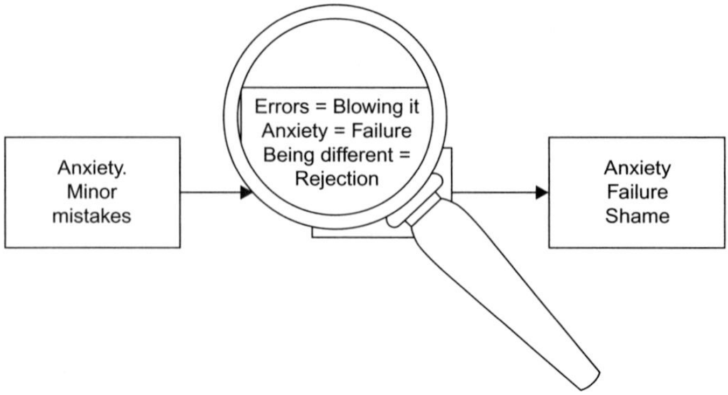

FIGURE 22.2 A cognitive behavioral model of social phobia. *(From M. W. Otto, Cognitive-behavioral therapy for social anxiety disorder: Model, methods, and outcome. Journal of Clinical Psychiatry, 60(Suppl 9) (page 15), 1999. Copyright 1999, Physicians Postgraduate Press. Reprinted by permission.)*

for social situations may be directly reduced, further attenuating the cycle of anticipatory anxiety and negative interpretations detailed in Figure 22.2.

Some of these hypothesized mechanisms of the action of pharmacotherapy are open to empirical testing. Given that fears of anxiety sensations appear to form their own factor on social anxiety measures (Safren et al., 1998), the time course of changes on this factor, relative to other aspects of social anxiety fears, can provide insight about the degree to which pharmacotherapy has initial, specific effects on catastrophic interpretations of anxiety sensations, and whether other changes in negative cognitions change more slowly over time. Likewise, examination of the effects of antiexposure instruction during the early phase of pharmacological treatment of SAD would help elucidate which cognitive changes may be a more direct effect of medications, and which are dependent on successful exposure to social situations for change. Finally, examination of residual levels of fears of negative evaluation, relative to residual anxious distress or avoidance, offers the potential of clarifying which changes are most important for maintenance of treatment gains from medication.

MECHANISMS OF TREATMENT: CBT

Research provides good evidence that the outcome of CBT is not dependent on expectancy or nonspecific effects alone, although positive expectancies are positively associated with treatment benefit (Safren, Heimberg, & Juster, 1997). Furthermore, CBT has been shown to offer efficacy over nonspecific treatment effects alone, such as group support and time with a caring therapist (Heimberg et al., 1990; Heimberg et al., 1994).

Cognitive behavioral treatments for SAD focus directly on the modification of patterns hypothesized to maintain the disorder. Informational, cognitive restructuring and exposure interventions are central to most current treatment packages. These interventions are combined, at times, with social skills training or anxiety management interventions. Informational components are designed to provide the patient with a model of the disorder, a rationale for treatment procedures, and a guide for collaborative treatment efforts. Cognitive restructuring focuses directly on the modification of the anxiogenic cognitions and core beliefs associated with the disorder. It has, relative to the model presented in Figure 22.2, at least four interrelated targets for modification: (1) the negative expectancies that are present before and during exposure to social situations; (2) failure-focused attention to and overestimation of the cost of social failures; (3) amplifying cognitions and associated dysfunctional interpretations of social performance and anxiety affect; and (4) maladaptive self-evaluations following performance in social situations.

In typical cognitive restructuring, thoughts are treated as hypotheses, and emphasis is placed on the development of more-accurate thinking patterns. Cognitive-restructuring strategies include guided discussions, Socratic questioning, and self-monitoring, although distinctions between cognitive and exposure procedures are blurred by the additional use of behavioral experiments to test the validity of specific beliefs using an exposure format. Indeed, the use of behavioral experiments to effect cognitive change is consistent with evidence that exposure treatments alone achieve cognitive changes in the same range as those achieved by traditional cognitive-restructuring procedures used alone (e.g., Hope, Heimberg, & Bruch, 1995; Mattia et al., 1993; Mattick, Peters, & Clark, 1989; Newman, Hofmann, Trabert, Roth, & Taylor, 1994). However, cognitive change appears to be only one component of the benefits offered by exposure. Mattick et al. (1989) found that exposure trailed cognitive-restructuring interventions in achieving cognitive changes, but it outperformed cognitive restructuring for overall improvement of social anxiety. In a meta-analysis conducted by Gil and colleagues (2001), no statistically significant differences in effectiveness were found between exposure techniques, cognitive restructuring, and social skills training. What then are the additional mechanisms of action of exposure?

A traditional perspective is that exposure breaks learned associations by a process of habituation to anxiety-provoking stimuli within an exposure session. Extinction of the fear response over repeated exposures (for review, see Barlow, 1988) has received central attention as a mechanism of exposure treatment. As long as patients are not resensitized by the actual occurrence of feared outcomes, fear reduction should occur fairly naturally with prolonged exposure. However, this perspective ignores the powerful role that cognitive conceptualizations play in determining whether the feared outcome occurs. Danger in social situations is not an objective phenomenon but a subjective evaluation dependent on the cognitive biases detailed, in part, in Figure 22.2.

Two case examples illustrate this point. The first is provided by Heimberg (1991) in his treatment manual for CBGT. He describes an exposure session in which a woman was asked to pour water into a cocktail glass as part of a mock cocktail party exposure. Although the patient's performance was objectively successful, the patient was aware that she spilled a few drops of water during the exposure and concluded that she had failed and was a hopeless case. An unsuccessful suicide attempt followed.

Although such extreme reactions are rare, this example illustrates the importance of cognitive interpretations in determining whether exposures are sensitizing or anxiolytic. Likewise, a recent patient in our treatment program reported that he went to a party and started a conversation with three new people, exceeding his exposure goal of talking to one person during the evening. However, the patient considered this experience a failure because of his belief that this task would be hard only for someone who is "truly inadequate."

These examples illustrate the powerful role of cognitive interpretations on defining whether feared outcomes have occurred and how exposure treatments must take into account the "cognitive set" of patients during exposure. Indeed, simple instruction to attend to task-relevant rather than internal (anxiety) stimuli appears to increase the effectiveness of social exposure (Wells & Papageorgiou, 1998). Recently, Furukawa et al. (2009) examined the role of self-focused attention and engagement in safety behaviors; the results indicated that the degree to which patients reduced their level of self-focused attention predicted observer ratings of their visible anxiety as well as the degree of reduction in beliefs in feared outcomes.

In addition, research has begun to focus more closely on changes in judgmental bias as a possible cognitive mechanism (Foa, Franklin, Perry, & Herbert, 1996; Foa, Huppert, & Cahill, 2006; Hofmann, 2004; McManus, Clark & Hackmann, 2000; Smits, Rosenfield, McDonald, & Telch, 2006). More specifically, judgmental bias in SAD can be broken down into a probability bias – the tendency to associate feared stimuli or responses with an unrealistically high estimation of harm – and a social cost bias – the tendency to exaggerate the negative consequences of a harmful event. Thus far, research has been mixed regarding which of these two biases plays a more prominent role in the maintenance of SAD. Studies conducted by Foa and colleagues (1996) as well as Hofmann (2004) support the notion that changes in cost bias account for a significant proportion of the variance in treatment outcome while research conducted by McManus and colleagues (2000) asserts that changes in cost bias did not account for a significant proportion of variance in outcome when probability bias was statistically controlled. Additionally, in studying the contribution of each of these biases, Smits and colleagues (2006) found that reductions in probability bias lead to a reduction in fear whereas the reduction in cost bias was a consequence of fear reduction. As the data in this area are still mixed, a treatment approach that addresses both may be warranted. Traditional cognitive reappraisal can be used to correct overestimation of threat, and social cost exposure, a type of exposure in which the patient purposely causes a social mishap to occur, can allow the patient to more correctly asses the true threat when that social mishap does happen (e.g., Hofmann & Otto, 2008).

The question remains, however, whether exposure is simply the weakening of fear associations in the context of corrective experiences, or whether much more active learning of safety is involved. Recent findings in the animal learning literature support the latter view. Rather than reflecting unlearning, exposure-based extinction appears to reflect the learning of alternative associations. As a result of exposure trials, fear cues may take on a much more ambiguous meaning (e.g., no longer signaling danger). Such extinction effects also appear to be sensitive to the context of learning, in which the presence of external or internal (e.g., emotional) contextual cues may influence whether fear or safety associations are recalled upon re-exposure to a phobic stimulus (for review, see Bouton & Nelson, 1998; Bouton & Swartzentruber, 1991). Morissette, Spiegel, and Barlow (2008) examined the role medication can play as a contextual cue in exposure procedures and found that state-dependent learning effects are possible when combining exposure and pharmacotherapy.

A useful heuristic for conceptualizing the nature of exposure treatment is provided by information-processing theories of emotion that focus on fear networks. According to Lang's (1977) bioinformational theory of emotion, fear networks consist of: (1) stimulus elements that represent sensory cues associated with the feared event; (2) response elements that include cognitive, affective, physiological, and behavioral responses to these cues; and (3) interpretive elements that include information about the meaning of the event and the nature of the association between the stimulus and response elements. Once the network is formed, cues associated with the network (e.g., either stimulus or response cues) can activate the fear network and consequently activate anxiety and urges to avoid or escape.

Regarding treatment, Foa and Kozak (1986) have argued that two conditions are necessary for fear reduction via exposure: activation of the fear network and incorporation of new information into that network. Foa and Kozak emphasize four issues associated with accessibility to and modification of fear networks: (1) the match between the fear network and exposure cues; (2) the medium in which the exposure is delivered; (3) the duration of exposure; and (4) adequate attention to fear cues.

Fear evocation appears to be maximized by realistic exposure scenarios. These can be achieved by role-play social situations, which are easily instrumented in group treatment settings (see Heimberg, 1991; Hope & Heimberg, 1994). In addition, to ensure realistic exposure conditions, clinicians should consider the need to include response cues in exposure sessions. For example, for patients who fear speaking because they catastrophically interpret the potential consequences of having a dry throat or feeling dizzy during the presentation ("They will think I am crazy; I will be unable to continue"), authors of exposure assignments may well want to include procedures for inducing these feared symptoms in conjunction with speaking exposures (e.g., the exposure would be conducted only after the patient induced symptoms using interoceptive exposure techniques, in this case hyperventilation).

Regarding the medium of exposure, SAD treatments often rely on *in vivo* exposure formats that are likely more powerful than approximated methods including verbal descriptions, imaginal exposure, and role-play situations that may be used in other disorders (e.g., PTSD).

The duration of the exposure session has received consistent attention in the treatment of phobic conditions. A decrease in anxiety during the exposure session is thought to allow integration of new information into the fear network, in part because exposure to the cues is not accompanied by current threat or incessant anxiety. Longer exposure sessions provide greater opportunities for habituation, and, correspondingly, prolonged exposure (e.g., 50 minutes or more) has been found to be superior to short exposure for more-severe phobic conditions (Foa & Kozak, 1986). In addition to duration, Berry, Rosenfeld, and Smits (2009) found that extinction retention, the extent to which fear reduction is maintained between two separate exposure sessions, is also associated with improvement in fear and avoidance.

Work by Moscovitch, Hofmann, Suvak, and In-Albon (2005) further clarified the relationship between SAD and major depression, providing support for the notion that differential underlying treatment mechanisms are at work. Their results indicate that, while 91% of the variance in decreases in depressive symptoms can be accounted for by changes in social anxiety, the reciprocal is not true. This provides support for the notion that improvement in SAD is distinct from direct mood effects of interventions.

Finally, as discussed previously, objective presentation of phobia cues does not ensure that these cues will be processed. Patients may modulate their emotional responses to exposure by minimizing their attention to exposure stimuli or using a variety of safety cues or behaviors. In addition to those detailed by Wells et al. (1995), safety cues may include being accompanied to social events by a person who is less phobic or having a beverage in hand while talking. Safety behaviors may also include cognitive strategies such as "acting" the part of another while in a social situation. Accordingly, Wells et al. (p. 160) have suggested guidelines for maximizing the effectiveness of exposure by taking into account safety behaviors and cognitive biases that may insulate patients from corrective feedback and thus interfere with anxiety reduction:

1. Patients' feared catastrophes and their perceived likelihood should be assessed.
2. Safety behaviors that are rationally linked to these feared catastrophes should be identified.
3. A cognitive set focusing on active disconfirmation of negative beliefs should be established.
4. Safety behaviors should be eliminated or reversed during exposure.
5. The outcome of the assignment should be discussed in information-processing terms.

In particular, the therapist should ask whether the feared catastrophe happened. If it did not, what is the patient's explanation? Is the nonoccurrence simply attributed to residual safety behavior, or has the exercise produced a more profound change in belief?

All of these considerations suggest that exposure is an active process that must take into account information-processing biases. Moreover, the goal of exposure is more than the simple loosening of fear associations; it is the active relearning of safety in the phobic situation. Consequently, effort needs to be applied to ensure that this learning is not conditional (e.g., "I will be OK only if I do not sweat, if I use safety behaviors, or if I am with my partner," etc.) by providing unambiguous exposure practice.

Given the overlap in methods between cognitive and exposure interventions, it is perhaps not surprising that combined cognitive and exposure interventions sometimes fail to produce results significantly better than exposure alone (compare Gil et al., 2001; Hope et al., 1995). Relative to the model of SAD presented here, cognitive restructuring provides a means to challenge and reduce the negative expectations and self-defeating amplifying cognitions associated with SAD. This process is aided by monitoring of thoughts during naturally occurring anxiety episodes, and specific practicing of cognitive restructuring during exposure procedures. The combination of exposure and cognitive restructuring also provides patients with an opportunity to develop alternative cognitive skills in the context in which these skills are needed most, including more-accurate self-evaluation of performance.

As a consequence, exposure combined with cognitive restructuring provides a context for correcting dysfunctional thoughts, redirecting failure-focused attention, and the elimination of safety behaviors. The construction of clear behavioral goals for exposure and reviews of objective goal attainment provide a context for challenging dysfunctional, subjective evaluations of performance. In particular, with repeated exposure patients learn that they tend to meet objective performance goals despite their subjective experience of anxiety. As confidence rises with subsequent exposures, negative expectations and evocation of anxiety in social situations is further reduced. Successful exposure breeds more-positive memories and more-adaptive expectations for future performance. At the same time, patients learn to not fear minor social mishaps and to change evaluations of the "adequacy" of social performance. In short, fear memories are replaced by alternative, more-adaptive associations and beliefs.

There has also been a recent focus on using therapy-enhancing medications, such as DCS, to speed up the aforementioned learning process. A departure from typical pharmacotherapy for social anxiety, which generally provides medications meant to reduce anxiety, DCS is administered prior to exposure sessions as a means of enhancing behavioral learning. Studies to date have demonstrated that the use of DCS as an adjunct to exposure-based therapies enhances treatment outcomes for socially anxious patients when compared to those receiving the same therapy and a placebo (Guastella et al., 2008; Hofmann et al., 2006).

Our own view is that cognitive interventions are especially useful in reducing negative expectancies prior to exposure, inhibiting maladaptive information processing, guiding attention to actual performance demands during exposure, and aiding the accurate evaluation of objective performance after exposures. It is, however, experience in exposure situations that may provide the most useful learning, as suggested by the more optimal outcome for exposure techniques relative to cognitive strategies alone (see Gould et al., 1997; Heimberg & Juster, 1995; Taylor, 1996).

COMBINED PHARMACOTHERAPY AND CBT

One implication of the models of change detailed previously is that combinations of pharmacotherapy and CBT may have the additive benefits of physiologically mediated anxiety suppression combined with direct modification of anxiogenic cognitive and behavioral patterns. Research to date in this area has been mixed with some evidence for enhanced effects of combined treatments (Blomhoff et al., 2001) and some demonstrating no increased benefit for this treatment approach (Davidson et al., 2004; Foa, Franklin, & Moser, 2002). This one–two punch may have specific advantages early in treatment, but, due to the hypothesized role of medications serving as safety cues, it may interfere with unambiguous reductions in fear later in treatment. Consequently, patients continuing to take medications during the conclusion of short-term CBT would be expected to be at higher risk of relapse than patients who achieved similar treatment gains without medication. Moreover, both the animal-learning literature and treatment studies in humans (compare Bouton, Kenney, & Rosengard, 1990; Marks et al., 1993) provide evidence for the re-emergence of fears upon medication discontinuation, when extinction trials were conducted while subjects were medicated.

Concerns about the combination of pharmacotherapy and CBT are also voiced by Gray (1982a, 1982b). Pharmacological blockade of noradrenergic and serotonergic afferents to the septohippocampal system are hypothesized to provide only temporary blockade of anxiety, with a return of anxiety upon removal of medication. In contrast, exposure treatment is hypothesized by Gray to have more permanent effects on the septohippocampal system, eliminating the danger interpretation to phobic stimuli through a process of habituation. Gray emphasizes that the potential habituating effects of exposure on the septohippocampal system may be disrupted by medication use: With modulation of afferents to the septohippocampal system by medications, crucial biological effects of exposure ("biological toughening up") may not occur. One mechanism for the absence of strong additive effects between pharmacotherapy and CBT is that pharmacotherapy may block some of the natural memory-enhancing effects of cortisol release during exposure (Otto, McHugh, & Kantak, 2010), attenuating the degree to which therapeutic learning during CBT is retained. Additional research is needed to further examine these hypotheses and to further examine the nature of failures to obtain additive effects between CBT and pharmacotherapy (e.g., Davidson et al., 2004) as well as longer-term attenuation of CBT efficacy with combination treatment (e.g., Otto, Smits, & Reese, 2005).

SOCIAL SKILLS TRAINING

Inadequate social skills, as differentiated from the inhibition of extant skills due to social anxiety, may require additional interventions. Social skills training is designed to help patients develop a more adaptive social repertoire, eliminating patterns that may be leading to poor social performance and consequent anxiety about future interactions. Actual skill deficits are not assumed to be a necessary feature of SAD, and, accordingly, there is some support for a treatment-matching approach. Social skills training appears to be more efficacious for patients who are socially unskilled relative to socially overanxious patients (Heimberg & Barlow, 1991; Öst, Jerremalm, & Johansson, 1981), but this is clearly not always the case (see Mersch, Emmelkamp, & Lips, 1991; Stravynski, Kyparissis, & Amado, Chapter 6 this volume).

It is important to note that social skills training can easily incorporate exposure procedures as part of skill training and rehearsal, making it difficult to ascertain the effects of skill acquisition separate from exposure practice. Indeed, different conclusions on the efficacy of social skills training (compare Heimberg & Juster, 1995; Taylor, 1996) appear to be largely a function of the inclusion of studies utilizing social skills training in the context of exposure in estimates of the efficacy of social skills training.

ACCEPTANCE AND COMMITMENT THERAPY

Other behavioral treatments do not focus on restructuring maladaptive thoughts; rather, they focus on teaching patients to conceptualize thoughts as behaviors in their own right that should be considered as useful or not useful instead of correct or incorrect. This sort of perspective, represented prominently by ACT (Hayes, 1995), focuses on increasing adaptive behaviors by helping patients to focus on the contingencies at hand rather than elevating the importance of thoughts about what they must do in response to emotions. Using rich metaphors to help patients re-evaluate the nature of thoughts, ACT guides patients to accept emotions while targeting their behaviors toward relevant contingencies.

In our experience, the goals of ACT are similar to exposure therapy in many ways in our clinical and research applications of Heimberg's CBGT (Heimberg, 1991), as well as treatments emphasizing social cost exposures, and also traditional exposures (Hofmann & Otto, 2008). By midtreatment (e.g., sessions 5–7 of a 12-session treatment protocol), as patients complete exposures and objectively evaluate their performance, they begin to realize that objective goals are reliably met despite negative expectations and anxiety. In other words, patients learn that negative thoughts and the experience of anxiety do not match objective performance; goals are met despite these internal events. As treatment progresses, cognitive evaluations and affective experience come in line with these objective evaluations.

This process of change is consistent with some of the goals of ACT: to eliminate reliance on maladaptive cognitions or faulty emotional signals, to teach emotional acceptance, and to guide patients to respond to contingencies at hand. Emotional acceptance of anxiety in particular (e.g., treating anxiety as an emotional signal rather than a statement on the true danger of the situation or the personal effectiveness of the individual) is directly relevant to the modification of amplifying cognitions (see Figure 22.1). With both treatments, anxiety loses its ability to signify failure and becomes a sign of emotional arousal alone. Research into ACT's effectiveness with socially phobic populations in still in the early stages; however, several pilot studies have demonstrated potential promise in this area (Dalrymple & Herbert, 2007; Ossman, Wilson, Storaasli, & McNeil, 2006).

OTHER PSYCHOSOCIAL TREATMENTS

Despite the wealth of evidence for the effectiveness of CBT for anxiety disorders, relatively few patients appear to receive these treatments in clinical practice, and psychodynamic treatments continue to be commonly applied for anxiety disorders, at least in certain locales (Goisman et al., 1993). What are the likely effects of psychodynamic psychotherapy from the perspective of the model presented in Figure 22.2?

Based on the model, any treatment that leads patients to re-evaluate their negative and catastrophic interpretations of social situations and associated anxiety symptoms offers the potential to help patients enter social situations and further decrease subjective evaluations of danger (as long as performance deficits do not maintain actual poor performance). Accordingly, to the extent that psychodynamic treatments offer patients a historical explanation (narrative truth) for the anxiety elicited in social situations, new cognitions may be engendered, so patients can disattend to their catastrophic or amplifying cognitions and attend more to objective reality. Additional social confidence may be engendered by the accepting environments offered by therapists, in which patients have the opportunity to test aspects of their social selves without social punishment. However, such indirect, in-session "exposure practice" may generalize poorly to out-of-session social situations without specific practice. Indeed, completion of out-of-session homework tends to be a significant predictor of therapeutic change in CBT for SAD (Leung & Heimberg, 1996), and psychodynamic theories do not necessarily guide patients toward in-the-moment applications of historical insights or encourage re-entry into avoided situations. This is particularly true given that psychodynamic therapeutic relationships are frequently discussed as being "unlike any other relationship." This uniqueness suggests that generalization of skills learned in the context of the therapeutic interaction may be particularly hard to generalize to out-of-session interactions.

These hypotheses await empirical evaluation, with attention to both the efficiency as well as the ultimate outcome of psychodynamic interventions and the therapeutic interventions that appear to drive beneficial change. Interestingly, investigations of this kind are under way. For example, Ablon and Jones (2002) coded session transcripts of therapists doing IPT or cognitive therapy for depression in the context of the multicenter treatment trial for major depression (Elkin et al., 1989). Prototypic psychodynamic and cognitive behavioral therapist behaviors were coded, and scores were examined as predictors of treatment outcome. Despite the psychodynamic rationale for interventions in the manual-driven IPT, interventions that were coded as cognitive behavioral within this therapy (and within CBT) were those most linked with beneficial outcome.

SUMMARY

Throughout this chapter, we have argued that successful treatment of SAD is achieved by interruption of the ongoing cycle of the negative social expectations, and vigilance to negative outcomes, rising symptoms, negative interpretations of symptoms and outcomes, and avoidance and escape behaviors that characterize the disorder. Pharmacological, cognitive, and exposure-based interventions were hypothesized to intervene at different points in this cycle, attending to different "linchpins" in disrupting the self-perpetuating cycle of social anxiety. Both pharmacological and psychosocial interventions work. Exposure is obviously not the central element of change in pharmacotherapy as it is in CBT. Nonetheless, exposure as an important element of change has earned attention in both modalities of treatment. Exposure is designated in Gray's (1982a, 1982b) neuropsychologic theory of anxiety as a tool to achieve more enduring changes in neurophysiologic systems maintaining anxiety. Exposure also ranks as an important context for the application of pharmacological treatment (Sutherland & Davidson, 1995), and it is given central attention in various cognitive behavioral accounts of the disorder and its treatment (Hofmann, 2000; Hofmann & Otto, 2008).

Exposure effects were conceptualized as being far from a passive process of loosening fear associations. Instead, exposure was discussed as an active process involving the acquisition of safety in a phobic situation, which is richly dependent on the cognitive set that accompanies the processing of the exposure experience. Although the mechanisms of action presented here are consistent with the available data, the mere consistency between the model and available data does not rule out alternative accounts of the mechanisms of change. Whenever possible, we have suggested areas for future inquiry that may further clarify change mechanisms in SAD.

REFERENCES

Ablon, J. S., & Jones, E. E. (2002). Validity of controlled clinical trials of psychotherapy: Findings from the NIMH Treatment of Depression Collaborative Research Program. *American Journal of Psychiatry*, *159*, 775–783.

Alstrom, J. E., Nordlund, C. L., Persson, G., Harding, M., & Ljungqvist, C. (1984). Effects of four treatment methods on social phobic patients not suitable for insight-oriented psychotherapy. *Acta Psychiatrica Scandinavica*, *70*, 97–110.

Ball, S. G., Otto, M. W., Pollack, M. H., Uccello, R., & Rosenbaum, J. F. (1995). Differentiating social phobia and panic disorder: A test of core beliefs. *Cognitive Therapy and Research*, *19*, 473–482.

Barlow, D. H. (1988). Anxiety and its disorders: The nature and treatment of anxiety and panic. New York: Guilford Press.

Beck, A. T., Emery, G., & Greenberg, R. L. (1985). Anxiety disorders and phobias: A cognitive perspective. New York: Basic Books.

Berry, A. C., Rosenfield, D., & Smits, J. A. (2009). Extinction retention predicts improvement in social anxiety symptoms following exposure therapy. *Depression and Anxiety*, *26*, 22–27.

Blomhoff, S., Haug, T. T., Hellstrom, K., Holme, I., Humble, M., Madsbu, H. P., et al. (2001). Randomised controlled general practice trial of sertraline, exposure therapy and combined treatment in generalized social phobia. *British Journal of Psychiatry*, *179*, 23–30.

Bogels, S. M., & Mansell, W. (2004). Attention process in the maintenance and treatment of social phobia: Hypervigilance, avoidance, and self-focused attention. *Clinical Psychology Review*, *24*, 827–856.

Bouton, M. E., Kenney, F. A., & Rosengard, C. (1990). State-dependent fear extinction with two benzodiazepine tranquilizers. *Behavioral Neuroscience*, *104*, 44–55.

Bouton, M. E., & Nelson, J. B. (1998). The role of context in classical conditioning: Some implications for cognitive-behavior therapy. In W. O'Donohue (Ed.), *Learning and behavior therapy* (pp. 59–84). Needham Heights, MA: Allyn & Bacon.

Bouton, M. E., & Swartzentruber, D. (1991). Sources of relapse after extinction in Pavlovian and instrumental learning. *Clinical Psychology Review*, *11*, 123–140.

Bruch, M. A., Mattia, J. I., Heimberg, R. G., & Holt, C. S. (1993). Cognitive specificity in social anxiety and depression: Supporting evidence and qualifications due to affective confounding. *Cognitive Therapy and Research*, *17*, 1–21.

Clark, D. M., & Wells, A. (1995). A cognitive model of social phobia. In R. G. Heimberg, M. R. Liebowitz, D. A. Hope, & E. R. Schneier (Eds.), *Social phobia: Diagnosis, assessment, and treatment* (pp. 69–93). New York: Guilford Press.

Dalrymple, K. L., & Herbert, J. D. (2007). Acceptance and commitment therapy for generalized social anxiety disorder: A pilot study. *Behavior Modification*, *31*, 543–568.

Davidson, J. R. T. (2003). Pharmacotherapy of social phobia. *Acta Psychiatrica Scandinavia*, *108*, 65–71.

Davidson, J. R., Foa, E. B., Huppert, J. D., Keefe, F. J., Franklin, M. E., Compton, J. S., et al. (2004). Fluoxetine, comprehensive cognitive behavioral therapy, and placebo in generalized social phobia. *Archives of General Psychiatry*, *61*, 1005–1013.

Davidson, J. R. T., Tupler, L. A., & Potts, N. L. S. (1994). Treatment of social phobia with benzodiazepincs. *Journal of Clinical Psychiatry*, *55*(Suppl 6), 28–32.

Dohr, K. B., Rush, A. J., & Bernstein, I. H. (1989). Cognitive biases and depression. *Journal of Abnormal Psychology*, *98*, 263–267.

Elkin, I., Shea, T., Watkins, J. T., Imber, S. D., Sotsky, S. M., & Parloff, M. B. (1989). National Institute of Mental Health treatment of depression collaborative research program: General effectiveness of treatments. *Archives of General Psychiatry*, *46*, 971–982.

Fava, M., Bless, E., Otto, M. W., Pava, J. A., & Rosenbaum, J. E. (1994). Dysfunctional attitudes in major depression: Changes with pharmacotherapy. *Journal of Nervous and Mental Disease*, *182*, 45–49.

Fedoroff, I. C., & Taylor, S. (2001). Psychological and pharmacological treatments of social phobia: A meta-analysis. *Journal of Clinical Pharmacology*, *21*, 311–324.

Feske, U., & Chambless, D. L. (1995). Cognitive behavioral versus exposure only treatment for social phobia: A meta-analysis. *Behavior Therapy*, *26*, 695–720.

Foa, E. B., Franklin, M. E., & Moser, J. (2002). Context in the clinic: How well do cognitive behavioral therapies and medications work in combination? *Biological Psychiatry*, *52*, 987–988.

Foa, E. B., Franklin, M. E., Perry, K. J., & Herbert, J. D. (1996). Cognitive biases in generalized social phobia. *Journal of Abnormal Psychology*, *105*, 433–439.

Foa, E. B., Huppert, J. D., & Cahill, S. P. (2006). Emotional processing theory: An update. In B. O. Rothbaum (Ed.), *Pathalogical Anxiety: Emotional processing in etiology and treatment* (pp. 3–24). New York: Guilford Press.

Foa, E. B., & Kozak, M. J. (1986). Emotional processing of fear: Exposure to corrective information. *Psychological Bulletin*, *99*, 20–35.

Furukawa, T. A., Chen, J., Watanabe, N., Nakano, Y., Ietsugu, T., Ogawa, S., et al. (2009). Videotaped experiments to drop safety behaviors and self-focused attention for patients with social anxiety disorder: Do they change subjective and objective evaluations of anxiety and performance? *Journal of Behavior Therapy and Experimental Psychiatry*, *40*, 202–210.

Gil, P. J. M., Carrillo, F. X. M., & Meca, J. S. (2001). Effectiveness of cognitive behavioral treatment in social phobia: A meta-analytic review. *Psychology in Spain*, *5*, 17–25.

Goisman, R. M., Rogers, M. P., Steketee, G. S., Warshaw, M. G., Coneo, P., & Keller, M. B. (1993). Utilization of behavioral methods in a multicenter anxiety disorders study. *Journal of Clinical Psychiatry*, *54*, 213–218.

Gould, R. A., Buckminster, S., Pollack, M. H., Otto, M. W., & Yap, L. (1997). Cognitive-behavioral and pharmacological treatment for social phobia: A meta-analysis. *Clinical Psychology: Science and Practice*, *4*, 291–306.

Gould, R. A., & Otto, M. W. (1996). Cognitive-behavioral treatment of social phobia and generalized anxiety disorder. In M. H. Pollack, M. W. Otto, & J. F. Rosenbaum (Eds.), *Challenges in clinical practice: Pharmacologic and psychosocial strategies* (pp. 171–200). New York: Guilford Press.

Gray, J. A. (1982a). Precis of the neuropsychology of anxiety: An enquiry into the functions of the septo-hippocampal system. *Behavioral and Brain Sciences*, *5*, 469–534.

Gray, J. A. (1982b). The neuropsychology of anxiety: An enquiry into the functions of the septa-hippocampal system. Oxford, UK: Oxford University Press.

Guastella, A. J., Richardson, R., Lovibond, P. F., Rapee, R. M., Gaston, J. E., Mitchell, P., et al. (2008). A randomized controlled trial of D-cycloserine enhancement of exposure therapy for social anxiety disorder. *Biological Psychiatry*, *63*, 544–549.

Hayes, S. C. (1995). Acceptance and commitment therapy (ACT): A working manual for the treatment of emotional avoidance disorders. Unpublished manuscript. University of Nevada, Reno.

Heimberg, R. G. (1991). *Cognitive behavioral treatment of social phobia in a group setting: A treatment manual.* Unpublished treatment manual. Philadelphia, PA: Temple University.

Heimberg, R. G. (2001). Current status of psychotherapeutic interventions for social phobia. *Journal of Clinical Psychiatry*, *62*(Suppl 1), 36–42.

Heimberg, R. G., & Barlow, D. H. (1991). New developments in cognitive-behavioral therapy for social phobia. *Journal of Clinical Psychiatry*, *52*(Suppl), 21–30.

Heimberg, R. G., Dodge, C. S., Hope, D. A, Kennedy, C. R., Zollo, L., & Becker, R. E. (1990). Cognitive behavioral group treatment for social phobia: Comparison with a credible placebo control. *Cognitive Therapy and Research*, *14*, 1–23.

Heimberg, R. G., & Juster, H. R. (1995). Cognitive-behavioral treatments: Literature review. In R. G. Heimberg, M. R. Liebowitz, D. A. Hope, & F. R. Schneier (Eds.), *Social phobia: Diagnosis, assessment, and treatment* (pp. 261–309). New York: Guilford.

Heimberg, R. G., Juster, H. R., Brown, E. J., Holle, C., Makris, G. S., Leung, A.W., et al. (1994). Cognitive-behavioral versus pharmacological treatment of social phobia: Posttreatment and follow-up effects. Paper presented at the annual meeting of the Association for Advancement of Behavior Therapy, San Diego, CA.

Heimberg, R. G., Liebowitz, M. R., Hope, D. A., Schneier, E. R., Holt, C. S., Welkowitz, L. A., et al. (1998). Cognitive behavioral group therapy vs. phenelzine therapy for social phobia: 12-week outcome. *Archives of General Psychiatry*, *55*, 1133–1141.

Hofmann, S. G. (2000). Treatment of social phobia: Potential mediators and moderators. *Clinical Psychology: Science and Practice*, *7*, 3–16.

Hofmann, S. G. (2004). Cognitive mediation of treatment change in social phobia. *Journal of Consulting and Clinical Psychology*, *72*, 393–399.

Hofmann, S. G., Meuret, A. E., Smits, J. A., Simon, N. M., Pollack, M. H., Eisenmenger, K., et al. (2006). Augmentation of exposure therapy with D-cycloserine for social anxiety disorder. *Archives of General Psychiatry*, *63*, 298–304.

Hofmann, S. G., & Otto, M. W. (2008). Cognitive behavior therapy for social anxiety disorder: Evidence-based and disorder-specific treatment techniques. New York: Routledge.

Hope, D. A., & Heimberg, R. G. (1994). Social phobia and social anxiety. In D. H. Barlow (Ed.), *Clinical handbook of psychological disorders* (2nd ed.) (pp. 99–136). New York: Guilford Press.

Hope, D. A., Heimberg, R. G., & Bruch, M. A. (1995). Dismantling cognitive-behavioral group therapy for social phobia. *Behaviour Research and Therapy*, *33*, 637–650.

Ingram, R. E. (1989). Affective confounds in social-cognitive research. *Journal of Personality and Social Psychology*, *57*, 715–722.

Jorstad-Stein, E. C., & Heimberg, R. G. (2009). Social phobia: An update on treatment. *Psychiatric Clinics of North America*, *32*, 641–663.

Kim, E. J. (2005). The effect of decreased safety behaviors on anxiety and negative thoughts in social phobics. *Journal of Anxiety Disorders*, *19*, 69–86.

Lang, P. J. (1977). Imagery in therapy: An information processing analysis of fear. *Behavior Therapy*, *8*, 862–886.

Leung, A. W., & Heimberg, R. H. (1996). Homework compliance, perceptions of control, and outcome of cognitive behavioral treatment of social phobia. *Behaviour Research and Therapy*, *34*, 423–432.

Liebowitz, M. R, Campeas, R., & Hollander, E. (1987). Possible dopamine dysregulation in social phobia and atypical depression. *Psychiatry Research*, *22*, 89–90.

Marks, I. M., Swinson, R. P., Basoglu, M., Kuch, K., Noshirvani, H., O'Sullivan,, G., et al. (1993). Alprazolam and exposure alone and combined in panic disorder with agoraphobia: A controlled study in London and Toronto. *British Journal of Psychiatry*, *162*, 776–787.

Mattia, J. I., Heimberg, R. G., & Hope, D. A. (1993). The revised Stroop color-naming task in social phobics. *Behaviour Research and Therapy*, *31*, 305–313.

Mattick, R. P., Peters, L., & Clark, J. C. (1989). Exposure and cognitive restructuring for social phobia: A controlled study. *Behavior Therapy*, *20*, 3–23.

McEwan, K. L., & Devins, G. M. (1983). Is increased arousal in social anxiety noticed by others? *Journal of Abnormal Psychology*, *92*, 417–421.

McManus, F., Clark, D. M., & Hackmann, A. (2000). Specificity of cognitive biases in social phobia and their role in recovery. *Behavioural and Cognitive Psychotherapy*, *28*, 201–209.

McNally, R. J. (1996). *Cognitive biases in the anxiety disorders. Nebraska Symposium on Motivation*: *Vol. 43* (pp. 211–250). Lincoln, NB: University of Nebraska Press.

Mersch, P. P., Emrnelkamp, P. M. G., & Lips, C. (1991). Social phobia: Individual response patterns and the effects of behavioral and cognitive interventions. A follow-up study. *Behaviour Research and Therapy*, *29*, 357–362.

Miranda, J., Persons, J. B., & Byers, C. N. (1990). Endorsement of dysfunctional beliefs depends on current mood state. *Journal of Abnormal Psychology*, *99*, 237–241.

Morissette, S. B., Spiegel, D. A., & Barlow, D. H. (2008). Combining exposure and pharmacotherapy in the treatment of social anxiety disorder: A preliminary study of state dependent learning. *Journal of Psychopathology and Behavioral Assessment*, *30*, 211–219.

Moscovitch, D. A., Hofmann, S. G., Suvak, M. K., & In-Albon, T. (2005). Mediation of changes in anxiety and depression during treatment of social phobia. *Journal of Consulting and Clinical Psychology*, *73*, 945–952.

Newman, M. G., Hofmann, S. G., Trabert, W., Roth, W. T., & Taylor, C. B. (1994). Does behavioral treatment of social phobia lead to cognitive changes? *Behavior Therapy*, *25*, 503–517.

Ossman, W. A., Wilson, K. G., Storaasli, R. D., & McNeil, J. W. (2006). A preliminary investigation of the use of acceptance and commitment therapy in a group treatment for social phobia. *International Journal of Psychology & Psychological Therapy*, *6*, 397–416.

Öst, L.-G., Jerremalm, A., & Johansson, J. (1981). Individual response patterns and the effects of different behavioral methods in the treatment of social phobia. *Behaviour Research and Therapy*, *19*, 1–16.

Otto, M. W. (1999). Cognitive-behavioral therapy for social anxiety disorder: Model, methods, and outcome. *Journal of Clinical Psychiatry*, *60*(Suppl 9), 14–19.

Otto, M. W., McHugh, R. K., & Kantak, K. M. (2010). Combined pharmacotherapy and cognitive-behavioral therapy for anxiety disorders: Medication effects, glucocorticoids, and attenuated outcomes. *Clinical Psychology: Science and Practice, 17,* 91–103.

Otto, M. W., Pollack, M. H., Fava, M., Uccello, R., & Rosenbaum, J. F. (1995). Elevated Anxiety Sensitivity Index scores in patients with major depression: Correlates and changes with antidepressant treatment. *Journal of Anxiety Disorders*, *9*, 117–123.

Otto, M. W., Pollack, M. H., Gould, R. A., Worthington, J. J., Heimberg, R. G., McArdle, E. T., et al. (2000). A comparison of the efficacy of clonazepam and cognitive-behavioral group therapy for the treatment of social phobia. *Journal of Anxiety Disorders*, *14*, 345–358.

Otto, M. W., Pollack, M. H., & Sabatino, S. A. (1996). Maintenance of remission following cognitive behavior therapy for panic disorder: Possible deleterious effects of concurrent medication treatment. *Behavior Therapy*, *27*, 473–482.

Otto, M. W., Smits, J. A. J., & Reese, H. E. (2005). Combined psychotherapy and pharmacotherapy for mood and anxiety disorders in adults: Review and analysis. *Clinical Psychology: Science and Practice*, *12*, 72–86.

Peselow, E. D., Robins, C., Block, P., Barouche, F., & Fieve, R. R. (1990). Dysfunctional attitudes in depressed patients before and after clinical treatment and in normal control subjects. *American Journal of Psychiatry*, *147*, 439–444.

Potts, N. L. S., & Davidson, J. R. T. (1995). Pharmacological treatments: Literature review. In R. G. Heimberg, M. R Liebowitz, D. A. Hope, & F. R. Schneier (Eds.), *Social phobia: Diagnosis, assessment, and treatment* (pp. 334–365). New York: Guilford Press.

Rapee, R. M., & Heirnberg, R. G. (1997). A cognitive behavioral model of anxiety in social phobia. *Behaviour Research and Therapy*, *35*, 741–756.

Safren, S. A, Heimberg, R. G., Brown, E. J., & Holle, C. (1997). Quality of life in social phobia. *Depression and Anxiety*, *4*, 126–133.

Safren, S. A., Heimberg, R. G., & Juster, H. R. (1997). The relationship of patient expectancies to initial severity and treatment outcome in cognitive-behavioral group treatment of social phobia. *Journal of Consulting and Clinical Psychology*, *65*, 694–698.

Safren, S. A., Heimberg, R. G., & Turk, C. (1998). Factor structure of the Social Phobia Scale and the Social Interaction Anxiety Scale. *Behaviour Research and Therapy*, *36*, 443–453.

Smits, J. A., Rosenfield, D., McDonald, R., & Telch, M. J. (2006). Cognitive mechanisms of social anxiety reduction: An examination of specificity and temporality. *Journal of Consulting and Clinical Psychology*, *74*, 1203–1212.

Sutherland, S. M., & Davidson, J. R. T. (1995). Blockers and benzodiazepines in pharmacotherapy. In M. B. Stein (Ed.), *Social phobia: Clinical and research perspectives* (pp. 323–326). Washington, DC: American Psychiatric Press.

Sutherland, S. M., Tupler, L. A., Colket, J. T., & Davidson, J. R. T. (1996). A 2-year follow-up of social phobia: Status after a brief medication trial. *Journal of Nervous and Mental Disease*, *184*, 731–738.

Szentagotai, A., David, D., Lupu, V., & Cosman, D. (2008). Rational emotive behavior therapy versus cognitive therapy versus pharmacotherapy in the treatment of major depressive disorder: Mechanisms of change analysis. *Psychotherapy: Theory, Research, Practice and Training*, *45*, 523–538.

Tancer, M. E., Lewis, M. H., & Stein, M. B. (1995). Biological aspects. In M. B. Stein (Ed.), *Social phobia: Clinical and research perspectives* (pp. 323–326). Washington, DC: American Psychiatric Press.

Taylor, S. (1996). Meta-analysis of cognitive-behavioral treatments for social phobia. *Journal of Behaviour Therapy and Experimental Psychiatry*, *27*, 1–9.

Taylor, S., Koch, W. J., Woody, S., & McLean, P. (1996). Anxiety sensitivity and depression: How are they related? *Journal of Abnormal Psychology*, *105*, 474–479.

Telch, M. J., Agras, W. S., Taylor, C. B., Roth, W. T., & Gallen, C. (1985). Combined pharmacological and behavioral treatment for agoraphobia. *Behaviour Research and Therapy*, *23*, 325–335.

van Ameringen, M., Mancini, C., Patterson, B., & Simpson, W. (2009). Pharmacotherapy for social anxiety disorder: An update. *Israel Journal of Psychiatry and Related Sciences*, *46*, 53–61.

van der Linden, G. J. H, Stein, D. J., & van Balkom, A. J. L. M. (2000). The efficacy of the selective serotonin reuptake inhibitors for social anxiety disorder (social phobia): A meta-analysis of randomized controlled trials. *International Clinical Psychopharmacology*, *15*, 15–23.

Weeks, J. W., Heimberg, R. G., Rodenbaugh, T. L., & Norton, P. J. (2008). Exploring the relationship between fear of positive evaluation and social anxiety. *Journal of Anxiety Disorders*, *22*, 386–400.

Wells, A., Clark, D. M., Salkovskis, P., Ludgate, J., Hackmann, A., & Gelder, M. (1995). Social phobia: The role of in-situation safety behaviors in maintaining anxiety and negative beliefs. *Behavior Therapy*, *26*, 153–161.

Wells, A., & Papageorgiou, C. (1998). Social phobia: Effects of external attention on anxiety, negative beliefs, and perspective taking. *Behavior Therapy*, *29*, 357–370.

Westra, H., & Stewart, S. H. (1998). Cognitive behavioral therapy and pharmacotherapy: Complimentary or contradictory approaches to the treatment of anxiety? *Clinical Psychology Review*, *18*, 307–340.

Index

A

B

C

D

Q

R